RECOGNIZING THE PAST IN THE PRESENT

RECOGNIZING THE PAST IN THE PRESENT

New Studies on Medicine before, during, and after the Holocaust

Edited by
Sabine Hildebrandt, Miriam Offer, and Michael A. Grodin

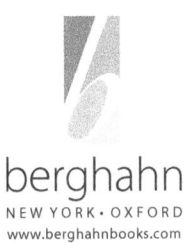

berghahn
NEW YORK • OXFORD
www.berghahnbooks.com

First published in 2021 by
Berghahn Books
www.berghahnbooks.com

© 2021, 2024 Sabine Hildebrandt, Miriam Offer, and Michael A. Grodin
First paperback edition published in 2024

All rights reserved. Except for the quotation of short passages
for the purposes of criticism and review, no part of this book
may be reproduced in any form or by any means, electronic or
mechanical, including photocopying, recording, or any information
storage and retrieval system now known or to be invented,
without written permission of the publisher.

Library of Congress Cataloging-in-Publication Data

Names: Hildebrandt, Sabine, editor. | Offer, Miriam, editor. | Grodin, Michael A., editor.
Title: Recognizing the Past in the Present: New Studies on Medicine before, during, and after the Holocaust / edited by Sabine Hildebrandt, Miriam Offer, Michael A. Grodin.
Description: New York: Berghahn Books, 2021. | Includes bibliographical references and index.
Identifiers: LCCN 2020048840 (print) | LCCN 2020048841 (ebook) | ISBN 9781789207842 (hardback) | ISBN 9781789207859 (ebook)
Subjects: LCSH: Human experimentation in medicine—Germany—History—20th century. | Medical scientists—Germany—History—20th century. | Medicine—Research—Germany—History—20th century. | Medical ethics—Germany—History—20th century. | Jews—Medicine—History—20th century. | Holocaust, Jewish (1939–1945)—Germany. | World War, 1939–1945—Atrocities—Germany.
Classification: LCC R853.H8 R425 2021 (print) | LCC R853.H8 (ebook) | DDC 174.2/80943—dc23
LC record available at https://lccn.loc.gov/2020048840
LC ebook record available at https://lccn.loc.gov/2020048841

British Library Cataloguing in Publication Data

A catalogue record for this book is available from the British Library

ISBN 978-1-78920-784-2 hardback
ISBN 978-1-80539-335-1 paperback
ISBN 978-1-80539-444-0 epub
ISBN 978-1-78920-785-9 web pdf

https://doi.org/10.3167/9781789207842

This book is dedicated to Hersch Bergner, who was born on 10 December 1907 in Dabrowka-Ruska, Poland, and worked as a laborer in nearby Sanok. He was deported to Auschwitz on 12 December 1941 and died only twelve days later, on 24 December 1941. It is not known if Hersch Bergner was a victim of medical experimentation at Auschwitz. However, he stands for the millions of victims of Nazi medicalized murder.

We must not see any person as an abstraction. Instead, we must see in every person a universe with its own secrets, with its own treasures, with its own sources of anguish, and with some measure of triumph.

—Elie Wiesel, "Foreword," in George J. D. Annas and Michael A. Grodin, *The Nazi Doctors and the Nuremberg Code: Human Rights in Human Experimentation* (New York, Oxford: Oxford University, 1992), ix.

Contents

	List of Illustrations	X
	Acknowledgments	XII
	Foreword William E. Seidelman	XIII
Introduction	Recognizing the Past in the Present Sabine Hildebrandt, Miriam Offer, and Michael A. Grodin	1

Part I. The Past

Chapter 1	Non-mechanistic Explanatory Styles in Interwar German Racial Theory: A Comparison of Hans F. K. Günther and Ludwig Ferdinand Clauß Amit Varshizky	21
Chapter 2	From "Racial Surveys" to Medical Experiments in Prisoner-of-War Camps Margit Berner	44
Chapter 3	"Der Doktor": The Writings of Mordechai Lensky during the Interwar Period Miriam Offer	59
Chapter 4	Rabbinic Responsa during the Holocaust: The Life-for-Life Problem Johnathan I. Kelly, Erin L. Miller, Rabbi Joseph Polak, Robert Kirschner, and Michael A. Grodin	82
Chapter 5	Un(B)earable: Pregnant Bodies and Obstetrical Genocide Annette Finley-Croswhite	103
Chapter 6	"Complete Mastery of the Subject": The Connection between Forced Sterilization and Gynecological Fertility Research in National Socialism Gabriele Czarnowski	125

Chapter 7	Deference, Pragmatism, Ideology: The Medical Student Kurt Gerstein and the Predicament of Ethical Conduct under National Socialism *Mathias Schütz*	140
Chapter 8	Ludwig Stumpfegger (1910–45): A Career at the Interface of Hitler, Himmler, and Ravensbrück Concentration Camp *Stephanie Kaiser and Mathias Schmidt*	154
Chapter 9	Between Participation in National Socialist Medicine and Everyday Administrative Action: On the Economic Argument of the Psychiatric Planning Commission (1941–45) *Felicitas Söhner*	172
Chapter 10	Dentists in National Socialist Germany: A Fragmented Profession *Matthis Krischel*	190
Chapter 11	Only Following Orders? Aviation Medicine in Nazi Germany *Alexander von Lünen*	204
Chapter 12	Blood and Bones from Auschwitz: The Mengele Link *Paul J. Weindling*	222

Part II. The Present: Postwar Continuities, Legacies, and Reflections

Chapter 13	Renewed Trauma: Abraham de la Penha's Testimony against Dr. Franz Lucas in the Frankfurt Auschwitz Trial *Andrew Wisely*	241
Chapter 14	"Schluss mit der Rassenschande!" From Separation to Extermination: The Fate of Jewish Mentally Ill Patients in Germany and Occupied Poland, 1939–42 *Kamila Uzarczyk*	257
Chapter 15	"Since She Was in Auschwitz, the Patient Feels That She Is Being Persecuted": Holocaust Survivors and Austrian Psychiatry after World War II *Herwig Czech*	276
Chapter 16	"To Prevent Further Unfounded Aly Constructions" *Götz Aly*	298

Chapter 17	Baneful Medicine and a Radical Bioethics in Contemporary Art *Andrew Weinstein*	327
Chapter 18	The History of the Vienna Protocol *Sabine Hildebrandt, Rabbi Joseph Polak, Michael A. Grodin, and William E. Seidelman*	354
	Appendix: Excerpts from Recommendations for the Handling of Future Discoveries of Human Remains from Victims of Nazi Terror and Vienna Protocol	363
Conclusion	The Past in the Present and the Future *Sabine Hildebrandt, Miriam Offer, and Michael A. Grodin*	373
	Index	377

Illustrations

Figures

Figure 8.1	Portrait of Ludwig Stumpfegger, taken from a handwritten CV, undated.	157
Figure 14.1	View of Zofiówka, 2019, interior.	266
Figure 14.2	View of Zofiówka, 2019, exterior.	267
Figure 17.1	Internet meme, ca. 2019.	330
Figure 17.2	The Tissue Culture & Art Project (Oron Catts and Ionat Zurr), *Semi Living Worry Dolls*, 2000.	331
Figure 17.3	Eduardo Kac, *GFP Bunny*, 2000. Transgenic rabbit.	332
Figure 17.4	Eduardo Kac, *GFP Bunny—Paris Intervention*, 2000.	333
Figure 17.5	Eduardo Kac, *Free Alba!*, 2001–02.	334
Figure 17.6	Eduardo Kac, *Rabbit in Rio*, 2004. Rio de Janeiro, Brazil.	335
Figure 17.7	Verena Kaminiarz, *may the mice bite me if it is not true*, installation detail: *Habitat*, 2008.	336
Figure 17.8	Verena Kaminiarz, *may the mice bite me if it is not true*, installation detail: *Felix*, 2008.	337
Figure 17.9	Verena Kaminiarz, *may the mice bite me if it is not true*, installation detail: *Gilles and Joseph*, 2008.	338
Figure 17.10	Verena Kaminiarz, *death masks (mus musculus)* (details), 2008.	339
Figure 17.11	Jake and Dinos Chapman, *Zygotic Acceleration, Biogenetic Desublimated Libidinal Model (Enlarged × 1000)*, 1995.	341
Figure 17.12	Jake and Dinos Chapman, *Ubermensch*, 1995.	344
Figure 17.13	Jake and Dinos Chapman, *Fucking Hell*, 2008.	345

FIGURE 17.14 Jake and Dinos Chapman, *The Sum of All Evil* (detail), 2012–13.   346

FIGURE 17.15 Jake and Dinos Chapman, *Hell* (detail), 1999–2000.   347

FIGURE 17.16 Jake and Dinos Chapman, *Arbeit McFries*, 2001.   348

Table

TABLE 9.1 Documented visits by the planning commission.   179

Acknowledgments

The authors are very grateful to all those without whose personal assistance and institutional support this volume would not have been possible:

- Division of General Pediatrics, Department of Pediatrics, Boston Children's Hospital / Harvard Medical School
- Center for Health Law, Ethics & Human Rights, Boston University School of Public Health
- The Project on Medicine and the Holocaust at the Elie Wiesel Center for Jewish Studies, Boston University
- The United States Holocaust Memorial Museum, Washington DC
- Holocaust Studies Program, Akko Israel, Western Galilee College
- Israel Ministry of Science and Technology
- Professor Dan Michman, Head of The International Institute for Holocaust Research and Incumbent of the John Najmann Chair of Holocaust Studies, Yad Vashem
- Azrieli Foundation
- Erin L Miller, medical student at New York University Long Island School of Medicine
- Gargi Panday, student at Boston University

Foreword

William E. Seidelman

The profession of medicine proclaims an ancient ethic based on the Greek physician/philosopher Hippocrates of the Aegean island of Kos, who pronounced that the physician must do no harm. The Oath of Hippocrates was sworn to the Greek god Apollo. In the centuries since Hippocrates, the field of medicine, despite the limitations of knowledge of illness and disease, still attempted to follow those precepts. Regardless of their ignorance of the causes of diseases and death, and the limitations of their craft, physicians attempted to practice medicine based on the ancient Hippocratic precept to avoid harm.

Over two millennia after the death of Hippocrates, the twentieth century marked a turning point in which medicine came to be practiced as a consequence of revolutionary discoveries into the causes of death and disease; infectious agents in particular. Medical science discovered ways of preventing and treating disease by methods that included X-rays, diagnostic tests of blood and body fluids, pasteurization, asepsis, and immunization, as well as therapies and interventions such as anesthesia, surgery, antimicrobials, transfusion of blood, and even the replacement of body parts and organs such as joints, heart, lung, liver, and kidney.

Most of the pioneering discoveries that gave birth to this scientific revolution took place in nineteenth- and twentieth-century Europe, Germany in particular. The German-language universities and clinics, which included those in Austria and Czechoslovakia, were the destination of hundreds of physicians from all parts of the world who sought to advance their skills. Knowledge of the German language was considered a requirement in order to understand the scientific and clinical advances that emanated from German-language institutions and were published in German-language journals. The influence of German medical science and the German university was such that the United States, led by influential industrialists/philanthropists such as Andrew Carnegie and John Rockefeller, through their respective foundations, undertook to bring medical education in the United States and Canada to a new level of quality, a standard based principally on the German system that merged the academic stringency of the German university with the enormous discoveries emanating from the German clinics and laboratories that were revolutionizing medical practice.

The name most often associated with these changes is that of the American educator Abraham Flexner, who undertook a study of medical education on behalf of the Carnegie Foundation, which became known as the Flexner Report.[1] Flexner subsequently played a critical role in the implementation of his ideas and recommendations as an officer of the Rockefeller Foundation, which dispensed funds to support the changes Flexner himself had proposed. According to a biography of Abraham Flexner by Thomas Bonner, Flexner also sought to include the English model of clinical education along with the academic and scientific rigor of the German universities, laboratories, and clinics.[2]

While these revolutionary changes in medical education were being implemented in North America, Europe was experiencing the consequences of World War I and the emergence of fascism, which, by 1933, had overtaken Germany and would eventually wreak havoc on most of Europe and much of the world. The Nazi state oversaw the death of the Hippocratic principle of "do no harm" with its replacement by a political and professional ethos in which harm was permissible, where the state defined an individual or a group as "unworthy" or "undesirable," without any rights or protections. The role of the physician changed from being a person who protected an individual from harm to a practitioner who could exercise harm on behalf of the Hitler state. The overriding principal was the promotion of the "Health of the People," known as *Volksgesundheit*. Excluded from the *Volk*—the German people—were the disabled, ethnic groups such as the Sinti and Roma, homosexuals, religious dissenters such as Jehovah's Witnesses, and, above all, Jews. Officially defined as "subhuman" or *Untermenschen*, the aforementioned categories of human beings were stripped of any and all protections; even of those protections that were afforded by official statute to protect animals from experimentation. Certain human "animals," numbering in the millions, did not qualify.[3]

With the end of World War II and the realization of the enormity of human and physical destruction, such as the Jewish Holocaust or Shoah, it was difficult to comprehend the role played by medicine. How could a profession based on the ethos of preventing harm, a profession that had only recently played such a critical role in the advancement of medical science, treatments, and interventions that had revolutionized healthcare and saved literally millions of lives, have played a role in such a catastrophic program of exploitation and slaughter of millions of innocent human beings? How could it have been possible? How could such distinguished professors have been involved? How could esteemed universities and research institutions, some the beneficiaries of Rockefeller Foundation largesse, have played a role? It seemed beyond belief. But it was true. All of it.

It has taken a long time to begin to discover the truth and document the facts. Indeed, seventy-five years after the end of World War II we are still at the beginning of documenting the full extent of the involvement of medical science and the health professions, including world-renowned academic institutions and research organizations, in the design, implementation, and exploitation of the greatest program of organized human destruction in the history of mankind.

This volume is an important link in a chain of documentation on the critical role of medicine in achieving the policies, practices, and crimes of the Hitler regime. While there was an awareness of egregious medical crimes, the breadth and depth were not fully appreciated in the early period after the war. The Nuremberg Doctors Trial was an important step, but it involved very few perpetrators and focused on inhuman experimentation. The difficult reality is that the transgressions of the medical profession during the Hitler regime encompassed virtually the entire healthcare system, all personnel and institutions, including leading professional organizations and internationally renowned academic and research institutions.

Documenting the history has been a challenging exercise. Revelations of the bestial brutality of the Shoah and abuses such as the "euthanasia" programs of mass murder of the so-called "mentally ill" and handicapped were gradually revealed, and some criminal trials were eventually held. However, there was another reality, namely one of "business as usual" by the majority, of whom many were complicit in crimes, if discovered. Institutions and organizations that had heretofore prided themselves on investigation, documentation, and communication adopted a position of silence. Mouths were closed, archives sealed, and secrets hidden. Scientific and clinical discourse was replaced by intimidation of those who dared to tell the truth. Professors who held important roles during the Hitler regime were able to preserve their distinguished careers after the war and protect their colleagues. The German doctors' organization, the Bundesärztekammer (BÄK), was led for decades after the war by physicians who had been associated with the Nazi regime: Dr. Karl Haedenkamp, Professor Ernst Fromm, and Professor Hans Sewering, the latter two former members of the SS.[4] So successful was the subterfuge of the BÄK, it assumed de facto control of the World Medical Association (WMA), an organization that purportedly represents national medical organizations in the promotion of standards in bioethics. The 1993 candidate for president of the WMA, the aforementioned Professor Hans Sewering, had been linked to the death of a neurologically impaired adolescent girl, Babette Fröwis, murdered in the child "euthanasia" program at the killing center of Eglfing-Haar.[5] The audacity of the BÄK is best exemplified by the professional excommunication of a young German physician, Dr. Hartmut Hanauske-Abel, who had the temerity to document German medicine's role in the Holocaust in an article published in the renowned medical journal *The Lancet* in August 1986.[6]

While a number of courageous German scholars documented the history of German medicine's role from within Germany in the postwar years, it wasn't until the 1980s that major scholarship based on archival research began to appear in the English language. With two notable exceptions, most of the credible publications were from scholars based outside Germany. The two exceptions were the English-language translations of German-language works by the molecular biologist/historian Professor Benno Müller-Hill: *Murderous Science*,[7] and the anthology *Cleansing the Fatherland*, with contributions from the German historians Götz Aly, Christian Pross, and Peter Chroust.[8] Professor Michael Kater, while born in Germany, was based in Canada, with most of his major work being published in English.[9] With the new millennium, younger scholars from within Germany and Austria began to follow the example of their courageous predecessors exemplified by the journalist/historian Aly. For a comprehensive listing of important German-language publications from the 1980s see Roelke.[10]

This was also a time of institutional reflection and examination exemplified by the Max Planck Society's five-year (1999–2004) research project on the history of its antecedent, the Kaiser-Wilhelm Society, and research institutes during the Hitler period, followed by endeavors focusing on the German Association for Psychiatry and Psychotherapy in 2010 and the Anatomische Gesellschaft (Anatomy Association) in 2011. In 2012, the Bundesärztekammer, after almost seven decades of suppression, repression, and intimidation, issued an official declaration formally acknowledging the role of Germany's physicians in the criminal activities of the Hitler period.[10] However, the BÄK's historic declaration arose, not from within the organization, but as the result of "an appeal from historians of medicine and members of the German branch of the IPPNW (International Physicians for the Prevention of Nuclear War)."[11] Neither the BÄK nor the putative protector of medical ethics, the World Medical Association, has officially acknowledged the role of their former leader and SS alumnus, Professor Hans Sewering, in the death of Babette Fröwis at Eglfing-Haar.

The German historian of medicine Professor Volker Roelcke has provided what is probably the most detailed accounting of the role of the BÄK in that organization's attempts to avoid addressing the historical truths of the critical role played by the German medical profession it represents. Roelcke's paper is a detailed account of the struggles to document the reality despite the resistance of the BÄK.[12]

This volume adds important knowledge to what will be a long, complicated history. First, it graphically describes obstacles, exemplified by the experience of Dr. Götz Aly, that scholars have faced in documenting this painful history. Second, many of the contributors are from a younger generation of European scholars, working in a more open environment than their predecessors did. Third, the subjects include important areas that had not previously been explored in detail. They include, among other topics, the exploitation of women for gynecological experiments, the fate of pregnant women and their newborn children in ghettos and concentration camps, and the agonizing questions asked of physicians and rabbis by doomed captives in ghettos and concentration camps. There is also an account of coming to grips with the moral challenges of the continuing legacy as exemplified by the infamous Pernkopf atlas of human anatomy and ongoing discoveries of the remains of possible victims.

Some scholars in the field have emphasized the importance of teaching the subject of the Holocaust and medicine within the undergraduate curriculum for students in the health professions. The Second International Scholars Workshop on Medicine during the Holocaust and Beyond held in Northern Israel (Western Galilee College, Galilee Medical Center, the Bar-Ilan Faculty of Medicine in the Galilee—Safed) in May 2017, at which a number of the papers in this volume were originally presented, also produced the "Galilee Declaration," which proposes a model framework for such a curriculum. The Galilee Declaration is further supported by a scholarly monograph titled "The Holocaust, Medicine and Becoming a Physician: The Crucial Role of Education" by Professor Shmuel Reis of the Hadassah/Hebrew University Faculty of Medicine, Dr. Hedy Wald of Brown University in the United States, and Professor Paul Weindling of Oxford-Brookes University, the noted scholar of the history of medicine in Nazi Germany.[13] Strong support for the Reis/Wald/Weindling proposal is provided by the eminent editor in chief of *The Lancet*, Professor Richard Horton, in a commentary that builds on the apparent rise in anti-Semitism that has recently embroiled the British Labor Party and is becoming increasingly apparent in European countries that, not too long ago, saw their Jewish communities destroyed in the Holocaust.[14] Horton's powerful and timely commentary had a profound impact that was soon reflected in a 24 November 2019 decision of the Council of the Ontario Medical Association (OMA), the largest province of Canada, "that OMA endorse and promote the recent call by the editor of *The Lancet* to 'include the Holocaust in the curriculum of health professionals.'"[15]

As important and worthwhile as such proposals may be, they face significant challenges. Despite the impressive documentation elucidated in the Reis/Wald/Weindling paper, the fact is that research and scholarly publication on the subject of medicine and the Holocaust, for reasons elucidated here, is in its infancy. Despite a growing group of young scholars, there is far from a critical mass required for a base of *informed experts* to teach the subject to every undergraduate course in medicine. There is as yet no agreed-upon curriculum based on established historical evidence. There is no agreed-upon basic bibliography. There is no established academic center, with formal links to the academic medical community, that has the scholarly and administrative resources or funding commitments to *support and sustain* such an effort. The subject of medicine and the Holocaust has not been a major priority of Holocaust documentation centers. Serious scholarly publications on the subject only began to appear in the 1980s. The acceptance of responsibility for their roles in the Holocaust by major German medical organizations only began at the beginning of this century. Research into the institutional history of German academic institutions such as universities and medical faculties has been problematic.[16]

In addition to these factors, the challenge of curriculum change and adaptation in an increasingly complex medical environment may make such a goal difficult to achieve. The actualization of such a change will be facilitated by documentation of the most significant curriculum revolution in the history of medical education, namely the transformation of academic medicine under the Hitler regime and the death of the Hippocratic proscription against doing harm. Knowing the end result of the calamity of the Hitler regime, any detailed scholarly examination of what really happened within the hallowed halls of German academia promises to be a sobering experience. There is certainly much to be learned by examining the pathology of power in medicine as exemplified by the German university and clinics that gave rise to modern medical science AND the perversion of medicine during the Nazi regime. Once we have a clearer understanding of the pathology, then we will have a better, evidence-based platform to formulate a curriculum based on a perspective of how it began. The first "learners" need to be the leaders and teachers, the professional successors to those who wrought such terrible havoc on medicine and humanity and remain, for the most part, ignorant of what actually happened and how their forbears played a critical role.

The chapters in this volume will be valuable for scholars, teachers, historians, students, and anyone who is interested in the history of the Holocaust and the history of medicine in the twentieth century, and how they are interrelated. The texts represent an important contribution to extending a path that is far from complete and will continue to be constructed for many years, indeed generations, to come. Hopefully, they will become part of the bibliography of an informed curriculum for the education of future leaders of the healthcare system and students of the health professions—an evidence-based curriculum taught by informed teachers that is sustained by strong and steady institutional support and reinforced by continuing scholarly research into a field that we are only beginning to properly explore free of impediments.

Acknowledgments

I wish to acknowledge the invitation of the editors to contribute this foreword and their generous responses to this submission. I am especially grateful to Professor Volker Roelcke, the director of the Institute for the History of Medicine of the Justus-Leibig University of Giessen, Germany, for his critical review of the preparatory manuscript for this foreword and his constructive suggestions that I have attempted to incorporate in the final revision.

Dr. William E. Seidelman, an emeritus professor of family medicine at the University of Toronto, has been involved for the past four decades in researching the role of academic and scientific elite medical institutions associated with the crimes of the Third Reich. His focus has been on the exploitation of the bodies of victims of Nazi terror, some of which remained in institutional collections for decades after the war. In 1995, Professor Seidelman joined Professor Howard Israel, a specialist in oral and maxillofacial surgery in New York, who together with Yad Vashem: The World Holocaust Remembrance Center, brought pressure to bear on the University of Vienna for a full examination of their collections of human specimens after the Anschluss. Professor Seidelman chaired the 17 May 2017 Special Symposium at Yad Vashem on the subject of discovered remains of possible victims of the Holocaust.

Notes

1. Flexner 1910.
2. Bonner 2002.
3. Seidelman 1986.
4. Kater 1987.
5. Hohendorf 2009; Seidelman 2014; Hohendorf 2014.
6. Hanauske-Abel 1986; Stock 1987; Roelcke 2014.
7. Müller-Hill 1988.
8. Aly et al. 1994.
9. Kater 1989.
10. Reis 2012.
11. Roelcke 2010; 2014.
12. Roelcke 2014.
13. Reis et al. 2019.
14. Horton 2019.
15. Dr. Frank Sommers (Toronto), email to W. Seidelman, 26 November 2019.
16. Roelcke 2010.

References

Aly, Götz, Peter Chroust, Christian Pross. 1994. *Cleansing the Fatherland: Nazi Medicine and Racial Hygiene*. Foreword by Michael H. Kater. Translated by Belinda Cooper. Baltimore: Johns Hopkins University Press.

Bonner, Thomas N. 2002, *Iconoclast: Abraham Flexner and a Life in Learning*. Baltimore: Johns Hopkins University Press.

Flexner, Abraham. 1910. "Medical Education in the United States and Canada: A Report to the Carnegie Foundation for the Advancement of Teaching." *Bulletin No. 4*. Retrieved 30 July 2020 from http://archive.carnegiefoundation.org/publications/pdfs/elibrary/Carnegie_Flexner_Report.pdf.

Hanauske-Abel, Hartmut. 1986. "From Nazi Holocaust to Nuclear Holocaust: A Lesson to Learn?" *The Lancet* 2: 271–73.

Hohendorf, Gerrit. 2009. "The Sewering Affair." *Korot: The Israel Journal of the History of Medicine* 19 (for 2007/2008): 83–104.

———. 2014. "The Sewering Affair." In *Silence, Scapegoats, Self-Reflection: The Shadow of Nazi Medical Crimes on Medicine and Bioethics*, edited by Volker Roelcke, Sascha Topp, and Etienne Lepicard, 131–46. Göttingen: V&R unipress.

Horton, R. 2019. "Offline: Medicine and the Holocaust—It's Time to Teach." *The Lancet* 394: 105.

Kater, Michael.H. 1987. "The Burden of the Past: Problems of a Modern Historiography of Physicians and Medicine in Nazi Germany." *German Studies Review* 10(1): 31–56.

———. 1989. *Doctors under Hitler*. Chapel Hill: University of North Carolina Press.

Müller-Hill, Benno. 1988. *Murderous Science: Elimination by Scientific Selection of Jews, Gypsies, and Others Germany 1933–45*. Translated by George R. Fraser. Oxford: Oxford University Press.

Reis, S. 2012. "Reflections on the Nuremberg Declaration of the German Medical Assembly." *Israel Medical Association Journal* 14: 529–30.

Reis, Shmuel, Hedy S. Wald, and Paul Weindling. 2019. "The Holocaust, Medicine and Becoming a Physician: The Crucial Role of Education." *Israel Journal of Health Policy Research* 8(55): 1–5.

Roelcke, Volker. 2010. "Medicine During the Nazi Period: Historical Facts and Some Implications for Teaching Medical Ethics and Professionalism." In *Medicine after the Holocaust: From the Master Race to the Human Genome and Beyond*, edited by Sheldon Rubenfeld, 17–28. New York: Palgrave McMillan.

———. 2014. "Between Professional Honor and Self-Reflection: The German Medical Association's Reluctance to Address Medical Malpractice during the National Socialist Era, ca. 1985–2012." In *Silence, Scapegoats, Self-Reflection: The Shadow of Nazi Medical Crimes on Medicine and Bioethics*, edited by Volker Roelcke, Sascha Topp, and Etienne Lepicard, 244–278. Göttingen: V&R unipress.

Seidelman, William E. 1986. "Animal Experiments in Nazi Germany." *The Lancet* 1(8491): 1214.

———. 2014. "*Requiescat Sine Pace*: Recollections and Reflections on the World Medical Association, the Case of Prof. Dr. Hans Joachim Sewering and the Murder of Babette Fröwis," In *Silence, Scapegoats, Self-Reflection: The Shadow of Nazi Medical Crimes on Medicine and Bioethics*, edited by Volker Roelcke, Sascha Topp, and Etienne Lepicard, 281–300. Göttingen: V&R unipress.

Stock, Ulrich. 1987. "Deutsche Ärzte und die Vergangenheit." *Die Zeit*, 12 June. Retrieved 4 February 2015 from http://www.zeit.de/1987/25/deutsche-aerzte-und-die-vergangenheit.

Introduction
Recognizing the Past in the Present

Sabine Hildebrandt, Miriam Offer, and Michael A. Grodin

The past matters, as it continues to reach into the present and influence the future. The acknowledgment that this holds true for the legacies of medicine in the Holocaust has long been denied by the medical professions after World War II, to the point that systematic research into this history only began in the 1980s.[1] Too easy was it to point to the results of the Nuremberg Doctors Trial and claim that only a criminal few had been responsible for the atrocities committed by physicians in the extermination of those considered unworthy of life and the European Jewry.[2] Too easy was it to claim that medicine itself had been abused by the criminal regime of National Socialism.[3] Research into the complicity of medical scientists, physicians, nurses, midwives, and other health personnel gained momentum only after the perpetrators of crimes—and in academic medicine often their pupils too—had left their positions that they had reclaimed after the war. And the potential failings of the theory of scientific medicine itself have come into the focus of historical analysis only late.[4] Many threads of this history are currently under investigation, their roots traced back to the time before 1933, and they need to be placed in the larger framework of *continuities* of persons, thought patterns and epistemology, and *legacies* that include the trauma of victims, the published results, and the physical remains of Nazi research.

These continuities and legacies are encountered in many forms—at this point no longer in the person of the postwar psychiatrist, who is the same as the one complicit in a "euthanasia" verdict, evaluating a Nazi victim,[5] but in the publication of a neuroanatomist who used the brains of "euthanasia" victims for his research after the war.[6] Continuities from the past are also encountered in the specimens of "euthanasia" victims that are still held in scientific collections or in the bones of potential Holocaust victims that are found inadvertently.[7] They are encountered in journal articles and books that were created from research on Nazi victims and are still in use.[8] They are encountered in medical practices such as sterilization techniques that were perfected by Nazi gynecologists.[9] More intangibly, continuities from this history are encountered in persistent thought patterns of objectifying medicine, misogyny, and anti-Semitism. Importantly, they are also present in the intergenerational trauma of families of Holocaust survivors.[10]

A largely unexplored legacy from the history of medicine during the Holocaust concerns the practice of Jewish physicians during this time, as well as rabbinical responses to ethical dilemmas concerning medical aspects of victims' suffering under the Nazis.[11] Here Jewish medical ethics may aid in a productive interaction with the legacies of Nazi medicine, as in the example of the Vienna Protocol on what to do with Jewish or possibly Jewish human remains.[12] The fact that ultimately all aspects of human life are affected by patterns from the past in the present is most obviously reflected in contemporary artwork that engages with current and potential future challenges in bioethics.[13]

However, the ability to recognize the patterns of the past in the present relies on two prerequisites: on continued scholarly historical research on medicine during the Holocaust and on the teaching of this history in medical curricula.[14] Why more historical research? Here the example of Josef Mengele is instructive: while he is arguably the most notorious perpetrator of Nazi medical crimes, hardly any archival research of his scientific activities in Auschwitz exists, and Paul Weindling's chapter in this volume presents entirely new results. Thus this volume contributes new studies of the wide spectrum of the history of medicine before and during the Holocaust, and then illustrates postwar continuities from this history in another set of new studies that discusses examples of the legacies from this history.

Situating Medicine within the General History of the Holocaust

Looking at patterns from the past in the present is all the more relevant in times of resurging anti-Semitism, and in light of Dan Michman's analysis, which places the origin of the Holocaust in Hitler's goal of the elimination of the *Jüdischer Geist*—literally the "Jewish spirit," that is, Jewish life and Jewish thinking—and sees medicine as a main driving force of the Holocaust. He presented these thoughts in a keynote lecture at a conference of medical historians in Akko, Israel, in 2017,[15] thereby setting a milestone in the historiography as the first historian of the Holocaust to assign a major role for medicine in the destruction of European Jewry. This is all the more significant as Professor Michman is one of the foremost scholars in the field of Holocaust research and holds the position of head of the International Institute for Holocaust Research and incumbent of the John Najmann Chair of Holocaust Studies at Yad Vashem.

Michman laid out his thoughts on resituating the place of medicine in the grand picture of the Holocaust within the context of a review of the historiography of the Holocaust.[16] He observed that the Holocaust was often missing in narratives of the history of medicine, and at the same time medicine was missing from the historiography of the Holocaust, appearing only as a marginal phenomenon if at all. However, he stated, the history of medicine had increasingly become a field of study for historians and not—as previously—only medical professionals, and thus medicine had been placed in its "political, social and cultural context."[17] Based on a critique of intentionalist, functionalist, and synthetic approaches in the historiography of the Holocaust, Michman proposed a new interpretation of this history in situating the origin of the Holocaust in the complete annihilation of the *Jüdischer Geist* as defined by the National Socialists. Drawing from, among others, historian Johann Chapoutot's explanation of Nazi thinking and acting,[18] Michman described Hitler as "activating" the preexisting anti-Semitism in the German population, as Germans sought relief from the economic and mental trauma following World War I. In implementing the "total removal of Jews" as carriers of the "Jewish spirit," the National Socialists availed themselves of "legal" means of exclusion that included economic spoliation and expropriation; de-Judaization/self-purification of art, language, sciences, and humanities; and medicine. The National Socialists sought the support from the medical profession in the theory and practice of medicalized killing. Thus, in Michman's reinterpretation of the origin of the Holocaust, medicine was one of the integrated and essential factors contributing to the purge of the "Jewish spirit." He sees NS medicine in clear contrast to Jewish medicine practiced at the same time in the ghettos created by the National Socialists, as Jewish medicine counteracted NS medicine by working to save Jewish life and Jewish spirit.

Michman's interpretation represents a significant transition in the perspective of major scholars of the Holocaust and Holocaust documentation centers. Heretofore the subject of medicine and the Holocaust was considered, for the most part, as a marginal subject, separate from the mainstream of traditional Holocaust scholarship and research. Michman's interpretation opens a new, intellectually and philosophically legitimizing context for the importance of medicine within studies on the Holocaust.

The chapters included in this volume reflect many aspects of Professor Michman's reinterpretation of the origins of the Holocaust and the place of medicine with it. They also confirm the observations on the historiography of medicine in the twentieth century made by Huisman et al. in 2017[19]: the studies present a variety of actors and show medicine in its sociopolitical context. Among the authors are not only scholars specialized on the history of medicine but also those from different fields of history and other professional disciplines altogether, established and emerging scholars. They discuss medical perpetrators, racial hygiene theorists, and NS bureaucrats, as well as Jewish physicians practicing before and during the war, and record the histories of victims. It will become clear that medicine in National Socialism is a particularly glaring example of the fact that "social and ideological conflicts were often transported into the medical domain and that, conversely, medical arguments were used to support a variety of political opinions."[20] These chapters allow new insights into the continuity of medical thinking, practice, and societal impact from before the NS period, throughout this time, and into the postwar period and the present.

The Origins of Medicine during the Holocaust

The roots of medicine during the Holocaust go back to the nineteenth-century history of eugenics, racial anthropology, and racism, and their continuities reach to what today may be called "othering."[21] Physicians and biological scientists were always part of this history. By the time the National Socialists attained government power in Germany in 1933, the biological sciences had provided foundational arguments for NS ideology and were on the verge of facilitating NS policies of positive and negative eugenics. In 1934, anthropologist Otto Aichel could proudly write in a tribute to the leader of the field of racial hygiene, Eugen Fischer,

> We stand at the turn of an era. For the first time in world history the Führer Adolf Hitler puts into practice the knowledge of the biological foundations of the development of peoples—race, heritage, selection. It is no coincidence that Germany is the place of this event: the German science put the tools into the hands of the politician.[22]

A few months earlier, Fischer—an anatomist, trained physician, and newly elected president of the Friedrich-Wilhelm-Universität in Berlin—had given the anniversary address for the foundation of this institution, which had opened in 1811.[23] He looked back on Germany in the nineteenth century, as the political union of the German Empire in 1871 followed decades of strife between individual German states, but this new nation-state—in Fischer's consideration—lacked the unifying appreciation for shared blood and race. Fischer described the biological and technical advancements in hygiene and medicine in this period and held them responsible for differential population growth, as well as cultural and moral decline. Believing that "we feel our own race, and are conscious of being our one and own people [Volk],"[24] he claimed that this sense of "racial identity" had been lost, especially after the devastation of World War I and in the interwar period, but had been regained through his own field of work, racial hygiene and hereditary biology, which provided the scientific basis for the "eugenic-racial hygienic-people-based" state.[25] Fischer declared that it was only the NS Party that from the start had integrated regulations on genetic health and racial purity in its political program, and thus the NS state was now a *"völkisch"* one, that is, based on the biological and racial unity of its people. An inclusion of other races, namely Jews, in the German people was to be denied. Fischer saw the new German state insofar as a "socialist" entity, as every healthy person of German race was considered to be of equal worth. In essence Fischer formulated here the basis for what historian Claudia Koonz called "the Nazi Conscience."[26]

Fischer touched in his speech on many pertinent aspects of German political and social history of the nineteenth century, a history that in certain parts was shared internationally: the rise of nationalism, racial ideology, the development of medicine as a biological science with its many new disciplines, and particularly the transferal of concepts of Darwinism to the social and political context, leading to the international movement of eugenics.[27] German biological and medical scientists had gained internationally recognized status as leaders in research and first practical applications of research results. This included not only the foundational sciences of bacteriology, immunology, histology, and embryology but also new technological developments such as radiology. Specific to the German context was particularly the implementation of ideas of preventative medicine based on insights from social hygiene—today's public medicine—in institutions supported by the German state as early as 1871. These included compulsory health insurance for the whole population, licensing of panel doctors, and state-run health offices, which were supported by German governments through all their different political manifestations from the Imperial German State to the Weimar Republic.[28] The administrative institutions of healthcare and the interactions between state and healthcare provider were manifold and well established at the time of the NS takeover of the government, and were then adapted according to NS policies. Within the time span of only a few years, these policies progressed from exclusion, forced sterilization, and "euthanasia" of children and adults to the extermination of those not considered part of the German people.[29] As late as 1943, at a time when Fischer should have fully understood the murderous intent of the NS regime as mass deportations of Jews to the east had started all over Germany, he published a newspaper article in which he wrote, "It is a special and rare good fortune for theoretical research, when it falls into a time in which it receives recognition by the world. A time, in which even practical research results are welcomed as the basis for public policies."[30]

Fischer was one of many scientists in medicine who lived and worked in a symbiosis with the NS regime, to use historian Sheila Weiss's term.[31] For the racial hygienists, interactions with the National Socialists had already started in the 1920s, when Hitler came across the Baur-Fischer-Lenz, the standard work on racial hygiene and human heredity, in the prison library during his incarceration in Landsberg in 1923—he subsequently integrated reasoning from racial hygiene with his own anti-Semitism in his book *Mein Kampf*.[32] In 1931 geneticist Fritz Lenz—Fischer's coauthor and colleague at the Berlin Kaiser Wilhelm Institute for Anthropology, Human Heredity and Eugenics—called the politics of National Socialism "applied Biology,"[33] a term repeated by Hitler's deputy Rudolf Hess in 1934.[34] Psychiatrist Ernst Rüdin had helped draw up the 1933 Law for the

Prevention of Hereditarily Diseased Offspring, which was patterned on decades-old similar laws in the United States,[35] and he, with Fischer and many other racial hygienists, served as a judge on the hereditary health courts.[36] At the same time, many other medical disciplines profited from the new NS policies: gynecologists honed their technical skills in ever new ways of sterilization; pathologists, forensic physicians, and anatomists had access to ever-increasing numbers of bodies of dead NS victims; and those from all fields of medicine interested in experimenting on the living could either do so in their own hospital setting—as long as their experimental subjects were considered as not belonging to the healthy German *Volk*—or they could apply to SS leader Heinrich Himmler for access to prisoners in concentration camps.[37] The techniques of mass murder were developed by physicians within the escalating "euthanasia" killing programs and employed in the psychiatric hospitals in Germany, then those in Poland and other occupied territories, ultimately arriving in the gas chambers of the extermination camps.[38]

The Bauer-Fischer-Lenz text not only influenced Adolf Hitler in the development of *Mein Kampf*, its impact also extended internationally through an English-language edition that proved very popular. Copies of the English-language edition of the Bauer-Fischer-Lenz text can be found to this day on the shelves of university libraries in North America. Eugen Fischer also represents an important transitional figure through not only his coauthorship with Baur and Lenz but also his career with the Kaiser Wilhelm Institute for Anthropology, Human Heredity and Eugenics in Berlin-Dahlem and advocacy for his successor, Otmar von Verschuer. The internationally renowned institute and its member scientists had received support not only from organizations in Germany but also from distinguished foundations such as the Rockefeller Foundation.[39] Fischer was succeeded as director by Verschuer, the internationally noted expert on twin studies. Verschuer played a key role as the principal investigator for his former student and acolyte Josef Mengele, who was the holder of two doctorates, a PhD in anthropology from the University of Munich and an MD from the University of Frankfurt. After the war, Fischer protected Verschuer, who had been under suspicion from the Allied authorities. Because of Fischer's support, Verschuer was eventually appointed professor and chair of genetics at the University of Muenster, where Verschuer became the most influential geneticist in postwar Germany[40] and drew admiration from his Italian colleague, Professor Luigi Gedda of the Gregor Mendel Institute of Genetics in Rome and the founding editor of the journal *Acta geneticae medicae et gemellogiae: Twin studies*. In 1956 Gedda published a special *Festschrift* on the occasion of Verschuer's sixtieth birthday. The lead article (in Italian) by Gedda paid tribute to Verschuer as "Un Maestro et Un Esempio" (a teacher and an example).[41] The examples of Fischer and Verschuer show that the history of medicine during the Holocaust can be traced through the work of individual persons from before the Nazi period to the postwar decades, and that their influence was international.

The Past

Systematic investigations of the collaboration between physicians, medical scientists, academic institutions, and professional organizations with the National Socialist regime began in the 1980s, often against severe opposition from the existing German medical establishment, which continued to include many historical actors from the Third Reich and their apologists.[42] Since then, researchers have presented a wide array of studies that span from historical investigations of the leading scientific institutions, individual universities, and medical care facilities to in-depth perpetrator biographies, collections of victims' biographies, and studies of the actions of professional organizations.[43] In essence, these studies revealed that much, if not all, of German medical science and practice had been affected by the political conditions of National Socialism, and also that they had interacted with the regime. Anybody who was not persecuted and remained in Germany collaborated in some form or other with the National Socialist government, as only few individuals opted for overt political resistance. Instead, many of those who worked in the field of medicine actively sought the collaboration with the regime, either out of conviction or to advance their careers. And most of these scientists, physicians, nurses, midwifes, health educators, and administrators continued to work in their respective fields after the war, usually following an only short phase of so-called denazification. Thus, in the last decade, topics of postwar consequences of medicine during the Third Reich have been the focus of several studies by medical historians and ethicists that assess the continuities and legacies from this time.[44]

The collection of essays presented here sees itself in line with such studies and is organized in two parts. Part I, "The Past," begins with a focus on the theory and practice of the racial sciences before 1933, continues with the underresearched topics of Jewish medicine before and during the war, as well as gendered victimization that will be put in focus, and concludes with present studies that reflect the wide spectrum of medical perpetrators and their motivations. Part II, "The Present: Postwar Continuities, Legacies, and Reflections," includes postwar narratives of the continuing anguish of victims and the denial of medical professionals to deal with this suffering or their own potential guilt. However, legacies of the past not only include the continued presence and influence of former NS physicians and the fate of the surviving victims but also the search for traces of the vanished victims, including the identification of human remains from the Holocaust era. And apart from these physical legacies, there are moral ones: how should we remember the dead, how do we honor their memory, how should we reflect on human dignity in today's world?

The contributions in this volume come from an international and interdisciplinary group of authors, a unique collaboration insofar as it includes not only philosophers and historians of science, medicine, and art but also anthropologists, psychiatrists, and anatomists, and among them not only established but also emerging new scholars of medicine and the Holocaust. Overall, this collection presents a widening of the perspective and a maturation of the scholarship in this field of historical inquiry. Topics that were once deemed "unmentionable"— such as gendered victimization or the, however misplaced, "idealism" of Nazi perpetrators—are here systematically analyzed. Throughout it will become apparent that the past that is discussed here in its various aspects is still very much present and relevant for today's medicine, thus substantiating clinical psychologist Michael Wunder's observation: "No modern bioethics or medical ethics discussion is possible without the knowledge of history and lines of development."[45] It is our goal as editors of this volume to make these "lines of development" from the past to the present visible.

The first chapters of this volume discuss the theory and practice of racial science, which provided the so-called scientific basis for many of the manifestations of medical discrimination in the Third Reich. Israeli historian of science Amit Varshizky explores the different explanatory styles in German racial anthropology through a comparison of the work of Hans F. K. Günther and Ludwig Ferdinand Clauß, then the leading theorists of race, including an exploration of extra-scientific factors influencing their thinking. Varshizky calls for a reevaluation of the place of genetic science in German racial anthropology, showing how German racial ideas were built on detailed concepts of biology, heredity, and genetics that went beyond the traditions of naturalistic enquiry and causal explanations. Austrian anthropologist Margit Berner then investigates examples of the application of such racial theories in anthropological fieldwork during World War II. She describes how her predecessors in the Department of Anthropology at the Natural History Museum Vienna undertook extensive "racial" surveys of Jews and prisoners of war under the leadership of Josef Wastl, the director of the Department of Anthropology. Another anthropologist from the museum later moved on to collaborate in physiological and medical experiments on color vision and cerebrospinal fluid from prisoners of war in collaboration with a camp physician in the Kaisersteinbruch POW camp, thereby clearly transgressing an ethical boundary traditionally observed by his colleagues. As curator of the bone collection of the anthropological department of the museum, Berner herself had to deal with the physical legacies of her predecessor's work.[46]

Racial science also provided a framework for National Socialist medical ethics,[47] and the examples of Jewish medicine and medical ethics presented in the following chapters can be interpreted as illustrating a concept that ran diametrically counter to National Socialist medical ethics. Jewish physicians active during the Third Reich left a wealth of scientific, publicist, literary, and personal writings from the interwar period, the Holocaust, and the time afterward. However, as Israeli historian Miriam Offer points out in her chapter, these writings have rarely been investigated to expose the physicians' professional, spiritual, and ethical worlds, even though such studies could facilitate a deeper understanding of the history of Jewish physicians and Jewish medicine during that period. She explores this potential of physicians' writings in an exemplary manner with the study of Dr. Mordechai Lensky, who survived the Warsaw ghetto, describing his medical practice and ethics as established before World War II. Whereas Offer focuses her chapter on the biography of one physician, philosopher of religion Johnathan Kelly and his coauthors explore through the lens of rabbinic responsa—scholarly legal and ethical evaluations in the Jewish tradition that rabbis provide in answer to specific questions posed to them—a specific set of ethical problems in medical decision-making caused by NS persecution during World War II. Using the example of life-for-life choices during the Holocaust, the authors study here a set of documents rarely examined by historians or bioethicists. The rabbinic responsa provide a rare glimpse into the ways Jews were able to follow the principles of Jewish law and ethics in response to the attacks on their lives. The responsa also powerfully demonstrate the breadth and resiliency of the Jewish legal-ethical tradition in facing the most difficult ethical decisions in medicine. Fittingly, a question arising from postwar legacies of NS medical atrocities will be answered through the rabbinic responsum the Vienna Protocol (see chapter 18).

Many of the rabbinic responsa discussed by Kelly and colleagues concern questions that specifically address the plight of women. The topic of gendered victimization during the Holocaust has long been avoided in studies of this history, as US historian Annette Finley-Croswhite points out in her chapter. She argues that the "Jewish womb" became a killing field for the destructive forces of National Socialism, and she presents information that allows for a quantification of the loss of lives due to gender-specific forms of violence. This discriminatory assault on the female body is also the topic of the chapter by German historian Gabriele Czarnowski, a pioneer in the field of the history of gendered victimization in the Third Reich. She investigates the self-concept of Nazi gynecologists, who dealt out medical violence on one set of women through forced sterilization while at the same time living a medical ethos of help and care for another set with sterility problems. The postwar suffering of these women is addressed in medical historian Herwig Czech's contribution to this volume (chapter 15), and deserves further systematic exploration.

The theme of the self-conception and motivation of perpetrators will be further explored in a group of chapters that present a wide spectrum of historical actors in NS medicine, a spectrum reaching from a concerned medical student to notorious medical criminals exemplified by Dr. Josef Mengele. Studies of the motives and actions of these individuals not only show a surprising range but also reveal some unexpected findings. One of the latter is presented by German historian Mathias Schütz, who has studied the early career of SS officer Kurt Gerstein, which included a brief period as a medical student at the University of Tübingen.

During that time, Gerstein authored a highly unusual memorandum on ethics in anatomy that was in many respects decades ahead of its time. Schütz places this memorandum within the context of Gerstein's biography and the wider historical background. In another biographical study, German medical historians Stephanie Kaiser and Mathias Schmidt present a typical Nazi careerist in their detailed exploration of Hitler's physician Ludwig Stumpfegger's life. This reveals not only his medical activities but also his medical ethics and political aspirations. However, it was not only physicians who had decisive roles as perpetrators in Nazi medicine, as German historian Felicitas Söhner's report on the actions of bureaucrat Ludwig Trieb reveals. Based on archival documents, she presents and discusses his role within the Nazi "euthanasia" program as administrative manager of the Günzburg mental hospital by determining the mechanisms and objectives of administrative decision-making processes.

Likewise productive are analyses of groups and networks of perpetrators, as even eight decades after the Third Reich many of the professional associations have not been investigated, much less in detail. German medical historian Matthis Krischel presents a group portrait of German dentists as a fragmented profession. He describes the ready self-alignment of this professional group with Nazi politics and their willing collaboration in matters of hereditary health policies in order to advance their professional agenda. In another group portrait, UK historian Alexander von Lünen studies the dynamics within the scientific community of aviation medicine in Nazi Germany. His conclusion—based on new interpretations of the Milgram experiments—is that these physicians were not just blindly obedient but acted out of idealism. And while they did not perform inhumane experiments themselves, they had great interest in the results of the deadly studies performed by physician Sigmund Rascher in the name of aviation medicine at the concentration camp Dachau. Indeed, perpetrators like Rascher did not work alone but did so within a network of colleagues and interests. Such a network is at the center of the chapter by Paul Weindling, pioneer historian in the field of medicine and National Socialism. Weindling presents an in-depth look at the professional relationship between Dr. Josef Mengele and Professor Otmar von Verschuer. And while both individuals are well known if not notorious, Weindling's archival investigation reveals a depth of criminal action and connections that has not been known so far.

The Present

Recent work by Weindling and his group has shown that coercive medical experimentation and research by Nazi physicians was much more extensive and involved many more victims than previously thought.[48] Few of the medical perpetrators were ever held responsible for their deeds, and even fewer were brought to trial after the war. Their victims, however, had to live with their experiences forever and were often re-traumatized in the process of trying to give testimony to the atrocities committed on them.

The legacies of the past in the postwar period are explored in part II of this volume, which includes chapters that trace these continuities and their interpretations into the present. From the United States, German studies scholar Andrew Wisely discusses an example of such re-traumatization in his chapter on Abraham de la Penha's testimony against Dr. Franz Lucas in the Frankfurt Auschwitz Trial. He describes how memory failure, miscommunications, and factual errors rendered de la Penha's testimony invalid. Wisely argues convincingly that, even with its forensic contradictions, this eyewitness account deserves reconsideration as conveying a message of trauma that transcends mere facts. He concludes that the naming and describing of the trauma of victims may be more important than proving the guilt of the perpetrator.

Using similar eyewitness accounts, Polish historian of medicine Kamila Uzarczyk explores the so far neglected history of the destruction of Jewish psychiatric patients in occupied Poland. She anchors her research in the case study of the Jewish psychiatric hospital Zofiówka in Otwock, near Warsaw, and describes not only the fate of its patients but also the postwar denial of any memory of this past and its victims. The postwar lives of victims are then also at the center of Austrian medical historian Herwig Czech's contribution to this volume. He investigates the history and politics of Austrian psychiatry after the war and the fate of survivors of Nazi persecution. By describing the postwar landscape of various schools of psychiatric thinking, their proponents, and the effects on victim patients, Czech provides insights into the tragic continuities that led to the re-victimization of many, including sterilization victims.

However, it is not only the postwar fate of the victims themselves that is an important field of research in need of further illumination. There are also the legacies of "books, bones, and bodies" from coercive experimentation and research that have to be considered. German historian and journalist Götz Aly shares in his chapter a personal account of his effort to locate and identify the physical remains of "euthanasia" victims in the archives of various institutes of the Max-Planck-Society. His chapter provides an example of the struggles of one dedicated researcher in dealing with an institution that for many years shied away from taking on the responsibility for the legacies it had inherited from its predecessor, the Kaiser Wilhelm Society. US art historian Andrew Weinstein then widens the perspective of reflection on Nazi medicine by not only including the perspective of the artist but also by reflecting on the meaning of Nazi medical ethics for the unprecedented challenges society faces from bioengineering and other new technologies in the field of medicine. He discusses examples of important recent artistic representations that reflect on Nazi ethical transgressions, based on Adorno's concept of "identity" as a stereotypical image of a group—stereotypes that are reminiscent of Nazi racial categorizations. Weinstein argues that art offers an approach to "truth" that is a productive alternative to the scientific one and allows for flexible answers to and reflections on a changing reality. In his conclusion he states that many artists promote a deceptively simple antidote to the array of transgressions: they ask that biomedical researchers embrace responsibility and even cultivate love—or at least a recognition of the dignity of the Other—for the lives, human and nonhuman, with which they work and create.

Taking on responsibility for the past is at the center of the last chapter of this volume. Here anatomist Sabine Hildebrandt, Rabbi Joseph Polak, and medical historians Michael Grodin and William Seidelman point to the future by discussing the history of the Vienna Protocol, a set of guidelines on how to deal with the many physical remains from victims of Nazi atrocities that continue to emerge either inadvertently, e.g. through routine construction excavations, or through systematic searches in university collections or archeological digs. And it is not only "bones and bodies" that reappear, but books and publications based on research on these "bones and bodies," which continue to exist in the worldwide literature. The Vienna Protocol includes recommendations on how to deal with these "books, bones, and bodies," the first such set of which features an authoritative Jewish responsum on the subject. Thus the Jewish perspective of medical ethics becomes a valuable tool in responding to the question of how to deal with physical remains from Holocaust victims and data derived from them. The protocol is a universal, ecumenical document with potential application where the remains of victims of human rights violation may be found, irrespective of their national, ethnic, or religious origin.

Recognizing Patterns

The past does not repeat itself in the same form, but patterns are repeated. This volume of new studies on medicine before, during, and after the Holocaust aims to render such patterns recognizable and motivate the reader to further explore topics that are presented here for the first time. Bioethicists Barron Lerner and Arthur Caplan state that

> good history transports those studying and practicing bioethics to an earlier time, figuratively putting them in the shoes of their predecessors and teaching them how these past individuals rationalized choices they made—choices that now seem clearly ethically dubious. Learning how societal values, scientific zeal, ideological beliefs, and the desire for personal achievement influenced these persons reveals how similar factors can and often still remain in play, even in our supposedly more "enlightened" era.[49]

In this sense it is hoped that readers of this volume will learn to recognize reflections of the past in present-day medical theory and practice, thus becoming more critical and at the same time more productive in this world.

Sabine Hildebrandt, MD, is an associate professor of pediatrics at Boston Children's Hospital and an anatomy educator at Harvard Medical School. Her research interests are the history and ethics of anatomy. She also works on the restoration of biographies of victims of the Holocaust. Her book *The Anatomy of Murder: Ethical Transgressions and Anatomical Science during the Third Reich* was published in 2016, paperback in August 2017, and is the first systematic study on this topic. The biography *Käthe Beutler, 1896–1999: Eine jüdische Kinderärztin aus Berlin* was published in June 2019.

Miriam Offer, PhD, is an expert on Jewish medicine in the Holocaust. Her book *White Coats inside the Ghetto: Jewish Medicine in Poland during the Holocaust* was published in Hebrew in 2015 by Yad Vashem; English edition forthcoming. Miriam has researched the history of medicine (organization, science, ethics) in ghettos in Poland and Lithuania. Her current focus is Jewish medical activity immediately before, during, and after the Holocaust, and medicine/Holocaust gender issues. Miriam is a senior lecturer in the Holocaust Studies Program, Western Galilee College, and teaches medicine and the Holocaust in the Sackler Faculty of Medicine, Tel Aviv University.

Michael A. Grodin, MD, is professor of health law, bioethics, and human rights at the Boston University School of Public Health, and professor and director of the Project on Ethics and the Holocaust at the Elie Wiesel Center for Jewish Studies. Dr. Grodin has served on national and international commissions focusing on medical ethics, human rights, and the Holocaust. He has received a special citation from the United State Holocaust Memorial Museum for "profound contributions—through original and creative research—to the cause of Holocaust education and remembrance," and is the author of over two hundred articles and the editor or coeditor of seven books.

Notes

1. For a review of the historiography of medicine in the Third Reich, see Hildebrandt 2016, chapter 1.
2. Peter 1994.
3. Roelcke 2010.
4. Baader 1999; Roelcke 2014.
5. E.g. Dr. Werner Catel, see Klee 2001; see also chapter by Czech in this volume.

6. See chapter by Aly in this volume.
7. See chapters by Aly and Hildebrandt et al. in this volume.
8. As a most notable example: the Pernkopf *Atlas of Topographical and Applied Human Anatomy*, Yee et al. 2019.
9. See chapter by Czarnowski in this volume; also Hildebrandt et al. 2017.
10. Kellermann 2009.
11. See chapters by Offer and Kelly et al. in this volume.
12. Seidelman et al. 2017.
13. See chapter by Weinstein in this volume.
14. Reis et al. 2019; on the question of medical curricula, see foreword to this volume by Seidelman.
15. The Second International Conference and Medicine and the Holocaust and Beyond in the Western Galilee, Israel, 7–11 May 2017.
16. Michman 2017.
17. Michman quoted here, Wolffram 2017, 1.
18. Chapoutot 2018.
19. Huisman et al. 2017.
20. Huisman et al. 2017, 5.
21. Morrison 2017.
22. Original: "Wir stehen in einer Zeitenwende. Der Führer Adolf Hitler setzt zum ersten Male in der Weltgeschichte die Erkenntnisse über die biologischen Grundlagen der Entwicklung der Völker- Rasse, Erbe, Auslese- in die Tat um. Es ist kein Zufall, dass Deutschland der Ort dieses Geschehens ist: Die deutsche Wissenschaft legt dem Politiker das Werkzeug in die Hand." Aichel and Verschuer 1934, vi.
23. Fischer 1933.
24. Fischer 1933, 5: original: "Die eigene Rasse wird gefühlt und ist als eigenes Volkstum bewusst."
25. Fischer 1933, 6: original "eugenisch-rassenhygienisch-völkisch."
26. Koonz 2003.
27. Cocks 1997; detailed history for Germany in Weindling 1989a, 1989b; international aspects in Kaupen-Haas and Saller 1999.
28. Labisch 1997.
29. Süss 2003.
30. Hofer and Leven 2003, 27.
31. Weiss 2010.
32. Fangerau 2000, 38.
33. Proctor 2000, 341.
34. Lifton 1986, 54.
35. Black 2003.
36. Proctor 1988.
37. For an overview, see Weindling 2017.
38. Proctor 1994.
39. Sachse and Massin 2010.
40. Kröner 1998.
41. Gedda 1956.
42. Examples can be found in this volume: Aly; also: Hohendorf 2014; Seidelman 2012.
43. Reviews of the large scope of literature can be found—however incomplete—in Jütte et al. 2011; Eckardt 2012.
44. E.g. Rubenfeld 2010; Rubenfeld and Benedict 2014; Roelcke et al. 2014; Czech et al. 2018.
45. Wunder 2014.
46. Berner 2005.

47. Bruns 2009; Bialas and Fritze 2014; Gross 2010; Chapoutot 2018.
48. Weindling et al. 2016; Weindling 2017.
49. Lerner and Caplan 2016, 6.

References

Aichel, Otto, and Otmar von Verschuer. 1934. "Festband Eugen Fischer zum 60. Geburtstag gewidmet." *Z Morph Anthr* 34: v–vi.
Baader, Gerhard. 1999. "Die Erforschung der Medizin im Nationalsozialismus als Fallbeispiel einer Kritischen Medizingeschichte." In *Eine Wissenschaft emanzipiert sich: Die Medizinhistoriographie von der Aufklärung bis zur Postmoderne*, edited by Ralf Bröer, 113–20. Pfaffenweiler: Centaurus-Verlagsgesellschaft.
Berner, Margit. 2011. "'Die haben uns behandelt wie Gegenstände': Anthropologische Untersuchungen an jüdischen Häftlingen im Wiener Stadion während des Nationalsozialismus." In *Sensible Sammlungen: Aus dem anthropologischen Depot*, edited by Margit Berner, Anette Hoffmann, and Britta Lange, Britta, 147–67. Hamburg: Philo Fine Arts.
Bialas, Wolfgang, and Lothar Fritze (eds.). 2014. *Nazi Ideology and Ethics*. Newcastle upon Tyne: Cambridge Scholars Publishing.
Black, Edwin. 2003. *War against the Weak: Eugenics and America's Campaign to Create a Master Race*. New York: Four Walls Eight Windows.
Bruns, Florian. 2009. *Medizinethik im Nationalsozialismus*. Stuttgart: Franz Steiner Verlag.
Chapoutot, Johann. 2018. *The Law of Blood: Thinking and Acting as a Nazi*. Cambridge, MA: The Belknap Press of Harvard University Press.
Cocks, Geoffrey. 1997. "Introduction." In *Medicine and Modernity: Public Health and Medical Care in Nineteenth- and Twentieth-Century Germany*, edited by Manfred Berg and Geoffrey Cocks, 1–17. Cambridge: Cambridge University Press.
Czech, Herwig, Christiane Druml, and Paul Weindling. 2018. "Medical Ethics in the 70 Years after the Nuremberg Code, 1947 to the Present." *Wiener Klinische Wochenschrift* 130(3).
Eckart, Wolfgang Uwe. 2012. *Medizin in der NS-Diktatur: Ideologie, Praxis, Folgen*. Wien: Böhlau Verlag.
Fangerau, Heiner. 2000. "Das Standardwerk zur menschlichen Erblichkeitslehre und Rassenhygiene von Erwin Baur, Eugen Fischer und Fritz Lenz im Spiegel der zeitgenössischen Rezensionsliteratur 1921–1941." Medizinische Dissertation Bochum.
Fischer, Eugen. 1933. Rektoratsrede "Der Begriff des völkischen Staates, biologisch betrachtet." Retrieved 6 December 2019 from https://www.digihub.de/viewer/image/BV040483545/7/LOG_0006/.
Gedda, Luigi. 1956. "Un maestro e un esempio." *Acta geneticae medicae et gemellologiae* 5: 241–48.
Gross, Raphael. 2010. *Anständig geblieben: Nationalsozialistische Moral*. Frankfurt am Main: Fischer Verlag
Hildebrandt, Sabine. 2016. *The Anatomy of Murder: Ethical Transgressions and Anatomical Science during the Third Reich*. New York: Berghahn Books.
Hildebrandt, Sabine, Susan Benedict, Erin Miller, Michael Gaffney, and Michael A. Grodin. 2017. "'Forgotten' Chapters in the History of Transcervical Sterilization: Carl Clauberg and Hans-Joachim Lindemann." *Journal of the History of Medicine and Allied Science* 72(3): 272–301.
Hofer, Hans Georg, and Karl Heinz Leven. 2003. *Die Freiburger Medizinische Fakultät im Nationalsozialismus: Katalog einer Ausstellung des Instituts für Geschichte der Medizin der Universität Freiburg*. Frankfurt am Main: Peter Lang.
Hohendorf, Gerrit. 2014. "The Sewering Affair." In *Silence, Scapegoats, Self-Reflection: The Shadow of Nazi Medical Crimes on Medicine and Bioethics*, edited by Volker Roelcke, Sascha Topp, and Etienne Lepicard, 131–46. Göttingen: V&R unipress.

Huisman, Frank, Joris Vandendriessche, and Kaat Wils. 2017. "Introduction: Blurring Boundaries: Towards a Medical History of the Twentieth Century." *BMGN—Low Countries Historical Review* 132(1): 3–15.

Jütte, Robert, Wolfgang U. Eckart, Hans-Walter Schmuhl, and Winfried Süss. 2011. *Medizin im Nationalsozialismus: Bilanz und Perspektiven der Forschung*. Göttingen: Wallstein Verlag.

Kaupen-Haase, Heidrun, and Christain Saller (eds.). 1999. *Wissenschaftlicher Rassismus: Analysen einer Kontinuität in den Human- und Naturwissenschaften*, Frankfurt am Main: Campus Verlag.

Kellermann, Natan P. F. 2009. *Holocaust Trauma: Psychological Effects and Treatment*. New York: iUniverse.

Klee, Ernst. 2001. *Deutsche Medizin im Dritten Reich: Karrieren vor und nach 1945*. Frankfurt am Main: S. Fischer Verlag GmbH.

Koonz, Claudia. 2003. *The Nazi Conscience*. Cambridge, MA: The Belknap Press of Harvard University Press.

Kröner, Hans-Peter. 1998. *Von der Rassenhygiene zur Humangenetik*. Stuttgart: Gustav Fischer Verlag.

Labisch, Alfons. 1997. "From Traditional Individualism to Collective Professionalism: State, Patient, Compulsory Health Insurance, and the Panel Doctor Question in Germany, 1883–1931." In *Medicine and Modernity: Public Health and Medical Care in Nineteenth- and Twentieth-Century Germany*, edited by Manfred Berg and Geoffrey Cocks, 35-55. Cambridge: Cambridge University Press.

Lerner, Barron H., and Arthur L. Caplan. 2016. "Judging the Past: How History Should Inform Bioethics." *Annals of Internal Medicine* 164: 553–557.

Lifton, Robert Jay. 1986. *Ärzte im Dritten Reich*. German Edition 1998. Berlin: Ullstein Buchverlag GmbH&Co KG.

Michman, Dan. 2017. "Medicine in the Grand Picture of the Holocaust: Critical Reflections on Mainstream Holocaust Historiography." The Second International Scholars Workshop on Medicine in the Holocaust and Beyond, Western Galilee College, Akko, 8 May 2017. Retrieved 1 December 2019 from https://www.youtube.com/watch?v=omtwu_-Cpho.

Morrison, Toni. 2017. *The Origins of Others*. Cambridge, MA: Harvard University Press.

Peter, Jürgen. 1994. *Der Nürnberger Ärzteprozess im Spiegel seiner Aufarbeitung anhand der drei Dokumentensammlungen von Alexander Mitscherlich und Fred Mielke*. Münster: Lit-Verlag.

Proctor, Robert N. 1988. *Racial Hygiene: Medicine under the Nazis*. Cambridge: Harvard University Press.

———. 1994. "Racial Hygiene: The Collaboration of Medicine and Nazism." In *Medical Ethics and the Third Reich: Historical and Contemporary Issues*, edited by John J Michalczyk, 35–41. Kansas City, MO: Sheed & Ward.

———. 2000. "Nazi Science and Nazi Medical Ethics: Some Myths and Misconceptions." *Perspectives in Biology and Medicine* 43(3): 335–46.

Reis, Shmuel P., Hedy S. Wald, and Paul Weindling. 2019. "The Holocaust, Medicine and Becoming a Physician: The Crucial Role of Education." *Israel Journal of Health Policy Research* 8(1): 55. doi: 10.1186/s13584-019-0327-3.

Roelcke, Volker. 2010. "Medicine during the Nazi Period: Historical Facts and Some Implications for Teaching Medical Ethics and Professionalism." In *Medicine after the Holocaust: From the Master Race to the Human Genome and Beyond*, edited by Sheldon Rubenfeld, 17–29. New York: Palgrave MacMillan.

———. 2014. "Sulfonamide Experiments on Prisoners in Nazi Concentration Camps: Coherent Scientific Rationality Combined with Complete Disregard of Humanity." In *Human Subjects Research after the Holocaust*, edited by Sheldon Rubenfeld and Susan Benedict, 51–66. Cham: Springer.

Roelcke, Volker, Sascha Topp, and Etienne Lepicard (eds.). 2014. *Silence, Scapegoats, Self-Reflection: The Shadow of Nazi Medical Crimes on Medicine and Bioethics*. Göttingen: V&R unipress.

Rubenfeld, Sheldon. 2010. *Medicine after the Holocaust: From the Master Race to the Human Genome and Beyond*. New York: Palgrave MacMillan.

Rubenfeld, Sheldon, and Susan Benedict (eds.). 2014. *Human Subjects Research after the Holocaust*. Cham: Springer.

Sachse, Carola, and Benoit Massin. 2000. *Biowissenschaftliche Forschungen an Kaiser-Wilhelm-Institute und die Verbrechen des NS-Regimes: Informationen über den gegenwärtigen Wissensstand*. Retrieved 4 February 2020 from https://www.mpiwg-berlin.mpg.de/KWG/Ergebnisse/Ergebnisse3.pdf.

Seidelman, William E. 2012. "Dissecting the History of Anatomy in the Third Reich—1989-2010: A Personal Account." *Annals of Anatomy* 194: 228–36.

Seidelman, William E., Lilka Elbaum, and Sabine Hildebrandt (eds.). 2017. "How to Deal with Holocaust Era Human Remains: Recommendations Arising from a Special Symposium. Recommendations/Guidelines for the Handling of Future Discoveries of Human Victims of Nazi Terror / 'Vienna Protocol' for When Jewish or Possibly-Jewish Human Remains are Discovered, by Rabbi Joseph A. Polak." Elie Wiesel Center for Jewish Studies. Retrieved 30 January 2020 from https://www.bu.edu/jewishstudies/research/medicine-and-the-holocaust/recommendations-for-the-discovery-of-jewish-remains-project/.

Süss, Winfried. 2003. *Der "Volkskörper" im Krieg. Gesundheitspolitik, Gesundheitsverhältnisse und Krankenmord im nationalsozialistischen Deutschland 1939-1945*. München: Oldenbourg.

Tenenbaum, Joesph. 1956. *Race and Reich: The Story of an Epoch*. New York: Twayne Publishers.

Weindling, Paul. 1989a. *Health, Race and German Politics between National Unification and Nazism, 1870–1945*. Cambridge: Cambridge University Press.

———. 1989b. "The 'Sonderweg' of German Eugenics: Nationalism and Scientific Internationalism." *British Journal for the History of Science* 22: 321–33.

Weindling, Paul (ed.). 2017. *From Clinic to Concentration Camp: Reassessing Nazi Medical and Racial Research, 1933–1945*. Oxon: Routledge.

Weindling, Paul, Anna von Villiez, Aleksandra Loewenau, Nicola Farron. 2016. "The Victims of Unethical Human Experiments and Coerced Research under National Socialism." *Endeavour* 40(1): 1–6.

Weiss, Sheila. 2010. *The Nazi Symbiosis: Human Genetics and Politics in the Third Reich*. Chicago: University of Chicago Press.

Wolffram, Dirk Jan. 2017. "From the Editors." *BMGN—Low Countries Historical Review* 132(1): 1–2.

Wunder, Michael. 2014. "Learning with History: Nazi Medical Crimes and Today's Debates on Euthanasia in Germany." In *Silence, Scapegoats, Self-Reflection: The Shadow of Nazi Medical Crimes on Medicine and Bioethics*, edited by Volker Roelcke, Sascha Topp, and Etienne Lepicard, 301–12. Göttingen: V&R unipress.

Yee, Andrew, Demetrius Coombs, Sabine Hildebrandt, William E. Seidelman, Henk Coert, and Susan E. Mackinnon. 2019. "Nerve Surgeons' Assessment of the Role of Eduard Pernkopf's Atlas of Topographical and Applied Human Anatomy in Surgical Practice." *Neurosurgery* 84(2): 491–98.

Part I

THE PAST

CHAPTER 1

NON-MECHANISTIC EXPLANATORY STYLES IN INTERWAR GERMAN RACIAL THEORY
A Comparison of Hans F. K. Günther and Ludwig Ferdinand Clauß

Amit Varshizky

The profound involvement of German physicians and biomedical scientists in Nazi eugenic and racial policy has been the subject of an impressive number of studies in the past two and a half decades. These studies have demonstrated the widespread complicity of particular scientists and institutions in Nazi crimes, indicating the ways in which opportunistic motives and ideological fanaticism have played a role in implementing racial hygiene measures against allegedly biologically "unfit" individuals and populations. While the concepts of race and racism are often used in a broad sense to encapsulate the rationale, ambitions, and underlying logic of the Nazi medical crimes, recent studies have undermined the coherency of racial thought, pointing at the diffuse nature of "race" and the contested and competing meanings it entailed within scientific, cultural, and political discourses of the time.[1] This chapter joins the recently growing scholarly attempts to comprehend Nazi racial ideas from new perspectives by challenging the coherence and the comprehensiveness of the category of "race," exemplifying how Nazi racial theoreticians sought new ways to conceptualize race beyond the limits of natural science and causal explanations, thereby creating new paths for political, cultural, and ethical renovation.

This chapter adds to the understanding of the complex relationship between scientific and extra-scientific factors within the framework of racial theory in interwar Germany. While some studies have emphasized racial scientists' dilemmas regarding the questions of science and politics, they often describe the subjugation of science to politics in an "extra-scientific" manner, ascribing it to personal, professional, or political motivations that gained new traction following the Nazi seizure of power.[2] As much as these factors indeed played an important role in the nazification of science, this chapter clearly shows that the conception of politicized science was already prevalent in racial discourse as early as the 1920s and inherent to the way in which *Rasseforscher* (literally: researcher of race) approached the core problems of science and life. By addressing their philosophical argumentations, the chapter highlights the culturally laden ideas, which became an integral part of racial theoreticians' "theoretical tool-box" as early as the 1920s, and shows how they were used to rationalize their scientific "deviations," justifying the obedience of science to politics. Histories of racial science and eugenics in interwar Germany often mark the rise of genetics as the main feature behind the formation of a new biological, racist, and ideologically driven racial theory (*Rassenkunde*) in the early 1920s. Alongside political, institutional, and professional factors, historians have emphasized the role of Mendelian inheritance (in addition to the continuing influence of Darwinism) in the process of transforming German anthropology from the physical and liberal discipline of the late nineteenth century into the racist and nationalistic racial science of the 1920s.[3] Even though much of the research has demonstrated the complexity, incoherence, and diversity of the scientific fields that came to be known as racial science, very few have undertaken a thorough investigation of the antipositivist trends within German race theory and the growing influence of holistic and non-mechanistic explanatory styles, which, alongside genetics, contributed to the shape of German *Rassenkunde* in the interwar years.

Although one cannot overestimate the contribution of genetics to the formation of interwar German racial science, it seems that its impact upon German anthropologists, eugenicists, and *Rassenforscher* should be reexamined within the intellectual and epistemological context of postwar Germany and the overall sense of cultural crisis and intellectual insecurity. Even though genetics offered endorsement for eugenic and racial-social claims, it also spurred a series of new problems that exposed the inherent tensions between the practical aspects of eugenics and its ideological and ethical imperatives. As will be shown, some problems had to do with the Mendelian method itself, including the difficulty in bridging the gap between genotype and phenotype and the insufficiency of genealogical methods in verifying mental heredity, whereas other problems referred much broader philosophical and ethical questions that evolved around contemporary debates over science and value.

This chapter seeks to reexamine the place of genetics in German racial thought by drawing on the work of two of the most prominent and outspoken representatives of interwar racial theory: Hans F. K. Günther and Ludwig Ferdinand Clauß. Both achieved a dominant voice within the racial scientific discourse of the day and played a central role in the formation and popularization of German racial theory during the 1920s and the 1930s. Although fundamentally differing in their approaches and methods, both were motivated by the will to provide a new understanding of human biology and to break down the barriers between the spiritual and the physical, between scholarship and worldview (*Weltanschauung*), and between science and "life." Their works illustrate how contemporary holistic, vitalist, and phenomenological ideas colored racial classifications and were implemented within the framework of interwar racial theory. By implementing non-mechanistic models of explanation, they sought to transform racial science into an enterprise rooted in both reason and intuition, capable of uniting its insights with those of empirical knowledge, aesthetics, and metaphysics.

Whereas Günther formulated his racial typology on physiognomic and ethnohistorical models, Clauß cultivated a new racial psychology (*Rassenseelenkunde*) based on phenomenological principles, rejecting the importance of anatomical and morphological characteristics in favor of bodily-emotional expressions of the living "racial soul." Although clearly differing in their approaches and methods, Günther and Clauß represent some of the underlying currents that shaped the direction of German racial theory during the interwar years. As will be shown, in taking up the call for a new racial science, they were not only challenging the traditional outlines of physical and liberal anthropology and its division between the physical and the mental but were also undermining the very foundations of scientific positivism and its sharp distinction between facts and values, science and politics.

The Biological Turn in German Anthropology and the Question of Mental Heredity

In the early 1920s racial scientists shared a common feeling that they were part of an innovative transformation and revolutionary breakthrough, as they celebrated the triumph of genetics over the morphological and descriptive anthropology of the nineteenth century. The rediscovery of Mendelian laws in 1900 and their successful implementation within the field of human heredity intensified the belief that natural heredity, and not environmental factors, was the main force behind racial differences. The category of race was reconceptualized from a physical and anatomical category, as had been the norm in the descriptive and morphological vein of nineteenth-century anthropology, to a "group of identical genetic traits, which constitute physical, anatomical, and mental characteristics."[4]

Nonetheless, they all agreed that the discipline was still making its first steps and had to bypass some major obstacles on its way to consolidation. Crucial to this point was the question of mental heredity and the difficulty of verifying mental racial differences. Günther stressed as early as 1922 that "if human races differed only according to their physical characteristics, then the study of the racial phenomenon would be of much lesser importance."[5] Mendelian genetics provided for the first time a significant scientific evidence for the correlation between physical constitution and mental faculty. Yet, applying Mendelianism to racial anthropology led racial scientists to a fundamental problem that forced them to employ alternative strategies for validating racial-mental differences. According to Mendel's second law—known also as "the law of independent assortment"—different genes independently separate from one another when reproductive cells develop. Racial scientists were fully aware of the fundamental difficulty of proving the distribution of mental traits according to the Mendelian scheme, particularly of proving the correlation between phenotype—that is, the genetic potentials actually realized in the individual—and between the genotype, the overall, nonactualized, and "invisible" genetic "code" that constitutes the same individual. This way Mendelian genetics impeded any possibility to draw conclusions about man's racial essence from his external and empirical appearance.

Since phenotypic characteristics could no longer serve as a criterion for the study of human races, racial scientists had to abandon traditional anthropometric methods and adopt new methods that were based on the genealogical strategies of tracing and mapping hereditary traits and their modes of transmission. A main strategy was the drawing of family trees (*Ahnentafel*) and the use of mathematical and statistical tools to prove the distribution of certain features over time. This method enabled tracing the appearance of certain phenotypic traits in parents and offspring, testing them according to the Mandelian model, and verifying their genotypical sources. Nonetheless, whereas these measures could provide certain insights about the distribution of physiological traits, they were unable to provide any insight regarding the inheritance of mental traits. To address this problem, genealogical methods were applied to the hereditary-mental history of lineages. Thus, genealogical trees of famous families, known for producing geniuses in multiple instances over the generations, were used alongside genealogical trees of families characterized by severe mental illness or intergenerational tendencies for criminality. However, this method was arbitrary, and its weakness was obvious.

Beside it being a matter of crucial importance, proving the existence of mental-racial diversity was also the most complex and problematic issue, and it continued to evoke harsh controversies between racial scientists during the 1920s and 1930s. Fritz Lenz, one of Germany's prominent racial hygienists and the coauthor of the 1921 Baur-Fischer-Lenz volume, the standard work on racial hygiene and inheritance of its time, stated in 1921 that mental inheritance, while being of the utmost importance to the racial science, poses many difficulties, since "the measurable mental qualities are so few and so difficult to grasp."[6] In 1925, Walter Scheidt, a leading spokesman for the new biological anthropology and the first director of the "institute for racial and cultural biology" at the University of Hamburg, proclaimed that "as far as the characteristics of mental inheritance are concerned, we often find it difficult to define what we are dealing with."[7] Nine years later, in 1934, he stated that "racial psychology has not yet been fully consolidated."[8] The anthropologist Theodor Mollison also admitted that same year that "to date, we lacked the appropriate means to establish exact and quantitative racial psychology on the basis of methods detached from previous [environmental] influences."[9]

Thus, the problem of mental heredity and the basic difficulty of proving the distribution of mental traits according to the Mendelian scheme drove many racial scientists to appropriate alternative strategies that corresponded with contemporary trends within German life and mind sciences, and coincided with the overall climate of intellectual and cultural crisis.

Holism, Vitalism, and the Rise of a New Biocentric Thought in Postwar Germany

Fin de siècle Germany was afflicted by an increasing mood of restless, antimodernist, and cultural despair. Large segments of the educated classes felt threatened by a vision of a mechanistic–technocratic society and feared a growing materialization of life. In response, an inchoate and scattered intellectual movement took shape, raising the banner of holism, which was introduced as an antidote to the sweeping sense of spiritual and existential decay. The rebellion against the fortress of rationalism was the hallmark of an epoch that saw rapid changes in all spheres of life and was deeply absorbed in social anxieties and a widespread antagonism toward liberalism, secularism, and industrialism.[10]

This vigorous intellectual climate manifested itself in multiple ways, including but not limited to political ones. The widespread popularity of the so-called "life philosophy" (*Lebensphilosophie*) among various intellectual circles, the revival of vitalism and romantic nature philosophy (*Naturphilosophie*) in biology (primarily through the works of the embryologist Hans Driesch), and the prevailing status of *Gestalt* psychology and the emergence of phenomenological psychology pioneered by Franz Brentano were all hallmarks of a epistemological bias and a deep antagonism to reductionist positivism, mechanistic science, and materialist philosophy, and these reflected an intellectual yearning for new paths in sciences that will also bring on a cultural and spiritual renovation.

The humiliating military defeat, the punitive Treaty of Versailles, and the sudden leap into a new democratic system all made for a situation of crisis and uncertainty. These postwar political and social upheavals added to the already prevailing mood of "cultural despair" and the hostility of many German intellectuals to materialism and utilitarianism that were attributed to the liberal "mechanization" and "atomization" of society. As several historians have shown, aspirations to establish holistic science as part of the general reaction to nineteenth-century materialism and mechanism became rooted in all fields of knowledge, particularly in the life and mind sciences.[11]

According to historian Anne Harrington, this holistic turn "was really more a family of approaches than a single coherent perspective. The need to do justice to organismic purposiveness or teleological functioning—to questions of 'what for?' and not merely 'how'—was central in all cases."[12] Central to this thinking was the premise of the irreducibility of the organism to a machine. Hence, "biology" was perceived as an ontological totality, which cannot be reduced to the generalizing and classificatory categories of natural science. Within the increasing existential and epistemological uncertainty of the postwar years, biology gained a unique and authoritative status and was embraced as a potential strategy for overcoming what Edmund Husserl termed the "crisis of the European sciences."[13] Biology was considered a potential mediator between the natural sciences (*Naturwissenschaften*) and the humanities (*Geisteswissenschaften*) and thereby could provide a much more meaningful picture of human existence that is rooted both in the physiological and the psychological manifestations of life.

This biocentric propensity, accompanied by its holistic and anti-mechanistic impetus, trickled into the renewed postwar anthropological discourse, where it helped to reshape scientific definitions and categories as evidenced in the works of Hans Günther and Ludwig Ferdinand Clauß.

Hans F. K. Günther and the Idealistic Imperative of Race

One of the events that marked the most significant turning point of the German racial thought was undoubtedly the publication of Hans F. K. Günther's *Rassenkunde des deutschen Volkes* in 1922. Immediately after its appearance, this work gained unprecedented circulation, and by 1942 its sales reached 124,000 copies.[14] Günther's book is of particular importance, mainly due to its great popularity among the general public in the twenties and thirties, and the author's prestige in the eyes of the National Socialist ideological elite. Additionally, it was widely accepted by younger anthropologists and, as noted the anthropologist Bernhard Struck, it was highly appraised by prominent figures in the field, including Eugen Fischer, Erwin Baur, Theodor Mollison and Carl Toldt.[15] A shortened, popularized, version of the book, published in 1929 under the name *Kleine Rassenkunde des deutschen Volkes*, was compulsory reading in all schools in the Third Reich. In 1942 alone, it sold 295,000 copies.[16]

Günther's rapid rise in German academia was greatly aided by his extensive contacts with senior Nazi officials, who saw him as a faithful representative of their views. In May 1930, following the intervention of Wilhelm Frick, Günther was appointed to professor of social anthropology at the University of Jena, and in 1932 he joined the ranks of the Nazi Party. A year later he became a member of the Interior Ministry's advisory committee on race policy, and in 1935 he served as director of the Institute for the Study of Race, Ethnic Biology and Political Sociology (Anstalt für Rassenkunde, Völkerbiologie und ländliche Soziologie) in Dahlem, Berlin. From 1939 he served as professor at the University of

Freiburg.[17] During the 1930s and 1940s, Günther won various prizes and awards, including the Nazi Science Prize, given to him by Alfred Rosenberg at the 1935 Party Day celebrations, and the Goethe Medal of Art and Science, which Hitler himself presented him in 1941. During the 1920s and 1930s Günther was one of the prominent voices of the Nordic Movement (*Die Nordische Bewegung*), and edited influential and widely circulated journals such as the *Nordische Ring* and *Rasse*.[18] His work gained primacy in the Third Reich, and his racial typology was embraced by the political establishment and became, in many cases, a stamp of ideological correctness.[19]

The Physiognomic Gaze and the Search for Racial *Gestalt*

Günther's *Rassenkunde* was a first attempt to analyze the racial makeup of the German people, and marked racial anthropology's break from the "liberal" physical tradition. The book constituted a direct attack against the principles of physical anthropology and its descriptive methods, as formulated during the second half of the nineteenth century. His critique addressed not only the traditional disciplinary division between anthropology and ethnology, the natural sciences and the humanities, but also the "liberal" distinction between science and value, and between scholarship and ideology. In this sense, Günther's writing was an explicit call for political and social action, an attempt to shake the discipline out of its descriptive neutrality and "abstract" objectivism and to usher in a politically oriented and "life-enhancing" mode of thought.

At the core of Günther's racial teaching stood the rejection of the exclusive authority of natural sciences. This he sought to replace with a racial classification based on a more holistic and interdisciplinary approach, combining physiognomic-photographic techniques with ethnological and historical analyses. Following Houston Stewart Chamberlain, Günther ascribed the Goethean conception of *Anschauung*, or intuitive perception, with a specifically racial (Nordic) way of observing the world, employing an "intuitive seeing" as a means to overcome what he defined as the contemporary "non-pictorial" (*Unbildlichkeit*) natural-scientific world-picture.[20] A real and substantial racial science, he argued, must be based on a "racial-scholarly gaze" (*Rassenkundliche Blick*) that encompassed the whole "human *Gestalt*" (*Menschengestalt*) and not just partial physical or morphological features.[21]

Although Günther believed that *Rassenkunde* should "attribute a special weight to the study of racial biology and hereditary health,"[22] he utterly rejected biological reductionism in favor of a more holistic and "synthetic" approach that combines empirical analysis with intuitive observation and allows—as he puts it—the attainment of "human being as it really is." According to him, "given the current state of research, we can say very little today about the racial-genetically transmission of mental traits. [However,] what is most likely is that the human being does indeed 'appear to be what he actually is' (*der Mensch ist, wie er aussieht*) [Schopenhauer]."[23] By appealing to Schopenhauer's postulate, which proclaims a total identity between being and appearance, Günther sought to reinforce his holistic and physiognomic premises, putting forward the presumption that "all people, unconsciously or consciously, are convinced that mental characteristics are racial-genetically transmitted."[24]

Drawing on eighteenth-century German physiognomic tradition, Günther sought to establish his racial typology on the basis of intuitive perception, supported by the empirical, quantifying techniques of natural science.[25] However, unlike traditional physiognomics, such as that of Lavater or Lichtenberg, who were concerned with the individual, Günther's physiognomy was oriented toward racial classification and aimed at attaining "the essential racial core" (*rassisch bedingter Wesenskern*) of a person.[26] He defined his typology as being based, "first of all, [upon] the physical characteristics (*körperlichen Merkmale*), [and only] then [upon] the mental traits (*seelischen Eigenschaften*)]while acknowledging that] the mental and physical aspects of the race are of equal importance to race theory."[27] Accordingly, Günther's physiognomics aimed at drawing conclusions from the racial physical (empirical) characteristics about the (non-empirical) psychological and mental qualities, and thus, with the additional support of cultural-ethnological and historical analyses, it aspired to verify racial mental differences.

Since, according to Günther, perception, observation, and contemplation are predetermined by specific mental biological predispositions, they are also inherently relative and differ fundamentally from one race to another. Accordingly, any intellectual activity, including science, is the necessary result of a particular racial *Anschauung*, and is therefore always partial and can never be "universal," "objective," or "neutral." This logic stood at the core of Günther's call for establishing *Rassenkunde* not on positivist, value-free science but on a new epistemological and ethical ground.

Racial Theory between Science and *Weltanschauung*

In his *Rassenkunde*, Günther not only challenged the traditional outlines of physical and liberal anthropology, with its division between the physical and the mental, the biological and the cultural, but also undermined the very foundations of scientific positivism and its sharp distinction between fact and value, science and ideology. His conception of science must be seen in the light of contemporary polemics on "value-free science" (*Wertfreie Wissenschaft*), which were promoted in the years preceding World War I by figures like Max Weber and Werner Sombart.[28] During the 1920s, Weber's well-known statement that science can say what there is (*das Seiende*) but not what ought to be (*das Seinsollende*) was largely manipulated by prominent racial scientists, who used it as ideological ammunition to mobilize scientific racism in the service of national politics.[29]

As early as 1922, Günther declared that any attempt to establish racial science on the principles of naturalistic, positivistic, and value-free methods was doomed to failure, since the racial question was itself a question of value. As such, it could not be measured by the quantitative methods of exact science.[30]

Günther firmly rejected the materialist and deterministic premises underlying genetics and demanded that *Rassenkunde* be given a special status that exceeded the limited framework of empirical and descriptive science. In his view, it was not enough for racial teaching to merely describe reality—it must also shape it. In other words, racial thinking must strengthen German racial awareness, as well as German morals, values and collective will, thereby launching Germany on a new path toward national renovation. This explains Günther's critique of some contemporary attempts to establish racial theory exclusively on the basis of positivistic science and genetics. In 1922 he stated that "all those 'biological' and 'biologistic' worldviews, positioned today at the forefront of racial science, . . . are damaging to German [national] renewal. . . . Biology as an autonomous science will never be able to serve as a basis for a *Weltanschauung*."[31]

Underlying this declaration was the assumption that science cannot determine values, and therefore it cannot provide the groundwork for a moral and national renovation. In other words, science can only describe processes but never essences; it can explain the "how" but never the "what," or the "what for." For Günther, genetics, and natural sciences in general, were based on causal mechanistic principles that explain life through physicochemical processes of cause and effect, resulting in a determinism that rules out any possibility of free will or moral choice.

The objective reality of racial mixture in Europe, and within the German people in particular, in addition to the inability of biological anthropology to draw clear outlines of racially pure types, led Günther to embrace an idealistic view in which pure racial types were regarded as "ideas in their Platonic sense."[32] The German people, whom Günther perceived as being in an advanced state of racial decline, must strengthen the Nordic elements within it—a process that Günther called "re-Nordification" (*Wiedervernordnung*)—and eradicate the genetically mixed or racially inferior elements within it, a process described as *Aufnordung*. The idea of "re-Nordification" was thus a call for a total transvaluation of values that would be generated through "re-education" of the German people.[33] But Germany's "re-Nordification" was also meant as a tool for national integration and for the establishment of a new national belonging, based on what Günther termed "the Nordic ideal" (*Der nordische Gedanke*). In this manner he called for "a worldview . . . that would, above all else, reflect a spirit of responsibility in relation to all questions related to blood. Only a worldview that is 'idealistic' in the sense of Plato, Kant and Fichte may bring this about."[34]

In his programmatic 1925 book *Der nordische Gedanke unter der Deutschen* (The Nordic ideal among the Germans), Günther elaborated his racial-based idealism further, emphasizing Germany's need to employ strict educational and pedagogical means, alongside an uncompromising eugenic policy, in order to make the Nordic vision a viable reality. In other words, the realization of the Nordic ideal was not to be achieved merely through racial selection and hygiene but also through the personal obedience of all Germans to the aesthetical and ethical imperatives embedded in the "Nordic ideal." This inner commitment, which Günther also named the "heroic idea," was aimed at arousing the inner moral responsibility of the individual for the collective purposes of enlarging and strengthening the Nordic racial stocks of the German people. The Nordic ideal was to guide individuals in choosing the right spouse, and in restraining or increasing the number of offspring, in accordance with their racial fitness. To foreground this, Günther reformulated Kant's categorical imperative to accord with his idealistic-eugenic message: "Act only according to that maxim whereby you can, at the same time, will that it should become a Nordic-racial law."[35]

Günther conceived the Nordic ideal as a model (*Vorbild*) and a target vision (*Zielbild*) of a utopian horizon to be continuously pursued: "The strengthening of a people is possible only through the sense of internal tension between the existing reality and the model of purpose. Every nation must fulfill something if it wishes to keep on reproducing."[36]

But for Günther, the Nordic ideal was perceived not only as an educational instrument and indoctrination tool but also as empirical evidence of the existence of Nordic mental traits among the German people: "The unconscious, or partly conscious, pursuit of Nordicism, provides firm evidence of the existence of a mental direction [*eine seelische Richtung*] particular to the German people, and of the memory of an earlier model, one that is still alive, and manifests itself through the [German] people."[37] According to Günther, the hallmark of a Nordic "mental direction" was the aesthetic urge toward ontological wholeness and the desire for harmony between the external and the internal, between form and essence. In this way, Günther drew a straight line between Germanic paganism, the *kalokagathia* of the ancient Greeks, German Romantic pantheism, and Nazi racial ideas.[38] In order to strengthen his position, Günther collected a wealth of historical evidence from the ancient world and Germanic history, which, he argued, proved the naturally inherited tendency of the Germanic peoples to the "Nordic" aesthetic model of psychosocial unity.

In this way, "race" became an aesthetic ideal that embodied the primal image of a pure Germanhood, and striving after the realization of the Nordic ideal became both a goal and a means. On the one hand, it served as a pedagogic instrument to inculcate in the younger generation the importance of a eugenic society, but on the other hand it served as phenomenological and trans-historical evidence of the existence of a "racial-mental direction" among its carriers and cultivators. Since each race possesses a unique aesthetic ideal that corresponds with its inherent racial-mental tendencies, striving for the realization of this ideal was perceived as an existential evidence of mental-racial predispositions. Günther outlined the idealistic and non-materialistic nature of his racial thought as follows:

> The Nordic ideal is not a thought that stems—as many mistakenly presume—from the material (materialism), but rather perceives itself as a Spirit [Geist], seeking to shape itself through the body, and by shaping its actual body, it sees the materiality of its world as a physical component. The Nordic ideal is a spirit that strives to be realized in the noblest body, hence the conception of racial selection (Zuchtgedanke) that underlies it: Plato's thought. The Nordic movement comes from the spirit, but it is not lost in the spirit; it penetrates reality . . .[39]

Günther here explicitly acknowledged the supremacy of the sprit, or the will, over material corporality while simultaneously emphasizing their essential unity. Underlying this exposition was a bio-vitalist position that sees "life" as a dynamic morphological manifestation of a nonphysical element, of an essential interior, encoded in organic matter itself. Conceptualizing race in vitalist terms allowed Günther to bypass the problem of mechanistic biology while nonetheless substantiating his racial teaching on biological predispositions. Yet, in contrast to the biological determinism inherent in genetic science, Günther attributed a key role to the human ability to induce change through willpower and self-training. These qualities held a central place in his racial ethics, which he grounded on the willpower of the individual and his inner moral ability to overcome the inferior elements in his blood.

Since the Nordic ideal constitutes a phenomenological and trans-historical evidence of a psycho-racial reality, the quest for its affirmation becomes an introspective process of self-discovery and internal refinement. Günther's theory posited that most Germans were racially mixed, a fact that forced them to struggle with their inferior racial traits and to overcome themselves by the virtue of their will and creative personality. In this way, the process of racial-anthropological inquiry shifted to the subjective realm of the individuum, becoming a psychodynamic process of self-awareness and self-affirmation and involving the sublimation of mental conflicts in the direction of active and creative action for the common good.[40]

Günther designated the ability of self-overcoming as the "Faustian element" residing in the Nordic soul, which enables "placing all uncertain, non-Nordic mental characteristics at the service of advancing this direction."[41] Goethe, Dante, Beethoven, Schiller, and Nietzsche were all Nordic-Dinaric, and therefore exemplified the ability to transcend the inferior features of their blood and their internal mental conflicts. According to Günther, "tension, conflict, [and] overcoming, are at the foundation of the great works, and among people who are racially mixed, there may be more tensions and conflicts than among racially-pure people."[42]

In toto, Günther's conception of race was based on a deep ambivalence toward scientific genetics and a firm rejection of its biological determinism. It promoted a vitalist conception of human psychophysics and called for a national-spiritual revival based on inner striving and an aesthetic urge, aimed at arousing the collective-racial responsibility of all Germans and channeling their individual wills for the purpose of national renewal in the spirit of the Nordic ideal. While his idealistic Nordicism was praised by prominent geneticists such as Fritz Lenz and Eugen Fischer,[43] it was also criticized for its lack of scientific basis. One of the most vehement attacks launched against Günther's theory came from the botanical geneticist Friedrich Merkenschlager, the head of the Botanical Laboratory in the Biological Reich Institute for Agriculture and Forestry in Berlin-Dahlem, and an early member of the NSDAP and the SA. In his 1927 *Götter, Helden und Günther: Eine Abwehr der Güntherschen Rassenkunde* (Gods, heroes, and Günther: A repudiation of Günther's racial ethnology), Merkenschlager criticized Günther's "shockingly low level of biological knowledge."[44] Alongside the anthropologist Karl Saller, he launched a campaign against Günther's Nordicism, putting forward the concept of a "German race" while emphasizing the malleable and dynamic nature of races and the equilibrant interaction of hereditary and environmental factors. This view gained a certain political support from senior Nazi officials such as Achim Gercke, Gerhard Wagner, and Fritz Bartels; however, it was silenced as early as 1934, after a decisive intervention by Walter Groß, head of the Nazi Party's Office of Racial Policy.[45]

Whereas Günther formulated his racial typology on physiognomic and ethnohistorical models, other theoreticians of race went even further in diminishing the role of naturalistic and anthropometric methods, firmly rejecting the relevance of phenotypical characteristics for racial classification. One of the leading representatives of such an approach was Ludwig Ferdinand Clauß.

Ludwig Ferdinand Clauß and Racial Phenomenology

Ludwig Ferdinand Clauß studied philosophy, psychology, and philology at the University of Freiburg, and between 1917 and 1920 he served as assistant to Edmund Husserl. Despite Clauß's later attempts to shake off his teacher's intellectual legacy, for reasons of political correctness and careerist opportunism, he owed a significant intellectual debt to Husserl's phenomenology. In May 1933, Clauß joined the National Socialist Party, and in July of that year he assisted Jakob Wilhelm Hauer in founding the "German faith movement" (*Deutsche Glaubensbewegung*). In 1934, together with Günther, he founded the journal of the Nordic Movement, *Rasse*, of which he was the coeditor. From 1936 to 1941, he served as a professor of racial psychology at the University of Berlin, and in 1941 he was appointed professor of racial science and politics at the University of Posen. In 1942, after a protracted legal struggle in the Supreme Party Court with Walter Groß, Clauß was expelled from the Nazi Party and lost his academic position.[46]

From the Material Body to the Living Body: Race as a "Style of Experience"

The problem of mental heredity drove Clauß to develop a new racial psychology (*Rassenseelenkunde*) based on phenomenological principles, rejecting the importance of anatomical and morphological characteristics in favor of bodily and facial expressions, that were seen as the corporal side of a latent inner "racial soul."

Clauß proclaimed race to be a phenomenological manifestation of an internal "style of experience" (*Stil des Erlebnisses*), which takes the form of a "living Gestalt."[47] The body, Clauß argued, is a site (*Schauplatz*) for the soul to express itself; it is a "something-for-soul" (*Etwas-für-Seele*), a medium for the realization of the racial-mental qualities.[48] According to this view, the human psyche manifests itself through the movements and the expressions of the "living body" (*Leib*), and thus represents a particular racial style. Such expressions of the living body cannot be captured by scientific quantitative methods that reduce "life" through physicochemical processes and narrow it to its material components, as postulated by material monism. Thus, the Claußian conception of race shifted the focus of racial inquiry from the material, corporal, and static body (*Körper*), which is the object of natural science, to the living, moving body (*Leib*), which is the object of a new racial psychology based on phenomenological and humanistic methods.[49]

According to Clauß, the natural sciences, including physical and biological anthropology, in their pursuit of abstract and definite generalizations, distort life as they really are, namely a dynamic process of formation and becoming, by imposing upon them the static, descriptive, and classificatory logic of the exact sciences. In Clauß's view, it is not the measurement, comparison, or statistical quantification of racial characteristics that reveals the laws of race but rather the investigation of the "fields of movements" (*Bewegungsfelder*), of the bodily and facial lines. These expose the racial-mental "style" that constitutes the human *Gestalt*. Hence his statement that "when talking about race, we do not mean a collection of characteristics [*eine Sammlung von Eigenschaften*], as can often be falsely understood from scientific terminology, but rather something that encompasses the entire essence of a living being and exposes an internal law [*ein inneres Gesetz*]."[50]

Clauß embraced Husserl's view, according to which the living body is the medium through which the spirit (*Geist*) expresses itself and becomes objectified. In this sense, movements, gestures, and facial expressions are seen as phenomenological manifestations of the spirit that come into realization through the body. Clauß racialized Husserl's universal insights, reformulating them into his psycho-racial typology. Therein, he argued that the psychological diversity of races can be classified systematically according to the principles of phenomenology, since each race possesses a particular psychic predisposition that empirically expresses itself in its encounter with the world. Accordingly, each race can be classified by fixed criteria, such as its interaction with its environment, its relationship to human beings, its vitality, sensitivity, temperament, ultimate value, and more. Clauß used these criteria to compose a comparative perspective on the different racial styles of experience.

Within this framework, each race was defined according to the style of its conscious intention toward the objects with which it was surrounded. Different races might possess the same mental characteristics, yet identical characteristics manifest themselves differently in different styles, which are determined by racial predispositions. Thus, while "character" (*Charakter*) dictates the presence or absence of certain mental attributes in an individual, it is his racial "style" that determines the way in which these attributes manifest themselves. As Clauß propounded, "racial mental traits cannot be discerned in the fact that a person is lying or not lying, but rather in the style of his lying: a Nordic liar lies differently than an eastern [*ostische*] Mediterranean or Middle Eastern liar."[51]

Hence, it is possible to understand why Clauß attributed a decisive weight to environmental factors, particularly to culture and education, in the shaping of individuals and society: "Neither the racial *Gestalt* alone nor the style of experience alone, determine the value of man as a participant in a community, but rather what wraps his *Gestalt* and the style and dictates whether his qualities are good (or bad). In one word: his character."[52] While "style," or race, was perceived as a priori, fixed, and unchanging, then "character" was merely a flexible mental strata that could be shaped and improved through education and self-cultivation.[53]

Since the moral and the ethical value of a person is determined by his character and not by his race, eugenics' claim to improve society by "purifying the Nation's blood" is meaningless. Much like Günther, Clauß also attributed a decisive role to the individual's ability to overcome the foreign racial elements that had become mingled with it over the generations, to transcend its inner racial conflicts, and to create new "cultural values." In Clauß's view, this inner struggle was only fruitful if it ended in the undisputed victory of the Nordic style laws. The inner moral obligation of the individual was therefore clear: "to confront himself and lead the Nordic within him to victory."[54]

Racial Psychology beyond Natural Science

Clauß's relativism led him to adopt a more flexible and pluralistic approach than Günther did. Both men believed that racial science could not be "universal" or "objective," since racial differences dictated and regulated in advance the very boundaries of conception, thereby rendering different ways of looking upon the world. However, unlike Günther, Clauß emphasized the need to implement a relative approach while avoiding any hierarchical conception of races.[55] For this reason, Clauß also demanded abandoning "exact" and quantitative methods, which measure the various races by objective means and general schemes, in favor of more humanistic, holistic, and qualitative methods, which could assess the subjective nature of the human psyche.

Against this background, it is easy to understand Clauß's critique of biological and physical anthropology and its pretention of drawing general conclusions about racial mental differences. In the preface to his 1929 book *Von Seele und Antlitz der Rassen und Völker* (Of soul and face of races and peoples), he stated that "the soul is not an object of nature [*Naturding*] and therefore cannot be measured or weighed. . . . If naturalistic anthropology is to remain methodologically decent, it must avoid talking about the soul."[56] In his view, the failure of *Rassenkunde* in validating racial mental differences, whether based on physiognomic expositions such as Günther's or on genealogical and genetic methods, was due to the fact that its objectives and methods were in the field of natural science, which deals with the world of physical phenomena but allows no access to the psychic terrain.

Clauß mocked racial scientists who, ensconced in their laboratories, purport to investigate the various races in their "naturalness," while the objects of their research are detached from their natural environment. As an alternative, he proposed a method described as the "mimetic method" (*Mimische Methode*), or the "participation method" (*Methode des Mitlebens*), which studies racial objects by "visiting the world in which they live, and participating in their lives as much as possible."[57] Clauß developed a unique photographic technique defined by him as the "mimetic series," which aimed at capturing the "racial object" in its natural environment, fulfilling its daily tasks and engaging in spontaneous behavior. In his books, Clauß published a series of body and facial photographs from different angles, usually presenting a sequence of expressions, actions, and movements. Their purpose was to expose the expressional lines of the moving body to the camera and to trace the emotional style that dictates its movements. The decision of presenting a series of photographs of the same object rather than a single picture, as was customary in the literature of the period, expresses Clauß's general criticism of the racial classification used in the writings of Günther and other contemporary racial researchers. In his books, Clauß demonstrated how a particular face may look "Nordic" from one angle and "Mediterranean" from another, or "Oriental" from the front and "phallic" from the profile. Alongside the "mimetic method," and the use of photographs, Clauß made use of ethnological tools, particularly linguistics, which served to illustrate the supposed cognitive gaps between the different races and the modes in which they perceive and contextualize reality.

Clauß's *Rassenseelenkunde* signified a systematic and severe attack on contemporary biological anthropology and its naturalistic conception of race. It provided a way out of the paradoxes underlying scientific racism. By moving away from biological and physiological definitions of race and implementing a phenomenological approach based on vitalist understanding of human psychophysics, Clauß was able to bypass some of the major problems that troubled the minds of interwar racial anthropologists.

As expected, the obvious empirical weakness of the Claußian method, and its excruciating challenge to biological anthropology, gave rise to criticism from racial scientists and eugenicists, who viewed it as a speculative position that did not conform to critical science. Some, such as Fritz Lenz, praised Clauß's contribution to the understanding of racial-mental differences, but regarded it as an unfinished task.[58] Others, such as the psychologist Bruno Petermann, pointed to a series of logical and methodological failures that stripped the Claußian system of all its scientific pretensions.[59]

But Clauß's theory was also ideologically problematic: Firstly, Clauß's relativism was in sharp contrast to the Nazi movement's admiration of Nordic chauvinism and elitism. Secondly, Clauß's rejection of biological and anthropometric methods, and his exclusive reliance on humanistic and phenomenological methods, undermined the scientific pretensions of Nazi racial theory that sought to anchor its ideological claims to solid empirical ground. Thirdly, Clauß's attacks on biological anthropology revealed its methodological and theoretical weaknesses and strengthened its critics, both those who cast doubt on its scientific credibility and those who viewed it as a too-rigid materialist science.[60] Finally, the theoretical complexity of the Claußian theory made Nazi racism less accessible to the masses. Unlike Günther's aesthetical idealization of the Nordic race, the theoretical complexity of the Claußian doctrine, and the grounding of the concept of race on "stylistic" and movement-related principles, made it difficult to promulgate. Claußian theory made the visual representation of racial ideals impossible, for how could standard artistic tools capture an aesthetic ideal that was not based on clear formal physical architecture but on movement, body language, and facial expressions? As a result, race became an elusive, complex, and at times amorphous object, whose diagnosis and labeling required professionalization and depth, and was not easily accessible to the common eye. All these served as an ammunition at the hands of Walter Groß, who launched in 1941 a severe attack on Clauß ideas, which ended, a year later, in his expulsion from the Nazi Party and his removal from his academic position.

Conclusion

The racial theories of Günther and Clauß demonstrate the idiosyncratic nature of German racial thought during the interwar years. They illustrate how biological racism was formulated not only in accordance with the latest discoveries in the field of genetics but also in correspondence to contemporary debates over value-free science and biological determinism. Although they differed fundamentally in their disciplines, methods, and conceptual frameworks, their work was nonetheless influenced by a deep hostility to materialism, mechanism, and reductionism, and was driven by a prevailing mood of severe cultural crisis and intellectual uncertainty. The critique of positivistic and mechanistic thinking had become an obligatory intellectual imperative for these thinkers who sought to overcome what they saw as the pressing problem of modern nihilism and the downfall of absolute values, by reference to biological-determined "living experience" as the ultimate basis of knowledge and ethics, thereby upholding the intrinsic "organic" values supposedly residing beyond empirical objectivity. The distinction between fact and value, between "is" and "ought," which has been the mainstay of positivism, motivated these thinkers to employ a new biological reasoning that undermined mechanistic and causal explanations. Appropriating a notion of biological totality enabled them to overcome the obstacles raised by Mendelian genetics, to bypass mechanistic biology, and to invest biology with "value." This laid the foundation for a new conception of race, which was no longer bound to the descriptive and reductionist categories of scientific (materialistic) biology but rather was defined holistically and saturated virtually all areas of thought. Thus, their attempts to promote holistic and vitalist understanding of human psychophysics stood at the center of their theoretical and scientific endeavors, underpinning their motivation to break down the barriers between theory and praxis, scholarship and politics, and more generally between science and "life." This new science was no longer aimed solely at describing reality; it also strove to shape it anew in accordance with the national Germanic spirit and its Nordic vision.

As far as this scientific mode of thinking must be regarded in its normative and context specifics, it possesses significance that is not merely historical but is also relevant for essential questions concerning science and ideology existing in the present day. Facing the increasing ethical and moral challenges arising from new scientific fields such as biotechnology or artificial intelligence, we must direct our criticism not only toward the possible dangers of enlisting science for political and extra-scientific agendas but also to the scientist's tendency to reduce human experience and value-creating to biological and evolutionist explanations and thus to rule out, albeit never explicitly, any feasibility of moral choice. Science and ethics should maintain their autonomy as two separated fields of knowledge that conduct a free and fruitful, although nevertheless restraining, dialogue. Only then can we benefit from the blessed fruits of human progress without abandoning our responsibility to future generations.

Amit Varshizky, PhD, is a postdoc fellow of the Minerva Stiftung at the Friedrich-Schiller-University in Jena. He is the Goldberg Prize winner for an excelling, original, theoretical manuscript for 2019. The manuscript *The Metaphysics of Race: Science and Faith in the National-Socialist Worldview* will be published by the Open University of Israel Publishing House and the Yad Vashem International Institute for Holocaust Research. His current research deals with the philosophy and psychology of religion of Erich Rudolf Jaensch.

Notes

1. See, for example, the recently published volume *Beyond the Racial State: Rethinking Nazi Germany*, edited by Devin O. Pendas, Mark Roseman, and Richard Wetzell. Dan Stone also discusses the inappropriateness of reducing Nazism to biologism in chapter four of his *Histories of the Holocaust*. Christopher Hutton, in his *Race and the Third Reich*, explains why the Nazi leadership wanted to replace the concept of *Rasse* with that of *Volk* in a way that bypassed racial scientific inconsistency.

2. The works of Paul Weindling, Robert Proctor, Hans-Walter Schmuhl, Veronika Lipphardt, Volker Roelcke, and Uwe Hoßfeld provide excellent examples of historical analyses that are both very sensitive to the scientific work itself and aware of the scientists' complex relations with ideological, political and social factors. However, none of them have addressed the growth of alternative explanatory styles in the life and mind sciences, and the ways they provided new justifications for the *politicization* of science. See Weindling 1993; Schmuhl 2005; Lipphardt 2009; Hoßfeld 2016; Roelcke 1997.

3. Studies that support this view are many and diverse. Some prominent works in this field include Proctor 1988; Weindling 1993; Zimmerman 2001; Schmuhl 2005; Evans 2010.

4. Fischer 1927, 11. Unless otherwise noted, all translations of the German original are the author's.

5. Günther 1925a, 156.
6. Günther 1925a, 661.
7. Scheidt 1925, 433.
8. Scheidt, 1934a, 7.
9. Mollison 1934, 35–36.

10. As Fritz Ringer notes, many German intellectuals never distinguished between the industrialization process and the erosion of fundamental morals and values. As a result, "they linked commerce with commercialism, machine with mechanistic conceptions, and the new economic organization with rationalism and utilitarianism." Ringer 1969, 221.

11. Following Paul Forman's pioneering and controversial thesis about Weimar's physics, scholars have attempted to trace the connection between German science and Weimar cultural values, exploring the relationship between the German irrational "hunger for wholeness," in Peter Gay's words, and the emergence of indeterministic, anti-mechanistic, and acausal scientific paradigms. Thus, the work of Anne Harrington, Mitchell G. Ash, Jonathan Harwood, and Carsten Timmerman has provided a highly detailed picture of the various ways in which holistic ideas influenced the hard theoretical core of scientific knowledge in the Weimar era. See Forman 1971; Harwood 1993; Ash 1995; Harrington 1996; Timmerman 2001.

12. Harrington 1996, xvii.
13. Husserl 2012, 5–7.
14. Weingart, Kroll, and Bayertz 1992, 452.
15. Evans 2010, 213.
16. Lutzhöft 1971, 32.
17. Klee 2013, 208
18. Breuer 2008, 115.
19. Weingart, Kroll, and Bayertz 1992, 452; Lutzhöft 1971, 41–45; Gray 2004, 267–71. In a 1937 speech, Alfred Rosenberg characterized Günther's contribution to the formulation of the National Socialist race theory with these words: "National-socialist racial thought finds in the works of Professor Hans Günther a seal which we all welcome today because they provide a broad summary of past studies in a realistic and valuable way for the German people." Rosenberg 1937, 3.
20. It should be noted that despite Chamberlain's considerable influence, Günther believed that racial objects can indeed be validated and verified by scientific means, and that the striving for the "Nordification" of the German people is to be based on as solid empirical evidence as possible. In his view, the development of the study of genetics and human heredity reinforces Chamberlain's ideas and provides for the first time practical means for realizing the Nordic vision. See Günther 1926, 76–77.
21. Günther 1925a, 1–2. Thus Günther writes in the opening page of his *Rassenkunde des deutschen Volkes*, "The gaze of contemporary man is unbalanced. Perhaps it is the natural sciences, in part or in full, that have contributed to the diffusion of the unimaginative of vision and imagination. The purpose of science is—and must be—the transfer of all phenomena through a numerical expression of knowledge. But the danger is that because of our scientific approach, the *Gestaltung*, our formation of image, namely the physical-tangible essence of the phenomenon, will be lost. . ." Günther 1925b, 1.
22. Günther 1925b, 414.
23. Günther 1925b, 262.
24. Günther 1925b, 264.
25. For further reading see Gray 2004, 219–73.
26. Günther 1925b, 2.
27. Günther 1925b, 8.
28. For a comprehensive discussion of the "value-neutrality" debate and the prevalent call for the exclusion of politics and morals from science in late nineteenth-century and early twentieth-century Germany, see Proctor 1991; Beiser 2011, 511–68; Gert 2010; Glaeser 2014.
29. Günther 1925a, 81. Leading racial scientists such as Fritz Lenz and Walter Scheidt also cited this statement in their writings, using it to justify their calls for subjecting science to politics. Lenz 1932, 9; Scheidt 1934b, 13.
30. Günther 1925a, 81.
31. Günther 1925b, 414.
32. In 1928 Günther published a book titled *Platon als Hüter des Lebens: Platons Zucht und Erziehungsgedanken und deren Bedeutung für die Gegenwart* (Plato as the protector of life: Plato's ideas of breeding and education and their meaning for contemporary times) in which he claimed Plato to be the first and the most authentic forerunner of racial theory and the eugenic worldview. According to Günther, Plato was the first to reorganize the state in accordance to the hierarchical principles of inherited natural qualities.
33. Günther 1925b, 400.
34. Günther 1925b, 414.
35. Günther 1935, 191.
36. Günther 1925a, 56.
37. Günther 1925a, 55.

38. In a lecture delivered in February 1933, Günther emphasized this line of thought: "What has been called 'Lebensphilosophie' more or less bypasses the school of German Idealism, moves from Goethe and some of the impulses derived from Romanticism's so-called philosophy of nature, via Schopenhauer to Nietzsche and, as many people believe, ultimately to Ludwig Klages. We recognize in all of these thinkers . . . a firm belief in the very body-soul unity that was prevalent in the thought of the ancient Indogermanic peoples, a unity that is also confirmed by present-day biology." Quoted in Gray 2004, 271–72.

39. Günther 1925a, 72.

40. Günther described the immense creative potential inherent in the conflicted soul of a racially mixed man and the advantages of his creative powers over those of a pure-blood man. According to him, "The active discontent underlying racial mixing creates in the individual the tension required to create a special spiritual achievement." He relies on the examples of Goethe and Beethoven: two German geniuses who succeeded in their will to overcome their inferior racial traits, to transcend the racial-psychological conflict taking place within them, and to extract the powerful creative force embodied in the Nordic race. Goethe, who was racially mixed (his facial lines are evident to Nordic-Danish traits but his physical structure points at "oriental influences"), is a striking example of how "a person who accepts himself fully can bundle all the internal conflicts within him and sublimate the energy they generate toward a certain direction." Günther 1925a, 63.

41. Günther 1925a, 63.

42. Günther 1925a, 683.

43. Lenz, for instance, praised Günther's achievement of shaping a realistic image of the Nordic race, avoiding the risk of arbitrary speculation by systematic comparison of intuitive gaze and material evidences provided by ethnology and history. He backs up Günther's view by stressing that the image of the Nordic race is in fact not "physical" (*körperliche*) but rather "spiritual" (*geistige*), for it is contingent upon the actual psychobiological prism through which natural phenomenon are being observed and constructed. Baur, Fischer, and Lenz 1936, 714–15.

44. Günther, in Töppel 2018, 89.

45. See Wetzell 2017, 154–57.

46. On Clauß, see Weingart 1995; Wiedemann 2009; Gray 2004, 273–333.

47. Clauß 1937b, 17.

48. Clauß 1929, 73–74.

49. Based on similar assumptions, Wehrmacht psychologists sought to develop new methods that would enable the measuring of willpower, considered to be a highly important feature because of the nature of the tasks required of soldiers on the battlefield. Because, according to this view, the human psyche manifests itself through the movements and expressions of the living body, Wehrmacht psychologists developed new methods for analyzing mental qualities and emotional expressions by means of body language, gestures, facial expressions, muscle tension, and voice. See Geuter 1992, 94–98.

50. Clauß 1929, x.

51. Clauß 1937a, 235.

52. Clauß 1935b, 460.

53. See Clauß 1936, 79.

54. Clauß 1935a, 13.

55. Clauß maintained this emphasis throughout his professional career, including during his activities under the auspices of the Nazi Party. For example, in the preface for the sixteenth edition of his book *Rasse und Seele* (1939), Clauß used an apologetic tone while responding to the Catholic critics on his racial theory: "It is illogical and unscientific to look at the Mediterranean race with a Nordic eye and judge it according to Nordic standards, as much as it is unscientific to do the opposite." Clauß 1939, 16.

56. Clauß 1929, viii.

57. Clauß 1939, 21.
58. Lenz 1932, 760–61.
59. Petermann 1935.
60. See, for example, Walter Groß's accusations against Clauß in Weingart 1995, 84.

References

Ash, Mitchell G. 1995. *Gestalt Psychology in German Culture, 1890–1967*. Cambridge: Cambridge University Press.
Baur, Erwin, Eugen Fischer, and Fritz Lenz. 1936. *Menschliche Erblehre und Rassenhygiene*. München: J. F. Lehmanns Verlag.
Beiser, Frederick C. 2011. *The German Historicist Tradition*. New York: Oxford University Press.
Breuer, Stefan. 2008. *Die Völkischen in Deutschland: Kaiserreich und Weimarer Republik*. Darmstadt: Wissenschaftliche Buchgesellschaft.
Clauß, Ludwig Ferdinand. 1929. *Von Seele und Antlitz der Rassen und Völker: Eine Einführung in die vergleichende Ausdrucksforschung*. München: J. F. Lehmanns Verlag.
———. 1935a. "Rassenseele und Volksgemeinschaft." *Rasse: Monatsschrift der Nordischen Bewegung*: 3–19.
———. 1935b. "Die innere Landschaft." *Rasse: Monatsschrift der Nordischen Bewegung* 3, Heft 12: 457–60.
———. 1936. *Rasse und Charakter*. Frankfurt am Main: Diesterweg.
———. 1937a. "Asbjörn, Wirfils Sohn, und das 'Glück' des nordischen Helden." *Rasse: Monatsschrift der Nordischen Bewegung*: 234–43.
———. 1937b. *Rasse ist Gestalt*. München: Zentralverlag der NSDAP, Franz Eher Rachf.
———. 1939. *Rasse und Seele: Eine Einführung in den Sinn der Leiblichen Gestalt*. 16th ed. Berlin: Büchergilde Gutenberg.
Evans, Andrew D. 2010. *Anthropology at War: World War I and the Science of Race in Germany*. Illinois: University of Chicago Press.
Fischer, Eugen. 1927. *Rasse und Rasse-Entstehung beim Menschen*. Berlin: Ullstein.
Forman, Paul. 1971. "Weimar Culture, Causality, and Quantum Theory, 1918–1927: Adaptation by German Physicists and Mathematicians to a Hostile Intellectual Environment." In *Historical Studies in the Physical Sciences* vol. 3, edited by R. McCormmach, 1–115. Oakland: University of California Press.
Gert, Albert. 2010. "Der Werturteilsstreit." In *Soziologische Kontroversen*, edited by Georg Kneer and Stephan Moebius, 14–45. Frankfurt am Main: Suhrkamp.
Geuter, Ulfried. 1992. *The Professionalization of Psychology in Nazi Germany*. Cambridge: Cambridge University Press
Glaeser, Johannes. 2014. *Der Werturteilsstreit in der deutschen Nationalökonomie: Max Weber, Werner Sombart und die Ideale der Sozialpolitik*. Marburg: Metropolis.
Gray, Richard T. 2004. *About Face: German Physiognomic Thought from Lavatar to Auschwitz*. Detroit: Wayne State University Press.
Günther, Hans F. K. 1925a. *Der nordische Gedanke unter den Deutschen*. Munich: J. F. Lehmanns Verlag.
———. 1925b. *Rassenkunde des Deutschen Volkes*. 7th ed. München: J. F. Lehmanns Verlag.
———. 1926. *Adel und Rasse*. Munich: J. F. Lehmanns Verlag.
———. 1928. *Platon als Hüter des Lebens: Platons Zucht und Erziehungs-Gedanken und deren Bedeutung für die Gegenwart*. München: J. F. Lehmanns Verlag.
———. 1935. *Ritter, Tod und Teufel: Der heldische Gedanke*. 4th ed. München: J. F. Lehmanns Verlag.

Harrington, Anne. 1996. *Reenchanted Science: Holism in German Culture from Wilhelm II to Hitler*. Princeton, NJ: Princeton University Press.

Harwood, Jonathan. 1993. *Styles of Scientific Thought: The German Genetics Community, 1900–1933*. Chicago: University of Chicago Press.

Hoßfeld, Uwe. 2016. *Geschichte der Biologischen Anthropologie in Deutschland: Von den Anfängen bis in die Nachkriegszeit*. Stuttgart: Franz Steiner Verlag.

Husserl, Edmund. 2012 [1936]. *Die Krisis der europäischen Wissenschaften und die Transzendentale Phänomenologie*. Hamburg: Felix Meiner Verlag.

Hutton, Chrisopher. 2005. *Race and the Third Reich*. Cambridge: Polity Press.

Klee, Ernst. 2013. *Das Personenlexikon zum Dritten Reich: Wer war was vor und nach 1945*. Frankfurt am Main: Fischer Taschenbuch.

Lipphardt, Veronika. 2009. *Biologie der Juden: Jüdische Wissenschaftler über "Rasse" und Vererbung 1900–1935*. Göttingen: Vandenhoeck und Ruprecht Verlag.

Lenz, Fritz. 1932. *Menschliche Auslese und Rassenhygiene (Eugenik)*. 3rd ed. Published as vol. 2 of *Grundriß der Menschliche Erblichkeitslehre und Rassenhygiene*, edited by Erwin Baur, Eugen Fischer, and Fritz Lenz. Munich: J. F. Lehmanns Verlag.

Lutzhöft, Hans-Jürgen. 1971. *Der Nordische Gedanke in Deutschland 1920–1940*. Stuttgart: Ernst Klett Verlag.

Mollison, Theodor. 1934. "Rassenkunde und Rassenhygiene." In *Erblehre und Rassenhygiene im völkischen Staat*, edited by Ernst Rüdin, 35–36. Munich: Lehmanns Verlag.

Pendas, Devin, Mark Roseman, and Richard Wetzell (eds.). 2017. *Beyond the Racial State: Rethinking Nazi Germany*. Cambridge: Cambridge University Press.

Petermann, Bruno. 1935. *Das Problem der Rassenseele: Vorlesungen zur Grundlegung einer allgemeinen Rassenpsychologie*. Leipzig: Verlag von Johann Ambrosius Barth.

Proctor, Robert. 1988. "From 'Anthropologie' to 'Rassenkunde' in the German Anthropological Tradition." In *Bones, Bodies, Behavior: Essays on Biological Anthropology*, edited by George W. Stocking Jr., 138–79. Madison: University of Wisconsin Press.

———. 1991. *Value-Free Science? Purity and Power in Modern Knowledge*. Cambridge, MA: Harvard University Press.

Ringer, Fritz K. 1969. *The Decline of the German Mandarins: The German Academic Community, 1890–1933*. Cambridge, MA: Harvard University Press.

Roelcke, Volker. 1997. "Biologizing Social Facts: An Early 20th Century Debate on Kaerpelin's Concepts of Culture, Neuroasthenia, and Degeneration." *Culture, Medicine and Psychiatry* 21: 383–403.

Rosenberg, Alfred. 1937. "Weltanschauung und Wissenschaft." *Weltanschauung und Wissenschaft: 5 Vorträge der dritten Reichsarbeitstagung der Dienststelle für Schrifttumspflege bei dem Beauftragten des Führers für die gesamte geistige und weltanschauliche Erziehung der NSDAP; Und der Reichstelle zur Förderung des deutschen Schrifttums*, 1–7. Bayreuth: Gauverlag Bayerische Ostmark.

Scheidt, Walter. 1925. *Allgemeine Rassenkunde: Als Einführung in das Studium der Menschenrassen*. Munich: J. F. Lehmann.

———. 1934a. *Die Lebensgeschichte eines Volkes: Einführung in die rassenbiologische und kulturbiologische Forschung*. Hamburg: Richard Hermes Verlag.

———. 1934b. *Die Träger der Kultur*. Berlin: Alfred Metsner Verlag.

Schmuhl, Hans-Walter. 2005. *Grenzüberschreitungen: Das Kaiser-Wilhelm-Institut für Anthropologie, menschliche Erblehre und Eugenik, 1927–1945*. Göttingen: Wallstein Verlag.

Stone, Dan. 2010. *Histories of the Holocaust*. New York: Oxford University Press.

Timmerman, Carsten. 2001. "Constitutional Medicine, Neoromanticism, and the Politics of Antimechanism in Interwar Germany." *Bulletin for the History of Medicine* 75: 717–39.

Töppel, Roman. 2018. "Volk und Rasse: In Search for Hitler's Sources." In: *Hitler—New Research*, edited by Elizabeth Harvey and Johannes Hürter, 71–111. Berlin: De Gruyter.

Weindling, Paul. 1993. *Health, Race and German Politics between National Unification and Nazism 1870–1945*. New York: Cambridge University Press.

Weingart, Peter. 1995. *Doppel-Leben: Ludwig Ferdinand Clauss; Zwischen Rassenforschung und Widerstand*. Frankfurt am Main: Campus.

Weingart, Peter, Jürgen Kroll, and Kurt Bayertz. 1992. *Rasse, Blut und Gene: Geschichte der Eugenik und Rassenhygiene in Deutschland*. Frankfurt am Main: Suhrkamp.

Wetzel, Richard, F. 2017. "Eugenics, Racial Science, and Nazi Racial Policy: Was There a Genesis of the 'Final Solution' from the Spirit of Science?" In *Beyond the Racial State: Rethinking Nazi Germany*, edited by Devin Pendas, Mark Roseman, and Richard Wetzell, 147–76. Cambridge: Cambridge University Press.

Wiedemann, Felix. 2009. "Der doppelte Orient: Zur völkischen Orientromantik des Ludwig Ferdinand Clauß." *Zeitschrift für Religions- und Geistesgeschichte* 1: 1–24.

Zimmerman, Andrew. 2001. *Anthropology and Antihumanism in Imperial Germany*. Illinois: University of Chicago Press.

CHAPTER 2

From "Racial Surveys" to Medical Experiments in Prisoner-of-War Camps

Margit Berner

Historiographic studies have demonstrated that "racial studies" were often conducted in a situation of oppression, such as in prisons, police stations, or military institutions, which were characterized by colonial or National Socialist power structures and the power of definition of scientists and authorities.[1] In these studies, ethical, personal, and religious boundaries of the investigated men, women, or children were often transgressed.[2]

"Racial science" was, as Benoit Massin has pointed out, "not a new invention of the Nazis, but came from established academic science and medicine." Social Darwinism and "racial hygiene" were essential components of Nazi ideology, and anthropology and "racial science" were among those disciplines that flourished under the Nazis; new research institutes were founded; research projects were increased; and applied science was promoted. This development was initiated predominantly by the anthropologists themselves out of professional concerns and scientific persuasion.[3] It was thus physical anthropology as a discipline that played an affirmative role—a reality that should not be underestimated—in connection with the promotion of "racial ideology" during the Nazi period.

Between 1939 and 1943, the Department of Anthropology of the Natural History Museum Vienna undertook extensive "racial surveys" on Jews and prisoners of war.[4] These investigations were carried out under the leadership of the anthropologists Josef Wastl and Robert Routil.[5] Already at the beginning of 1939, Wastl initiated and established the anti-Semitic exhibition "Das körperliche und physische Erscheinungsbild der Juden" (The physical and spiritual appearance of the Jews).[6] In 1942, the department purchased skulls and death masks of concentration camp victims, Jews, and Polish resistance fighters from the Anatomical Institute of the Reich University Posen under the chair Hermann Voss.[7] Between 1942 and 1943, 220 Jewish skeletons were unearthed in a Viennese cemetery. In addition, between 1941 and 1945, Wastl composed several hundred records of "racial" and paternity assessments for courts or for the Reich Office of Genealogy (Reichssippenamt) in unclear or disputed ancestry.[8]

From 1939 onward, research and collection interests focused especially on Jews and prisoners of war; in other words, on expanding the museum's collections with "material" that had never before been available. Wastl emphasized the unique opportunity to collect material such as measurement sheets, photographs, hair samples, hand- and fingerprints, and plaster facemasks. These collections would be of considerable value and would greatly enrich the holdings of the museum.[9] The anthropologists also took advantage of the war situation, as they saw great advantages there over the difficulties encountered in civilian investigations. In the military camps, enforced discipline facilitated their activities due to the "need for all nude photos, measurements on naked bodies, plaster casts of the head and other body parts."[10]

With the prisoner-of-war studies, the museum's anthropologists aimed to investigate "racial morphology and racial types" of and within national and ethnic groups. The studies followed the methods and procedures developed during similar investigations in World War I, where German and Austrian anthropologists, linguists, and ethnologists undertook extensive research in prisoner-of-war camps.[11] However, during World War II, some of the "racial investigations" of the Viennese anthropologists in the prisoner-of-war camps changed over time and turned to medical research and experiments.

Joint investigations of anthropologists and medical doctors were not a new phenomenon in German physical anthropology. This is partly due, firstly, to the roots of the discipline, where many early representatives were anatomists or other medical professionals, and, secondly, to the interest of exploring normal variation, which implies a delineation of pathological forms. In the first half of the twentieth century and especially during the Nazi period, the interest in the differences between humans was no longer limited to the investigation of morphology, but extended to internal anatomical, physiological, and neurological differences. Subsequently, questions of different mental characteristics also became the subject of investigations. Moreover, during the interwar period anthropologists gained an increased interest in applied science, resulting in close cooperation with medical institutions, courts, criminologists, and other disciplines.[12]

Based on the Department of Anthropology's collections at the museum, this chapter focuses on the research and context of the prisoner-of-war studies in World War II. Based on an overview of the subject, the question will be explored as to how the situation of the war influenced the research and collecting activities. It will become apparent that for the anthropologists the camps represented "ideal" conditions to conduct so-called "racial" studies. The research studies and collecting activities were influenced by the relation and interaction between the researched and the researcher, as well as by the different treatment of nationalities in the camps. Moreover, the studies can be seen as an example of how personal contact, ideology, and the special situation of the war influenced motivations and activities of the scientists during the Nazi period.

The Prisoner-of-War Studies of the Viennese Anthropologists

Immediately after the start of the war, the museum's anthropologists began with "racial" studies on Jews of Polish origin imprisoned in the Viennese soccer stadium in September 1939. Shortly after, the museum gained permission to conduct "racial" research on prisoners of war from the High Command of the German Armed Forces (Oberkommando der Wehrmacht) and the Ministry of Internal and Cultural Affairs (Ministeriums für innere und kulturelle Angelegenheiten).[13]

The "racial" investigations were carried out in the prisoner-of-war camps Kaisersteinbruch (Stalag XVII A) in Lower Austria and Wolfsberg (Stalag XVIII A) in Carinthia between 1940 and 1943. Kaisersteinbruch was one of the first and, until 1941, also one of the largest prisoner-of-war camps in the territory of the German Reich. With the transformation of the officers camp (*Oflag* or *Offizierslager*) into main camps (*Stalags* or *Mannschaftslager*), many inmates of Kaisersteinbruch passed into the administration of Stalag XVIII A, Wolfsberg, and XVIII B, Spittal an der Drau.[14] In the camps, prisoners of war were separated by nationality, as in all camps there existed a hierarchy among the prisoners of war, according to "specially developed ranking scales" by the Oberkommando der Wehrmacht.[15] The positioning within this "prisoners hierarchy depended, on the one hand, on the fixed position of the individual ethnic groups, and, on the other hand, on the power-political calculation of possible reprisals against German prisoners detained by the respective enemy state."[16] At the top of the hierarchy were the British, the Americans, and the French. Greeks and Serbs represented a separate category. Until 1941, Poles were at the bottom of the hierarchy, and after the beginning of the German-Soviet War, the Soviet prisoners of war took that position.[17] For the Soviet prisoners of war, "the Stalags of the 'Ostmark' became 'death camps.'"[18]

The "racial" surveys started in January 1940 in Kaisersteinbruch. Within a month, the team investigated more than one thousand Polish prisoners of war, who were divided into groups such as ethnic Germans (*Volksdeutsche*), Poles, Ukrainians, Belarusians, and Jews. In effect, these studies began with the investigations of Jewish prisoners of war, as Jews always were considered as a separate group. In April 1940, Wastl's team investigated another 130 Polish prisoners of war. From the Nazi point of view, Poland had ceased to exist as a sovereign state following the occupation by the German Reich, and for that reason the application of the Geneva Convention was considered unnecessary. From the beginning of January 1940, reports and lists were no longer sent to the International

Committee of the Red Cross in Geneva, and in May 1940, as a result of Hitler's decree (*Führererlass*), about nine-tenths of Polish prisoners of war had been forcibly converted into the "status of civilian workers." This meant that Polish prisoners of war were transferred from the *Stalags* to "camps for laborers of the East" (*Ostarbeiterlager*), and thus came from "the custody of the Wehrmacht into that of the Gestapo."[19]

In 1940, the surveys continued in July and August and later in September and November. From this time on, the anthropologists conducted measurements on French prisoners of war, who constituted the majority of inmates in the Kaisersteinbruch camp at that time.[20] Wastl enthusiastically wrote to the museum's director, "We feel that probably no anthropologist has ever seen the racial representatives of European France in such a colorful mixture as we do."[21] Comparatively privileged, the captured French soldiers formed, as Hubert Speckner wrote, "soon a kind of 'camp elite' who shaped camp life through the French-dominated self-administration of the prisoners of war."[22] Even within the prisoners of a country there existed different categorizations. For instance, among Belgian prisoners of war the Flemish were treated better—for political reasons—than the Walloons.[23] Colored soldiers were often recorded separately, as shown in a document from July 1940, which listed over one thousand colored prisoners of war for Kaisersteinbruch.[24] There are no records from Kaisersteinbruch regarding the situation and treatment of Jewish-French prisoners of war or of French colonial soldiers, who came mainly from Morocco, Algeria, Tunisia, and French Indochina.[25] Finally, by the end of 1940, the team of anthropologists had investigated 4,795 men.

The plan to continue the surveys in the POW camps in 1941 could not be realized, just as a plan to study Jews in the Netherlands had similarly failed. During that year, the anthropologists conducted "racial" investigations on families and people in villages of the Bohemian Forest and in Upper Austria.[26]

One year later, in the spring and autumn of 1942, the prisoner-of-war studies were continued in Wolfsberg. From this time on, the anthropological team encountered several difficulties regarding the organization and practicalities of the research. For example, during the day most prisoners of war worked outside the camp in forced labor. In addition, team members no longer received exemptions from their military duties. Wolfsberg was chosen because there were prisoners of war from different nationalities among them, including Frenchmen, Belgians, Soviets, and about fifty-one hundred British prisoners.[27] The anthropologists were particularly interested in conducting "racial" investigation on British colonial soldiers, especially from Australia and New Zealand. However, referring to the Geneva Convention, the British prisoners refused the investigations, and Wastl and his team had to accept their protest.[28] Nevertheless, the anthropologists continued to study other prisoner-of-war groups, including Serbs, Soviets, and Frenchmen, further sick prisoners, and members of the regional defense unit (*Landesschützen-Battaillon*) of the camp. Altogether seven hundred men were investigated in Wolfsberg. In addition, Soviet prisoners of war in the nearby Stalag XVIII B in Spittal an der Drau were examined. Soviet prisoners of war lived in the camps under catastrophic circumstances. According to Speckner, Stalag XVIII B was "the only pure 'Russian camp' in annexed Austria." It existed from December 1941 to October 1942; the highest occupancy rate of over eleven thousand men was recorded in August 1942. A high percentage of men died, and around six thousand Red Army soldiers were buried in mass graves.[29]

During the investigations in Wolfsberg, Wastl had started to extend his work to Soviet prisoners of war. In June 1943, the anthropologists continued the "racial" studies in Kaisersteinbruch, and at that time they started with medical research. In May 1943 there were 23,209 French, 2,012 Belgian, 103 Polish, 8,669 southeasterners from the Balkans, and 13,480 Soviet prisoners of war in the camp.[30] However, by then the war situation had changed fundamentally for the German Reich. Due to recruitment of all others for the military war effort, only a small team consisting of Wastl, Routil, and two staff members of the museum came to the camp and conducted "racial" research on 355 Russian, Serb, and Ukranian prisoners of war. The terrible situation and treatment of Soviet prisoners of war is reflected in the high mortality rate. Besides 216 citizens of all other nations, over 9,500 Soviet prisoners of war were buried in the camp cemetery of Kaisersteinbruch.[31] In addition to poor medical and nutritional care, forced labor, and the terrible living conditions, the Soviet prisoners of war were constantly reminded of their inhumane treatment by seeing the better situation of the British, Americans, and French.[32]

The prisoner-of-war studies received funding in the amount of 5,000 Reichsmark from the State Administration General Section for Art Funding, State Theater, Museums and Public Education of the State Administration of the Reichsgau in Vienna (Generalreferat für Kunstförderung, Staatstheater, Museen und Volksbildung der Staatlichen Verwaltung des Reichsgaues Wien),[33] also 2,500 Reichsmark from the Reich Research Council in Berlin[34] and 1,400 Reichsmark from the Academy of Sciences in Vienna.[35] Supported by the Academy of Sciences, the museum's director planned to establish the working group as an official commission of the Wehrmacht (*Wehrmachtsamtliche Kommission*) for anthropological and "racial" investigations in the camps, including ethnographic studies and determination of blood group types. The museum's director Hans Kummerlöwe had hoped for financial support and an exemption from military service for the team members, but the Wehrmacht declined the request.[36]

"Racial" Research and Personal Consent

The "racial" studies were carried out in teams following a tradition established in previous studies, namely the studies on prisoners of war during World War I.[37]

After the recording of the biographical data, the actual survey began. One anthropologist studied the morphological traits of the head and took notes of tattoos, cauterizations, other body modifications, as well as pathologies or variations. One investigated the color and structure of the hair, eyes, and skin. Others took measurements of head and body. At one station, finger- and handprints were taken. Wastl himself supervised the photographic stations. Several photographs were taken of the prisoners of war: both black-and-white and colored portrait photos, further stereo photographs, and photographs of the study subject in the nude. Finally, some prisoners of war were chosen for taking plaster casts of the face. Some prisoners of war were assigned to work with the team for technical assistance and data collection, but instead of monetary compensation they received cigarettes.

The investigations were carried out in a situation of oppression and military discipline. From official correspondence and the protocol books it is evident that permission to conduct "racial" studies was granted by military and civilian authorities. While being measured and observed is not painful per se and without apparent health risk, such a procedure may transgress bodily, personal, and ethical borders. For some measurements and photographs, the soldiers had to undress. Depending on personal attitude and experiences, the men chosen for investigations might have felt uncomfortable, ashamed, and humiliated. At any rate, the procedure of mask-taking was an uncomfortable, uncanny, and sometimes painful and dangerous process.[38]

As mentioned above, in Wolfsberg British prisoners of war generally refused to be investigated, citing the Geneva Convention. There is no information as to what extent the prisoners of war of other countries were obligated instead, or whether individual men could refuse the investigation. Occasional records in the protocol books testify to the fact that not all prisoners of war agreed to the anthropological examinations—e.g., "with the exception of a Koran and scripture teacher, there is no opposition to any kind of investigation."[39] Elsewhere, Routil noted that some Bosnians refused the investigations and photographs of the naked body for religious reasons.[40]

The anthropologists were aware of the different treatment and extremely bad care of the Soviet prisoners of war. During the investigations in Wolfsberg, Routil documented that compared to the German soldiers, the "difference in physical capability" of the Soviet prisoners of war is based mainly on severe malnutrition and weakened condition.[41] Routil had visited the "Russian Hospital" in Spittal an der Drau, Stalag XVIII B, where 133 Soviet prisoners of war were stationed, who were "mostly suffering from progressive TB or convalescents after typhus fever."[42] He must have noticed the catastrophic conditions in the camp.

Although there is no evidence of direct coercion by the anthropologists on the prisoners of war whose faces and body parts were cast in plaster, notes mention punishment in case of rejection. In Kaisersteinbruch, Serbian prisoners of war refused to have plaster masks taken of their faces in summer 1943. Wastl wrote, "While all the previous groups willingly submitted to having their plaster casts taken, most Serbians find some excuse, they all simply reject it."[43] However, another entry of July 1943 testifies to the use of coercion on Soviet prisoners of war: "Of the Russians, two prisoners of war refused having their plaster casts taken. After sergeant Kummer of camp commando 1 was called, one of the two was taken away and presented to the doctor for a decision. The Russians apparently received the message that Serbians who refused taking plaster casts remained unpunished. After this incident, the Russians allowed the plaster casting."[44]

The photographs, masks, and anthropological data reflect the relation and interaction between the researched and researcher. Moreover, the differential treatment and ranking scales of the prisoners of war in the camps influenced the behavior and interaction with the scientists, and thus the possibility to refuse the anthropological investigations and making of casts. While in some cases prisoners of war might have participated out of curiosity, boredom, and indifference or because of the chance to receive some cigarettes, as mentioned above some notes refer to the anthropologists' expectation of having to convince or coerce their research subjects.

From "Racial" Studies to Medical Experiments

Officers and doctors visited the investigations regularly. Wastl and Routil made daily notes of the numbers of men measured, activities of the anthropologists, and sometimes observations. Occasionally somebody else wrote an entry; e.g., one doctor suggested to expand the studies "by at least a partial intelligence test, albeit in the simplest form."[45]

First interactions with medical studies are known from summer 1940. Around the same time when Wastl and his team conducted their research in Kaisersteinbruch, the physician and eugenicist Robert Stigler, together with four doctors and one medical student, carried out "racial" physiological investigations on French and French colonial prisoners of war.[46] The physicians took blood samples, performed sternal punctures, took respiratory measurements, and administered hearing and eyesight tests. Stigler also performed tests on the psychological reaction time and made comparative observations of secondary sexual characteristics. In a subsequent publication, Stigler mentioned the negative attitude of the prisoners toward the investigations.[47] It is not clear whether Wastl's and Stigler's research teams overlapped in time. The physiological studies were not mentioned in Wastl's documentation. Moreover, so far no documentation of Stigler's research is known that might allow the identification of the prisoners of war in his studies. According to Stigler's article, it is quite likely that his investigations were carried out on the same prisoners of war that were investigated by the anthropologists.

In the same year, the president of the Academy of Science, Heinrich Srbik, wrote in a letter to the museum's director Hans Kummerlöwe "that it would be of unique value if there existed a possibility of bringing the corpses of Africans, who died in Kaisersteinbruch, to the Anatomical Institute of the University of Vienna for scientific investigation." Srbik emphasized, "There exists very little research on the extent to which racial variation finds its expression in internal organs."[48] Informed by the academy, the head of the Anatomical Institute, Eduard Pernkopf, expressed also his interest in the "examination of prisoners of war of exotic races" and a possible transfer of deceased prisoners of war to his institute.[49] Nevertheless, so far no documents were found indicating transports of corpses of colonial prisoners of war to the Viennese anatomical institute.

While it is known that in 1942 Routil had visited the military hospital for Soviet prisoners of war in Spittal an der Drau, there is no evidence of a cooperation or involvement of the anthropologists in medical studies or experiments with medical doctors for this time. The only direct cooperation is documented for the year 1943, when the military physician (*Stabsarzt*) Robert Exner and the anthropologists carried out physiological and neurological studies under "racial" aspects, seemingly more a random project than a planned one. In spring 1943, Wastl wrote to the commanding officer of Kaisersteinbruch that he wanted to continue his "racial studies on Eastern European and Asian people," but he did not mention medical surveys. Wastl considered the "racial, psychological and ethnological investigations" on Soviet prisoners of war as a "scientifically and politically important work."[50] However, already one day after the arrival in the camp, Wastl, Routil, and Exner had a meeting concerning the cooperation in physiological medical examinations such as "recordings of color perception and lumbar punctures."[51]

The physiological studies were carried out predominantly on Soviet prisoners of war and aimed to determine possible "racial" differences in color perception. In their postwar publications, Routil and Exner referred to "51 members of the Allied armies."[52] The investigations were carried out in darkened rooms. Using a special device, the examined person had to look through a tube toward a gypsum board at colored glasses and "indicate or describe the seen color." The investigations were based on the studies of color sensitivity (*Farbempfindlichkeit*) carried out by Eduard Haschek in the 1920s.[53] Exner's intention was to "study the characteristics of the color Gnosis via the detour of the color phases."[54] Later, Exner continued these studies on patients who suffered from headshot wounds in the reserve hospital XVI (*Reservelazarett*) and until 1947 on private patients. Exner and Routil regarded the studies as a pilot project, which they felt should be extended with better equipment and quantitative analyses on a large group.[55]

At the same time, Exner and Routil started with lumbar punctures to study cerebrospinal fluid. The medical interventions were most likely carried out in the camp clinic (*Krankenrevier*). Lumbar puncture is a medical procedure in which a needle is inserted into the spinal canal, most commonly to collect cerebrospinal fluid for diagnostic testing. Nine Soviet prisoners of war were subjected to this experiment. In two cases—one man with "meningitis and tuberculosis" and one with "epilepsy, debilitas"—the removal of cerebrospinal fluid may also have served for diagnostic purposes. Seven other prisoners of war of the Soviet Army (classified as Azerbaijanis, Armenians, Uzbeks, Lezgians, and Russians), however, had to undergo this procedure for racist reasons and without any medical indication.[56]

Later Exner, an officer, and the Russian physician Dr. Pnischuk examined together the crystallization of the cerebrospinal fluid under the microscope. The microscopic observations with moderate magnification and using a blue and green filter were noted in the protocol book. Routil and Exner thought they had found distinct "racial" differences and described for Europeans a "distinctly greater formation of crystals with a moderate density," while "Orientalid-Near-Asian peoples exhibit a rich, small-scale crystal formation," and "Mongolids" showed "rich, almost streaky-cloudy crystalline formation." Finally, they concluded, "the analysis of cerebrospinal fluid crystals could be a physiologically valuable method, which may lead to new findings in both normal biology and pathology."[57]

While the color perception studies can be regarded as a medical physiological study, the procedure of lumbar punctuation is clearly an intervention without a medical indication. Exner and Routil's interest was "racial" research and did not serve the purpose of medical diagnosis and therapy.

Conclusion

The medical studies were planned to continue, and by 1944, Exner had already assembled a list of Caucasian and Tatar prisoners of war.[58] However, due to an illness befalling Routil, the plan failed, and no further investigations took place. After the war, Wastl was suspended from museum service as a "minor National Socialist" and sent into retirement in 1948. Like many in his field, however, he continued to work on a freelance basis until his death in 1968, providing well-remunerated paternity evaluations. In 1949, after his denazification, Routil became head of the Anthropological Department of the Natural History Museum Vienna until his death in 1955.[59]

The wartime activities of the museum's anthropologists were characterized by an increased interest in collecting anthropometric data, photographs, and plaster casts of Jews and prisoners of war. Viennese anthropologists were not the only ones who conducted or planned "racial" investigations in prisoner-of-war camps. Eugen Fischer, director of the Kaiser Wilhelm Institute for Anthropology, Human Heredity and Eugenics, supported the Viennese prisoner-of-war studies and recommended "taking advantage of the unique opportunity to study anthropologically many thousands of people of foreign racial origins."[60] He further argued, "A racial investigation of such diverse people of the numerous tribes of the Asian, and partly also of the European Soviet territories would also be of great interest for the elucidation of certain anthropological problems in the whole of Europe and thus also in Germany. Such an insight into the anthropological conditions of Russia as the prison camps now offer will never come again for the German scholars."[61]

Fischer's assistants, Otto Baader and Wolfgang Abel, were also involved in prisoner-of-war investigations. Baader examined North African soldiers, and the Vienna-born Wolfgang Abel examined French colonial soldiers in prisoner-of-war camps in France.[62] In the winter of 1941–42, Abel conducted "racial" surveys on Soviet prisoners of war for the Oberkommandos der Wehrmacht. The purpose of these investigations was, as Hans-Walter Schmuhl and Benoit Massin have pointed out, the "future treatment" of the Russian population. In 1942, based on his analysis of the "racial composition of the Soviet prisoners of war," Abel suggested in all seriousness "either the extermination of the Russian people or the Germanization of the Nordic elements of the Russian people."[63] Abel continued later with extensive surveys of Soviet prisoners of war. Therefore, he tried to cooperate with the SS-Ahnenerbe in order to get several scientists temporarily assigned. The exact circumstances of these investigations and the extent to which this cooperation actually came about cannot be clarified by the written sources.[64]

Scientific investigations in prisoner-of-war camps were also requested by other institutions. For example, letters from the Wehrmacht to the Academy of Science as well as to the Institute for German Work in the East (Institut für Deutsche Ostarbeit) reveal that according to a decree of 1941, "scientific research in prisoner-of-war camps is supported only after recommendation by the Reich Ministry of Science, Education and Public Instruction."[65] This measure was taken to "restrict the scientific work on prisoners of war to the extent of what is necessary and manageable for the administration of prisoner of war camps."[66] In addition to military organizations, the ministries for science and the interior, organizations of "racial," national, and health research, and ethnological and "racial" university and museum institutions are mentioned among the places that deal with scientific work in prisoner-of-war camps.[67]

While in the first years the studies in the prisoner-of-war camps were clearly devoted to physical "racial" characteristics, i.e. the collection of measurement sheets, photographs, hair samples, hand- and fingerprints, and facemasks, they were later extended to experimental and medical studies. With this collaboration, the anthropologists took one step further away from physical anthropological investigations toward invasive studies and medical experiments. The investigations of the cerebrospinal fluid are clearly to be understood as coerced research. Lumbar puncture is a procedure that—although rare—bears risks of complications and potential danger for the patients.[68] In addition, it should be remembered that in 1943 the health situation and nutrition, especially of Soviet prisoners of war, was extremely bad and precarious, and any additional unwarranted medical procedures were prone to harm patients.

In comparison to medical research, coerced research, and medical experiments in concentration camps, the knowledge of anthropological and medical studies in prisoner-of-war camps is less well documented and researched.[69] In the context of exploitative research without or with questionable consent, the "racial" studies of prisoners of war performed by Viennese museum anthropologists constitute another example of the transgressions of ethical borders in science during the National Socialist regime.

The many changes of medical research ethics after World War II extend to the field of anthropology, where a process had started with the formulation of guidelines for clinical research at the Nuremberg Trials in 1947 and led to national and international bioethical recommendations and declarations.[70] In the last decades, societies of physical and biological anthropology are stressing the responsibilities for the conduct of research or are implementing ethic committees (see for example the committee of the American Association of Physical Anthropology).[71] Moreover, in museum associations such as the International Council of Museums (ICOM) or national associations such as the German Museums Association, new guidelines for care of human remains, including ethical issues, have been released.[72] Ethical issues are intended to be an integrated and essential part of research projects and publications. Gaining consent and information of participants has become a requirement in research.

Margit Berner, PhD, studied physical anthropology at the University of Vienna, and is a curator and scientist at the Department of Anthropology, Museum of Natural History Vienna. Her research and publications are in the field of history of anthropology and physical anthropology, and she cooperates and participates in various scientific projects and exhibitions.

Notes

1. The term "race" and "racial" are used as a historical concept throughout the text.
2. E.g. Zimmerman 2001; Schmuhl 2005; Hoffmann 2009; Johler, Marchetti, and Scheer 2010; Berner, Hoffmann, and Lange 2011.
3. See Proctor 1988; Massin 2004.
4. Teschler-Nicola and Berner 1998; Pawlowsky 2005; Spring 2005; Berner 2009.
5. Josef Wastl had been employed in the museum since the 1920s, in 1938 he became head and in 1941 director of the Department of Anthropology. Wastl joined the NSDAP as early as 1932 and remained an "illegal" member when the party was banned in Austria between 19 June 1933 and 13 March 1938. In September 1939, Robert Routil had been released from his assistantship at

the University of Vienna to participate in the museum's "racial" investigations of Jews in the soccer stadium. In 1941 he received a position in the museum, and in 1943 he was appointed curator. Routil too had joined the NSDAP in 1933 as an "illegal" member but stopped payments in 1934; his later requests of reentry were rejected.

6. Purin 1995.
7. Aly 1987; Heimann-Jelinek 1999.
8. Teschler-Nicola and Berner 1998, 336–39, 345–49; Pawlowsky 2005, 71–72, 75–76.
9. Naturhistorisches Museum, Anthropologische Abteilung (NHM, AA): Korrespondenz 1939, 218, 21 December 1939.
10. NHM, AA, Somatologische Sammlung, Inv. Nr. 2735; Korrespondenz Kaisersteinbruch, Kummerlöwe to the High Command of the German Armed Forces, 16 April 1941.
11. Berner 2005; Lange 2011.
12. E.g. Massin 2004; Hoßfeld 2005; Schmuhl 2005.
13. Pawlowsky 2005; Spring 2005.
14. Speckner 1999, 2003; Klösch 2013.
15. Stelzl-Marx 2000, 40.
16. Stelzl-Marx 2000, 40–41.
17. Speckner 1999, 262–84.
18. Stelzl-Marx 2000, 43.
19. Speckner 1999, 262–64.
20. Speckner 1999, 301; in September 1940 there were 40,077 French, 3,536 Belgian, and 176 Polish prisoners of war in Kaisersteinbruch.
21. NHM, AA, Somatologische Sammlung, Inv. Nr. 2735; Korrespondenz Kaisersteinbruch, Wastl to Kummerlöwe, 31 July 1940.
22. Speckner 1999, 305.
23. Stelzl-Marx 2000, 44.
24. Martin and Alonzo 2004, 585.
25. Speckner 1999, 244–49.
26. Maria Teschler-Nicola and Margit Berner 1998; Pawlowsky 2005.
27. Klösch 2013, 51–60; Speckner 1999, 368–70. In spring 1942, there were about 24,000 prisoners of war in the Wolfsberg camp including 16,224 French, 5,096 English, 915 Belgian, 151 Southeast Europe, and 1,583 Soviet prisoners. By October, the number of Soviet POWs rose to 3,883.
28. NHM, AA, Korrespondenz 1941–1947; Wastl, 6 May 1942, an (Kummerlöwe).
29. Speckner 1999, 392.
30. Speckner 1999, 302.
31. Speckner 1999, 309.
32. Stelzl-Marx 2000, 43.
33. NHM, AA, Somatologische Sammlung, Inv. Nr. 2735, Korrespondenz Wolfsberg, Staatliche Verwaltung des Reichsgaues Wien to Kummerlöwe, 7 August 1940.
34. NHM, AA, Somatologische Sammlung, Inv. Nr. 2735; Korrespondenz Wolfsberg, Reichsforschungsrat to Kummerlöwe, 22 August 1940.
35. Archiv der Akademie der Wissenschaften (AÖAW), Subventionen, math.-nat., K.12, 264/1940; Kummerlöwe to the president of the academy, request for financial support, 5 July 1940; Hochstetter to the Treitlkommission, 13 July 1940, Srbik to Kummerlöwe, financial support was granted in the amount of RM 1,400, 18 July 1940; for the Academy of Sciences in Vienna 1938 to 1945 see Feichtinger, Matis, Sienell, and Uhl 2013.
36. NHM, AA, Somatologische Sammlung, Inv. Nr. 2735; Korrespondenz Kaisersteinbruch, Kummerlöwe to the High Command of the German Armed Forces, 16 April 1941; see also AÖAW, Subventionen, math.-nat., K.12, 264/1940; Kummerlöwe to Srbik, 11 August 1941 (219/1941); High Command of the German Armed Forces to the president of the Academy, 10 September 1941.

37. Berner 2005.
38. Two men who had been subjected to the "racial studies" in the Viennese soccer stadium remembered the racist investigations; see Evan 2000, 53–54; Berner 2011, 147–67.
39. NHM, AA, Somatologische Sammlung, Inv. Nr. 2735; Protokollbuch 3, p. 3, note 18 July 1940.
40. NHM, AA, Somatologische Sammlung, Inv. Nr. 2735; Korrespondenz Wolfsberg, handwritten report of Routil, n.d., p. 2.
41. NHM, AA, Somatologische Sammlung, Inv. Nr. 2735; Korrespondenz Wolfsberg, handwritten report of Routil, n.d., p. 3.
42. NHM, AA, Somatologische Sammlung, Inv. Nr. 2735; Korrespondenz Wolfsberg, handwritten report of Routil, n.d., p. 5.
43. NHM, AA, Somatologische Sammlung, Inv. Nr. 2735; Protokollbuch 11, p. 192, entry of Wastl, 14 July 1943.
44. NHM, AA, Somatologische Sammlung, Inv. Nr. 2735; Protokollbuch 11, p. 20, entry of Wastl, 15 July 1943.
45. NHM, AA, Somatologische Sammlung, Inv. Nr. 2735; Protokollbuch 11, entry of Lang, p. 4.
46. Berner 2004; Stigler 1943; beside Stigler the physicians Hanns Fleischhacker, W. Gillesberger, Hans Kolin, and Karl Schuhecker, along with the student Helmut Poindecker, were participating.
47. Stigler 1943, 49.
48. AÖAW, Subventionen, math.-nat., K.12, Nr. 264/1940, Srbik to Kummerlöwe, 9 July 1940.
49. NHM, AA, Somatologische Sammlung Inv. Nr. 2735, Korrespondenz Kaisersteinbruch, Pernkopf to Mühlhofer, 17 July 1940, to Pernkopf and the Anatomical Insitute see Hildebrandt, 2016.
50. NHM, AA, Somatologische Sammlung, Inv. Nr. 2735; Korrespondenz Kaisersteinbruch, Wastl an Kommandantur Kaisersteinbruch, 19 May 1943.
51. NHM, AA, Somatologische Sammlung Inv. Nr. 2735, Protokollbuch 11, p. 2.
52. Exner and Routil 1950; Exner and Routil 1949/50.
53. Haschek and Hattinger 1936.
54. Exner and Routil 1950, 22.
55. Exner and Routil 1950, 23.
56. NHM, AA, Somatologische Sammlung Inv. Nr. 2735, Protokollbuch 11, p. 11.
57. NHM, AA, Somatologische Sammlung Inv. Nr. 2735, Protokollbuch 11, p. 11.
58. NHM, AA, Somatologische Sammlung, Inv. Nr. 2735; Korrespondenz Kaisersteinbruch, letters of Exner, 3 April 1944, and Wastl 7 April 1944.
59. Pawlowsky 2005.
60. NHM, AA, Somatologische Sammlung, Inv. Nr. 2735, Korrespondenz Kaisersteinbruch, Fischer to Kummerlöwe, 3 October 1941.
61. NHM, AA, Somatologische Sammlung, Inv. Nr. 2735, Korrespondenz Kaisersteinbruch, Fischer to Kummerlöwe, 3 October 1941.
62. Schmuhl 2005, 442–43.
63. Schmuhl 2005, 455–57; Massin 2004.
64. Schmuhl 2005, 458–63.
65. AÖAW, Subventionen, math.-nat., K.12, 264/1940 High Command of the German Armed Forces to the Academy of Sciences, 10 September 1941.
66. AÖAW, Allgemeine Akten, Nr. 225/1941; Reichsminister für Wissenschaft, Erziehung und Volksbildung, 25 August 1941.
67. AÖAW, Allgemeine Akten, Nr. 225/1941; Reichsminister für Wissenschaft, Erziehung und Volksbildung, 25 August 1941; AUJ, Institut für Deutsche Ostarbeit
68. Greenlee and Caroll 2004, 10–12.
69. Weindling 2017.
70. Czech, Druml, and Weindling 2018.

71. https://physanth.org/about/committees/ethics/.
72. See, for example, https://icom.museum/en/resources/standards-guidelines/code-of-ethics/; or https://www.museumsbund.de/wp-content/uploads/2017/04/2013-recommendations-for-the-care-of-human-remains.pdf.

References

Aly, Götz. 1987. "Das Posener Tagebuch des Anatomen Hermann Voss." In *Biedermann und Schreibtischtäter: Materialien zur deutschen Täter-Biographie* (=Beiträge zur Nationalsozialistischen Gesundheits- und Sozialpolitik 4), edited by Götz Aly, Peter Chroust, H. D. Heilmann, and Hermann Langbein, 15–66. Berlin: Rotbuch.

Berner, Margit. 2004. "Rassenforschung an kriegsgefangenen Schwarzen." In *Zwischen Charleston und Stechschritt: Schwarze im Nationalsozialismus*, edited by Peter Martin and Christine Alonzo, 605–13. Hamburg and München: Dölling and Galitz.

———. 2005. "Forschungs-'Material' Kriegsgefangene: Die Massenuntersuchungen der Wiener Anthropologen an gefangenen Soldaten 1915–1918." In *Vorreiter der Vernichtung: Eugenik, Rassenhygiene und Euthanasie in der österreichischen Diskussion vor 1938*, edited by Heinz Eberhard Gabriel and Wolfgang Neugebauer, 167–98. Wien, Köln, and Weimar: Böhlau.

———. 2009. "The Nazi Period Collections of Physical Anthropology in the Museum of Natural History, Vienna." In *"Col Tempo" The W. Project. Catalog of the Installation in the Hungarian Pavilion of the 53rd International Art Exhibition in Venice—La Biennalia di Venezia Péter Forgács's installation. Curator: András Rényi*. Edited by András Rényi, 34–48. Budapest: Masterprint.

———. 2011. "'Die haben uns behandelt wie Gegenstände': Anthropologische Untersuchungen an jüdischen Häftlingen im Wiener Stadion während des Nationalsozialismus." In *Sensible Sammlungen: Aus dem anthropologischen Depot*, edited by Margit Berner, Anette Hoffmann, and Britta Lange, 147–67. Hamburg: Philo.

Berner, Margit, Anette Hoffmann, and Britta Lange. 2011. *Sensible Sammlungen: Aus dem anthropologischen Depot*. Hamburg: Philo.

Czech, Herwig, Christiane Druml, and Paul Weindling. 2018. "Medical Ethics in the 70 Years after the Nuremberg Code, 1947 to the Present." *Wiener Klinische Wochenschrift* Suppl. 130: 159–253.

Evan, Gershon. 2000. *Winds of Life: The Destinies of a Young Viennese Jew*. Riverside: Ariadne.

Exner, Robert, and Robert Routil. 1949/50. "Studien zur Farbentheorie." *Annalen des Naturhistorischen Museums in Wien* 57: 6–11.

———. 1950. "Von der Lichtwelle zum Farbbegriff. Ein Beitrag zu menschlicher Art." *S.A.S Bolettino del Comitato Internazionale per l' Unificazione dei Metodi e per la Sintesi in Antropologia ed Eugenica* 20–21: 1–84.

Feichtinger, Johannes, Herbert Matis, Stefan Sienell, and Heidemarie Uhl (eds.). 2013. *The Academy of Sciences in Vienna 1938 to 1945*. Wien: Österreichische Akademie der Wissenschaften.

Greenlee, John E., and Karen C. Caroll. 2004. "Cerebrospinal Fluid in Central Nervous System Infections." In *Infections of the Central Nervous System*, edited by W. Michael Scheld, Richard J. Whitley, and Christina M. Marra, 5–30. 3rd ed. Philadelphia: Lippincott Williams & Wilkins.

Haschek, Eduard, and Max Hattinger. 1936. *Farbmessungen: Theoretische Grundlagen und Anwendungen: Monographien aus dem Gesamtgebiete der Mikrochemie*. Wien and Leipzig: Haim.

Heimann-Jelinek, Felicitas. 1999. "Zur Geschichte einer Ausstellung. Masken. Versuch über die Schoa." In *"Beseitigung des jüdischen Einflusses . . .": Antisemitische Forschung, Eliten und Karrieren im Nationalsozialismus* (Jahrbuch 1998/99 zur Geschichte und Wirkung des Holocaust), edited by Fritz Bauer Institut, 131–46. Frankfurt am Main: Campus.

Hildebrandt, Sabine. 2016. *The Anatomy of Murder: Ethical Transgressions and Anatomical Science during the Third Reich*. New York: Berghahn Books.
Hoffmann, Anette (ed.). 2009. *What We See: Reconsidering an Anthropometrical Collection from Southern Africa: Images, Voices and Versioning*. Basel: Basler Afrika Bibliographien.
Hoßfeld, Uwe. 2005. *Geschichte der biologischen Anthropologie in Deutschland: Von den Anfängen bis in die Nachkriegszeit*. Stuttgart: Franz Steiner.
Johler, Reinhard, Christian Marchetti, and Monique Scheer (eds.). 2010. *Doing Anthropology in Wartime and Warzones: World War I and the Cultural Sciences in Europe*. London: Transcript.
Klösch, Christian. 2013. *Lagerstadt Wolfsberg: Flüchtlinge—Gefangene—Internierte*. Edition Museum im Lavanthaus 1. Wolfsberg: Theiss.
Lange, Britta. 2013. *Die Wiener Forschungen an Kriegsgefangenen 1915–1918: Anthropologische und ethnografische Verfahren im Lager*. Wien: Österreichischen Akademie der Wissenschaften.
Martin, Peter, and Christine Alonzo (eds.). 2004. *Zwischen Charleston und Stechschritt: Schwarze im Nationalsozialismus*. Hamburg and München: Dölling and Galitz.
Massin, Benoit 2004. "The 'Science of Race.'" In *Deadly Medicine: Creating the Master Race*, edited by Susan Bachrach and Dieter Kuntz, 89–126. Washington, DC: United States Holocaust Memorial Museum.
Pawlowsky, Verena. 2005. "Erweiterung der Bestände: Die Anthropologische Abteilung des Naturhistorischen Museums 1938–1945." *Zeitgeschichte* 32: 69–90.
Proctor, Robert. 1988. "From Anthropology to Rassenkunde in the German Anthropological Tradition." In *Bones, Bodies, Behavior: Essays on Biological Anthropology*, edited by George W. Stocking, 138–79. Madison: University of Wisconsin.
Purin, Bernhard. 1995. *Beschlagnahmt: Die Sammlung des Wiener Jüdischen Museums nach 1938*. Wien: Jüdisches Museum der Stadt Wien.
Schmuhl, Hans-Walter. 2005. *Grenzüberschreitungen: Das Kaiser-Wilhelm-Institut für Anthropologie, menschliche Erblehre und Eugenik 1927–1945*. Geschichte der Kaiser-Wilhelm-Gesellschaft im Nationalsozialismus 9. Göttingen: Wallstein.
Speckner, Hubert. 1999. *Kriegsgefangenenlager in der "Ostmark" 1939–1945: Zur Geschichte der Mannschaftsstammlager und Offizierslager in den Wehrkreisen XVII und XVIII*. Dissertation, Universität Wien.
———. 2003. *In der Gewalt des Feindes: Kriegsgefangenenlager in der "Ostmark" 1939 bis 1945*. Wien and München: Oldenburg.
Spring, Claudia. 2005. "Vermessen, deklassiert und deportiert: Dokumentation zur Anthropologischen Untersuchung an 440 Juden im Wiener Stadion im September 1939 unter der Leitung von Josef Wastl vom Naturhistorischen Museum Wien." *Zeitgeschichte* 32(2): 91–110.
Stelzl-Marx, Barbara. 2000. *Zwischen Fiktion und Zeitzeugenschaft: Amerikanische und sowjetische Kriegsgefangene im Stalag XVII B Krems-Gneixendorf*. Tübingen: Gunter Narr.
Stigler, Robert. 1943. "Rassenphysiologische Untersuchungen an farbigen Kriegsgefangenen in einem Kriegsgefangenenlager." *Zeitschrift für Rassenphysiologie* 13(1–2): 26–57.
Teschler-Nicola, Maria, and Margit Berner. 1998. "Die Anthropologische Abteilung des Naturhistorischen Museums in der NS-Zeit, Berichte und Dokumentationen von Forschungs- und Sammlungsaktivitäten 1938–1945." In *Senatsprojekt der Universität Wien: Untersuchungen zur Anatomischen Wissenschaft in Wien 1938–1945*, edited by Akademischen Senat der Universität Wien (project leader Gustav Spann), 333–58. Wien: Universität Wien.
Weindling, Paul (ed.). 2017. *From Clinic to Concentration Camp: Reassessing Nazi Medical and Racial Research, 1933–1945*. New York: Routledge.
Zimmermann, Andrew. 2001. *Anthropology and Antihumanism in Imperial Germany*. Chicago: University of Chicago Press.

CHAPTER 3

"DER DOKTOR"

The Writings of Mordechai Lensky during the Interwar Period

Miriam Offer

> I have written for those who have shed tears over the fresh grave of a beloved parent or over the grave of a younger brother or sister who died.
> I have written this book for parents who sat by their sick child's bed, night after night, tortured by the thought that their only hope may suddenly be extinguished.
> I have written also for those already in despair and who wish to grasp a warm spark of life.
> —Mordechai Lensky, *The Modern Family Doctor*[1]

The supreme importance of the sanctity of human life as a value in the Torah and the commandment in Halakhah (Jewish Law) to preserve life have led to the highly esteemed status of the medical profession in Jewish society.[2] Throughout the generations, Jewish physicians have distinguished themselves through their medical activities and achievements, beyond their relative numerical proportion in the population.[3] In the modern era, influenced by the enlightenment and secularization, and significantly during the interwar period, this process accelerated, and a particularly high number of Jews completed their medical studies.

Alongside their professional work, many Jewish physicians took on public roles in the community. They excelled in scientific writing in their fields, in addition to recognizing the importance of publishing their views on journalistic platforms. They published in leading journals, in the Jewish and the general press, and contributed both prose and poetry to literature and culture. The vast majority perished during the Holocaust along with the rest of their fellow Jews.[4]

A substantial number of physicians who died during the Holocaust, as well as some of those who survived, left behind diverse types of writings, authored over a lengthy period: between the two world wars, during the Holocaust, and, in the case of survivors, later as well. These writings were left in archives, libraries, and private collections at the homes of their descendants. A study of them, along the time continuum, reveals the professional, spiritual, and ethical world of these physicians and provides deeper insight into the study of the history of doctors, medicine, and the Jewish society during this critical period.

Many of the writings have received no attention whatsoever to date. In the few cases where this body of work has been addressed, no reference has been made to the abundance of written documents by doctors throughout this time period. Reference has been made to research of the Jewish world during the interwar period,[5] to the study of medicine and Jewish doctors during the Holocaust,[6] and to the development of this field after the war.[7] However, very little has been mentioned about the writings by Jewish physicians along the timeline of this fateful era for the Jewish people, before, during, and after the Holocaust.[8]

This chapter focuses on one example: the writings of Dr. Mordechai Lensky (1890–1964), a physician, who practiced during the interwar period in Warsaw and Włocławek, and during the Holocaust in the Warsaw Ghetto. Dr. Lensky survived the war. Alongside his work as a physician, he wrote incessantly from the early 1920s until his death in 1964. Due to the immense scale of the material, this chapter is devoted only to his writings during the interwar period, which reflect his personality, worldview, professional identity as a physician, and activities in historical context. The historical picture that emerges from a study of these writings presents deeper insight into the professional and ethical values of the Jewish doctors deported to the ghettos, whence they drew the strength to establish professional medical systems under unprecedented, inhumane conditions.

Most of Dr. Lensky's writings were found in the private archive of his son, the late Professor Yaacov Lensky.[9] They include letters, a personal diary, newspaper cuttings, writings on his personal philosophy, opinion pieces, unpublished monographs, and many handwritten manuscripts and typewritten material. The texts are varied, incorporating different genres: some adhere to the various definitions of ego documents (writings about the author's actions, thoughts, and emotions),[10] some to microhistory[11]; some were written as professional medical literature, and a large proportion was devoted to public health. Later in life, Lensky focused on classical historical research of Jewish history in ancient and modern times. He combined populist history or "history from below," which focuses on the daily lives of ordinary people in society, with elitist history or "history from above," focusing on political movements, politicians, policy, etc.

Dr. Lensky is not an unknown figure. His memoirs as a physician inside the Warsaw Ghetto, written toward the end of the war and in its aftermath, were published as a Hebrew book in 1961, with a second Hebrew edition in 1983.[12] The English translation was published in 2009.[13] However, most of his writings from before and after the Holocaust, except for a few brief references, have not been published—evidence of the research gap and latent potential and priceless value of the genre of the doctors' writings.

Dr. Mordechai Lensky: Prewar Activities and Writings, 1890–1939

From Warsaw to Moscow, and Back

Dr. Mordechai Lensky was born on 23 November 1890 in Warsaw, to Pesah and Haya (daughter of R' Yosef Hever).[14] At that time, Warsaw was the largest Jewish community in Poland. During the nineteenth century, particularly during the Congress Poland period (1815–63), the city's Jewish population expanded and established the social frameworks and ideological streams that continued to exist until the bitter end during the Holocaust. After Russia's economy opened to the Poles, and following the industrialization of the country, Warsaw developed rapidly. The Jews fulfilled an important and sometimes leading role in this development. The city attracted many Jews from areas of Russian settlement, who contributed to the social and spiritual awakening among the Jews of Poland and of Warsaw in particular. Nationalistic ideology, revolutionary unrest, the revival of Hebrew literature, and the emergence of Yiddish literature, as well as publicist and journalistic writings in both languages, came into being during this period.[15] On the eve of World War I, 337,000 Jews lived in Warsaw, constituting more than 38 percent of the entire population in the city.[16]

Mordechai Lensky was raised and educated in Warsaw in the spirit of Jewish culture and Jewish tradition. He studied medicine in Moscow, qualifying as a physician in 1917. His first professional post was as a doctor in the Russian army until the end of World War I, and on demobilization he practiced as a physician in Leningrad. There, in 1919, he married Dr. Ida Mapu, a dentist. She was the great-granddaughter of the Hebrew novelist Abraham Mapu, of the *Haskalah* (Enlightenment) movement and famous for publishing the first Hebrew novel, *Ahavat Zion* (For the love of Zion) and for the romantic, nationalistic ideas in his books that served as the ideological basis for the Zionist movement. The newlyweds lived with Ida's family in Leningrad. Lensky specialized in internal medicine, and Ida practiced dentistry. In 1921, their first child, a daughter, Emelia (Mila) was born. In 1923, Lensky moved from Leningrad to Warsaw with his family, where they lived at the home of his parents, Pesah and Haya, at 28 Miła Street.[17]

In a 30 January 1923 letter from Mordechai Lensky in Warsaw to his cousin Yitzhak Hacarmeli, who had emigrated from Poland to Eretz Israel (the Land of Israel), we learn something of Lensky's family life and his writing pursuits. Lensky begins his letter by thanking his cousin for sending him the address of the Israeli medical journal *Harefuah*. "My dear Yitzhak! I received your recent letter. Many thanks for the information about the publisher of *Harefuah*. I will contact them." *Harefuah*, the Israeli Medical Association journal, began to take shape in the Jewish *Yishuv* (the body of Jewish residents) in Eretz Israel, which, at that time, numbered approximately 80,000 people, including only about 190 Jewish doctors.[18] In 1924, *Harefuah* was officially established as a journal, and Lensky had articles published there.[19] The later part of the letter portrays Lensky as a warm family man, enthusiastic about his two-year-old daughter's developmental progress. He gives a lengthy description of the infant's play, in an atmosphere influenced by her parents' professional fields: "The child is growing up and her speech is advancing rapidly. She writes a lot. . . . She plays at being a dental practitioner. . . ." In this letter, Lensky's sense of responsibility and concern for his extended family is apparent through his report, to his cousin, that his mother, who was living in Warsaw, had been ill. Lensky believed that she would benefit from a vacation in the country: "Your mother was seriously ill last week, but has now recovered. . . . I recommend a refreshing month's rest, by summer pastures . . . she could breathe the fresh summer air to rejuvenate her weakened lungs. . . ."[20] Clearly, the idea of curative visits to the countryside were on Lensky's mind, as he published an article on the importance of summer holiday villages for young people's health in the Yiddish newspaper *Der Moment* two months later, in March 1923.[21]

Dr. Lensky's Work as Physician of the Office for Eretz Israel in Warsaw: 1923–26

On Lensky's arrival in Warsaw, he worked as a physician at the Office for Eretz Israel in the city. This office was the executive branch of the Zionist Organization in Eretz Israel, whose main function was the promotion of settlement in the Land of Israel. These offices existed in many European countries, providing medical checkups for members of youth organizations applying for certificates to immigrate to Eretz Israel as pioneers.[22] These checkups were fraught with tension. During the 1920s, the Zionist enterprise in Mandatory Palestine was developing, and fundamental questions regarding the rate and modes of immigrant absorption were on the agenda. The Zionist Organization leadership struggled with the question of whether the institutions of the Jewish *Yishuv* were adequately prepared to receive great numbers of Diaspora Jews, or whether immigration should be selective, granted only to those with the appropriate skills and capabilities for preparing the necessary infrastructure for the establishment of a Jewish state. In the end, British Mandate policy, which limited the number of certificates and entry into the country, forced the Zionist Organization to set criteria for selective and gradual immigration, giving preference to healthy immigrants who were able to contribute to building the homeland. [23]

From 1923 to 1926, Lensky served as a doctor in the Office for Eretz Israel in Warsaw and was appointed head physician. This was the organization's largest office in Europe, where doctors performed medical checkups on great numbers of Jews on their way to Eretz Israel. Lensky's worldview, work, and character, as manifest during that time, is reflected in an 18 November 1926 letter that he wrote to *Ha'aretz*—established as a daily newspaper in Eretz Israel in 1918. In this letter, he raised concerns about the medical checkup procedure in the Office for Eretz Israel. He called for change—for clear, professional, and objective criteria. At the beginning of the letter, he stated the importance of his job and the responsibility it involved:

> Whoever holds the issues of Eretz Israel close to his heart should know that its development depends largely on the quality of the human resources that enter the land. If the new immigrants, whether spiritually or with regard to their physical health, will truly qualify for their certificates, since it is on their shoulders that history has placed the transcendent burden of manually building up the land, it is our hope that their actions will be blessed. . . . Regarding eugenics,[24] we must invest in the idea of a healthy nucleus of new immigrants from which a living and courageous people will develop, in accord with how we imagine the Jews in Eretz Israel in the future.[25]

In their research of the medical screening of potential immigrants to Eretz Israel during the interwar period, historians of science Eyal Katvan and Nadav Davidovitch described Lensky as "a figure representing the sociopolitical background of the period in the context of health and Zionism."[26] Indeed, the physicians involved in the medical checkups in the Offices for Eretz Israel saw their mission as serving both medicine and Zionism. As physicians, they acted according to public health principles, and from the Zionist point of view, they did not authorize certificates for applicants who, for health reasons, would be unable to withstand the contemporary hardships in Eretz Israel and the physical strength required to build Jewish settlements.

The Immigration Office in Eretz Israel repeatedly complained to Dr. Lensky and the other physicians performing the examinations in Poland that, despite the checkups, many sick immigrants were entering the country. Lensky criticized the Immigration Office in Eretz Israel for failing to determine a clear procedure and criteria for assessing potential immigrants. Several months after his letter appeared in the press, Lensky was dismissed from his post in the shadow of this controversy. Lensky was criticized for apparently failing to adhere to the meticulous standards required by the medical checkups and was even accused of making biased decisions based on political affiliation.

Dr. Noach Davidson, an ophthalmologist and active leader of the Zionist institutions in Warsaw at that time, supervised the physicians' activities in the Office for Eretz Israel. He spoke out in defense of Dr. Lensky, resolutely contradicting the unfounded accusations. In an article in the Yiddish daily newspaper *Haynt*, distributed among the Jews of Eastern Europe, Davidson claimed that Lensky had conducted himself professionally with no hint of political nepotism. He wrote that Lensky had acquired the examinees' trust and "stood steadfast as a rock" against pressure exerted by political parties, who sometimes intervened, attempting to arrange certificates for their members who were ill and thus did not fit the criteria.[27]

Dr. Lensky's Work as a Teacher of Anatomy and Physiology in Tarbut Schools

In addition to his work as physician in the Office for Eretz Israel, Dr. Lensky taught anatomy and physiology in *Tarbut* schools in Warsaw. *Tarbut* was a network of Jewish Zionist schools throughout Eastern Europe during the interwar period. Its comprehensive education system included kindergartens, elementary schools, secondary schools, teacher-training seminars, pedagogical courses, adult evening classes, and more. The vision was to establish secular, Jewish, Zionist schools, integrating Jewish and general subjects, humanities, and science, using modern education methods. Hebrew was the language of instruction, to assist its revival, and the staff educated the students toward the ideals of *Aliyah* (immigration to Israel) as the ultimate goal.[28]

Dr. Lensky's Writings during the Interwar Period: The People's Health

Articles in the Daily Yiddish Press

Parallel to his work as physician and lecturer, scientific and publicist writing were an inseparable part of Dr. Lensky's life, and he continued to write until his dying day. Between 1923 and 1933, Lensky published more than fifty articles on medicine in the Warsaw Yiddish press, mainly in daily newspapers *Haynt* and *Der Moment*. Notwithstanding his specialization in internal medicine, a field in which he published scientific articles, Lensky felt it to be his mission, as a physician, to promote public health and to disseminate medical knowledge to the Jewish community at large. *Haynt* (1908–39) and *Der Moment* (1910–39) reflected the flourishing of Yiddish journalism in Jewish society in Eastern Europe in general, and in Poland in particular. Approximately twenty-five thousand copies of *Haynt* appear to have been printed during the 1930s. Since they were passed around to others who could not afford to buy a newspaper, Lensky's articles would have been read by literally thousands of Jews in Warsaw and other Jewish communities in Poland.[29] Lensky's articles dealt with individual and societal aspects of healthcare and medicine, and in Jewish society in particular, based on his personal experience. Under the headline "Preventive Medicine," his articles included guidance and information on disease prevention, up-to-date information about prevalent illnesses and remedies, recommendations for a healthy lifestyle, and more. The content of the articles was adapted for all readers and had a substantial focus on "social medicine." Lensky kept the public informed of new developments in hygiene and sanitation, in addition to publishing his thoughts on issues that interested the Jewish society as a minority in their countries of residence.[30]

Books by Lensky during the Interwar Period

Besides his articles in the daily press, Lensky used his expertise to write books (in Yiddish) on specific medical subjects that he considered important to inform the public about. In 1927, the year he stopped working in the Office for Eretz Israel in Warsaw, two of his books were published: *The Epidemic of Influenza*[31] and *The Modern Family Doctor*.[32] It is noteworthy that, after World War I, the "Spanish flu" influenza pandemic became the most deadly epidemic recorded in the modern era, which claimed millions of lives. It was most active from 1918 to 1920, and Lensky, as a family physician, had doubtlessly treated many influenza patients and considered it vital to disseminate information about the illness and its treatment.[33]

The Modern Family Doctor was a success, and in the first year, hundreds of copies were sold throughout Poland.[34] This book, like many of Lensky's writings, was intended for the wider public, focusing on a description of various illnesses based on state-of-the-art scientific studies in the medical field. For accessibility to the lay public, the book included informative illustrations and pictures. In the foreword, Lensky explained his motives and goals in writing the volume. He perceived his work as a physician as mediator of medical information for the general public. Lensky imagines an archetypical doctor advocating public health and waving the banner of social medicine, who asks the author, "Why a book on family medicine? Is there a need for medical books for lay people who, when in trouble, can turn to the doctor for advice, who will write a prescription and, when necessary, will refer them to the most suitable convalescent home? Why torture the brain and the eyes by reading a medical book?"[35] Lensky responds that these questions genuinely apply to some people, who are preoccupied with anxieties of the full working day and whose little free time is spent at cultural or social events. "I confess that my book was not written for those people. May they continue to enjoy their recreation time. I have no desire to disturb their repose."[36] Instead, Lensky explains, he wrote his book for those who had personally experienced serious illness and were all too familiar with the consequences for the patient:

> [It is] for those people and those around them who witnessed their suffering and torment and the psychological upheaval for the patient during the malady. I have written for those who have shed tears over the fresh grave of a beloved parent or over the grave of a younger brother or sister who died. I have written this book for parents who sat by their sick child's bed, night after night, tortured by thoughts that their only hope may suddenly be extinguished. I have written also for those already in despair and who wish to grasp a warm spark of life. Those people will

easily understand my book since they know about illness from personal experience. They have felt the disease deep under their skin and wish to know the reasons for it and methods of cure.[37]

Lensky explained that his book was not intended merely as a practical guide or as an alternative to the doctor but to give readers an idea of the efforts by medical researchers to produce therapies and help for patients and to protect humanity from disease. Thus, he included in the book new studies of diseases and treatments, which he referred to as "the last word of medicine." He gave much thought to the book's presentation, avoiding dry descriptions of disease symptoms. "To my mind, a medical book designed for the people needs to be written in a descriptive manner. Pictures undoubtedly assist readers to absorb the idea of serious medical problems. I have attempted . . . to write my book in a gentle and even an interesting way, as reading material accompanied by illustrations, and if I have succeeded in doing this, I will dare to say that I have not wasted my time."[38]

On 13 February 1927, Lensky wrote another letter to his cousin who, in the meantime, had immigrated to the United States. He asked for help with the sale of *The Modern Family Doctor* across the Atlantic: "I am sending you two examples of my book . . . maybe you can arrange the marketing of my book in America." From a letter written a year later, it appears that Lensky continued his efforts to sell his book in America. The letter reflects the increasing economic difficulties in Poland of the late 1920s, on the eve of the global economic crisis with the Wall Street crash of 1929.[39] Among other things, Lensky wrote that the family in Poland received financial help for tuition fees from family members in the United States, and he expressed the hope that they would complete their studies, thus "ending the requests and appeals to relatives in America, and the letters from here will no longer have the stamp of beggars asking for donations."[40]

Lensky continued to write articles for the press and for scientific journals, and to market his books. It can be assumed that his work and its dissemination, which were a way of life for him, were due not only to his talents and economic considerations but also to his professional self-perception as a physician. Lensky wholeheartedly adopted the public health principles that were prevalent during this period, placing emphasis on the need for medical activity particularly among the poor. In 1927, the first year after successful sales throughout Poland of *The Modern Family Doctor*, Lensky wrote, "I am certain that about a thousand books a year could be sold in America, since in poor Poland, which cannot afford to buy books, about 700 copies were sold in the first year."[41]

He continued to publish scientific articles in the monthly journal *Harefuah* but complained that "they pay me nothing."[42] Lensky was informed about the development of medical journals in the Jewish world and tried to have his articles published there. In a letter to his cousin, he mentioned having heard of

Harofe Haivri (The Hebrew Physician) journal, but did not know if it was already being published or whether it was merely a proposal for the future. Indeed, it was founded in 1927 by Dr. Moses Einhorn and Dr. Asher Goldstein, in Hebrew and English.[43] Lensky was concerned that the new journal, too, would not grant royalties to its authors: "Who knows whether writing for *Harofe Haivri* will be more lucrative than my articles in *Harefuah* in Jerusalem?" He understood that writing for these journals could not earn him a living, but despite his precarious economic situation, he wanted to be informed and asked, "Please send me one [new issue of *Harofe Haivri*] at my expense." Dr. Lensky, Zionist physician who did not migrate overseas, had a keen sense of having missed out on "the American dream," with its door to wealth and promotion, and expressed his frustration: "If only he [his cousin, M. O.] knew the editors of the Yiddish press in America or Canada and they would print my medical articles for the people, just as I publish them regularly in Warsaw's *Haynt*. Unfortunately, I have no connections in those circles . . ."[44]

Four years later, in 1931, Lensky published his third volume: *A Guide for Circumcisers*.[45] In his foreword, he writes that he wrote the book at the request of Moshe Feldstein, the chairman of the Warsaw Jewish community's publishing house. He clarified that there was no need to discuss the importance of this book since "everyone fully understands the importance that *Mohalim* [circumcisers], in whose hands we place our babies in the first days of their lives, will have a thorough understanding of the human organism, and especially of the principles of disinfection." According to Lensky, this book was one of the first steps in introducing standards and order into "the general problem of *Mohalim*" and was intended to improve the knowledge and performance of *Brit Milah* (Jewish ritual circumcision). The book contains information that every *Mohel* (circumciser) needs to know about the surgical procedure that he is about to perform, and "it is hoped that *Mohalim* will put the principles of sterilization into practice."[46]

In the introduction to the book, the publisher wrote that the book consists of research published by the Warsaw Jewish community's department of culture as an elementary guide, for the *Mohel* to understand the necessary scientific knowledge for his profession. The chapters of the book provide the reader with the basic information on cells, tissue, the heart, the circulatory system, the kidneys, urine, the penis, microbes, antisepsis, sterilization, and standards for *Mohalim*, as well as a list of illustrations. The publisher signed off the introduction while emphasizing the responsibility imposed on *Mohalim*, in regard to performing circumcision, to read the book and the instructions derived from it in detail: "Any *Mohel* with intelligence and a conscience must learn from this book how to recognize the structure of the human organism. Every *Mohel* must strictly adhere to the instructions for hygiene and sterilization. . . . The book is, in fact . . . compulsory reading for *Mohalim* who, only in this way, can honestly and faithfully perform their duty."[47]

This book is an example of how Lensky combined his work in science and research with his medical activities in the public health field in which he was particularly engaged. Lensky tried to ensure the improvement of the work of the *Mohalim* to safeguard the health of the babies undergoing circumcision.

The Economic Crisis: The Lensky Family Moves from Warsaw to Ciechocinek and Włocławek

On finishing his work in the Office for Eretz Israel and in view of the economic difficulties in Poland that could not but affect Warsaw's Jews during the late 1920s, the Lensky family moved to the Ciechocinek, where they lived from 1927 to 1929. During that time, they faced adjustment difficulties in their new places of employment. Ida worked in a dentist's clinic in Nieszawa, approximately 180 kilometers northwest of Warsaw, and Mordechai worked as a physician in Włocławek, about 30 kilometers from there. Ida lived in Nieszawa with Emelia, and the family met in Włocławek on weekends. It was only in 1937 that the family reunited to live under the same roof in Włocławek. This period was stressful for Mordechai and Ida. In a letter to his cousin, Lensky wrote, "Forgive me for scarcely writing to you lately and for not replying to your last two letters. *Miscellaneous worries and troubles have prevented me from writing to you* . . ."[48]

In 1929, their second child, Yaacov, was born—a brother for Mila. The family rented rooms in the home of Mr. Zilke, an ethnic *Volksdeutscher* in Nieszawa. In one of them, Ida set up a dental clinic. In 1934, they were forced to move to another apartment in the town's market square, where Ida once again set up her clinic.[49] From 1931 to 1939, the family home and Dr. Lensky's clinic were situated in Włocławek. From 1933 to 1939, Dr. Lensky worked at the St. Anthony district hospital in Włocławek. According to one of the documents found in his private archive, during this time he published fifteen scientific articles based on research in the field of his hospital work.[50] From 1929 to 1933, Lensky devoted himself to a special initiative: the establishment of a Yiddish journal in general medicine for lay persons.

Der Doktor (The Doctor: A Biweekly Newspaper for Public Education in Medicine and Hygiene)

One of the most impressive projects in Dr. Lensky's legacy was *Der Doktor* (*The Doctor: A Biweekly Newspaper for Public Education in Medicine and Hygiene*).[51] It was a one-man project. Lensky was publisher, editor, head journalist, and disseminator rolled into one. Written by Lensky, every issue included one major column in addition to the editorial, critiques, notices, questions and answers, a medical glossary, and more. The newspaper was run from Lensky's home due to the lack of funding. He also published booklets on medical topics by other writers to be awarded as prizes for the readers of Der Doktor.[52]

This newspaper was launched on 1 July 1929 as a biweekly. Because of its high quality and success within its first six months, it became a weekly publication and gradually expanded its format to contain a larger amount of material. Publication continued until 1933. Each issue included twelve A3-size pages crammed with print. More than forty issues survived in the archive, holding rich information about the general history of medicine and medical practice in the daily life of the Jewish communities during the interwar period.

In the first issue of Der Doktor, Lensky explained the newspaper's goal: "We are planning to publish a medical question and answer journal for the general public. Everyone will be able to understand what is written in the paper; it doesn't matter which part of the population you belong to. We will present you with all the latest ideas and research in medical science." He went on to say that even though the various communities of Diaspora Jews were renowned for their interest in medicine, they had little understanding of questions of health and hygiene. The goal of this newspaper was to change that. Lensky set forth the focal areas of the newspaper to his readers: a large section for women's questions on hygiene, pregnancy, etc.; childrearing, especially during the early years; childhood illnesses and innovative cures; and "ways of protecting children from trouble." In addition, he stated that special attention would be given to research on the physical and the spiritual. Sexual problems would be approached according to advanced modern science. He clarified that the newspaper would cover not only serious illnesses that leave people bedridden but also everyday complaints in their early stages of development to which people usually pay no attention, even though they limit their activity. Lensky's aim was to disseminate medical knowledge and to discuss serious problems in a simple and engaging way. "We provide this medical knowledge for the general public, who spend long days hard at work and burdened with worries . . ."[53]

The newspaper set out to realize a vision of imparting medical knowledge to the public at large, with the intention of enhancing the quality of life of all parts of society. Its aim was to promote the health of women and children; in other words, its focus was on public health, social medicine, and attention to preventative medicine and to the "minor" bothersome daily problems. Every month, the newspaper received many letters from readers seeking advice for their problems. The framework and format were too narrow to respond to all of the readers' requests. Even after the format was expanded, it was still too small to contain everything that interested the readership, resulting in Lensky's decision to publish Der Doktor weekly. Issue no. 15, on 9 January 1930, was the first of the weekly publications. In his editorial, Lensky wrote that after six months of grueling work, Der Doktor had achieved a large circulation, and he emphasized that the weekly publication would remain faithful to its goals of being "a guide for all aspects of health, and for the healthy to maintain their youthful energy. Many people easily become depressed and lose their drive with any small ailment. I want to show them that while in a state of illness, people are not helpless. Using their reserves of energy, the patients themselves can overcome the illness and continue a normal life."[54] It was written parenthetically in the editorial that, over the coming year, a series of articles would be published on erectile dysfunction, sexual problems in women, and more. It is possible that, as well as making the public aware of ways to improve their sexual lives, the "sensational" element played a part in the decision to include such topics in *Der Doktor* to increase its circulation. This was a common phenomenon in the daily tabloids of the period, including those published and read by Jews.

Each issue of the newspaper dealt with a variety of subjects, authored by Lensky and a few other physicians whom he had recruited. It contained thirteen regular columns: an editorial by Mordechai Lensky; a review of a well-known physician, describing his specialization and achievements; a discussion of a medical problem (diagnosis and treatment methods); marital counseling; innovations in therapy, including surgical methods; information about "taboo" sexual subjects; children and hygiene, childrearing problems, gynecology, and information on convalescent resorts; safety and hygiene in the workplace; and a section of "miscellaneous items," readers' letters and responses, and, of course, advertisements. Thus, for example, in *Der Doktor* issue no. 1, Lensky wrote an article on diseases of the heart: "One of the greatest heart specialists in Europe, Prof. Ramberg from Berlin, recently proved that, in the last four years, the number of serious heart problems of the type known as angina pectoris has increased. Due to the importance of this question, we will briefly describe the disease."[55] Then continues a description of the location and frequency of the pain, the cause of angina pectoris, the medication that can be taken during an attack, etc. "Of course, these medications must be given only by a doctor, and should not be self-administered," warned Lensky. He went on to explain that, once the attack has passed, the patient is prescribed eight to fourteen days of bed rest at home before returning to work.

In the same issue, an article by Dr. Apper contained the headline, "What is the recommended age to get married?"[56] He wrote, "From a medical point of view, it is very important to clarify the question of the best age to get married." His article focused on the question of the most desirable age for a woman and her fetus to undergo pregnancy and childbirth. Following a review of the age of menstruation among women of different population groups, he stated that the acceptable recommended age for the first pregnancy is five years after the woman's first period, i.e., between the ages of eighteen and twenty. However, he noted in his column that "many specialists think that one should marry over 20 but no later than age 24." On the question of "when a man should marry,"

Dr. Apper mentioned the well-known fact that men remain fertile to an advanced age and that "in many cases, men aged 70 and 80 have married and their wives have borne children. However, subject to a long list of psychological and ethical factors relating to the woman's interests to prevent disharmony, the age gap between her and her husband should not be too large. The man should be older than the woman, but no more than by 10 or 12 years." Regarding the recommended age for marriage, the writer of the article stated that "this question has been addressed by philosophers in ancient times and through the ages. Aristotle recommended up to age 37, Plato recommended 30 to 35. However, the recommended age is about 25."

In the "On Taboo Subjects" column, Dr. L. Friedland wrote "A Physician's Report on Sexual Problems."[57] He wrote that he did not profess to cover all sexual problems, but would limit the content to discussing several areas of sexuality that could improve quality of life. He shared his experience with his readers as a result of conversations with patients on the breakdown of romantic and family relationships following a crisis. Despite claiming that he dared not blame the problem on the quality of the couple's sexual relations, he felt obliged to emphasize that a bad sex life was the cause of conflict in most cases. In addition, he wrote that the couples are often very young and immature. He saw the role of his newspaper column to make the public aware of the development of these difficulties in life. The column was written as a story, in a series of installments in consecutive issues. The story addressed various problems pertaining to relationships and sexual intercourse, medical and erotic issues, and philosophical outlooks on the pleasures of life, among other things.

The initiative to publish *Der Doktor* is the jewel in the crown of Lensky's writings during the interwar period. As described above, he engaged in this impressive project while working as a physician in private practice and simultaneous to his engagement with other public work. The publication expenses were presumably covered by the modest income from sale of the journal and from advertisements, but mainly from his physician's income. Thus, Lensky became a doctor for the people, and public education in medicine became his life's work. Lensky continued to publish the newspaper for approximately five years. The issues held in the archive contain knowledge that sheds light on diverse topics pertaining to society in general and the Jewish society in particular during the interwar period.

Lensky's Fate during the Holocaust

In 1933, the year of Hitler's rise to power, Lensky stopped publishing the newspaper. Unfortunately, the latest copy in the archive is from September 1932. An effort is warranted to locate the final issue, which may shed light on the reasons for the project's closure. No reference has been found in Lensky's writings to factors that may have led to the abandonment of *Der Doktor*. Could it have been the sense of foreboding when Hitler came to power? Were financial constraints the cause? Or was it the influence of his employment at the St. Anthony district hospital in Włocławek? Neither was any hint found in the archive of the discontinuation of this impressive medical project for the people.

With the outbreak of World War II, Dr. Lensky, then forty-nine years old, was enlisted as a physician in the reserves of the Polish army. Shortly before the Germans invaded Włocławek, on 14 September 1939 he was discharged. Once back home, he was brutally dragged away by the SS and forced, under abuse by the soldiers, to run several kilometers to the prison, together with another thousand or so Jewish prisoners. Lensky was injured by the German soldiers' violence, but he treated the injuries of Jews around him to the best of his ability. Two days later, due to the seriousness of his injury, he was released and returned home. After some time, he and his family escaped to Warsaw by paying a large sum of money to an ethnic German woman who owned a car with a German license plate, and she was able to drive them past all the German guards stationed between Włocławek and Warsaw. In the Warsaw Ghetto, Dr. Lensky worked at Czyste Hospital, in the refugee centers that sheltered tens of thousands of Jews who had been deported to the ghetto from the surrounding towns and villages, and in clinics in the ghetto operated by the *Judenrat* and the TOZ health organization. In spring 1943, shortly before the liquidation of the ghetto, Lensky, his wife, and his two children escaped to the Polish side of the city and went into hiding under a false identity. In fall 1944, after the surrender of the Armia Krajowa (Home Army) resistance fighters, Lensky was deported by the Germans to a village near Krakow and then released. He, his wife, and their two children were miraculously saved from all but certain death, but they experienced great suffering in the Warsaw Ghetto and later on the "Aryan" side.

In the Shadow of the Holocaust 1945–64

For a short time after the war, Lensky continued to work in the hospital in Włocławek. From 1945–48, he and his wife lived in Łódź, where Polish Jewish Holocaust survivors had gathered, and he took part in activities of the association of Jewish writers and journalists. In addition to writing his articles in the medical field,[58] Lensky was immersed in researching, documenting, and memorializing the Holocaust. He reflected on the "new epidemic of destruction in Europe"[59] and documented episodes from the Warsaw Ghetto. During that period, he was a literary critic of Modern Hebrew poetry and prose and became interested in the study of Tanakh (the Hebrew Bible).

Intending to immigrate to Israel, the Lenskys left Łódź for Paris, where they stayed from May 1948 until September 1949. They sailed to Israel on the *Kedma* to join their children, who had preceded them. *The Black Notebook* was found in Lensky's posthumous collection—thirty-three handwritten pages bound in a black cover.[60] In it, he described the objective difficulties of integration into the young State of Israel and how the events of the Holocaust continued to haunt him day and night. Lensky's notebook is evidence of the mental suffering of so many Holocaust survivors.[61]

In 1961, his book of memoirs, *A Physician inside the Warsaw Ghetto*,[62] was published in Hebrew, and an English translation appeared in 2009.[63] His book is an important contribution to the study of the lives of Jews in the Warsaw Ghetto and of the various organizational, professional, and ethical aspects of medical activity in the ghetto. In the same year, Lensky's book *Who Brought Hitler to Power? Or the Weimar Republic in Germany and Hitler's Rise to Power* was published, discussing the different aspects that led Hitler to power and the sources that inspired Nazi ideology.[64] Lensky then immersed himself in another study focusing on scientific racism and its thinkers, in which he described the ideological development of the fathers of scientific racism and their writings.

Lensky also became involved in questions of policy regarding interactions between the State of Israel and public figures and political entities associated with the Holocaust. For instance, he wrote an article on the composer Richard Wagner that brought to public notice Wagner's hatred of Jews and his hope for their total annihilation, and Lensky attempted to influence the decision-makers to have Wagner's music banned in Israel.[65] Another central political and ethical concern was the question of diplomatic relations between the State of Israel and the German Federal Republic. Lensky left an extensive opinion piece in his archive addressing the subject, in which he supported the forming of such relations.[66] It is interesting to note that Lensky's argument refers to the values of compassion and *tikun olam* (repairing the world), following forefather Abraham's attempts to save the city of Sodom. Thus, even after the Holocaust, Lensky appears not to have lost his faith in human beings and in the possible social repair that is required to maintain peace.

Lensky's yearning to understand the meaning of the rise of the Nazis and the significance of the Holocaust gave him no rest. Alongside his work as a devoted physician in Jerusalem, he continued his research and publicist writings on the Holocaust until his dying day.

Conclusion

World War II and the Holocaust of the Jewish people put an end to Jewish life in Poland and, likewise, to the Jewish physicians' activities and writings. Of the thirty-five hundred Jewish physicians practicing in Poland on the eve of the Holocaust and the thousands of Jewish physicians practicing in other European countries that also suffered this cruel fate, only very few survived. The invaluable works of these physicians have been mostly forgotten by history. However, while no one can bring these physicians back, their ideas, their scientific and social accomplishments, and the moral values that motivated them can still be learned from archival studies. These writings are valuable in themselves, but a close reading of them reveals professional and ethical values behind the development of Jewish medicine during the interwar period. These principles later also withstood the medical challenges of Jewish medicine in the ghettos and camps. The exploration of these writings is an essential background to the analysis of the Jewish medical reaction during the Holocaust, which created a set of moral values diametrically opposed to those of the German physicians, despite working under extreme, unprecedented conditions of genocide.[67]

This review of Dr. Mordechai Lensky's writings between the two world wars paints a picture of a devoted family physician who also worked tirelessly as a proponent for public health. The writings reveal the picture of a Jewish physician in Poland, involved in the life of his community and in the Zionist activity that was forming during this period. As a physician, besides being a family doctor and a specialist in internal medicine, he focused his activities on preventative medicine. He actively disseminated state-of-the-art medical knowledge to the general Jewish population. A large proportion of his writings were intended to promote the people's health, expressed through his books that were published during this period. They were designed to spread medical knowledge, to deepen awareness of safeguarding health, to disseminate the importance of hygiene, to aid the prevention of disease, to teach coping strategies for first aid and alertness to symptoms of various illnesses, and to improve quality of life for individuals and for the weaker parts of the Jewish populace. His initiative to publish *Der Doktor*, a newspaper on public education in medicine and hygiene, was an impressive independent enterprise, the masterpiece of his writings for the sake of the Jewish society's health.

Dr. Mordechai Lensky is usually identified with Holocaust research, mainly in light of his memoirs about Jewish life in the Warsaw Ghetto from the perspective of a physician. However, as illustrated in this chapter, Lensky left behind many other writings, from before and after the Holocaust. The exploration of his writings from during the interwar period indicates his perception of medicine as a public mission and his sensitivity and feeling of social obligation toward the weak sectors of society. These perceptions and values were expressed also in the medical services that he provided in the Warsaw Ghetto. His pre-Holocaust writings and activities provide insight into the ethical dilemmas that he encountered, as described in his memoir *A Physician inside the Warsaw Ghetto*.[68] His desire to work in the refugee centers, the most hazardous health areas of the ghetto, is entirely consistent with the social perception expressed in *Der Doktor*.

Lensky continued to write prolifically after the Holocaust until his death in 1964. In these writings, briefly mentioned here, Lensky deeply researched the fundamental issues pertaining to the Holocaust and its causes, and addressed subjects that raised controversies in Israeli society in its aftermath. As the scope of his other writings exceeds the space constraints of this chapter, the postwar publications will need to be addressed in a future investigation.

Dr. Lensky's diverse writings shed light on the thoughts and actions of one Jewish physician out of the thousands who either perished during the Holocaust or who survived but remained unrecognized. His work also provides insights into the history of the "ordinary life" of Jewish people in the first half of the twentieth century. This investigation of Dr. Lensky's writings illustrates the productive outcomes of such a historic study and indeed the need for further explorations of the writings of other Jewish physicians.

The discussion of the history of medicine during the Holocaust requires a broad perspective, one that explores the factors and processes that led to the crimes committed by physicians in the Third Reich and their influence after the Holocaust. No less important, and under the same umbrella, is the study of the activities of the thousands of Jewish physicians. Many of them upheld the ethical values of the medical profession despite the conditions of genocide that prevailed in the ghettos and camps. A study of writings left from before, during, and after the Holocaust may contribute to the study of these values, perceptions, and beliefs that led the physicians, as victims, to remain faithful to professional medical values in an unprecedented historical situation, and motivated those who survived to engage in research and public activity for the sake of memorialization as well as for the emerging ethical significance of this history for the present and the future.

Miriam Offer, PhD, is an expert on Jewish medicine in the Holocaust. Her book, *White Coats in the Ghetto: Jewish Medicine in Poland during the Holocaust*, was published in 2020 by Yad Vashem (Hebrew edition, 2015). Miriam has researched the history of medicine (organization, science, ethics) in ghettos in Poland and Lithuania. Her current focus is Jewish medical activity immediately before, during, and after the Holocaust, and medicine/Holocaust gender issues. Miriam is a senior lecturer in the Holocaust Studies Program, Western Galilee College, and teaches medicine and the Holocaust in the Sackler Faculty of Medicine, Tel Aviv University.

Notes

1. Lensky 1927a.
2. In Jewish tradition, human life is a supreme value, and health preservation and healing is of the highest importance. Influenced by biblical and talmudic writings, by the commandment "choose life" (Deuteronomy 30:19), and inspired by the saying of the talmudic sages, "Whoever saves one life saves a whole world" (Tractate Sanhedrin 4:5), medicine is seen as a sacred art in Jewish culture and ethics.
3. *Encyclopedia Judaica* 1971–72, 1178–211.
4. Levin 2001, 165.

5. E.g., Menuhin 2016.
6. Several comprehensive studies have been written on this topic, e.g., Roland 1992; Offer 2020; von Villiez 2009; Schwoch 2018; van den Ende 2014; Ciesielska 2017. For an important collection of articles on this topic, see Grodin 2014.
7. E.g., Herzog 2020.
8. Examples of partial attempts in this direction: Jenss and Reinicke 2014; Golden 2018.
9. My heartfelt thanks to the late Professor Yaacov Lensky and to Miri Lensky for generously placing the archive in my care for the sake of research.
10. The term "ego document" was coined in the 1950s by the Dutch historian Jacques Presser. Much literature has been written to define and characterize the genre, which refers to written sources on the author's personal life experience or events, such as autobiographies, diaries, letters, etc. See Baggerman and Dekker 2006; Herzig 2006; Fulbrook and Rublack 2010.
11. The term "microhistory" was coined in the 1980s by the Italian historian Carlo Ginzburg. It focuses on writing "history from below," from the perspective of the daily life of individuals.
12. Lensky 1961 and 1983.
13. Lensky 2009.
14. Lensky 1983, "Introduction."
15. Rubinstein 1959.
16. Gutman 1990; Pinkas Hakehillot 1979, 1, 38–39, 64.
17. Lensky 2009, 200.
18. Levy and Levy 2012, 34.
19. E.g., Lensky 1927o; Lensky 1928a.
20. Lensky 1923a.
21. Lensky 1923b.
22. On this subject, see Katvan and Davidovitch 2010–11.
23. On the British Mandate period and aspects of the Jewish *Yishuv*, see Shapira 2012; Bareli and Karlinsky 2003.
24. Eugenics—a sociobiological philosophy, which focused on the study of the influence of heredity on human mental and behavioral characteristics with the aim of finding and implementing ways of "improving" the human race. The origin of the word "eugenics" is in Greek (*eu* = "well" or "good"; *genēs* = "born").

This school was popular at the beginning of the twentieth century in the United States and Western Europe, and some of the Jewish physicians also adopted the concept. Lensky's use of the expression should be read in the context of the situation in British Mandate Palestine with the limitations placed on the number of Jews allowed to immigrate and the resulting selective criteria; out of objective concern that ill or weak immigrants would be unable to withstand the difficult living conditions that prevailed there at the time.

After World War II, eugenics was defamed for its attempts to distinguish civilians of "good" or "normative" heredity from those with "defective" heredity. In Nazi Germany, the theory had developed to extremes, leading to the forced sterilization of approximately four hundred thousand people with serious diseases considered to be hereditary, and to the "euthanasia" project with the outbreak of the war, involving the murder of about two hundred thousand Germans with serious illnesses. On eugenics, see Redvaldsen 2017.

25. Lensky 1926b.
26. Katvan and Davidovitch 2010–11.
27. Katvan and Davidovitch 2007; Davidson 1927.
28. Lensky 1983; Plantowsky Peniel 1946; Bar-El 2008.
29. Novershtern, retrieved 2019; Cohen, retrieved 2019; Bareket Glanzer 2018; Nalewajko-Kulikov 2015.

30. Lensky 1925b; Lensky 1925e; Lensky 1926a; Lensky 1927d; Lensky 1927f; Lensky 1927h; Lensky 1927k; Lensky 1927m Lensky 1927i; Lensky 1930b; Lensky 1930f; Lensky 1930d; Lensky 1923b; Lensky 1925a; Lensky 1927j; Lensky 1933; Lensky 1925f; Lensky1925c; Lensky 1927c; Lensky 1928c; Lensky 1929b; Lensky 1929c; Lensky 1930e; Lensky 1925d; Lensky 1927e; Lensky 1927g; Lensky 1927b; Lensky 1923c; Lensky 1924; Lensky 1929a; Lensky 1927l; Lensky 1930c.
31. Lensky 1927n.
32. Lensky 1927a.
33. Barry 2005; Phillips and Killingray 2003; Beiner 2015.
34. Lensky 1928b.
35. Lensky 1927a, "Introduction."
36. Lensky 1927a, "Introduction."
37. Lensky 1927a, "Introduction."
38. Lensky 1927a, "Introduction."
39. On economic difficulties for the Jews during the interwar period, in Warsaw and Poland in general, see, e.g., Mahler 1969, 12–17, 37, 59; Pinkas Hakehillot 1979; Gutman 2001, 624–25.
40. Lensky 1928b.
41. Lensky 1928b.
42. Lensky 1928b.
43. For a brief biographical summary of Dr. Moses Einhorn, see, e.g., Beit Hatfutsot, retrieved 9 January 2020.
44. Lensky 1928b
45. Lensky 1931.
46. Lensky 1931.
47. Lensky 1931.
48. Lensky, not dated. Emphasis mine.
49. Lensky 2009, "Epilogue."
50. Anonymous 1964(?). I assume that this was the foreword to a book intended for publication after Lensky's death, to be dedicated to his research on the history of National Socialism and racial anti-Semitism; a book that he had not managed to publish during his lifetime.
51. Lensky 1929–33.
52. Lensky 1929–33. The document lacks a full explanation of how these prizes were distributed, but they were presumably intended to encourage subscription to the newspaper.
53. Lensky 1929d, 2.
54. Lensky 1930a.
55. Lensky 1929d, 3.
56. Apper 1929, 4.
57. Lensky 1929d, 5–9.
58. Lensky 1946.
59. Lensky 1947.
60. Lensky 1949–50.
61. Bamo'etza 1965.
62. Lensky 1983.
63. Lensky 2009.
64. Lensky 1961.
65. Lensky 1963; Barash 1966.
66. Lensky circa 1962.
67. Ethical issues were not removed from the agenda of the Jewish physicians in the different areas under Nazi occupation. The collective reaction of the Jewish leadership and the medical staff in the ghettos indicates the establishment of professional and humane medical systems by the Jews, as

victims, despite the extreme conditions enforced upon them by the Germans. See, e.g., Grodin 2014; Offer 2018; Offer 2012.

68. Lensky 2009, 80–87.

References

Anonymous. 1964(?). *Mordechai Lensky: An Outline of His Personality (1890–1964)*. Lensky Family Archive, Rehovot. [Hebrew].
Apper, Dr. 1929. "What Is the Recommended Age to Get Married?" [Yiddish]. In Mordechai Lensky, *The Doctor: A Biweekly Newspaper for Public Education in Medicine and Hygiene* 1: 4. Warsaw. [Yiddish]. Rehovot: Lensky Family Archive.
Barash, Menachem. 1966. *Yediot Aharonot*, 1 July, 9. [Hebrew].
Bareket Glanzer, Hani. 2018. *The Yiddish Daily Newspaper Moment (1939–1910): The Newspaper's Presentation of Contemporary Events in Poland*. Jerusalem: Hebrew University. [Hebrew].
Bar-El, Adina. 2008. "Culture." In *The YIVO Encyclopedia of Jews in Eastern Europe*, edited by Gershon D. Hundert. New Haven, CT: Yale University Press.
Barry, John M. 2005. *The Great Influenza: The Epic Story of the Deadliest Pandemic in History*. New York: Penguin.
Baggerman, Arianne, and Rudolf Dekker. 2006. "Ego Documents and the Study of the History of Culture." In *The Past and Beyond: Studies in History and Philosophy Presented to Elazar Weinryb*, edited by Amir Horowitz, Ora Limor, Ran Ben-Shalom, and Avriel Bar-Levav, 245–63. Raanana: The Open University of Israel. [Hebrew].
Bamo'etza. 1965. Jerusalem Workers Council Journal. 2–3 March.
Bareli, Avi, and Nahum Karlinsky (eds.). 2003. *Economy and Society in Mandatory Palestine 1918–1948*. Iyunim Bitkumat Israel, Thematic Series. Be'er Sheva: Ben-Gurion University of the Negev. [Hebrew].
Beiner, Guy. 2015. "Out in the Cold and Back: New-Found Interest in the Great Flu." *Cultural and Social History* 3: 496–505. doi: 10.1191/1478003806cs070ra.
Beit Hatfutsot, The Museum of the Jewish People website. Retrieved 9 January 2020 from https://dbs.bh.org.il/luminary/einhorn-moses.
Ciesielska, Maria. 2017. *Lekarze getta warszawskiego*. Warsaw: Wydawnictwo Dwa Światy.
Cohen, Nathan. *Der moment*. National Library of Israel and Tel Aviv University on Yiddish newspapers: Retrieved 8 March 2019 from http://web.nli.org.il/sites/JPress/English/Pages/DahrMamanet.aspx.
Davidson, Noach. 1927. "An Answer Must be Given!" *Haynt* 58 (9 March). [Yiddish].
Encyclopedia Judaica. 1971–72. Vol. 11, "Medicine," 1178–211. Jerusalem: Keter.
Fulbrook, Mary, and Ulinka Rublack. 2010. "In Relation: 'The Social Self' and Ego-Documents." *German History*, 28(3): 263–72. Retrieved 27 July 2020 from https://academic.oup.com/gh/article-abstract/28/3/263/786165.
Golden, Juliet D. 2018. "'Show That You Are Really Alive': Sara-Zofia Syrkin-Binsztejnowa's Emergency Medical Relief and Public Health Work in Early Interwar Poland and the Warsaw Ghetto." *Medizinhistorisches Journal* 53: 125–62.
Grodin, Michael A. (ed.). 2014. *Jewish Medical Resistance in the Holocaust*. New York: Berghahn Books.
Gutman, Israel. 1990. *Encyclopedia of the Holocaust*. Vol. 2: 1601. New York: Macmillan.
———. 2001. "Jews–Poles–Antisemitism." In *The Broken Chain: Polish Jewry through the Ages*, edited by Israel Gutman, and Israel Bartal, 2:624–25. Jerusalem: Zalman Shazar Center. [Hebrew].

Herzig, Hanna. 2006. "A Personal Testimony of the Holocaust: History from a Different Perspective." In *The Past and Beyond: Studies in History and Philosophy Presented to Elazar Weinryb*, edited by Amir Horowitz, Ora Limor, Ran Ben-Shalom, and Avriel Bar-Levav, 283–317. Raanana: The Open University of Israel. [Hebrew].

Herzog, Rachel. 2020. *To Heal the Fractures: Integration of Holocaust Survivor Doctors in Israeli Health Care and Society, 1945–1957*. Jerusalem: Yad Vashem. [Hebrew].

Jenss, Harro, and Peter Reinicke (Hrsg.) 2014. *Der Arzt Hermann Strauß, 1868–1944: Autobiographische Notizen und Aufzeichnungen aus dem Ghetto Theresienstadt*. Berlin: Hentrich & Hentrich.

Katvan, Eyal, and Davidovitch, Nadav. 2007. "Health, Politics and Professionalism: Medical Inspection of Jewish Candidates for Immigration to Palestine (1925–1928)." *Israel: Studies in Zionism and the State of Israel—History, Culture and Society* 11(1): 41–47. [Hebrew].

———. 2010–11. "Medical Inspection of Immigrants to Eretz-Israel during the Interwar Period." *Korot: The Israel Journal of the History of Medicine and Science* 20: 19–36. [Hebrew].

Lenski, Marek. 1946. "Jad zmii Jako Srodek Przeciwbolowy." *Zoddzialu Chorob Wewnetrznych Szpitala sw. Antoniego Wloclawku, Lekarski Instytut Naukowo-Wydawniczy, Warszawa*.

Lensky, Mordechai. N.d. Letters to his Cousin Yitzhak Hacarmeli. Lensky Family Archive, Rehovot. [Hebrew].

———. 1923a. Letters to his cousin Yitzhak Hacarmeli. 30 January. Lensky Family Archive, Rehovot. [Hebrew].

———. 1923b. "On Holiday Camps for Jewish Youth." *Der Moment* 56 (6 March). Warsaw. [Yiddish].

———. 1923c. "Jews and Military Service." *Der Moment* 35 (9 February). Warsaw. [Yiddish].

———. 1924. "Hebrew in the Jewish Family." *Der Moment* 227 (26 September). Warsaw. [Yiddish].

———. 1925a. "Can the Elderly Restore Their Youth? From Medical Discussions." *Haynt* 228 (2 October). Warsaw. [Yiddish].

———. 1925b. "The New Way of Preventing Scarlatina." *Haynt* 233 (9 October). Warsaw. [Yiddish].

———. 1925c. "Acids as an Effective Cure for Disease. From Medical Discussions." *Haynt* 247 (27 October). Warsaw. [Yiddish].

———. 1925d. "A Report of the TOZ (Towarzystwo Ochrony Zdrowia Ludności Żydowskiej, Society for Safeguarding the Health of the Jewish Population) Sanitary Exhibition." *Haynt* 277 (1 December). Warsaw. [Yiddish].

———. 1925e. "How Can the Common Cold Be Prevented? The Cold Epidemic in Warsaw." *Haynt* 283 (8 December). Warsaw. [Yiddish].

———. 1925f. "New Findings for a Cure for Cancer." *Haynt* 288 (14 December). Warsaw. [Yiddish].

———. 1926a. "New/Modern Diseases. From Medical Discussions." *Haynt*. 10 (12 January), 19 (15 January). Publication in two parts. Warsaw. [Yiddish].

———. 1926b. "On the Question of the Medical Criticism of the Offices for Eretz Israel." *Haaretz* 3 (18 November). [Hebrew].

———. 1927a. *The Modern Family Doctor*. Warsaw.

———. 1927b. The International Sanitary Hygiene Conference in Warsaw. *Haynt* 146 (27 June). Warsaw. [Yiddish].

———. 1927c. "Sunbathing for Healthy People and Patients." *Haynt* 153 (10 July). Warsaw. [Yiddish].

———. 1927d. "Why Do So Many People Suffer from Headaches and How Can They Be Prevented?" *Haynt* 160 (18 July). Warsaw. [Yiddish].

———. 1927e. "The Polish Conference on Hygiene and How to Improve the Housing Crisis." *Haynt* 166 (25 July). Warsaw. [Yiddish].

———. 1927f. "How to Protect Children From Measles." *Haynt* 173 (2 August). Warsaw. [Yiddish].

———. 1927g. "Can Disinfecting the Home Prevent Infectious Diseases?" *Haynt* 189 (21 August). Warsaw. [Yiddish].

———. 1927h. "Why Do So Many People Suffer from Rheumatism?" *Haynt* 214 (19 September). Warsaw. [Yiddish].

———. 1927i. "What Is the Meaning of the Polio Epidemic?" *Haynt* 219 (25 September). Warsaw. [Yiddish].

———. 1927j. "How Can the Overweight Get Slimmer?" *Haynt* 225 (4 October). Warsaw. [Yiddish].

———. 1927k. "Is There a Cure for Blood Poisoning?" *Haynt* 240 (27 October). Warsaw. [Yiddish].

———. 1927l. "Jewish Medicine." *Haynt* 272 (4 December). Warsaw. [Yiddish].

———. 1927m. "How to Avoid Typhoid Fever—The Fight against Typhoid in France and Germany." *Haynt* 284 (18 December). Warsaw. [Yiddish].

———. 1927n. *The Epidemic of Influenza.* Warsaw. [Yiddish].

———. 1927o. "The Von Grafe Sign and Aschner Reflex in Polish Immigrants." *Harefuah* 20(2): 370. [Hebrew].

———. 1928a. "Early Onset Hypcrotonia essentialis in Polish immigrants." *Harefuah* 2(6): 105. [Hebrew].

———. 1928b. Letters to his Cousin Yitzhak Hacarmeli. 4 March. Lensky Family Archive, Rehovot. [Hebrew].

———. 1928c. "Dietary Treatment for People with Digestive Problems." *Haynt* 305 (30 December). Warsaw. [Yiddish].

———. 1929a. "Representation for Jewish Communities: Clarifications, Remarks, and Answers to Questions." *Haynt* 2 (2 January). Warsaw. [Yiddish].

———. 1929b. "Sugar as a Remedy." *Haynt* 157 (14 July). Warsaw. [Yiddish].

———. 1929c. "The Surprising Discovery That Diet Can Cure Tuberculosis." *Haynt* 175 (4 August). Warsaw. [Yiddish].

———. 1929d. *Der Doktor: A Biweekly Newspaper for Lay People on Medicine and Hygiene* 1 (1 July). Warsaw. [Yiddish]. Rehovot: Lensky Family Archive.

———. 1929–1933. *Der Doktor: A Biweekly Newspaper for Lay People on Medicine and Hygiene.* National Library of Israel,002127713 [Yiddish]. Lensky Family Archive, Rehovot..

———. 1930a. *Der Doktor: A Biweekly Newspaper for Lay People on Medicine and Hygiene* 15 (9 January). Warsaw. [Yiddish]. Rehovot: Lensky Family Archive.

———. 1930b. "Will We Be Rid of Tuberculosis Any Time Soon?" *Haynt* 28 (2 February). Warsaw. [Yiddish].

———. 1930c. "Miracle-Makers in the 20th Century." *Haynt* 76 (30 March). Warsaw. [Yiddish].

———. 1930d. "Of What Should Pregnant Women Take Note?" *Haynt* 127 (4 June). Warsaw. [Yiddish].

———. 1930e. "New Ways of Avoiding Diphtheria." *Haynt* 208 (7 August). Warsaw. [Yiddish].

———. 1930f. "How Can We Avoid Cancer?" *Haynt* 264 (19 November). Warsaw. [Yiddish].

———. 1931. *Moshe Feldstein, a Guide for Circumcisers: Brief Notes on Anatomy, Physiology, and Infection.* Warsaw: Jewish Community Department for Culture. [Yiddish].

———. 1933. "How to Take Advantage of the Summer and the Summer Vacation." *Haynt* 144 (25 June). Warsaw. [Yiddish].

———. 1947 "The New Epidemic of Destruction in Europe," *Der Tog* 7 (5 January): 3, 5 [Yiddish].

———. 1949–50. *The Black Notebook.* Lensky Family Archive, Rehovot.

———. 1961. *Who Brought Hitler to Power? Or the Weimar Republic in Germany and Hitler's Rise to Power.* Jerusalem: Holocaust Library. [Hebrew].

———. Circa 1962. *Ought Israel to Establish Relations with West Germany?* Lensky Family Archive, Rehovot.

———. 1963. "Wagner Enemy of the Jews." *Ha'uma* 2(6): 306–11. [Hebrew].

———. 1983. "Introduction." *The Life of the Jews in the Warsaw Ghetto, Memories of a Physician.* Jerusalem: Rubin Mass. [Hebrew]. First edition, 1961. Jerusalem: Sifriyat Hashoah.

———. 2009. *A Physician inside the Warsaw Ghetto*. Foreword by Samuel Kassow. Jerusalem: Yad Vashem; New York: The Holocaust Survivor's Memoirs Project.
Levin, Dov. 2001. "The Medical Array of Baltic Jewry in the Holocaust, 1941–1945." *Proceedings of the Twelfth World Congress on Jewish Studies*. Division 5: Contemporary Jewish Society. Jerusalem. [Hebrew]
Levy, Nissim, and Yael Levy. 2012. *Physicians of the Holy Land 1799-1948*. Zikhron Ya'akov: Itai Bahur. [Hebrew].
Mahler, Raphael. 1969. *Polish Jewry between the World Wars: A Socioeconomic History in the Light of Statistics*. Tel Aviv: Dvir. [Hebrew].
Menuhin, Naomi. 2016. "Dr. Israel Milejkowski: The World of a Jewish Intellectual in Poland between Two World Wars." PhD diss., Ben Gurion University of the Negev. [Hebrew].
Nadav, Daniel. S. 2009. *Medicine and Nazism*. Jerusalem: Hebrew University Magnes Press.
Nalewajki-Kulikov, Joanna. 2015. "'Di Haynt-mishpokhe': Study of a Group Picture." In *Warsaw: The Jewish Metropolis; Essays in Honor of the 75th Birthday of Professor Antony Polonsky*, edited by Glenn Dynner and François Guesnet, 252–70. Leiden: Brill.
Novershtern, Avraham. *The Yiddish Press Section*. National Library of Israel, Tel Aviv University. Retrieved 8 March 2019 from http://web.nli.org.il/sites/JPress/English/Pages/sec_idish.aspx.
———. *Haynt*. National Library of Israel, Tel Aviv University. Retrieved 8 March 2019 from http://web.nli.org.il/sites/jpress/hebrew/pages/haynt_.aspx.
Offer, Miriam. 2012. "Ethical Dilemmas in the Work of Doctors and Nurses in the Warsaw Ghetto." *Polin: Studies in Polish Jewry* 25: 449–67.
———. 2018. "Jewish Medical Ethics during the Holocaust—The Unwritten Ethical Code." *Wiener klinische Wochenschrift, the Central European Journal of Medicine* 130: 172–76.
———. 2020. *White Coats in the Ghetto: Jewish Medicine in Poland during the Holocaust*. Jerusalem: Yad Vashem.
Phillips, Howard, and David Killingray (eds.). 2003. *The Spanish Influenza Pandemic of 1918–19: New Perspectives*. New York: Routledge.
Pinkas Hakehillot, Encyclopedia of Jewish Communities: Poland. 1979. Vol. 4: "Warsaw and Its Region." Jerusalem: Yad Vashem. [Hebrew].
Plantowsky Peniel, Noah. 1946. *On the History of the Tarbut Educational Institutions in Poland*. Jerusalem: Kohelet. [Hebrew].
Redvaldsen, David. December 2017. "Recent Works of the History of Eugenics: A New Landscape." *East Central Europe* 44(2–3).
Roland, Charles Gordon. 1992. *Courage under Siege: Starvation, Disease and Death in the Warsaw Ghetto*. New York: Oxford University Press.
Rubinstein, Abraham. 1959. "The Warsaw Community." *Mahanayim* 120. October-November 1959. http://www.daat.ac.il/daat/history/kehilot/varsha.htm Retrieved 8 March 2019
Schwoch, Rebecca. 2018. *Jüdische Ärzte als Krankenbehandler in Berlin zwischen 1938 und 1945*. Frankfurt am Main: Mabuse-Verlag.
Shapira, Anita. 2012. *A History, Part II: 1918–1948; A State-in-the-Making*. Woltham, MA: Brandeis University Press.
van den Ende, Hannah. 2014. *Vergeet niet dat je arts bent: Joodse artsen in Nederland 1940–1945*. Amsterdam: Boom.
von Greyerz, Kasper. 2010. "Ego-Documents: The Last Word?" *German History* 28(3): 273–82.
von Villiez, Anna. 2009. *Mit aller Kraft verdrängt, Entrechtung und Verfolgung "nicht arischer" Ärzte in Hamburg 1933 bis 1945*. Hamburg: Dölling und Galitz Verlag.

CHAPTER 4

RABBINIC RESPONSA DURING THE HOLOCAUST
The Life-for-Life Problem

Johnathan I. Kelly, Erin L. Miller, Rabbi Joseph Polak,
Robert Kirschner, and Michael A. Grodin

In September 1941, three months into the German occupation of Lithuania, the German authorities ordered the Jewish Council of the Kovno Ghetto to distribute five thousand labor cards among the population of twenty-seven thousand Jews who lived there. With the recent deportations and killings still fresh in their memory, the Jewish Council could only assume that the Germans' plan was to deport and murder those who did not hold a labor card after the cards were distributed.[1] "The purpose was clear," Avraham Tory, the secretary of the Kovno Jewish Council, wrote in his diary.[2] And yet, if the council refused to participate in the Germans' scheme and distribute the cards, it was nearly certain that the Germans would respond with rounds of killing and cruelty on the entire community. According to Rabbi Ephraim Oshry, members of the Kovno Jewish Council approached him for advice, asking him whether Jewish law permitted them to comply with the order and distribute the cards. How should the council proceed, they asked Rabbi Oshry, when their decision would likely lead to the sparing of those who received a labor card and to the deportation and murder of the many of those who did not?[3]

In the ghettos and camps, individual Jews also sought out the counsel of rabbis to ask what Jewish law permitted or required them to do. In late 1944, on the eve of Rosh Hashanah, fourteen hundred boys of less than a certain height were singled out for death at Auschwitz. After the selection, word spread throughout the camp that the boys would be killed. To rescue their sons, some camp inmates attempted to ransom particular boys by bribing the guards. Knowing that his son could be ransomed only if another boy took his place, a father of one of the boys selected for death asked Rabbi Tzvi Hirsch Meisels whether Jewish law permitted such an action. As Rabbi Meisels records, the man approached him and said, "Rabbi! My only son, my dear one so precious to me, is over there among the boys condemned to be burned; and I have the ability to ransom him. Yet we know without a doubt that the kapos [the guards] will seize another in his place. Therefore I ask of the rabbi a question of law and practice: according to the Torah, am I permitted to save him? Whatever you decide, I will do."[4]

Tragic choices like the ones faced by the Kovno Jewish Council and the father at Auschwitz, choices that would likely determine who would be spared and who would die, were forced upon Jews throughout the ghettos and camps. In the case of the Kovno Ghetto, we know that the Jewish Council carried out the order to distribute the cards, but the process that led to this decision was by no means a simple one, as we will see in this chapter. Neglected in many accounts of Jewish life in the ghettos and camps, the writings of the rabbis we discuss in this chapter give us a new window into how decisions by individual Jews and by the Jewish Councils were made, what kinds of religious, ethical, and practical considerations were weighed, and how the Jewish community dealt with the burden of being forced to make decisions that would likely lead to the sparing of some and the death of others.

Facing such decisions, many Jews could not access the counsel and advice of rabbis, nor of anyone else, in pressing cases where life and death were at stake. Moreover, the rabbis themselves faced the same horrific circumstances as the rest of the community. Nevertheless, when there was a window to do so, some Jews in the ghettos and camps sought out the advice and counsel of the rabbis, as Jews always had throughout the generations. Responding to those who came to them for help and advice, rabbis looked to sources within Jewish law (Halakhah) to provide guidance even under such extreme circumstances as they had always done.

In line with a long rabbinic tradition, many rabbis during the Holocaust recorded the questions asked of them, the situations from which the questions arose, and what they judged should be done. The genre of Jewish law that these texts fit into is known as rabbinic responsa: the written decisions of rabbinic authorities on questions of law and practice in daily Jewish life.[5] Responsa, a Latin term meaning "answers," are the branch of rabbinical literature comprised of authoritative replies (traditionally in letter form) written by rabbis and noted Jewish scholars in response to questions sent to them. Rabbis record both question and answer in epistolary form—elaborating *she'elot* (questions) and offering *teshuvot* (answers). After receiving a question or perhaps formulating one for themselves, the author of a rabbinic responsum undertakes a study of the relevant sources in Jewish law, sometimes consults with other rabbis and scholars on the question and the sources, then composes a responsum that records the question to be decided on, identifies and discusses the relevant sources, argues for an application of the sources to the current case, and issues a decision. The skill in reaching the legal decision lay in the breadth of knowledge needed to marshal the relevant sources, integrate them, and then subject their application to rigorous logical scrutiny.

Since Jewish law addresses all aspects of daily life, the responsa literature has covered a very wide range of questions over its history. During the Holocaust, rabbis were asked a host of pressing questions, some concerning how to carry on with daily life under Nazi rule, others even involving urgent matters of life and death. Living under extreme deprivation, without the books or even the writing materials needed to compose a reply, the rabbis gave most of their decisions orally, in conversation. As a consequence, relatively few records of the decisions issued by rabbis have survived. But some of these decisions did. A set of documents rarely studied by historians,[6] Holocaust-era rabbinic responsa provide a close-up and rare glimpse into how Jews responded to attacks on every aspect of their lives, as well as a telling witness of the Germans' attempt to make European Jews the agents of their own destruction.[7] Much like diaries and memoirs have shaped and reshaped our perceptions of both the victim and the perpetrator, Holocaust-era responsa provide a window into the kinds of tragic choices forced upon Jews during the Holocaust and how they met such challenges.[8]

One of the main purposes of our study of these rabbinic texts is to shed light on an attitude held by many Jews during the Holocaust, but one very rarely explored: the outlook of those Jews for whom the Jewish legal tradition continued to structure the decisions they made, even in the ghettos and camps where they were daily confronted with seemingly irresolvable dilemmas.[9] In examining the questions brought to the rabbis and their responses, our aim is to demonstrate the degree to which the rabbis and ordinary Jews found within the Jewish legal tradition sufficient resources to face an unprecedented set of dilemmas and to confront an enemy fixed on their total destruction. What we ultimately hope to shed light on in this chapter is the nature of a profound form of Jewish resistance during the Holocaust: the mindset of those Jews who, by steadfastly seeking to determine and to do what Jewish law required of them, withheld from the Germans and their collaborators what they wanted most—the corruption and degradation of Jewish self-worth and identity.[10]

Rabbinic Responsa, Medicine, and the Holocaust

At first glance, rabbinic responsa may appear as a topic mainly of interest to specialists in Jewish law and history. However, as will become clear in this chapter, there are many close points of contact between the responsa we discuss and contemporary questions in the areas of medicine and the Holocaust as well as bioethics more generally. First, much like the community continued to look to rabbis for support in the ghettos and camps, the Jewish community also continued to look to physicians for care, support, and advice.[11] Second, there are many parallels that can be drawn and usefully explored in showing how rabbis and physicians in each of their realms faced a similar set of problems involving the risking and saving of lives under circumstances that pushed them to the reaches of their vocations. And in their own essential ways, the rabbis and the Jewish physicians in the ghettos and camps never ceased in their work to preserve the physical, psychological, and spiritual health of the community.[12]

Third, the conditions in the ghettos and camps led to innumerable situations where determining how to observe Jewish law, how to survive, and how to make decisions concerning the saving and surrendering of life were equally questions of Jewish law and of medicine. Many Holocaust-era responsa thus address issues of basic health and medical care, questions of reproduction, and end-of-life decisions. For example, many approached the rabbis with questions about the eating of non-kosher food, the circumcision of newborns, the performance of abortions or Cesarean sections, and ending one's life.[13] While we have not been able to find records of any Holocaust-era rabbinic responsa addressing a question raised by a physician, it is clear that rabbis and Jewish physicians were asked a similar set of questions concerning life-for-life cases and thus may very well have consulted with each other.

On a most fundamental level, the physicians' process of triage mirrors the rabbinic process in making decisions only after rigorous analysis of all the available alternatives. The process of triage is powerfully illustrated in the classic Talmudic story, discussed later in this chapter, of two men lost in the desert and the rabbinic debates that followed. The two men lost in the desert have only enough water to save one of them; if both drink both will die. What should they do? In short, a comparison of major questions in Jewish law, medicine, and bioethics demonstrates the ways that the life-for-life problem is also often a medical problem.[14]

The Life-for-Life Problem in Jewish Law

The responsa we have selected for discussion in this chapter address specific cases during the Holocaust concerning the sparing or surrendering of life. Such cases have been debated throughout the history of Jewish law. However, in the case of Nazi Germany's war against the Jewish people, the aim of the regime was to totally exterminate the Jewish people and, in the process, to force the Jews to participate in their own destruction. The unprecedented scope of the Nazi attack on the Jews of Europe forced the Jewish community to face round after round of seemingly irresolvable situations and led them to face such dilemmas as: Can some lives be surrendered in order to save the remainder of the community? Can one put another's life or one's own life in grave danger in order to spare the lives of others? Can one intervene to save one's own life or that of one's family knowing that as a result another life will be lost?[15]

Such moral dilemmas, where the saving of one or more lives will almost certainly result in the loss of other lives, are cases of the "life-for-life problem" in Jewish law.[16] Consistently maintained and argued in many rabbinic texts, only in very rare cases is the taking of a human life justified or sanctioned, for any reason, by a rabbi.

While our focus here will be on life-for-life responsa, Holocaust-era responsa address much more than the life-for-life problem. Since Jewish law covers all aspects of daily life, and since the Nazi occupation brutally targeted every element of Jewish existence, Jews brought a very wide range of questions to rabbis. Giving up on the commandments governing daily life was not an option. But in the face of death, hunger, disease, and an attack on their whole way of life, observant Jews across Europe were forced to grapple with how to preserve their own lives—of how to maintain the principle governing Jewish life that "one should live by the commandments, but not die by them." In doing so, they adhered to the principle in Jewish law of *pikuach nefesh*, "the preservation of life," which teaches that the preservation of human life takes precedence over nearly all other commandments. Thus, as a rule in Jewish law, life must be preserved, even if doing so requires the violation of other commandments.[17]

In the ghettos and camps, simple matters of everyday life put the average Jew into the terrible position of choosing between preserving their own lives and violating a commandment. During the Holocaust, many Jews thus went to the rabbis and asked, is it is permissible to eat non-kosher food? To eat on Yom Kippur? For a man to shave his beard? Many Jews also asked if they should give up their lives rather than violate the commandments. Thus, some asked if it is permissible to endanger one's life in order to avoid violating the Sabbath, while others asked if it is permissible to carry a Christian baptism certificate to save one's life.[18]

Responsum on the Risking of One's Own Life to Save Another

The first responsum we will examine in detail is one from Rabbi Oshry's collection of Holocaust-era responsa, *She'elot u-teshuvot mi-ma'amakim* (questions and answers from out of the depths).[19] Soon after the Germans occupied Kovno and began persecuting and seizing Jews throughout the city, Rabbi Oshry along with a group of fellow rabbis had to decide whether they were obligated or even permitted to risk their lives in order to rescue a group of yeshiva students who had been kidnapped by the Lithuanian militia.[20] This was not a simple decision in either practical or ethical terms, since it was a possibility if not a certainty that the kidnapping of the yeshiva students was aimed at luring more Jews, and especially Jewish religious leaders, into the hands of the Lithuanian militia.[21]

Out of this situation the following question arose for Rabbi Oshry and the others: Is it permissible, according to Jewish law, for one or more of the rabbis to go to the Lithuanians to attempt to persuade them to negotiate release of the yeshiva students? It was conceivable that the rescuers would themselves be seized and murdered in such an attempt.[22] Under such circumstances, the question ran, was it permissible, much less obligatory, to endanger their lives in order to save the lives of the students?

The case is thus one of what is permissible or obligatory when the life of another is in danger, a question discussed at great length throughout the history of Jewish law. Rabbi Oshry's discussion of the case focuses on two closely connected rabbinic teachings: (1) the principle of "do not stand idly by the blood of your neighbor," and (2) the principle of "who knows whose blood is redder?" In his responsum, Rabbi Oshry shows how rabbinic authorities agree that the principle "do not stand idly by the blood of your neighbor" affirms that a person is obligated to save another from danger.[23] The duty to rescue, to "not stand idly by," indicates that he and the others are indeed obligated to intervene to save the students from danger. In the central argument of his responsum, Rabbi Oshry argues that in the major rabbinic precedents, distinguishing between whether lives are in possible, likely, or certain danger determines how the two principles apply.

The relation between the two sets of rabbinic teachings mirrors in a clear way the two sides of the dilemma Rabbi Oshry saw facing the rabbis: whether to intervene, which could save the lives of the yeshiva students but could also easily lead to more loss of life; or to remain in hiding and not send an advocate, despite the likelihood that the yeshiva students would be killed if no one intervened on their behalf.

Rabbi Oshry proceeds by carefully interpreting the two teachings. "From where do we know," reads the first Talmudic text, "that if one sees one's fellow drowning in a river, or if one sees a wild beast ravaging [a fellow] or bandits approaching to attack him, that he is obligated to save [the fellow]? Scripture teaches: do not stand by the blood of your friend."[24]

Rabbi Oshry then observes that the duty to rescue those in danger is grounded on the more general duty in Jewish law to preserve life, including one's own. Thus, after discussing the duty to rescue, Rabbi Oshry turns to a text in the Talmud that affirms the value of all human life. In posing the question "who knows whose blood is redder?" and asserting that "nobody can determine whose life is more precious to God,"[25] this second text led to conflicting interpretations among rabbinic authorities. As Rabbi Oshry notes, many rabbinic authorities have interpreted this passage to mean that just as one should not kill another to save oneself, one should not give up one's own life in order to save someone else's, since it is possible that one's own life in fact has greater value. On this reading of the principle of "who knows whose blood is redder?" it might appear forbidden for the rabbis to approach the Lithuanians on behalf of the yeshiva students, since doing so could endanger more lives.

A difficult question thus emerges: whether it is permissible to gravely risk one's life to save another's. Rabbi Oshry argues that the "who knows whose blood is redder" teaching should not lead to indecision about whether to intervene in a given situation. Rather, he points to how the two passages indicate situations where the level of risk is much different. Rabbi Oshry argues that "do not stand idly by" refers to situations like the one imagined in the Talmud,[26] where to step into a river to save someone who is drowning involves little risk to oneself. It is in such a case, where the risk to one's own life by intervening is minimal, that the principle of "do not stand idly by the blood of your neighbor" applies and one is obligated to intervene, Rabbi Oshry concludes. He thus stresses the importance of determining the level of risk involved: is one putting oneself in possible, likely, or certain danger by intervening? In discussions of the cases of certain danger in rabbinic literature, it is considered forbidden for one to intervene. Martyrdom is thus placed within severe limits in the rabbinic tradition.[27]

With these distinctions set down, Rabbi Oshry argues that the case of rescuing the yeshiva students is a case of one person placing himself in possible but not certain danger to save others who are in certain danger and is thus permissible. In other words, there is well-justified fear but much uncertainty regarding whether the Lithuanians would seize them if approached. But there is near certainty that the lives of the yeshiva students will be lost unless an attempt to save them is undertaken.

Rabbi Oshry then takes on a final ethical-legal distinction, between what is obligatory and what is merely permissible. While it is clear to him that it is permissible to intervene on behalf of the students, he concludes by asking if there are times when a person is obligated to endanger himself to save others. To address the question, Rabbi Oshry cites a nineteenth-century rabbinic discussion and argues that situations should be carefully weighed, and yet it is not always desirable to be overly protective of oneself.[28] In other words, depending upon the gravity of the situation, it might be obligatory for a person to place himself at risk. Moreover, while one may not be obligated to place oneself in a dangerous situation in a particular case, it could be considered praiseworthy to do so. Additionally, Rabbi Oshry argues, it is right to feel a higher degree of responsibility when given the opportunity to save a life. Thus, one may rightly feel obligated to intervene even if the law may not explicitly obligate one to do so. These considerations bring Rabbi Oshry to the conclusion that, while one is not obligated to endanger himself, he may do so if he is a person of strong and serious character.

Rabbi Oshry's responsum on the case of the yeshiva students is an example of a rabbinic decision that helped to determine which course of action would be taken. In a postscript to his responsum, Rabbi Oshry notes that that Rabbi David Itzkowitz followed Rabbi Oshry's advice and approached the Lithuanians. Rabbi Itzkowitz succeeded in this brave effort, convincing the Lithuanians to release the students. He himself was unharmed in the process, and the students were freed. Tragically, Rabbi Itzkowitz himself was later deported and died at Theresienstadt.[29]

The Decision of Whether to Distribute Labor Cards and Thus Determine Who Would Be Spared Deportation

The next responsum we discuss is from Rabbi Oshry's first collection of responsa, *Divrei Ephraim*.[30] In this responsum, Rabbi Oshry addresses one of the most difficult decisions forced upon almost all Jewish communities in the ghettos during the Holocaust: whether to comply with orders from the German authorities that would likely determine who would remain in the ghetto and who would be deported and killed. In this particular case, Rabbi Oshry is asked whether it is permissible for the Jewish Council in Kovno to distribute labor cards given to them by the Germans, knowing that those who did not receive a card would likely be rounded up in a selection, deported, and murdered.[31] By the time the labor cards decision was forced onto the Jewish leadership, ten thousand of the Jews of Kovno, over a quarter of the population of the ghetto, had already been murdered.

In his responsum, Rabbi Oshry carefully formulates the dilemma faced by members of the Kovno Jewish Council in deciding whether they should comply with the order. Is it permissible for the Jewish Council to distribute the cards as the German commandant had ordered, knowing that those who did not receive a card would likely be deported and murdered? Or should they refuse to distribute the cards, perhaps putting even more lives at risk as a result?

Rabbi Oshry begins his responsum by situating the labor cards case alongside the long-standing rabbinic debate around surrender to an enemy authority. In interpretations of a major legal text on surrender in the Palestinian Talmud,[32] two conditions emerge in determining if surrender to an enemy authority is permissible: who is selecting who will be surrendered, and whether or not the one(s) specified by the enemy authority is guilty of a capital crime. In the first case, if complying would require the group to select one of its own, they would be condemning one of their group to death. But if the enemy specifies who should be surrendered, and if that person is guilty of a capital offense, the group is not forced to single out arbitrarily one of their own as deserving of death. Since complying may spare the lives of the others, surrendering the guilty person specified is permissible, for the majority of rabbinic authorities.

Maimonides, the rabbi, philosopher, physician, and author of the great code of Jewish law, the *Mishneh Torah*, interprets the Palestinian Talmud text on surrender to teach that even if a particular person is specified by the enemy authority, he may not be surrendered unless he committed a capital offense and is thus "deserving of death."[33] Unless there is one "deserving of death," the group should let the authority kill all of them rather than hand one over. Applying Maimonides's teaching, Rabbi Oshry argues that even if one considered the nonworkers in the Kovno Ghetto to be singled out by the German order, they still cannot be seen as "deserving of death." On this basis, Rabbi Oshry declares that it appears to be forbidden to comply with the Germans' orders to distribute the cards.

Rabbi Oshry then goes on to consider the possible implications if all Jews in Kovno are sentenced to death. He points to the Germans' goal of exterminating all Jews, a scenario not directly addressed in the classic teachings on surrender. Rabbi Oshry writes, "It is possible to say that our case is not analogous to the law that obtains to specifying an individual for, according to the intentions of the wicked ones, may their memory be blotted out—they wanted to murder everyone, so now a suggestion appears to save some of them insofar as the permits are being issued and therefore collecting and distributing the tickets is a matter of saving [people]." We must note that many rabbinic authorities interpret Maimonides's teaching much like Rabbi Oshry, but it is not clear that Maimonides's ruling applies to cases where the murder of the entire group or community is possible. Indeed, Maimonides is addressing the situation discussed in the Palestinian Talmud where the price to be paid for noncompliance will be for all to be killed. "All" could refer to a large community, as well as a small group, but it is not clear how the teaching addresses mass murder or genocide, i.e. the murder of an entire people. Thus, it should be acknowledged that none of the precedents on surrender, including Maimonides's teaching, directly address a case with an enemy authority like the Nazis, whose intention and capacity was to exterminate the whole of the Jewish people.

There is nevertheless some question about the extent to which Rabbi Oshry's calculus here would have been disturbed by the knowledge, which he does not yet seem to have, that all Jews, workers or nonworkers, were scheduled to be murdered by the Nazis—some sooner, some later. This knowledge meant that every Jew is eligible for trade to the enemy, since his fate has been decided at Wannsee or even earlier.

It also renders the question of "whose blood is redder" irrelevant. And finally, it just about cancels the question of martyrdom—if everyone is sentenced to death, there may be no dying for a cause, and as Terrence Des Pres has pointed out, under such circumstances the highest goal is not dying for any cause but rather survival.[34]

Rabbi Oshry finds a final source of support for seeing the distribution of the cards as permissible by citing a decision given earlier by Rabbi Avraham Kahane Shapiro, the chief rabbi of Kovno, whom Rabbi Oshry would later replace after Rabbi Kahane Shapiro's death in February 1943. Rabbi Oshry writes of a case shortly after the German invasion in October 1941 when Rabbi Kahane Shapiro was asked by the members of the Jewish Council how they should respond to a

German decree ordering them to post signs in the ghetto announcing that all men, women, and children were to assemble for a selection whose likely outcome would be deportation and death. The Jewish Council went to Rabbi Kahane Shapiro to ask him how they should act according to the laws of the Torah.[35] Rabbi Kahane Shapiro told the Jewish Council that when the Jewish community is targeted for total destruction, and a means by which to save a portion of it emerges, then it becomes mandatory for the community's leaders to attempt to save as many people as possible.[36]

Rabbi Oshry thus concludes that the distribution of cards in this case similarly appears to be an act of saving. Like Rabbi Kahane Shapiro's decision, Rabbi Oshry's decision is that the Jewish Council is not only permitted but obligated to distribute the cards among the community.

In concluding from a very careful study of the major legal sources that the distribution of the cards is forbidden in one sense and required in another, Rabbi Oshry powerfully demonstrates the difficult if not impossible nature of the decision faced by the Jewish Councils. One way to interpret Rabbi Oshry's responsum is thus to conclude that since no guilty party has been identified among the victims of the Germans' orders, the classic rabbinic texts on surrender appear to require noncompliance with the German orders. On the other hand, the exceptional circumstances—the Germans' intent of extermination—demand compliance. According to this reading, Rabbi Oshry employs legal language to argue that distributing the cards is obligatory, calling it "an act of rescue," but he does not provide a conclusive argument to render the basic teaching on surrender or the principle of specification inapplicable. In the closing lines of his responsum, Rabbi Oshry concludes that it is difficult to determine if the principle of specification applies in this case, but given the undeniable fact that the intent of the Germans was total extermination of all of the Jews of Kovno, distribution of the cards is an act of rescue and is therefore obligatory.

A problem facing anyone reading or writing about the Shoah should be noted here: the temptation to assume with a measure of certainty what members of the Jewish community knew (or should have known) at the time about what was to come. It is hard to establish whether Rabbi Oshry and the members of the Kovno Jewish Council knew or believed at the time that the Germans' intention was total extermination of the entire Jewish population. Had they made such a deadly calculation, the questions surrounding the substitution of one life for another seem to disappear. Another way of putting this is to say that if all are condemned to death, then the life-for-life problem does not arise, as all are "sentenced to death." What then, we might ask, is the consequence of knowing that one's doom and the doom of one's community is inevitable? Does that mean you have no choices regarding the saving and surrendering of lives? Or does it mean that any choice to save or surrender made under the circumstances is permissible?[37]

Inadvertently Killing an Infant in a Bunker: The *Rodef*

The responsum we next turn to involves the loss of one life in order to save others. Unable to escape, many Jews in the ghettos created underground shelters referred to as "bunkers." These shelters were most commonly used to hide during Nazi selections and deportations, but they became more permanent places of refuge as the war progressed. The slightest noise could attract attention by the Nazis, and discovery often meant death for all of the bunker inhabitants.

There exist tragic cases of crying infants in bunkers who were sometimes smothered in order to avoid mortally endangering the group. After the war, Rabbi Shimon Efrati was approached by a man about such a case, in which a pillow was placed over the mouth of an infant who could not be consoled. The pillow was removed after the Nazis completed their search. The infant had died.

In his responsum, Rabbi Efrati asks, first, whether it was permissible to place a pillow over the infant's mouth in order to avoid detection, knowing that doing so might endanger the infant's life; and secondly, if it was not permissible, does the man who actually placed the pillow over the infant need to atone?[38]

In working on his responsum, Rabbi Efrati was deeply aware of just such an event. A group had been hiding in a bunker during a search when a baby burst out crying. Rabbi Efrati's brother, present with his family in the bunker, forbade anyone from stifling the child's cries, lest the child be harmed. All of the people hiding in the bunker, together with Rabbi Efrati's brother, Rabbi Yitchak Zvi Efrati, were discovered and murdered.[39]

In responding to the man who came to him after the war, Rabbi Efrati carefully analyzes if and when it might be permissible to act in such a way that to spare the life of a greater number, the lives of some may be jeopardized or taken. Rabbi Efrati's analysis of the rabbinic sources related to this case is extensive.[40] Most relevant for our purposes are his discussions of two major teachings of Maimonides: the first, the ruling on surrender, which we've already discussed, and then Maimonides's classic discussion of the *rodef*, "the pursuer."

In his ruling on surrender, Maimonides's emphasizes that it is very rare for a rabbinic authority to rule that the taking or surrendering of life is permissible. Only under two very narrow conditions, as Rabbi Efrati notes and as we discussed earlier, does Maimonides suggest that it may be permissible to surrender a person to an enemy authority: (1) if the individual is singled out by the enemy authority, and (2) if the individual is already guilty of a capital crime, and in this way, indicted and eligible for capital punishment.[41] Interpreting Maimonides's ruling carefully, Rabbi Efrati argues that it most clearly applies to a case in which, regardless of the action taken, one person will live and one person will die. Rabbi Efrati then argues that the situation in the bunker is precisely such a case. Since the infant would certainly be killed by the Nazis together with everybody in the bunker if its cries and voice are heard, then it is as if the Nazis singled the infant out. In this case, all of the Jews have been sentenced to death by the Nazis, and there is no possibility of being saved. Rabbi Efrati thus asks, "Why is it forbidden to surrender him?" If it is clear that noncompliance would result in the death of everyone, including the intended victim, there would be no logical reason to prohibit surrender.[42]

Rabbi Efrati could have let his decision rest on this interpretation of the principle of surrender, but he chooses to also engage in a large discussion of the *rodef* principle. According to Jewish law, one should not take pity on the life of the *rodef*—a pursuer who threatens life—if killing the *rodef* is necessary to spare innocent life, as Maimonides formulates the commandment concerning the *rodef*.[43] On the basis of this understanding of the *rodef*, rabbis have maintained that when serious complications arise and a pregnant woman cannot give birth, it is permitted to abort the fetus in her womb. The fetus, according to Maimonides, is like a *rodef* of its mother.

Rabbi Efrati accepts Maimonides's teaching on the *rodef* but draws an important distinction between a voluntary *rodef* and an involuntary *rodef*. The involuntary *rodef* is a pursuer under compulsion and whose threat can only be stopped by outside force. In the case of an involuntary *rodef*, a pursuer under compulsion, the *rodef* may be destroyed in order to save a life since without intervention both will die. The infant in the bunker classifies as a *rodef* under compulsion, since its cries will likely lead to the death of the other bunker inhabitants. In addition, the infant's life will also be taken as a result of its cries. Thus, Rabbi Efrati rules that in this case, since all including the infant would be killed, it is permitted to place the pillow over the infant. Despite the danger to the infant's life, it is a *rodef* under compulsion endangering the whole group, and so it is permissible to place the pillow over the infant's mouth so that the group may be spared.[44]

Rabbi Efrati concludes his analysis by comparing the two different teachings on which he based his decision—the surrender teaching, and the *rodef* teaching. He suggests that it would appear that Maimonides's ruling regarding surrender would permit the sacrifice of a life, whereas his ruling regarding the *rodef* would *require* the sacrifice of a life, since, according to Maimonides, one "does not spare the life of the pursuer."[45] The requirement to kill the pursuer applies only to a willful *rodef*, but in the case of this responsum, where the *rodef* is involuntarily endangering the group by its cries, killing the infant is permissible but not mandatory.[46] Thus, Rabbi Efrati ends his responsum by concluding that both principles would justify quieting the infant even at risk to its life and the person who did it need not have a guilty conscience. Rabbi Efrati adds that if those trapped in the bunker had refused to risk the life of the infant and were discovered because of its cries, they should be considered martyrs.[47] Rabbi Efrati thus aims to prevent an unfair judgment on those who in similar situations refused to silence the infant and were discovered and killed.

Rabbi Efrati's extension of the *rodef* principle to an unintentionally threatening presence is not unprecedented, but he is the first to extend the *rodef* label to an innocent infant. This extension raises an important ethical question not dealt with by Rabbi Efrati: Is it right to ever label an innocent person, with no intent to harm, a *rodef*?

We have emphasized throughout this chapter that the taking of a life is very rarely permitted in rabbinic judgments. Rabbi Efrati's responsum may thus appear as an exception, but it must be kept in mind that his responsum was issued after the fact. His judgment would not determine if a person's life would be surrendered; it would primarily determine if the person who had already surrendered the infant's life was guilty of a transgression. It is possible, then, that Rabbi Efrati sought to justify the action so those who survived could live with their conscience. Perhaps he would have taken an entirely different approach if his decision was going to determine whether a life would be surrendered.

The Ransoming of One Life for Another

One of the most troubling life-for-life problems that Jews faced during the Holocaust arose with the possibility of having to choose one person at the expense of another. In 1944, such a situation was brought to Rabbi Tzvi Hirsch Meisels[48] in Auschwitz, by a father considering whether he should try to ransom his son from the guards after a selection.

As we discussed in the introduction to this chapter, Rabbi Meisels describes in his responsum a "selection" on the eve of Rosh Hashanah in which some fourteen hundred boys of less than a certain height were singled out for death. As word spread through the camp that the boys selected would be taken to the gas chambers, some camp inmates sought to ransom particular boys by bribing the guards. However, because the guards would be murdered unless all fourteen hundred boys were turned over, the guards would not release any of the boys without seizing another to take his place.[49]

The father of one of the condemned boys, aware that his son could be ransomed only at the expense of another life, asked Rabbi Meisels whether Jewish law permitted such an action in this terrible circumstance. In his responsum, Rabbi Meisels first considers whether the guilt in taking another boy to replace the one ransomed would be on the guards rather than on the man who pays them for ransom. In addition, it was possible that the guards would consider the Jewish prohibition against murder and not take another life in place of the ransomed one. Despite this possibility, Rabbi Meisels tells the father that the guards would most likely seize another boy from the camp before releasing the ransomed prisoner, in order to maintain their quota and save themselves.

After seeing that this possible justification for ransoming the son could not be maintained, Rabbi Meisels tells the father that he cannot give a ruling in the case or tell him what he should do. Rabbi Meisels tells him, "I do not decide either yes or no. Do as you wish as if you had not asked me at all."[50] But the father continues to plead with Rabbi Meisels to give him an answer. Rabbi Meisels repeats to the father that he not ask him this question and adds that he could not answer without proper Jewish law texts in such an extreme situation. The father understood Rabbi Meisels's refusal to answer to mean that he could not permit him to ransom his son. As Rabbi Meisels records in his responsum, the father replied, "Rabbi, I did what I could, what the Torah obligated me to do: I asked a question of a rabbi, and there is no other rabbi here. Since you cannot answer me that I am allowed to ransom my child, this is a sign that according to the law you may not permit it. . . . This is enough for me . . . and I will accept this with love and rejoicing."[51]

Rabbi Meisels then records what the father did that day: "So he carried out his words and did not ransom his son. All that day of Rosh Hashanah he walked around talking to himself, murmuring joyfully that he had the merit to sacrifice his only son to God . . . like the binding of Isaac."[52]

The question brought to Rabbi Meisels, in contrast with those brought to Rabbi Oshry and Rabbi Efrati, was a current matter of life and death in a moment of terrible extremis. Also in contrast to Rabbi Efrati and Rabbi Oshry, when Rabbi Meisels was asked this question by a fellow prisoner at Auschwitz, he had no access to sources or other rabbis to consult or the time or calm needed to issue a carefully considered decision.

What is most distinctive in Rabbi Meisels's responsum is thus his admission that he could not give a decision in this case. Far from shirking his duty, Rabbi Meisels acts from his conviction that he could not tell the father that he should or shouldn't allow his son to be killed. There is precedent that may support Rabbi Meisels's refusal to give the father an answer. While it is a positive commandment for a qualified rabbinic scholar to render decisions when asked, the great rabbinic authority Rashi ruled that it is forbidden to do so while intoxicated or otherwise disoriented.[53] It seems reasonable to consider that the circumstances facing Rabbi Meisels when the father approached him that day at Auschwitz left him sufficiently disoriented, as he indicates in his response to the father.

Rabbi Meisels's responsum thus points to limits that even a rabbi must recognize in determining what is in accordance with Jewish law, as difficult as this may be for the rabbi and the one bringing the question. Rabbi Meisels's responsum thus provides us with a window into the enormous task the rabbis were faced with, the great piety of those who came to the rabbis with their questions, and the compassion that guided the rabbis in issuing their decisions.

Conclusion: Rabbinic Responsa and Spiritual Resistance

Before concluding, we must pause to remember that very few written responsa from the Holocaust have survived. Many of the rabbis who did manage to give decisions during the Holocaust, a number that is difficult to quantify, were murdered. Nevertheless, the Holocaust-era responsa handed down to us comprise a precious record of the Jewish experience under Nazi rule: how the rabbis and their communities viewed the catastrophe as it occurred, how they responded, how they searched for precedents to a persecution whose magnitude was unprecedented, how they brought to bear the weight of Jewish law and tradition in an attempt to impose on the chaos some semblance of order, and how, afterward, they worked to recover from the decimation of their people. The responsa also demonstrate that employing the value structures of the Torah during the Jewish people's darkest hour provided context and coherence to the victims when nothing else did or could.

To provide witness of how rabbis, members of the Jewish Councils, and ordinary Jews responded to Nazi rule, the responsa give us a firsthand look at what many Jews did to preserve the physical and spiritual health of the Jewish community. Study of the responsa thus adds powerful support to our understanding that Jews were not merely passive victims or "like lambs going to the slaughter," and confirms that they acted with courage and strength to resist the Nazi assault on their way of being, much as Jews had done for millennia while living under oppressive rule.

The responsa also bring to light the solace found in discovering that even when there were no clear answers to the dilemmas that confronted the Jewish community, the Torah could nevertheless provide guidance. Of ultimate significance to many Jews, before and during the Holocaust, was the standard of conduct demanded by Jewish law. Their dignity lay in their relationship to God and to the Jewish community, expressed in day-to-day conduct, which Nazi rule could never fully control even in the ghettos and camps. By continuing to look to Jewish law to guide them, many Jews were able to somewhat sidestep the Nazi attack on the ways of Jewish life that had endured for centuries and continue to endure.[54] This abiding adherence to Jewish law and Jewish communal life, in defiance of Nazi prohibitions, should be understood as a form of active, though unarmed, resistance, perhaps in its ultimate form. As Rabbi Oshry stated in an interview with the *New York Times* in 1975, "One resists with a gun, another with his soul."[55]

Acknowledgments

We would like to acknowledge Rabbi Douglass Kahn for sharing with us his doctoral dissertation completed at Hebrew Union College–Jewish Institute of

Religion, a very careful study of life-for-life issues in Holocaust responsa. We also offer our thanks to the faculty of the Elie Wiesel Center for Jewish Studies at Boston University, and the center's director, Michael Zank, in particular, for long-standing support of our work on the responsa and of graduate student research.

Johnathan I. Kelly is a PhD candidate in religious studies at Boston University and the graduate student research associate for the Project on Ethics and the Holocaust at Boston University's Elie Wiesel Center for Jewish Studies.

Erin L. Miller, MPH, is an MD candidate at New York University Long Island School of Medicine. Previously, Erin was senior research associate for the Project on Ethics and the Holocaust at Boston University's Elie Wiesel Center for Jewish Studies. As an MPH student at the Boston University School of Public Health, she concentrated in maternal and child health with an emphasis on reproductive justice and reducing maternal morbidity.

Rabbi Joseph Polak, a child survivor of two Nazi concentration camps, is the chief justice of the Rabbinical Court of Massachusetts and adjunct associate professor of health law at the Boston University School of Public Health. His memoir, *After the Holocaust the Bells Still Ring* (Urim, 2015), won the National Jewish Book Award and is scheduled to appear in a Hebrew translation being prepared by Yad Vashem. For almost half a century he was a university chaplain, mostly at Boston University.

Robert Kirschner is the author of *Rabbinic Responsa of the Holocaust Era* (Schocken, 1985) and *Baraita de-Melekhet ha-Mishkan: A Critical Edition with Introduction and Translation* (Hebrew Union College Press, 1992). His articles have appeared in *Journal for the Study of Judaism*, *Journal of Semitic Studies*, *Encyclopedia Judaica*, and *Encyclopedia of the Bible and Its Reception*.

Michael A. Grodin, MD, is professor of health law, bioethics, and human rights at the Boston University School of Public Health, and professor and director of the Project on Ethics and the Holocaust at the Elie Wiesel Center for Jewish Studies. Dr. Grodin has served on national and international commissions focusing on medical ethics, human rights, and the Holocaust. He has received a special citation from the United State Holocaust Memorial Museum for "profound contributions—through original and creative research—to the cause of Holocaust education and remembrance," and is the author of over two hundred articles and the editor or coeditor of seven books.

Notes

This chapter was adapted from Grodin et al. 2019.

1. The text of the Germans' labor card order is preserved in the diary kept by Avraham Tory, the secretary of the Kovno Jewish Council. See Tory's entry for 15 September 1941 in Tory 1991. For more information on how the dilemma of the cards was eventually handled by the council, see Tory's entry for 4 October 1941 and the editor's endnotes, pp. 37–39.
2. Tory 1991, 36.
3. Rabbi Oshry discusses the order to distribute the labor cards in his memoir of the ghetto years. See Oshry 1995, 49. He also gives a detailed account of the labor card situation in a rabbinic ruling (responsa) we discuss in detail later in this chapter. See Oshry 1949, no. 1. Our discussion of Rabbi Oshry's responsa in this chapter is based, in part, on Robert Kirschner's unpublished English translations of a selection of Rabbi Oshry's responsa. Currently, the best source in English related to Rabbi Oshry's responsa is the collection of synopses of his responsa published in Oshry 2001.
4. Kirschner 1985, 1:7–9.
5. For a helpful history and overview of the responsa genre, see Ta-Shma 2007.
6. Extensive scholarly studies in English of Holocaust-era responsa include Guttmann 1975; Rosenbaum 1976; Zimmels 1977; Kirschner 1985; Farbstein 2007; Stern 2016. For a concise overview of Holocaust responsa literature, on which our account here builds upon, see Kirschner 2007.
7. The question of how much authentic history can be extrapolated from rabbinic responsa has been pursued by Jewish scholars since the Crusades. For a detailed discussion of treating responsa as historical sources, see Soloveitchik 1990, and his earlier essay, Soloveitchik 1978. In his doctoral dissertation, Moshe Tarshansky treats in detail the question of the historical status of Rabbi Oshry's collection of responsa. See Tarshansky 2016.
8. The sermons and diaries composed by rabbis are an equally important set of texts for understanding Jewish life during the Holocaust, and they have been the subject of much broader study than the responsa. Perhaps most well-known are the set of sermons and Torah commentaries that Rabbi Kalonymus Kalman Shapira gave in the Warsaw ghetto after the deaths of his son and his mother. For an English translation of Rabbi Shapira's texts, see Miller 2002. For an excellent exploration of Rabbi Shapira's life and texts, see Polen 2004.
9. Jewish religious life remained prominent throughout the ghetto years despite being a special target of persecution and destruction by the Nazis and their collaborators. Indeed, continued clandestine existence of religious life in the ghettos stood as a profound center of resistance for the Jewish community in part because religious Jews were singled out by having all forms of Jewish religious life forbidden to them. In addition to closing down all houses of worship, study, prayer, and ritual cleansing and prohibiting all religious gatherings, the Germans and their collaborators made religious Jews the most vulnerable to anti-Jewish persecution and violence.

As Rabbi Oshry and members of the Kovno Jewish Council recorded in their memoirs, Kovno's rabbis maintained good, active relations with the underground movement in Kovno, with the partisans, and with the community at large. A similar pattern can be traced throughout the ghettos, where the Jewish councils, the resistance, and individual Jews looked to rabbis for leadership and advice, and for comfort and a listening ear for their uncertainty, pain, and grief. Much as before, the rabbis continued to lead, sustain, and give hope to the Jewish community with courage and integrity.

10. See, more generally, Rosen 2019.
11. For a wide-ranging collection of essays on Jewish physicians and underground medical care in the ghettos and camps, see Grodin 2014.
12. See Kelly, Miller, and Grodin 2017.
13. See Kirschner 1985.
14. It is also worth considering particular cases like the one of the Kovno Jewish Council, where the doctor Elchanan Elkes was unanimously elected as head of the Jewish Council and conducted

himself with utmost integrity and fairness throughout the ghetto years, according to all accounts. A prominent physician in Kovno prior to the war, Elkes clearly brought his vocation as a doctor to bear on his term as head of the council. Although we have not been able to find in Elkes's letters a description of the very difficult series of decisions he and the council had to make, there is no question that he dealt with utmost care and rigor the set of difficult life-for-life problems faced by the council, as Tory and Rabbi Oshry attest in their accounts. For more about Elkes, see Elkes 1999.

15. Two important, far-reaching scholarly studies on the problem of surrender in Jewish law and the major analytic and interpretive questions involved are Daube 1965 and Schochet 1973. Both books contain excellent discussions of all the relevant legal sources, including numerous responsa and commentaries that have dealt with similar situations throughout Jewish history.

16. For a broad overview of the life-for-life problem in Jewish law and complex discussions of many problems in contemporary medical ethics, see Dorff 1998.

17. In the Jewish tradition, human beings are created in God's image, making human life sacred and necessitating protection. The principle of *pikuach nefesh* expresses this view of the importance of human life and thus requires the preservation of life to take precedence over nearly all other commandments. The principle of *pikuach nefesh* is derived from Leviticus 18:5: "Keep my decrees and laws, since it is only by keeping them that a person can [truly] live." This verse has been interpreted as a general principle that one should live by the commandments, but not die by them. As a consequence, concerning all prohibitions in the Torah, the law is that if one is told, "Transgress such-and-such a prohibition and you will not be killed, but if you refuse to do so, we will kill you," one should transgress the prohibition and not allow oneself to be killed, except when one is told to engage in idol worship, illicit relations, or murder. For more on *pikuach nefesh* see, "Pikku'ah Nefesh" 2007.

18. Rabbi Oshry discusses each of these questions and the circumstances under which they were brought to him in Oshry 2001. For a broader list of questions brought to Rabbi Oshry and other rabbis, see Kirschner 2007. The most extensive collection of Holocaust-era responsa in print is Levine 2002. In English translation, the most extensive collection of Holocaust-era responsa is Kirschner 1985.

19. See Oshry 1959–76 (5 vols.). Rabbi Oshry's first collection of Holocaust-era responsa is published in Oshry 1949.

20. The Slobodka Yeshiva, where the captured students had been studying, was one of the greatest centers of Jewish learning in Europe, the home of many of the greatest scholars and rabbis of the time. Only a few years earlier, Rabbi Oshry himself had been a student at Slobodka. For Rabbi Oshry's account of Slobodka and other yeshivas in Kovno, see Oshry 1995.

21. Oshry 1995, 21.

22. Oshry 1963. Our discussion of Rabbi Oshry's responsum relies on Robert Kirschner's unpublished English translations of a selection Rabbi Oshry's responsa, as noted above.

23. *Babylonian Talmud*, Sanhedrin 73a. Throughout this chapter, we rely on the texts and English translation of the *Schottenstein Edition of the Talmud* 1994 for our citation of texts in the *Babylonian Talmud* and *Jerusalem Talmud*.

24. *Babylonian Talmud*, Sanhedrin 73a.

25. *Babylonian Talmud*, Sanhedrin 74a.

26. *Babylonian Talmud*, Sanhedrin 74a.

27. The Christian notion of martyrdom (derived from the Greek term for "witness") can be compared with the principle in Judaism known as *Kiddush Hashem*, "sanctification of the Divine name," a general principle in Judaism but which has been given particular application to one who gives up their life rather than give up Jewish law or identity. Throughout the Jewish tradition, any action that brings honor to God's name, including martyrdom, is considered *Kiddush Hashem*. The three cardinal sins in Judaism—idolatry, murder, and forbidden sexual relations—require one to give up one's life rather than violate, thereby upholding *Kiddush Hashem*. For more information on *Kiddush Hashem* see, Lamm and Ben-Sasson 2007, 139–45.

28. Epstein 1884, 426:4.

29. Oshry 1995. See the records for D. Itzkowitz, "The Yad Vashem Central Database of Shoah Victims' Names," retrieved 4 October 2018 from https://yvng.yadvashem.org.

30. Oshry 1949.

31. As was the case throughout the ghettos, after the Germans occupied Kovno and established a ghetto they ordered the formation of the *Judenrat*, a "council of elders." Like other Jewish councils (*Judenrate*) the Kovno Jewish Council was held responsible for implementing Nazi orders and organizing basic services in the ghetto. For a brief overview of the structure and activities of the Kovno Jewish Council, see the introduction in Gilbert 1992.

32. *Palestinian Talmud, Terumot* 47a.

33. Maimonides 1989.

34. See Des Pres 1976, in particular the chapter "Excremental Assault."

35. For a more detailed account of the circumstances surrounding the order for all the Jews of Kovno to assemble, see Zimmels 1977, 50–51.

36. Also see Rabbi Oshry's account of Rabbi Kahane Shapiro's decision in Oshry 1995, 61.

37. Among the most thoughtful and important studies of this issue is Bernstein 1994. In a wide-ranging discussion of Holocaust historiography and of representations of the Holocaust in literature, Michael Andre Bernstein brings to light the ways that many writings on the Holocaust are controlled by the tendency of what he calls "backshadowing." In Bernstein's account, backshadowing is "a kind of retroactive foreshadowing in which the shared knowledge of the outcome of a series of events by narrator and listener is used to judge the participants in those events as though they too should have known what was to come" (Bernstein 1994, 16). In addition to distorting or simply ignoring the historical position of European Jews at the time, backshadowing operates according to the judgment that the Jews of Nazi-occupied Europe should have known that destruction was inevitable and should thus have acted otherwise than they did. The alternative to backshadowing, for Bernstein, is not to blind ourselves to what was to come but to refuse "to see the future as pre-ordained; and, as a direct corollary, not to use our knowledge of the future as a means of judging the decisions of those living before that (still only possible) future became actual event" (Bernstein 1994, 16).

38. Efrati 1961, in Kirschner 1985, 65–87.

39. Kirschner 1985, 66.

40. For a helpful synopsis of the major points of interpretation in Rabbi Efrati's responsum, see Kirschner 1985, 66–68.

41. Maimonides 1989.

42. Efrati 1961, in Kirschner 1985.

43. Maimonides 2000.

44. Kirschner 1985, 80.

45. Kirschner 1985, 81.

46. Kirschner 1985, 81.

47. Kirschner 1985, 81.

48. Rabbi Tzvi Hirsch Meisels (1902–74) was the chief rabbi of Veitzen, Hungary, before being deported in Auschwitz in 1944. There his wife and seven children were brutally murdered. See Kirschner 1985, 111.

49. Meisels 1955, in Kirschner 1985, 113–14. As noted in Kirschner 1985, at the trial of Adolf Eichmann in Jerusalem, Joseph Kleinman gave testimony about a selection at Auschwitz that bears many similarities to the account given by Rabbi Efrati. According to Kleinman, on Yom Kippur in 1944, all two thousand boys at the camp were ordered to gather at a soccer field at 3:00 p.m. that afternoon. After the boys were gathered at the field, Dr. Josef Mengele, the SS doctor infamous for his experiments on prisoners at Auschwitz, arrived on a bicycle and then proceeded to angrily grab one of the boys, one who had told Mengele he was eighteen years old, and march him to the goalpost on the field. Mengele then told a guard to nail a plank into the goalpost to line up with the top of the boy's head. Once the plank was nailed into the goalpost, Mengele gave orders for all of the boys to be lined up and then walk single file toward the post, with those whose heads passed under without

touching the plank to be separated from the rest. It was clear to all the boys that those who were too short for their heads to reach the plank would be killed. See Kleinman's testimony in State of Israel Ministry of Justice 1992–95: Session 68 (Part 2 of 9).

50. Kirschner 1985, 118.
51. Kirschner 1985, 118.
52. Kirschner 1985, 118.
53. For more information on the duty to render a decision, see Kirschner 1985, 122n8.
54. We discuss in more detail the acts of spiritual resistance by Jews who continued to follow Jewish law, celebrate the Jewish holidays, and maintain a flourishing religious life in Kelly, Miller, and Grodin 2017.
55. Shanker 1985, 33.

References

Babylonian Talmud: Tractate Sanhedrin. 1994. Translated by Asher Dicker and Michael Weiner. Edited by Hersh Goldwurm. Brooklyn: Artscroll Mesorah Publications.

Berenbaum, Michael. 2007. "Elkes, Elhanan." In *Encyclopaedia Judaica*, 2nd ed., vol. 3, edited by M. Berenbaum and F. Skolnik, 358–59. Detroit: Macmillan Reference USA.

Bernstein, Michael Andre. 1994. *Foregone Conclusions: Against Apocalyptic History*. Berkeley: University of California Press.

Daube, David. 1965. *Collaboration with Tyranny in Rabbinic Law*. Oxford: Oxford University Press.

Des Pres, Terrence. 1976. *The Survivor: An Anatomy of Life in the Death Camps*. Oxford: Oxford University Press.

Dorff, Elliot N. 1998. *Matters of Life and Death: A Jewish Approach to Modern Medical Ethics*. Philadelphia: Jewish Publication Society.

Efrati, Shimon. 1961. *Mi-Gei ha-Haregah*, no. 1. Translated by Robert Kirschner as "Whether a Jew in hiding from the Germans in a ghetto bunker must repent for inadvertently smothering a crying infant to avoid detection." In Robert Kirschner (ed.). 1985. *Rabbinic Responsa of the Holocaust Era*, 65–87. New York: Schocken Books.

Elkes, Joel. 1999. *Dr. Elkhanan Elkes of the Kovno Ghetto: A Son's Holocaust Memoir*. Brewster, MA: Paraclete Press

Epstein, Yechiel Michal. 1884. *Aruch Hasulchan, Choshen Mishpat* 426: 4.

Farbstein, Esther. 2007. *Hidden in Thunder: Perspectives on Faith, Halachah and Leadership During the Holocaust*. Spring Valley, NY: Feldheim Publishers.

Gilbert, Martin. 1992. "Introduction." In *Surviving the Holocaust: The Kovno Ghetto Diary*. Cambridge: Harvard University Press.

Grodin, Michael (ed.). 2014. *Jewish Medical Resistance in the Holocaust*. New York: Berghahn Books.

Grodin, Michael, Johnathan I. Kelly, Erin L. Miller, Robert Kirschner, and Joseph Polak. 2019. "Rabbinic Responsa and Spiritual Resistance during the Holocaust: The Life-for-Life Problem." *Modern Judaism—A Journal of Jewish Ideas and Experience* 39(3): 296–325.

Guttmann, Alexander. 1975. "Human Insights of the Rabbis Particularly with Respect to the Holocaust." *Hebrew Union College Annual* (46): 433–55.

Itzkowitz, D. "The Yad Vashem Central Database of Shoah Victims' Names." Retrieved 4 October 2018 from https://yvng.yadvashem.org.

Katz, Biderman, and Gershon Greenberg (eds.). 2007. *Wrestling with God: Jewish Theological Responses during and after the Holocaust*. New York: Oxford University Press.

Kelly, Johnathan, Erin Miller, and Michael Grodin. 2017. "Resistance or Complicity: Medical and Religious Responses to Law under the Third Reich." In *Nazi Law: From Nuremberg to Nuremberg*, edited by J. Michalczyk. New York: Bloomsbury Academic.

Kirschner, Robert (ed.). 1985. *Rabbinic Responsa of the Holocaust Era*. New York: Schocken Books.
———. 2007. "Holocaust: Responses, the Holocaust and the Halakhah." In *Encyclopaedia Judaica*, 2nd ed., vol. 9, edited by M. Berenbaum and F. Skolnik, 362–64. Detroit: Macmillan Reference USA.
Lamm, Norman, and Haim Hillel Ben-Sasson. 2007. "Kiddush Ha-Shem and Hillul Ha-Shem." In *Encyclopaedia Judaica*, 2nd ed., vol. 12, edited by M. Berenbaum and F. Skolnik, 139–45. Detroit: Macmillan Reference USA.
Levine, Itamar. 2002. *Otiot Shel Esh: Eduyiot Mitkufat Hashoa Misifrut Hilkhatit*. Tel Aviv: Yedioth Ahronoth.
Maimonides, Moses. 1989. *Mishneh Torah, Hilchot Yesodei HaTorah* [The laws which are the foundations of the Torah], 5:5. Translated by Eliyah Touger. Brooklyn: Moznaim Publishing.
———. 2000. "Sefer ha-Mitzvot, no. 293." *Maimonides: The Commandments, The 613 Mitzvoth of the Torah Elucidated in English*. Translated by Charles B. Chavel. New York: Judaica Press.
Meisels, Tzvi Hirsch. 1955. *Mekaddeshei ha-Shem*. Translated by Robert Kirschner. In Robert Kirschner (ed.). 1985. *Rabbinic Responsa of the Holocaust Era*, 113–21. New York: Schocken Books.
Miller, Deborah (ed.). 2002. *Sacred Fire: Torah from the Years of Fury 1939–1942*. Translated by J. Hershy Worch. New York: Jacob Aronson.
Oshry, Ephraim. 1949. *Divrei Ephraim*. New York: self-published.
———. 1959–76. *She'elot u-teshuvot mi-ma'amakim*. 5 vols. New York: self-published.
———. 1963. *She'elot u-teshuvot mi-ma'amakim*. Vol. 2. New York: self-published.
———. 1995. *The Annihilation of Lithuanian Jewry*. Translated by Y. Leiman. New York: Judaica Press.
———. 2001. *Responsa from the Holocaust*. Edited by Y. Leiman. New York: Judaica Press.
"Pikku'ah Nefesh." 2007. *Encyclopaedia Judaica*. Vol. 16, 2nd ed., 152–53. Detroit: Macmillan Reference USA.
Polen, Nehemia. 2004. *The Holy Fire: The Teachings of Rabbi Kalonymus Kalman Shapira, the Rebbe of the Warsaw Ghetto*. New York: Rowman and Littlefield.
Rosen, Alan. 2019. *The Holocaust's Jewish Calendars: Keeping Time Sacred, Making Time Holy*. Bloomington: Indiana University Press.
Rosenbaum, Irving. 1976. *The Holocaust and Halakhah*. New York: Ktav.
Schochet, Elijah J. 1973. *A Responsum of Surrender*. Los Angeles: University of Judaism Press.
Shanker, Israel L. 1985. "Responsa: The Law as Seen By Rabbis for 1,000 Years." *New York Times*, 5 May.
Soloveitchik, Haym. 1978. "Can Halakhic Texts Talk History?" *AJS Review* 3: 153–96.
———. 1990. *The Use of Responsa as Historical Source: A Methodological Introduction*. Jerusalem: Hebrew University Press. [Hebrew].
State of Israel Ministry of Justice. 1992–95. *The Trial of Adolf Eichmann: Record of Proceedings in the District Court of Jerusalem*. Session 68 (Part 2 of 9). Jerusalem: Trust for the Publication of the Proceedings of the Eichmann Trial, in cooperation with the Israel State Archives and Yad Vashem, the Holocaust Martyrs' and Heroes' Remembrance Authority.
Stern, Nehemia. 2016. "To Sanctify the Name of God: Ritual Precision and Martyrdom in Rabbi Ephraim Oshry's Holocaust Responsa." *Holocaust Studies* 22(1): 100–124.
Tarshansky, Moshe. 2016. "The Communal Activity of Rabbi Ephraim Oshry and the Importance of His Responsa *Mimaamakim* for the Development of a Religious Historiographical Narrative of the Holocaust." PhD diss., Bar-Ilan University. [Hebrew].
Ta-Shma, Israel Moses, Shlomo Tal, and Menahem Slae. 2007. "Responsa." In *Encyclopaedia Judaica*, 2nd ed., vol. 17, edited by M. Berenbaum and F. Skolnik, 228–39. Detroit: Macmillan Reference USA.
Tory, Avraham. 1991. *Surviving the Holocaust: The Kovno Ghetto Diary*. Edited by Martin Gilbert. Translated by Jerzy Michalowicz. Cambridge: Harvard University Press.
Yad Vashem Central Database of Shoah Victims' Names. https://yvng.yadvashem.org.
Zimmels, Hirsch Jacob. 1977. *The Echo of the Nazi Holocaust in Rabbinic Literature*. New York: Ktav.

CHAPTER 5

Un(b)earable
Pregnant Bodies and Obstetrical Genocide

Annette Finley-Croswhite

Atrocities involving assault on pregnant women, sterilization, forced abortion, and infanticide reflect specific gendered violence meted out to Jewish women during the Holocaust. The literature exploring the Nazi attack on Jewish wombs, however, is underdeveloped, especially in scholarship not specifically focused on women's studies, and detailed research into estimates for the number of Jewish lives aborted under duress, killed at birth, or shot or gassed in utero have never been undertaken. Jewish law further complicates the discussion of pregnancy and the Holocaust because it subordinates the fetus to the mother and assigns no identity to the child before it is born, even while disapproving of causing it deliberate harm. Evidence exists showing that the Nazi assault on Jewish reproduction involved targeting the pregnant body, meaning that Jewish women obtained abortions out of instincts for self-preservation and that Jewish healthcare specialists performed abortions in order to save Jewish women's lives. Many women suffered post-traumatic stress long afterward, while some survivors were permanently damaged and later unable to conceive or bear children.[1]

This chapter explores the assault on the Jewish pregnant body during the Holocaust and attempts some statistical analysis of deaths *in utero* or infants killed at birth. It does not engage in a moral debate about abortion but conceptualizes the elimination of the pregnant body as an intrinsic part of Nazi medical genocide that Jewish legal experts were subsequently called on to explore. Indeed, it argues that the Jewish womb was a "Holocaust landscape," another kind of killing field where the murderous Final Solution was deployed.[2] Finally, it recognizes the role of Jewish pregnant women and their caregivers not only as resisters to Nazi aggression but also as conveyers of humane treatment in the worst possible situations.[3]

A Specific Kind of Horror

Pregnant women during the Holocaust experienced a specific kind of horror that is not well recognized in the standard Holocaust narrative. Author Beverly Chalmers articulates that the direct means of killing Jews either by bullets, starvation, disease, gas chambers, or torture have been exhaustively covered in Holocaust literature, but the same cannot be said for the more indirect ways the Nazis pursued to eliminate Jewish reproductive lives.[4] These indirect means targeted the Jewish womb in a number of ways; the sterilization experiments in the camps in the 1940s were just one example revealed further in the wide range of consequences pregnant women experienced during the Holocaust, which sent some straight to the gas chambers or forced others to abort in order to save their lives in the camps, ghettos, or hiding places.[5] To annihilate the Jewish people, it was necessary for the Final Solution to emphasize an attack on the Jewish womb as the embodiment of worldwide Jewry. The womb was a killing field, an interior landscape where potential Jewish life was formed, and its destruction not only created another bloody battleground on which the Holocaust was fought but also affected seriously the demographic realities of Jewish people for generations to come. Adolf Eichmann believed that by destroying all Jewry in the East, world Jewry in general would never recover.[6]

Historian Tim Cole refers to the Holocaust as a multiscalar event.[7] The attack on the Jewish womb aimed at complete obliteration of the Jewish population; the womb associated with life became a key site of Jewish destruction. Nazi leaders envisioned a future world populated almost exclusively by those they determined to be of the Aryan race, and to create this specific demographic reality, Jewish childbearing had to cease. Historian Zoë Waxman states, "Simply put, for Jewish women becoming pregnant was a criminal offense."[8] Pregnant women were viewed as a threat to Nazi goals of total Jewish annihilation, and, as such, policies were developed to employ gynecological genocide, denying Jewish men and women reproductive lives. For the Jewish man, entering the interior landscape of the Jewish woman was fraught with danger, for if pregnancy resulted the mother might be killed. In many instances, a pregnant woman's husband, family, and/or doctor faced death as well. Policies involving mandatory abortion or sterilization and the destruction of newborns became a regular part of ghetto and camp life during the Holocaust.[9]

Attacks on reproduction had begun in Germany long before the Nazis came to power, however, and were rooted in nineteenth-century social Darwinism, the eugenics movement, and a concept called racial hygiene devised to purify German society by preventing the procreation of persons deemed inferior. To ensure a healthy *Volkskörper* (political body of the German people), German scientists advocated sterilization for members of the gene pool with physical or mental impairments. Once the Nazis took control, they passed the Law for the Prevention of Hereditarily Diseased Offspring in 1933, which led to the sterilization of persons with various real and imagined disorders as well as the establishment of Genetic Health Courts to adjudicate who could and could not procreate. The Nuremberg Laws enacted in 1935 prohibited marriage or sexual intercourse between Aryans and Jews. During the very same period, the Nazis promoted "positive eugenics" to encourage German women to produce as many healthy children as possible. Abortion was further criminalized for Aryan women unless a pregnancy was identified as "defective."[10]

Attempts to "cleanse" German society through racial hygiene initiatives resulted in the sterilization of some four hundred thousand men, women, and children between 1933 and 1939, inclusive of many determined to be racially inferior such as the Jews, Sinti, and Roma, or persons of mixed race.[11] By 1939 the T4 program was in place, a project that used sterilization and euthanasia to ensure that people the Nazis considered "life unworthy of life" were either rendered unable to reproduce or were killed, a process that psychiatrist and author Robert Jay Lifton calls the "forerunner of mass murder."[12] During the war the attack on reproduction was further weaponized when SS leader Heinrich Himmler charged gynecologist Carl Clauberg in 1942 to devise an effective method of mass sterilization. At Birkenau in Sector BIa, Barrack 30, Block 10 at the Auschwitz main camp, and later at Ravensbrück near the end of the war, Clauberg used chemical irritants and X-rays on the fallopian tubes of hundreds of women, including at least 350 Jewish women from Holland and Germany. Most died of complications, and those who survived were left permanently damaged, their ovaries and other reproductive organs having been removed. At the height of Clauberg's experiments, he envisioned being able to sterilize over one thousand women a day, fulfilling the Nazi ideal of transforming Jewish wombs into barren landscapes. Many studies exist of the work of Clauberg and that of Horst Schumann, who conducted sterilization experiments on male prisoners at Auschwitz as part of the broader Nazi attack on Jewish reproduction.[13] This chapter, nevertheless, focuses specifically on pregnancy, childbirth, and, most significantly, abortion, a procedure that physician and scholar Tessa Chelouche calls a "weapon of mass destruction."[14] It privileges the lesser-known voices and experiences of Jewish female victims over the well-documented voices and research of German male perpetrators.

Multiple Silences

Explanations for the silence surrounding the attack on Jewish wombs are obvious. The post-Holocaust narrative began at a time when women's history and feminist theory were in their infancy, and as such women's experiences are addressed less often in Holocaust literature than men's experiences. Early Holocaust scholars also shied away from differentiating male and female Holocaust suffering, fearing that to do so would diminish Jewish victimization overall by privileging female experiences.[15] Since Jewish wombs were targeted on the ramp at camps like Auschwitz-Birkenau, moreover, by sending pregnant mothers straight to the gas chambers, many pregnant victims did not live to tell their stories, and those who did often repressed their experiences or refused to share them out of guilt or post-traumatic stress. Jewish victims conducted or experienced abortions in secrecy, thus reducing the numbers of people aware of these procedures. The Nazis banned births in the Shavli Ghetto in Lithuania, for example, in 1942, but even efforts to warn pregnant women were concealed carefully so that according to a member of the ghetto *Judenrat*, the matter did not "reach ears that should not hear it."[16] Scholars also often purposefully overlook difficult narratives tied to gender. As recently as 2010, the eminent Holocaust scholar Christopher Browning explained that in exploring testimonies from the Starachowice slave labor camps in Poland, he felt uncomfortable discussing survivor experiences with "childbirth, infanticide, abortion, sex, and rape."[17] He calls this lacuna "a chapter that cannot be adequately written."[18] Refusal to explore gender-specific destruction, however, underestimates the totality of Nazi genocidal agency. Philosopher and historian Joan Ringelheim explains that when gender is made irrelevant, the results are "'ignored memories' which eventually also turn into forgotten memories."[19] As a result, multiple silences surround the subjects of abortion and deaths in utero during the Holocaust. This chapter thus seeks to join other works published in the last two decades that attempt to place gendered violence and specifically obstetrical genocide at the center of Holocaust discussion, especially in light of the frequency with which it occurred.[20] Pregnancy narratives force us to acknowledge the gender-based decisions Jewish women had to make in their fight for survival.

Abortion: A Question of Jewish Law

The Holocaust presented challenges to Halakhah or Jewish law. Rabbis were thus forced to confront and respond to particular questions during the Holocaust, including abortion. Abortion in Jewish law, while complex, is not considered murder, and as a result there are situations in which abortion is not only permitted but sometimes mandated.[21] Jewish legal scholars have incorporated the reality of particular Holocaust situations into their various opinions. Even so, many Holocaust scholars perceive a conflict between abortion and Jewish law, or they prefer to ignore the issue altogether in order to avoid enmeshing Holocaust history with contemporary abortion debates.[22] While participating in a seminar at a prestigious Holocaust research center in 2011, an eminent scholar warned the author of this chapter away from the abortion issue and what was perceived as the unwanted politicization of Holocaust history. At times, discussion of abortion and

Holocaust has led to angry exchanges at academic conferences and between colleagues emphasizing the taboo nature of the subject in general. Graduate students have also been advised that pursuing the topic could have negative career ramifications.[23] Moreover, for contemporary halakhic scholars and Jewish medical ethicists, especially among the Orthodox, the acceptability of when abortion is condoned remains a central point of conflict, past and present, a moral debate in which consensus is challenging.[24] Both inside and outside academia, therefore, abortion during the Holocaust is a controversial subject.

Judaism recognizes the sanctity of life and privileges procreation as a mitzvah, but halakhic law does not define life as beginning at conception. The only biblical reference to abortion occurs in Exodus 21:22–25 when a man strikes a pregnant woman and accidentally causes her to abort. In this situation, if the woman is unharmed, the scripture indicates, the man is simply fined, and the action only becomes a capital crime if the woman loses her life. The scripture thus establishes a clear distinction between the woman and the fetus and implies that killing the fetus is not murder.[25]

Jewish law, furthermore, does not identify a fetus as a living being before it is born; it is a potential life and should not be harmed, although exceptions are possible. The distinction is that the mother is a *nefesh*, a living being, while the fetus is not and cannot be before the greater part of its body has emerged from the birth canal. The Sanhedrin 72b specifically refers to the head coming out of the mother's body as the moment that denotes *nefesh* status on the child. This distinction is critical, because halakhic scholars reference the Talmud as permitting abortion in order to save a mother's life, but only so long as the child has not been born. "Once the fetus has emerged it has the same status as the mother and then, even if it threatens the mother's life, it may not be touched."[26] According to Jewish law, one life cannot be more valuable than another.[27]

To advance the argument further, halakhic scholars recognize the legitimacy of abortion if the fetus threatens the life of the mother or could damage her health, either physically or mentally. Her life is more important because she is a person and the fetus is not.[28] She has legal status, while the fetus is only a potential person with no legal standing. In the second-century Mishnah (*Oholot* 7:6) the fetus is subordinated to the mother. While it is recognized as a living being, in certain circumstances the Mishnah indicates the fetus can become a *rodef* or an "aggressor" that pursues the mother and therein threatens her life. Revered medieval physician and rabbi Maimonides held this view in articulating that the life of the mother always takes precedence over the life of the fetus. According to Jewish law, therefore, feticide is not a capital crime, nor is it a punishable offense.[29] Abortion is permissible, even in advanced stages of pregnancy, to save the mother's life because the mother's welfare is paramount, and as a result most rabbis condone abortion in specific situations.[30] The late rabbi and bioethicist David M. Feldman stated, "A principle in the Jewish view of the matter is *tza'ara d'gufah kadim*, that her welfare, avoidance of her pain, comes first."[31] This understanding is particularly relevant to the Holocaust, when the pregnant body marked Jewish women for destruction, when the unborn child through no fault of its own was cast in the role of the aggressor, although one that did not initiate the mother's plight.[32] Author Rachel Biale underscores, "[Halakhah] does recognize as a fundamental principle the right of a woman to protect her life by abortion. It is part of the right and duty of self-preservation."[33]

During the Holocaust, victims asked rabbis a multitude of legal questions, and the rabbis in turn applied a certain amount of leniency in their interpretations given the unusual situations the Holocaust created. Warsaw rabbi Shimon Efrati (1908–88), for example, was queried on many difficult subjects, including if it was permissible for Jews in hiding to smother a crying infant if its cries threatened Nazi detection and thus death of the entire group.[34] Abortion became a crucial matter for rabbinical thought in the Warsaw Ghetto as well after November 1941, when the SS mandated the forced termination of Jewish pregnancies.[35] In the Balkan regions in February 1942, an SS decree forbade all Jewish births; birth became a crime punishable by death often for the pregnant woman and her entire family. Such rulings were amplified on 8 September 1942 when the Germans declared that in the Kovno Ghetto, any woman perceived to be pregnant would be killed.[36] In this context, Lithuanian rabbi Ephraim Oshry (1914–2003) was questioned about abortion. He stated, "I was asked [about] a woman who became pregnant in the ghetto, whether it is permissible for her to abort . . ."[37] Rabbi Oshry was in a somewhat favorable situation in Kovno to make a ruling in this case, because he worked in a warehouse where Jewish goods were stored and had access to some biblical and legal texts emphasizing the priority of the mother's life during pregnancy. While he lacked colleagues with whom he could debate the issue, Oshry recognized the extreme danger to the mother and understood that without an abortion she would be murdered. He thus concluded that abortion was appropriate in such cases. Perhaps he had been influenced by the fact that one day in front of the hospital in the Kovno Ghetto he watched in horror as a German soldier targeted a pregnant Jewish woman and shot her dead. An obstetrician at the hospital delivered her child after she died and the baby was born alive, but the Germans quickly entered the hospital and smashed its skull.[38] Oshry and other rabbis witnessing these situations took into consideration the terrible choices that had to be made in the Holocaust context, in this instance with regard to abortion and infanticide. They employed a certain amount of sensitivity to social situations, assuaging the guilt and shame resulting from extreme actions.[39] In numerous settings, abortions were necessary to save Jewish mothers' lives; pregnancies endangered women and made them more vulnerable to being shot or sent to gas chambers. For female victims of "choiceless choices," the Holocaust transformed the meaning of abortion and made it a difficult but necessary survival strategy.

Abortions throughout the Bloodlands and Beyond

It is impossible to know how many abortions were performed during the Holocaust, but certainly thousands and thousands, and testimonial archives often reference the themes of pregnancy and abortion.[40] In Kovno, Shavli, and Vilna, in Lithuania and Riga in Latvia, ghetto records indicate that not only were pregnant women encouraged to have abortions, but the SS threatened obstetricians if they refused to perform them. Scholar Miriam Offer comments on Shavli: "After the decree had been proclaimed, abortions took place in the ghetto almost every day."[41] In Kovno, beginning in early 1942, staff gynecologists performed approximately fifty abortions per month.[42] In the Vilna Ghetto, hospital records indicate that 50 to 60 percent of the 420 women admitted to the gynecological ward in 1942 were seen for abortions.[43] Rafael Szadowski, a doctor who worked in the hospital at the time, recounted, "I remember cases of women in the last months of pregnancy whom the Ghetto Police would bring in by force to the hospital in order to terminate the pregnancy."[44] Another gynecologist in Vilna, Dr. Moshe Figenberg, spoke of being "loaded down with abortion cases," in the ghetto.[45] Ruth Foster (born Heilbronn) was a German Jew deported to the Riga Ghetto, where at the age of nineteen she worked in the ghetto hospital. Foster spent over a year at the hospital between 1941 and 1943, and during that time she witnessed numerous abortions, many performed in the later months of pregnancy via Caesarian section. She recollected that she knew of only one child born during that time in the hospital, a boy named Ben Ghetto, whom the SS killed by pressing on his fontanelle. Foster explained that in Riga one German-Jewish gynecologist perfected the art of extracting fetuses using forceps so as not to leave a scar and so that women could return to work more easily.[46] One might argue that just as Nazi doctors experimented on Jewish bodies in the camps with diseases like typhus, Nazi genocidal policy also stimulated "abortion epidemics" that made Jewish women's pregnancies unsustainable.[47] Abortion weaponized attacks on Jewish female reproduction and thus became a form of Nazi biological warfare.

Ethical conflict over abortion also led to intra-family and community debate, especially in dire ghetto situations in which medical doctors well understood the threats to pregnant women and encouraged them to terminate their pregnancies.[48] Survivor Bernard Freilich explained, for example, that during the war his mother was pregnant with her sixth child but his father forbade an abortion even though their neighbors in Drohobycz, Poland (Western Ukraine), including one doctor, encouraged him to reconsider and warned he was endangering his whole family. One day in 1942, when Freilich and his father were at work at a nearby oil refinery, the Ghetto Police came and took his mother away to the ghetto hospital for an abortion. That night the hospital was liquidated and Freilich learned his mother was sent to Belzec where she was murdered. Freilich's father suffered horrible guilt afterward for not permitting an abortion at a time when it might have saved his wife's life.[49]

Nazi directives were never consistent, however, and changes of protocol and leadership added to the confusion.[50] In Theresienstadt just as in Kovno and elsewhere, births were prohibited and abortions mandatory. Sources indicate that at least 350 abortions were performed at Theresienstadt where the birth of children conceived in the camp was expressly prohibited.[51] Yet survivor Ruth Elias remembered that in 1943, a regulation was passed that prohibited all abortions in Theresienstadt, and doctors caught performing them were subject to immediate deportation.[52] It is plausible that the change in Nazi policy later in the war was simply meant to hasten deportation of pregnant women to camps like Auschwitz-Birkenau, where they would be identified as pregnant and gassed on arrival. The new ruling thus denied pregnant women life-saving abortions. Gisella Perl, the Czech gynecologist who produced a post-Holocaust memoir recounting aspects of the thousands of abortions she says she performed while at Auschwitz, offers vivid testimony of the "special treatments" pregnant women received at the camp. She recollected one instance where she happened upon a group of recent pregnant arrivals, "They were beaten with clubs and whips, torn by dogs, dragged around by the hair and kicked in the stomach with heavy German boots. Then, when they collapsed, they were thrown into the crematory—alive."[53]

Auschwitz-Birkenau, the largest of the concentration/extermination camps, had a constant supply of pregnant women who either faced extermination, experimentation, sterilization, abortion, or delivery.[54] Stanisława Leszczyńska, a Polish midwife who spent two years at the camp, stated, "Among the numerous transports of women that arrived at the camp, there was no shortage of pregnant women."[55] Nazi guards often squeezed the breasts and bellies of new arrivals to search out pregnant women and send them to their deaths.[56] Many women were able to hide their pregnancies and abort or deliver in secret. Pregnant women tried to find large dresses amid the prison attire to cover their growing stomachs, while others scavenged rags to fashion into belts used to bind their bodies and conceal their pregnancies.[57] Barracks became abortion clinics and maternity wards, where doctors and midwives and others with birthing knowledge faced difficult ethical challenges in trying to save Jewish lives. Dr. Perl, a Holocaust victim herself, wrote, "It was up to me to save the life of the mothers, if there was no other way, then by destroying the life of their unborn children."[58] In the "dark corners of the camp," in the hospital blocks and sometimes on the concrete channels that connected the cold fireboxes on either end of the barracks, Jewish wombs were manipulated so that the taking of potential lives, the "aggressors" in the halakhic sense, protected and saved the lives of the mothers.[59] In this context, many children born live were quickly killed, often without the mother's knowledge, their lifeless bodies tossed on heaps of corpses outside the barracks. Other newborn infants were abandoned under bunks inside the barracks.[60] Lucie

Adelsberger, another Jewish doctor at Auschwitz wrote, "The child had to die so that the life of the mother might be saved."⁶¹ Writing of her experiences in April 1944, Sara Nomberg-Przytyk, a teacher and journalist from Lublin who was deported from the Białystok ghetto first to Stutthof and then to Auschwitz, explained, "In the hospital block it is impossible to conceal the birth of a child from the Germans. Our procedure now is to kill the baby after birth in such a way that the mother doesn't know about it."⁶² This consideration was not always possible, however. Dr. Alfred Fiderkiewicz, a prisoner at Auschwitz in 1943, testified at the trial of camp commandant Rudolf Höss that in his time working in a surgical block at Auschwitz, he witnessed nonsterile Caesarian sections performed on women who were six, seven, and even nine months pregnant. The babies were tossed into large buckets inclusive of the placentas where the infants "screamed and groaned until it ended in death."⁶³ The moral ramifications of such acts weighed heavily on Jewish healthcare workers as well. In discussing forced abortions and premature births, one doctor from the Shavli ghetto lamented, "And what will happen if despite everything the child is born alive? Shall we kill it? I cannot accept such responsibility on my conscience."⁶⁴

Mothers lost their babies in other cruel ways as well, since Auschwitz-Birkenau was also a medical experimentation camp where Dr. Josef Mengele had a particular interest in pregnant women. Ruth Elias, mentioned above, described delivering a baby girl in the hospital block who Mengele planned to watch starve to death. With the help of a dentist named Maca Steinberg, Elias secured morphine to take the infant's life, which she believed saved her own life.⁶⁵ Newborns were often killed with phenol injections to the heart if they did not die soon after birth.⁶⁶ Near the end of the war, orders came from Berlin that slowed or stopped the gassing of pregnant women at Auschwitz. A Polish Jew named Gena Ajdelman reported that as a result she found herself in a hospital block with at least fifty other pregnant women. Many were given abortions before being sent off on transports as the Germans prepared to abandon Auschwitz. Ajdelman delivered her son on 10 January 1945, but he died on 27 January, the day the camp was liberated by the Soviet army.⁶⁷ Ajdelman concluded, "I know for a fact, of the children born in this time, not one is alive. They all died soon after being born."⁶⁸ During the liberation of the camps, moreover, some observers commented that non-Jewish women exited with their infants while few Jewish survivors had babies in their arms.⁶⁹

The womb was also a Holocaust landscape in motion, and as such the issue of pregnancy touched the totality of the war as women tried to escape Nazi oppression or were caught up in the Nazi movement of pregnant bodies from place to place. At times the abortion issue stretched beyond the territories under Nazi control. In December 1939, for example, Ingelore Honigstein, a deaf Jewish teenager, was returning from her job as a domestic worker in Berlin. En route to her school for the deaf, she was attacked by two Nazi military students, who took her to their room and repeatedly raped her. She told no one and soon thereafter her family received the paperwork to immigrate to the United States, where they arrived on 22 February 1940. At the age of fifteen, Honigstein discovered that she was pregnant, a result of the rape in Germany, and she aborted the child with help of a Dr. Vogel in New York City. She did not want the child: "I knew that it would always haunt me," she stated, "that this had come to pass because of what the Nazis had done to me."[70] Interviewed in 2006, Honigstein explained in sign language that her abortion resulted from fear about her own mental anguish stemming from the traumatic memory of the rape, a rationale many halakhic scholars would accept.[71]

Nazi transports near the end of the war also included pregnant women, especially after abortion policies ended in camps like Theresienstadt, Ravensbrück, and Auschwitz in 1944. In January 1945 during the Nazi retreat, Bergen-Belsen was made a receiving camp for pregnant female inmates coming from other camps further east. The women had very little chance of survival, however, in Bergen-Belsen's extremely overcrowded and diseased environment. Pregnant women participated in the death marches as well, and many gave birth en route.[72] In a filthy coal car headed to Mauthausen from Freiberg, Rachel Abramczyk gave birth to a son, but "no one knew how to sever the umbilical cord that had connected the baby to the mother and kept him alive."[73] Eventually Abramczyk was given a dirty razor blade. Amazingly her child survived; many other infants born on these transports were not so lucky.

It is impossible to provide a precise accounting of the number of pregnant women who were killed in the death camps, shot by *Einsatzgruppen* or other Germans and their collaborators, who aborted a child, or who gave birth in the ghettos, camps, forests, or in hiding in a situation in which neither mother nor child survived. Such records were not kept, and the sheer secrecy involved in the birthing process meant infant deaths went unacknowledged. Judith Sternberg Newman remembered watching the drowning of a newborn in her block in Auschwitz in 1942. She states, "I wanted to shout 'Murderess!,' but I had to keep quiet and could not tell anyone."[74] In the case of survivors, we have no way of knowing how many Jewish women aborted or gave birth during the war and never spoke of the experience again. Nor can we ascertain how many Jewish women aborted fetuses more than once, although the Shavli *Judenrat* records refer to one woman aborting three times.[75] Sulia Rubin, a Jewish partisan from Nowogródek in Poland, furthermore, explained that she endured four abortions over the course of the war because the rules were that women who gave birth and tried to keep the child were banished from the group. It was a matter of partisan group preservation. She states, "I was horribly afraid of pregnancy because I faced a few friends who had abortions or had in the sixth month an abortion and this was already a formed baby and you had to bury it."[76]

Estimating "Gynecological Genocide"

To get a sense of the magnitude of "gynecological genocide," we can consider the crude birth rate or the number of births that would have occurred in a population of six million, the figure given for the number of Jewish deaths in the Holocaust. Measuring natality as the relationship between the number of pregnant women in any population involves determining the number of births per 1,000 or B/P × 1,000 of the midyear population and recognizing that three-quarters of women who give birth during a twelve-month period are pregnant. In 1938, birth rates in the Nazi-occupied countries ranged from a low of 13.9 births per thousand in the population in Austria to 37.5 in Russia.[77] If we use 15 to 30 as a plausible range, this implies that 90,000 to 180,000 births would have occurred in a year, and at any moment in time 67,500 to 135,000 females would have been pregnant. Even so, not all pregnant women died in the Holocaust, especially since many pursued abortions to save themselves, and some women managed to give birth to children who survived. As such, it might be best to base the calculations on the prewar Jewish population figure of 9.5 million. In this case, if we use 15 to 30 again as a plausible range, this implies that 142,500 to 285,000 births would have occurred in a year and at any moment in time 106,875 to 213,750 females would have been pregnant. While recognizing that this estimate is a gross oversimplification, and acknowledging that malnutrition, starvation, and the stress tied to war would have led to lower fecundity rates during the Holocaust, it would still be unlikely that the number of deaths in utero or babies killed at birth would have been lower than 60,000 and could have easily been as high as 200,000 in the context of the prewar population figure.[78] Demographer George Alter states, "Even though the arrests and murders occurred over a number of years, we have to assume that the process was the same as if they all died on the same day. So, the estimate is for the entire 1939–45 period."[79]

If This Is a Woman: Ignored Victims

Questions about the moral permissibility of abortion whether within halakhic law or revealed more broadly within medical ethics and societal debates on abortion in general have hindered analytical exploration of Jewish women's experiences with pregnancy during the Holocaust. Dr. Aaron Pik, a respected doctor in the Shavli Ghetto in Lithuania, reacted with horror to the 5 February 1942 ban on births in the ghetto. He recorded in his diary, "The world has never before heard such a decree and will never forget it."[80] In fact, the world not only forgot the decree but in large measure has never fully integrated the Nazi assault on Jewish wombs into the larger Holocaust narrative. With regard to pregnant women and fetuses, there is no "presence of absence" here but rather an absence of presence in the Holocaust literature where the gender-based dimension of the Holocaust experience is largely ignored. The Jewish womb was a Holocaust wasteland that was vast and empty even though it encompassed a potential range of 60,000 to 200,000 deaths in utero, aborted fetuses, and/or babies who lived at most a few days. These numbers are not included in official Holocaust statistics but reflect sources of intense pain to the mothers who experienced brutal mental and physical torture and so often death, the healthcare workers who faced unimaginable decisions while attempting to save women's lives, and the Jewish leaders, rabbis, and fathers who subsequently confronted enormous ethical questions created uniquely by the horror of the Holocaust.

Scholars exploring the travails of pregnant women during the Holocaust often refer to these women as resisters and their acts to save themselves and their families through abortion as acts of resistance.[81] It is also important to identify the Holocaust birth stories as indicating moments of intense humanity, where victims revealed their humane instincts to help those mothers in dire situations. Survivor Anna Sussmann explained that on arrival at Auschwitz-Birkenau from France, a Polish prison doctor warned her to hide her pregnancy. Later when she went into labor, "several women concealed me, covering me with dirty blankets."[82] Liana Millu told a similar story about a mother named Maria hidden under blankets during roll call after she had just given birth.[83] There were no sterilized instruments inside the dirty barracks, and the risk of infection was great. Once a child was born there were no clothes available for it. Women prisoners most often came together and helped each other through labor and to obtain materials to make simple diapers. After giving birth, mothers returned to roll call or work immediately, supported by their fellow inmates. Inmates comforted the mothers once the babies were taken away or died soon after birth. In a world where childbirth meant child death, the support of female friends helped mothers to endure the sheer physical pain of the experience and the mental anguish of the terrible loss.[84] No matter the horror of the situation, in moments of extreme maternal stress, acts of human kindness prevailed. Katarina Grünsteinova, a prisoner in Auschwitz-Birkenau in 1942, recounted an interesting story about three beautiful Jewish sisters who arrived from France. The oldest, Pola, managed to hide her pregnancy on arrival from Drancy and gained admittance to Birkenau, but soon thereafter she gave birth. The birth was reported and mother and child were sent to the crematorium. When an SS guard arrived to take them away, he hissed, "The Jewish whore gave birth to a child."[85] Immediately Pola's sisters came to her defense and shouted in response, "This is not a whore; this is a woman."[86] Pola was murdered within hours of giving birth, but some of the last words she heard reaffirmed her dignity and status as an honorable woman, not a *Häftling* (prisoner), and certainly not a whore.

Conclusion

"Obstetrical genocide" was a key component of the implementation of the Final Solution. This chapter calls for greater acknowledgment of the breadth and scale of Holocaust-related abortion and infanticide. As historian David Patterson states, "In the murder camps, pregnancy was neither a medical condition nor a blessing from God—it was the worst of crimes against the German Reich."[87] Pregnant women faced grim decisions during the Holocaust, casting some into the role of resisters as they opted for abortion or infanticide as strategies of survival for themselves and/or their families. Other Jewish mothers rejected the idea of harming their fetuses, but were then caught by the Nazi assault on female reproduction nevertheless. Many pregnant women in Western Europe, for example, chose deportation in order to avoid abortion, only to be sent into gas chambers when they arrived in the East.[88] Survivor testimony additionally indicates that for many Jewish women, remembering these pregnancies and abortions was unbearable; the recollections were their "most difficult memories."[89] These statements suggest that the female mind does not easily forget interrupted pregnancy. Vera Schiff, an inmate at Theresienstadt, remembered her abortion as "short in duration, but to me lasting an eternity."[90] A recent study of survivors revealed that depression and anxiety were greater in female survivors; one can hypothesize that this might be especially true for survivors who experienced abortions, miscarriages, or infant death during the Holocaust and the trauma associated with these events.[91] Postwar infertility often resulting from wartime gynecological procedures further carried on the Nazi assault on the Jewish womb long past war's end and influences Jewish population statistics even today.[92] By avoiding abortion and infanticide discussions, by deeming them unbearable, we consign these Holocaust pregnancies to oblivion, which is what the Nazis wanted. We also dishonor Jewish mothers in the process who fought for survival as well as those Jewish infants born alive who lived only a few minutes, hours, or days but never made it into official Nazi documentation and are thus absent from archives.[93] Recognizing the sheer magnitude of the scale of Nazi assault on the pregnant Jewish woman should make clear that gynecological genocide was an effective means of Jewish destruction during World War II and that the ramifications, both statistical and emotional, continue to be little understood.

This chapter reconceptualizes abortion as a gendered tool of war during the Holocaust, used to target, in particular, Jewish women. The Nazi racist agenda stimulated epidemics of abortions, deaths in utero via bullets or gas, and infanticide by locating the interior landscape of the Jewish womb as a crucial site of the Final Solution. Today abortion remains a controversial subject, so often politicized and thus avoided in many instances by scholars engaged in serious study of the Holocaust. Genocide, however, is a global reality, past, present, and future, as are distinctive kinds of gendered attacks in time of war, especially those meted out to women who are often the most vulnerable victims. The medical history of the Holocaust is thus incomplete without an understanding of the ways in which application of the Final Solution was gender specific and abortion as well as other forms of attack on the Jewish womb are crucial parts of Holocaust history.

Annette Finley-Croswhite, PhD, is professor of European history at Old Dominion University in Norfolk, Virginia, and focuses on religious and political violence. She has published three books and many articles, and has explored tuberculosis in relation to the Holocaust. She has served as a faculty fellow with the Auschwitz Jewish Center.

Notes

1. Hanna Bloch Kohner endured an abortion while at Auschwitz and later had great difficulty having children. Kohner and Kohner 2008; Pollak 1990; Amesberger 2010, 150.
2. To my knowledge, referencing the womb as a Holocaust landscape is my analytical invention; however, many scholars have influenced my thinking, including Cole 2016.
3. For an overview of gender and Holocaust, see Goldenberg and Shapiro 2013; Patterson 1999a.
4. Chalmers 2015, 2. Chalmers's book is a corrective to the lacuna on women's experiences during the Holocaust within the context of sex, reproduction, and female victimization.
5. Sweet and Csapó-Sweet 2012; Benedict and Georges 2006.
6. Quoted in Hess 1960, 242; Goldenberg 2013, 116.
7. Cole 2016, 6.
8. Waxman 2017, 11.
9. Von Kellenbach 1999, 20–32.
10. Lifton 1986, 22–101; Proctor 1992, 18–27.
11. Bock 1986, 8; Proctor 1992, 21; Weindling 2015, 25–31.
12. Lifton 1986, 22.
13. Iwaszko et al. 1995, 2:348–56; Yahil 1987, 369; Hildebrandt et al. 2017; Shelley 1991; Weinberger 2009; Sweet 2012; Weindling et al. 2016; Wilking 2001.
14. Chelouche 2007, 202.
15. For more on the differences between male and female Holocaust experiences, see Gottlieb 1990; Ringelheim 1985b; Pine 2008; Ephgrave 2016; Kremer 1999.
16. Arad, Gutman, and Margaliot 1981, document #204.
17. Browning 2010, 185.
18. Browning 2010, 185.
19. Ringelheim 1997a, 20.
20. For example, Hedgepeth and Saidel 2010.
21. Feldman 1995c, 80.
22. Helfand 1983. This chapter discusses the challenges the Holocaust posed to Halakhah.
23. Smith 2013. This undergraduate paper was quite good, but when the student pursued graduate work, her advisor warned her off the abortion issue. Other researchers have encountered similar criticism of abortion topics from scholars and archivists. I reference my own experiences in this paragraph. One well-known Holocaust scholar told me "to forget this material and never try to publish it."
24. Mordhorst-Mayer, Rimon-Zarfaty, and Schweda 2013.

25. Biale 1984b, 219–20; Schenker 2008, 272.
26. Biale 1984b, 221.
27. Kirschner 1985, 80.
28. Sinclair 2003, 12.
29. Biale 1984b, 219–38; Feldman 2012a; Feldman 1974b, 280; Bokser and Abelson 2000, 195; Bleich 2000, 167; Klein 1970; Weiss and Carmy 1979; Schiff 2002, 130; Guttmann 1975.
30. Schenker 2008, 274.
31. Feldman 1995c, 80.
32. Mordhorst-Mayer, Rimon-Zarfaty, and Schweda 2013, 6, 8.
33. Biale 1984a, 238.
34. Kirschner 1985, 65–87; Bemporad, Pawlikowski, and Sievers 2000, 237–38.
35. Ringelblum 1974, 230.
36. Tory 1990, 132; Beinfeld 1998a, 81.
37. Quoted in Schiff 2002, 130; Oshry 2001b, 82.
38. Oshry 1995a, 92; Schiff 2002, 129–30; Rosenbaum 1976, 14, 42. Oshry wrote, "[W]here it was clear that if the Germans discovered [a woman's] pregnancy neither the woman nor the fetus would survive, I ruled that it was permissible to abort the fetus in order to save the woman's life." Oshry 2001b, 82.
39. Horowitz 2017, 139.
40. For more on testimonies and pregnancy, see Friedman 2001a; Friedman 2002b.
41. Offer 2017, 170.
42. Brauns 2017, 161.
43. Beinfeld 1998a, 82; Beinfeld 2017b, 123.
44. Quoted in Beinfeld 2017b, 123.
45. Preiss 2006.
46. Foster 1996, #63.
47. The term "abortion epidemics" is taken from an article by Gisella Bock, although Bock was referring to German women in the 1930s. Bock 1983, 411.
48. Offer 2017, 169; Grodin 2017, xvii.
49. Freilich 1996, #101. Freilich isn't clear who took his mother away; the assumption is that it was the Ghetto Police. He also says it occurred in 1943; however, he was told she was sent to Belzec, and the transports to Belzec from his town ended in December 1942. As such, there may be some confusion on the date.
50. Bergen 2009, 176.
51. Adler 2017, 465.
52. Elias 1999b, 102.
53. Perl 1948, 80; Peleg 2005.
54. Adelsberger 1995, 100. Adelsberger states, "Pregnant women were frequently admitted to the camp; they included women from mixed marriages, who were generally spared the gas chamber, and childless full Jews whose pregnancy was not detected when they arrived. A number of them were subjected to induced miscarriages as late as the fourth and fifth month without regard for the fact that an operation at this point was a medical mistake and the artificially induced termination of pregnancy in healthy women is taboo all over the world" (100–101). See as well, Lengyel 1995, 113; Jacobs 2006.
55. Leszcyńska 2010, 35; Adelsberger 1995, 101.
56. Holden 2015, 145; Bruml and Bruml 1993, 1:16.29–1:18.
57. Schiller 2015.
58. Perl 1948, 81.
59. Ibid. Tessa Chelouche stresses that we do not pass judgment on doctors forced to act under Nazi duress. Their testimonies reveal that ethical values were utmost in their minds. Chelouche 2007; Ben-Sefer 2010, 162–64.

60. Grünsteinova n.d., 67. The German phrases are, "Die Juden Hure hat da ein Kind noch zur Welt gebracht," and, "Das ist keine Hure, das ist eine Frau."
61. Aldelsberger 1995, 101; See, as well, Ritvo and Plotkin 1998, 215.
62. Nomberg-Przytyk 1985, 69.
63. Deposition of Dr. Alfred Fiderkiewicz in Kubica 2010, 30.
64. Arad, Gutman, and Margaliot 1981, 452.
65. Elias 1999b, 150–51. There are numerous stories of women carrying their babies to term and delivering in secret in the barracks. Babies were killed at birth with phenol injections, drowning, and other methods. For example, see Vago 1998, 281; Perl 1948, 80–85. For an interesting article on Nazi doctors and medical ethics, see Colaianni 2012.
66. Kubica 2010, 11.
67. Deposition of Gena Ajdelman in Höss Trial, in Kubica 2010, 22–24.
68. Deposition of Gena Ajdelman in Höss Trial, in Kubica 2010, 24.
69. Weisz and Kwiet 2018, 4.
70. Honigstein 2006, 40:16.
71. Honigstein 2006, 17:25–43:16; Guttmann 1975.
72. Amesberger 2010, 143; Holden 2015, 223.
73. Holden 2015, 223.
74. Newman 1963, 43.
75. Arad, Gutman, and Margaliot 1981, 452.
76. Rubin 1995, #85.
77. Mitchell 1978, 90–96, 114–20.
78. Shryock, Siegle, and Stockwell 1976, 276; Calculations and language suggested by Dr. George Alter, professor of history, Population Studies Center, University of Michigan, Ann Arbor, personal communication with author, 31 March 2017, 6 April 2017, and 8 April 2017. Most women stopped menstruating in the ghettos and camps, and sexual relations became more difficult, so natality rates must have dropped steeply. A group of questionnaires exists that sheds some insight on pregnancy during the Holocaust. Female Hungarian survivors who were deported between 1944 and 1945 and spent at least one year in a camp completed questionnaires between 1985 and 1990, and these documents included questions about pregnancy. Of the 580 respondents, five women indicated that they were pregnant during internment. They reported one live birth, and four abortions. Five out of 580 is less than 1 percent, a figure that corresponds somewhat to the lower end of estimates in this chapter of Holocaust pregnancies. Caution is advised for numerous reasons. Firstly, as some of the final deportees, Hungarian Jews had endured long years of war before arrival, so perhaps birth rates fell earlier during the war. Secondly, approximately 500,000 Hungarian Jews died in the Holocaust; the figure of 580 thus captures only a tiny part of the typical experience. Thirdly, since the Nazis targeted pregnant mothers for extermination, one can assume that many died in this context, and their experiences are not reflected on the questionnaires. Finally, many survivors have shown reluctance to speak of their experiences with abortion and pregnancy during the war. As a result, some women may not have responded accurately on the questionnaires. Pasternak and Brooks 2007, 215. For an interesting article addressing the complications of understanding quantitative aspects of Nazi killing, see Stone 2019.
79. George Alter, quoted in email communication with author, 8 April 2017.
80. Quoted in Offer 2017, 168.
81. Von Kellenbach 1999. The biological fecundity of Jewish women in displaced persons' camps goes beyond the scope of this chapter, but we might also consider female resisters during the war in the same context as those Jewish women who after the war married and created families quite rapidly. The focus in both contexts was Jewish survival. Atina Grossman refers to such gendered action in the postwar period as "biological revenge." Grossmann 2002, 291–318.
82. Memoir of Anna Sussmann, printed in Strzelecka 2017, 129.
83. Millu 1986, 89.

84. Saidel 2006, 211.
85. Interview, Grünsteinova n.d., 67.
86. Interview, Grünsteinova n.d., 67.
87. Patterson 2013b, 171.
88. Bondy 1998, 316.
89. Friedman 2001b, 7; Adelsberger 1995, 101; Video testimonies often show a real change in emotion on the part of speakers as they approach the subject of pregnancy, abortion, and infanticide. Much testimony exists of women who express grief over their Holocaust pregnancy experiences. See Ruth Elias's body language, for example, in Elias 1979a, 3315 Camera Roll #10, 4:00–4:11.
90. Schiff 1996, 163.
91. Carmel et al. 2017.
92. Waxman 2017, 139. Waxman also addresses postwar feelings of worthlessness brought on by infertility, extending the impact of the Nazi attack on Jewish reproduction long after the war ended. Weindling 2015, 221.
93. It is interesting to note that, after the war, survivors asked Rabbi Oshry whether Jewish men should take back their wives who the Nazi perpetrators or their collaborators had raped. Oshry ruled that because refusing the rapists would have led to the death of victims, it was permissible for them to return to their husbands. He encouraged no gossip against them and in fact called it a "mitzvah" to recognize and praise their grief. He made no such ruling in the context of abortion (to my knowledge), but the same generosity might apply. Guttmann 1975, 447.

References

Adelsberger, Lucie. 1995. *Auschwitz: A Doctor's Story*. Translated by Susan Ray. Boston: Northeastern University Press.
Adler, H. G. 2017. *Theresienstadt 1941–1945: The Face of a Coerced Community*. Translated by Belinda Cooper. Cambridge: Cambridge University Press.
Amesberger, Helga. 2010. "Reproduction under the Swastika: The Other Side of the Glorification of Motherhood." In *Sexual Violence against Jewish Women during the Holocaust*, edited by Sonja M. Hedgepeth and Rochelle G. Saidel, 139–55. Lebanon, NH: Brandeis University.
Arad, Yitzhak, Yisrael Gutman, and Abraham Margaliot (eds.). 1981. *Documents on the Holocaust: Selected Sources on the Destruction of the Jews of Germany, Austria, Poland, and the Soviet Union*. Jerusalem: KTAV Publishing House.
Beinfeld, Solon. 1998. "Health Care in the Vilna Ghetto." *Holocaust and Genocide Studies* 12(1): 66–98.
———. 2017. "Health Care in the Vilna Ghetto." In *Jewish Medical Resistance in the Holocaust*, edited by Michael A. Grodin, 106–40. New York: Berghahn Books.
Bemporad, Jack, John Pawlikowski, and Joseph Sievers. 2000. *Good and Evil after the Holocaust: Ethical Implications for Today*. Hoboken, NJ: KTAV Publishing House.
Benedict, Susan, and Jane M. Georges. 2006. "Nurses and the Sterilization Experiments of Auschwitz: A Post-Modernist Perspective." *Nursing Inquiry* 13(4): 277–88.
Ben-Sefer, Ellen. 2010. "Forced Sterilization and Abortion as Sexual Abuse." In *Sexual Violence against Jewish Women during the Holocaust*, edited by Sonia Hedgepeth and Rochelle G. Saidel, 156–74. Lebanon, NH: Brandeis University.
Bergen, Doris. 2009. *War and Genocide: A Concise History of the Holocaust*. Lantham, MD: Rowman & Littlefield.
Biale, Rachel. 1984a. *Women and Jewish Law: The Essential Texts, Their History and Their Relevance for Today*. New York: Schocken Books.

———. 1984b. *Women and Jewish Law: An Exploration of Women's Issues in Halakhic Sources.* New York: Schocken Books.
Bock, Giesella. 1983. "Racism and Sexism in Nazi Germany: Motherhood, Compulsory Sterilization and the State." *Signs: Journal of Women in Culture and Society* 8(3): 400–421.
———. 1986. *Zwangssterilisation im Nationalsozialismus: Studien zur Rassenpolitik und Frauenpolitik.* Opladen: Westdeutscher Verlag.
Bokser, Ben Zion, and Kassel Abelson. 2000. "A Statement on the Permissibility of Abortion." In *Life and Death in Jewish Biomedical Ethics,* edited by Aaron L. Mackler, 195. New York: Jewish Theological Seminary of America.
Bondy, Ruth. 1998. "Women in Theresienstadt and the Family Camp in Birkenau." In *Women in the Holocaust,* edited by Dalia Ofer and Lenore J. Weitzman, 310–26. New Haven, CT: Yale University Press.
Braham, Randolph (ed.). 1983. *Perspectives on the Holocaust.* Boston: Kluwer Academic Publishers Group.
Brauns, Jack. 2017. "Medicine in the Kovno Ghetto." In *Jewish Medical Resistance in the Holocaust,* edited by Michael A. Grodin, 155–63. New York: Berghahn Books.
Browning, Christopher. 2010. *Remembering Survival: Inside a Nazi Slave-Labor Camp.* New York: W. W. Norton.
Bruml, Hana, and Charles Bruml. 1993. RG-50.751.0037, United States Holocaust Memorial Museum Oral History. Retrieved 1 December 2018 from https://collections.ushmm.org/search/catalog/irn560487.
Cargas, Harry James (ed.). 1999. *Problems Unique to the Holocaust.* Lexington: University Press of Kentucky.
Carmel, Sara, David King, Norm O'Rourke, and Yaacov G. Bachner. 2017. "Subjective Well-Being: Gender Differences in Holocaust Survivors—Specific and Cross-National Effects." *Aging & Mental Health* 21(6): 668–75.
Chalmers, Beverly. 2015. *Birth, Sex and Abuse: Women's Voices under Nazi Rule.* Surrey: Grosvenor House Publishing.
Chelouche, Tessa. 2007. "Doctors, Pregnancy, Childbirth and Abortion during the Third Reich." *Israel Medical Association Journal* 9: 202–6.
Colaianni, Alessandra. 2012. "A Long Shadow; Nazi Doctors, Moral Vulnerability and Contemporary Medicine." *Journal of Medical Ethics* 38(7): 435–38.
Cole, Tim. 2016. *Holocaust Landscapes.* New York: Bloomsbury.
Elias, Ruth. 1979. "Theresienstadt—Auschwitz." Claude Lanzmann Shoah Collection. Interview with Ruth Elias. United States Holocaust Memorial Museum. RG-60.5003, FV3118. Retrieved 23 February 2019 from https://collections.ushmm.org/search/catalog/irn1003912.
———. 1999. *Triumph of Hope: From Theresienstadt and Auschwitz to Israel.* New York: John Wiley and Sons.
Ephgrave, Nicole. 2016. "On Women's Bodies: Experiences of Dehumanization during the Holocaust." *Journal of Women's History* 28(2): 12–32.
Feldman, David. 1974. *Martial Relations, Birth Control, and Abortion in Jewish Law.* New York: Schocken Books.
———. 1995. "This Matter of Abortion." In *Contemporary Jewish Ethics and Mortality: A Reader,* edited by Elliot N. Dorff and Louis E. Newman, 79–90. New York: Oxford University Press.
———. 2012. "Abortion: A Jewish View." In *Life and Death Responsibilities in Jewish Biomedical Ethics,* edited by Aaron L. Mackler, 196–211. New York; Jewish Theological Seminary Press.
Fiderkiewicz, Alfred. 2010. "Deposition on the Subject of Procedures for Terminating Pregnancy." In *Pregnant Women and Children Born in Auschwitz,* Voices of Memory 5, edited by Helene Kubinca, 30. Translated by William Brand. Oświęcim: Auschwitz-Birkenau State Museum.
Foster, Ruth. 1996. "Visual History Archive Online." USC Shoah Foundation: The Institute for

Visual History and Education. Retrieved 27 November 2018 from http://vhaonline.usc.edu/viewingPage?testimonyID=11890&returnIndex=0.

Freilich, Bernard. 1996. "Visual History Archive Online." USC Shoah Foundation: The Institute for Visual History and Education. Retrieved 23 February 2019 from http://vhaonline.usc.edu/viewingPage?testimonyID=22984&returnIndex=0#.

Friedman, Jonathan. 2001. "Togetherness and Isolation: Holocaust Survivor Memories of Intimacy and Sexuality in the Ghettos." *Oral History Review* 28(1): 1–16.

———. 2002. *Speaking the Unspeakable: Essays on Sexuality, Gender, and Holocaust Survivor Memory*. Lanham, MD: University Press of America.

Fuchs, Esther (ed.). 1999. *Women and the Holocaust: Narrative and Representation, Studies in the Shoah*. Vol. 22. Lanham, MD: University Press of America.

Goda, Norman, J. W. (ed.). 2014. *Jewish Histories of the Holocaust: New Approaches*. New York: Berghahn Books.

Goldenberg, Myrna. 2013. "Sex-Based Violence and the Politics and Ethics of Survival." In *Different Horrors/Same Hell: Gender and the Holocaust*, edited by Myrna Goldenberg and Amy Shapiro, 99–127. Seattle: University of Washington Press.

Goldenberg, Myrna, and Amy H. Shapiro (eds.). 2013. *Different Horrors/Same Hell: Gender and the Holocaust*. Seattle: University of Washington Press.

Gottlieb, Roger S. (ed.). 1990. *Thinking the Unthinkable: Meanings of the Holocaust*. New York: Paulist Press.

Grodin, Michael A. (ed.). 2017. *Jewish Medical Resistance in the Holocaust*. New York: Berghahn Books.

Grossmann, Atina. 2002. "Victims, Villains, and Survivors: Gendered Perceptions and Self-Perceptions of Jewish Displaced Persons in Occupied Postwar Germany." *Journal of the History of Sexuality* 11(1–2): 291–318.

Grünsteinova, Katarina. N.d. Archives of the Auschwitz-Birkenau State Museum. *Oświadczenia*, 147.

Guttmann, Alexander. 1975. "Humane Insights of the Rabbis Particularly with Respect to the Holocaust: A Chapter in the History of Halakhah." *Hebrew Union College Annual* 46: 433–55.

Hedgepeth, Sonia M., and Rochelle G. Saidel (eds.). 2010. *Sexual Violence against Jewish Women during the Holocaust*. Lebanon, NH: Brandeis University.

Helfand, Jonathan I. 1983. "Halakhah and the Holocaust: Historical Perspectives." In *Perspectives on the Holocaust*, edited by Randolph Braham, 93–103. Boston: Kluwer Academic Publishers Group.

Hess, Rudolf. 1960. *Commandant of Auschwitz*. Translated by Constantine Fitzgibbon. Cleveland: World Publishing.

Hildebrandt, Sabine, Susan Benedict, Erin Miller, Michael Gaffney, and Michael A. Grodin. 2017. "'Forgotten' Chapters of the History of Transcervical Sterilization: Carl Clauberg and Hans-Joachim Lindemann." *Journal of the History of Medicine and Allied Sciences* 72(3): 272–301.

Holden, Wendy. 2015. *Born Survivors: Three Young Mothers and Their Extraordinary Story of Courage, Defiance, and Hope*. New York: Harper Perennial.

Honigstein, Ingelore. 2006. United States Holocaust Memorial Museum. Oral History. 2010.9.2, RG-50.609.0002. Retrieved 1 December 2018 from https://collections.ushmm.org/search/catalog/irn39660.

Horowitz, Sara R. 2017. "'If He Knows to Make a Child . . .': Memories of Birth and Baby-Killing In Deferred Jewish Testimony Narratives." In *Jewish Histories of the Holocaust: New Transnational Approaches*, edited by Norman J. W. Goda, 135–51. New York: Berghahn Books.

Iwaszko, Tadeusz, Helena Kubica, Franciszek Piper, Irena Strzelecka, Andrzej Srzelecki (eds.). 1995. *Auschwitz, 1940–45 Central Issues in the History of the Camp*. Vol. 2: *The Prisoners—Their Life and Work*. Oświęcim: Auschwitz-Birkenau State Museum.

Jacobs, Janet. 2006. "The Female Body as Atrocity Text: The Feminization of the Holocaust at Auschwitz." *English Language Notes* 44(2): 243–51.

Kirschner, Robert (ed. and trans.). 1985. *Rabbinic Responsa of the Holocaust Era*. New York: Schocken Books.

Klein, Isaac. 1970. "Abortion and Jewish Tradition." *Conservative Judaism* 24(3): 26–33.

Kohner, Hanna, and Walter Kohner. 2008. *Hanna and Walter: A Love Story*. Lincoln, NE: iUniverse Inc.

Kremer, S. Lillian. 1999. *Women's Holocaust Writing: Memory and Imagination*. Lincoln: University of Nebraska Press.

Kubinca, Helene. 2010. *Pregnant Women and Children Born in Auschwitz*, Voices of Memory 5. Translated by William Brand. Oświęcim: Auschwitz-Birkenau State Museum.

Lengyel, Olga. 1995. *Five Chimneys: A Women Survivor's True Story of Auschwitz*. Chicago: Academy Chicago Publishers.

Lentin, Ronit (ed.). 1997. *Gender and Catastrophe*. London: Zed.

Leszczyńska, Stanisława. 2010. "Report by a Midwife from Auschwitz." In *Pregnant Women and Children Born in Auschwitz*, Voices of Memory 5, edited by Helene Kubinca, 35–37. Translated by William Brand. Oświęcim: Auschwitz-Birkenau State Museum.

Lifton, Robert Jay. 1986. *The Nazi Doctors: Medical Killing and the Psychology of Genocide*. New York: Basic Books.

Mackler, Aaron L. (ed.) 2000. *Life and Death in Jewish Biomedical Ethics*. New York: Jewish Theological Seminary of America.

Millu, Liana. 1986. *Smoke over Birkenau*. Translated by Lynne Sharon Schwartz. Evanston, IL: Northwestern University Press.

Mitchell, Brian. 1978. *European Historical Statistics 1750–1970: Abridged Edition*. New York: Columbia University Press.

Mordhorst-Mayer, Melanie, Nitzan Rimon-Zarfaty, and Mark Schweda. 2013. "Perspectivism in the Halakhic Debate on Abortion between Moshe Feinstein and Eliezer Waldenberg—Relations between Jewish Medical Ethics and Socio-Cultural Contexts." *Women in Judaism: A Multidisciplinary Journal* 10(2): 1–55. Retrieved 1 December 2018 from http://wjudaism.library.utoronto.ca/index.php/wjudaism/article/view/20905.

Newman, Judith Sternberg. 1963. *In the Hell of Auschwitz: The Wartime Memoirs of Judith Sternberg Newman*. New York: Exposition Press.

Nomberg-Przytyk, Sara. 1985. *Auschwitz: True Tales from a Grotesque Land*. Translated by Roslyn Hirsch. Chapel Hill: University of North Carolina Press.

Ofer, Dalia, and Lenore J. Weitzman (eds.). 1998. *Women in the Holocaust*. New Haven, CT: Yale University Press.

Offer, Miriam. 2017. "Medicine in the Shavli Ghetto: In Light of the Diary of Dr. Aaron Pik." In *Jewish Medical Resistance in the Holocaust*, edited by Michael A. Grodin, 164–72. New York: Berghahn Books.

Oshry, Rabbi Ephraim. 1995. *The Annihilation of Lithuanian Jewry*. Translated by Y. Leiman. New York: Judaica Press, Inc.

———. 2001. *Responsa from the Holocaust*. Edited by B. Goldman. Translated by Y. Leiman. New York: Judaica Press, Inc.

Pasternak, Alfred, and Philip G. Brooks. 2007. "The Long-Term Effects of the Holocaust on the Reproductive Function of Female Survivors." *Journal of Minimally Invasive Gynecology* 14(2): 211–17.

Patterson, David. 1999. "The Moral Dilemma of Motherhood in the Nazi Death Camps." In *Problems Unique to the Holocaust*, edited by Harry James Cargas, 7–24. Lexington: University Press of Kentucky.

———. 2013. "The Nazi Assault on the Jewish Soul through the Murder of the Jewish Mother." In *Different Horrors, Same Hell, Gender and the Holocaust*, edited by Myrna Goldenberg and Amy H. Shapiro, 163–76. Seattle: University of Washington Press.

Peleg, Roni. 2005. "Gisella Perl: A Jewish Gynecologist in Auschwitz." *Journal of Women's Health* 14(6): 587–91.
Perl, Gisella. 1948. *I Was a Doctor in Auschwitz*. New York: International Universities Press.
Pine, Lisa. 2008. "Gender and Holocaust Victims: A Reappraisal." *Journal of Jewish Identities* 1(2): 121–41.
Pollak, Marcia. 1990. "Review of the Legacy of the Holocaust: Psychohistorical Themes in the Second Generation." *Psychoanalytic Psychology* 7(3): 445–91.
Preiss, Leah. 2006. "Women's Health in the Ghettos of Eastern Europe." *Jewish Women's Archive: Encyclopedia*. Jewish Women's Archive. Retrieved 1 November 2018 from https://jwa.org/encyclopedia/article/womens-health-in-ghettos-of-eastern-europe.
Proctor, Robert N. 1992. "Nazi Doctors, Racial Medicine, and Human Experimentation." In *The Nazi Doctors and the Nuremberg Code: Human Rights in Human Experimentation*, edited by George J. Annas and Michael A. Grodin, 17–31. Oxford: Oxford University Press.
Ringelblum, Emmanuel (ed.). 1974. *Notes from the Warsaw Ghetto*. Translated by Jacob Sloan. New York: Schocken Books.
Ringelheim, Joan. 1985. "Women and the Holocaust: A Reconsideration of Research." *Signs* 10(4): 741–61.
———. 1997. "Genocide and Gender: A Split Memory." In *Gender and Catastrophe*, edited by Ronit Lentin, 18–33. London: Zed.
Ritvo, Roger A., and Diane Plotkin. 1986. *Sisters in Sorrow: Voices of Care in the Holocaust*. College Station: Texas A&M Press.
Rosenbaum, Irving J. 1976. *The Holocaust and Halakhah*. New York: KTAV Publishing House, Inc.
Rosner, Fred, and J. David Bleich. (eds.). 2000. *Jewish Bioethics*. Hoboken, NJ: KTAV Publishing House, Inc.
Rubin, Sulia. 1995. Visual History Archive Online. USC Shoah Foundation: The Institute for Visual History and Education. Retrieved 30 November 2018 from http://vhaonline.usc.edu/viewingPage?testimonyID=5287&returnIndex=0.
Saidel, Rochelle G. 2006. *The Jewish Women of Ravensbrück Concentration Camp*. Madison: University of Wisconsin Press.
Schenker, Joseph G. 2008. "The Beginning of Human Life: Status of Embryo; Perspectives in Halakha (Jewish Religious Law)." *Journal of Assisted Reproduction and Genetics* 25: 271–76.
Schiller, Rivka. 2015. "How a Jewish Woman Survived Pregnancy in a Nazi Concentration Camp to Give Birth to a Son." *The Independent*, 12 November. Retrieved 5 December 2018 from https://www.independent.co.uk/news/world/europe/how-a-jewish-woman-survived-pregnancy-in-a-nazi-concentration-camp-to-give-birth-to-her-son-a6731816.html.
Schiff, Daniel. 2002. *Abortion in Judaism*. Cambridge: Cambridge University Press.
Schiff, Vera. 1996. *Theresienstadt: The Town the Nazis Gave to the Jews*. Toronto: Lugus.
Shelley, Lore. 1991. *Criminal Experiments on the Human Beings in Auschwitz and War Research Laboratories: Twenty Women Prisoners' Accounts*. San Francisco: Mellen Research University Press.
Shryock, Henry S., Jacob S. Siegle, and Edward G. Stockwell. 1976. *The Methods and Materials of Demography*. New York: Academic Press.
Sinclair, Daniel B. 2004. *Jewish Biomedical Law: Legal and Extra-legal Dimensions*. Oxford: Oxford University Press.
Smith, Jan (pseudonym). 2013. "Broken Dreams and Muted Memories: The Holocaust of Motherhood." Unpublished honors thesis, Old Dominion University, Norfolk, Virginia.
Stone, Lewi. 2019. "Quantifying the Holocaust: Hyperintense Kill Rates during the Nazi Genocide." *Science Advances* 5(1): eaau7292. DOI: 10.1126/sciadv.aau7292.
Strzelecka, Irena (ed.). 2017. *Women in Auschwitz*. Translated by William Brand. Oświęcim: Auschwitz-Birkenau State Museum.

Sussmann, Anna. 2017. "Memoir by Former Prisoner Anna Sussmann." In *Women in Auschwitz, Voices of Memory 12*, edited by Irena Strzelecka, 129–30. Translated by William Brand. Oświęcim: Auschwitz-Birkenau State Museum.

Sweet, Frederick, and Rita M. Csapó-Sweet. 2012. "Clauberg's Eponym and Crimes against Humanity." *Israel Medical Association Journal* 14: 719–23.

Tory, Abraham. 1990. *Surviving the Holocaust: The Kovno Ghetto Diary*. Edited by Martin Gilbert. Translated by Jerzy Michalowicz. Cambridge, MA: Harvard University Press.

Vago, Lidia Rosenfeld. 1998. "One Year in the Black Hole of Our Planet Earth." In *Women in the Holocaust*, edited by Dalia Ofer and Lenore J. Weitzman, 273–84. New Haven, CT: Yale University Press.

von Kellenbach, Katharina. 1999. "Reproduction and Resistance during the Holocaust." In *Women and the Holocaust: Narrative and Representation, Studies in the Shoah*, edited by Esther Fuchs, 22:20–32. New York: University Press of America.

Waxman, Zoë. 2017. *Women in the Holocaust: A Feminist History*. Oxford: Oxford University Press.

Weinberger, Ruth Jolanda. 2009. *Fertility Experiments in Auschwitz-Birkenau: The Perpetrators and Their Victims*. Saarbrücken: Südwestdeutscher Verlag für Hochschulschriften.

Weindling, Paul. 2015. *Victims and Survivors of Nazi Human Experiments: Science and Suffering in the Holocaust*. New York: Bloomsbury.

Weindling, Paul, Anna von Villiez, Aleksandra Loewenau, and Nichola Farron. 2016. "The Victims of Unethical Human Experiments and Coerced Research under National Socialism." *Endeavour* 40(1): 1–6.

Weiss, Roslyn, and Shalom Carmy. 1979. "Abortion and Halakhah." *Tradition: A Journal of Orthodox Jewish Thought* 17(4): 112–15.

Weisz, George M., and Konrad Kwiet. 2018. "Managing Pregnancy in Nazi Concentration Camps: The Role of Two Jewish Doctors." *Rambam Maimonides Medical Journal* 9(3): 1–6. E0026. doi:10.5041/RMMJ.1034.

Wilking, Silvia. 2001. "Engenischer Rassismus: Die Fortpflanzungsbiologie Carl Claubergs." In *Nationalsozialistische Familienpolitik zwischen Ideologie und Durchsetzung*, edited by Wolfgang Voegeli, 247–69. Hamburg: Boysen & Mauke.

Yahil, Leni. 1987. *The Holocaust and the Fate of European Jewry*. Translated by Ina Friedman and Haya Galai. Oxford: Oxford University Press.

CHAPTER 6

"COMPLETE MASTERY OF THE SUBJECT"
The Connection between Forced Sterilization and Gynecological Fertility Research in National Socialism

Gabriele Czarnowski

One of the earliest activities of the Nazi state to threaten the physical integrity of the citizens was the introduction of forced sterilization by the *Gesetz zur Verhütung erbkranken Nachwuchses* (Law for the Prevention of Hereditarily Diseased Offspring) from 14 July 1933. This law was executed at all university women's hospitals (surgical departments of hospitals for men), governmental hospitals, great and small city hospitals, and private hospitals. Though the latter "only" performed the coercive interventions, scientists at the university hospitals additionally exploited the opportunity of access to these involuntary patients to abuse them further for the study of research problems.

The starting point of the following investigation is a presentation by Felix von Mikulicz-Radecki (1892–1966),[1] the director of the University Women's Hospital in Königsberg (then East Prussia, now Kaliningrad, Russia), for the members of the Königsberger Gelehrte Gesellschaft (the Learned Society of Königsberg) in 1936. The topic was "the mechanism of ovum capture in the woman and its relevance for sterility." He reported on his use of the new opportunities presented by forced sterilization on "genitally healthy women"—victims of sterilization—for observations of the movements of the ovarian tube throughout the menstrual cycle to understand the organ's function. These results were not only of theoretical importance for him, but he also developed "new guidelines on sterility treatment for women who want to have children."

While it is appalling that Mikulicz-Radecki combined forced sterilization with sterility research in the same woman, it is also a paradox that demands explanation. Why was it that during the National Socialist period gynecologists on the one hand used the scalpel to render a woman infertile against her will, and then on the other hand went on to treat the next woman for sterility, sometimes in the same day? Why could medical violence through forced sterilization coexist with the medical ethos of help toward women with sterility problems? What was the self-concept of these gynecologists? These questions will be discussed using the example of Mikulicz-Radecki for methodological grounds. His writings give a clear insight into his work rationale and include two very different texts: the talk on the "ovum capture" as well as a widely distributed surgeons' guide on sterilization, for which he had authored the chapter on the sterilization of women. Here, "hereditarily defective, genitally healthy women" and "sterile women" appear strangely merged into each other—women as sterilization patients and as sterility patients are correlated inversely, functionally, and practically. Unlike some of his other colleagues, he did not understand the "hereditarily defective" person as also "constitutionally inferior" but considered sterilization patients healthy with respect to those parts of their body that he was interested in. The question why forced sterilization and sterility research could so easily exist next to each other will be answered through analysis of both texts. In addition, related publications on the subject by his mentees will be examined.

A Lecture in Königsberg

On 16 December 1936, in a session of the Königsberger Gelehrte Gesellschaft, Felix von Mikulicz-Radecki gave his lecture on "the mechanism of ovum capture in the women and its relevance for sterility."[2] He began in the following manner: "The problem we are concerned with here is the question of how and under which protective measures the egg is transferred from the ovary to the uterine tubes to be available for fertilization," remarking that as in animals, in humans, too, "no direct connection [between tube and ovary] is found, so that a priori there is the risk that during ovulation the ovum falls into the abdominal cavity, thus escaping insemination."[3] In his deliberations he placed himself in a tradition of "natural scientists" that reached from 1776 to the twentieth century. During his time as chief resident at the Women's University Hospital in Leipzig, he had conducted "Experimental Studies on Movements of the Uterine Tubes"[4] on the organs of rabbits and on the "surviving human tube," in the contemporary nomenclature for surgically removed fallopian tubes. The topic had been suggested by his mentor, the prominent gynecologist Walter Stoeckel (1871–1971), who "had provided him gladly"[5] with the surgical specimens, as Mikulicz-Radecki put it. This reflected the attitude of researchers at the time, who attributed specimens of human tissues to their colleagues and not to the patients from whom those tissues were taken. This study had been published in 1926, at a time when research opportunities had been rather restricted, as he noted in his 1936 Königsberg lecture: "Up to now ... the clarification of the ovum capture mechanism depended on analogical deductions from mechanisms in animals, on discoveries by anatomists or on incidental finding during surgery."

Thus he considered it "obvious that the laws ruling normal life could not have been found in this manner."[6] Mikulicz-Radecki referred with the formulation "up to now" to the times before National Socialism enabled a new gynecological-political era in 1933. He used the phrase a second time in his lecture when he started the main subject of his talk, following the long historical introduction of his scientific topic:

> The gynecologist up to now has very rarely had the opportunity to look at entirely normal genital organs during a laparotomy; this changed with the implementation of eugenic sterilizations.[7] Here we operate on women who are usually quite healthy with respect to their genital organs; we also are in the position to operate on them . . . at any point of the menstrual cycle, a welcome opportunity for the detailed study of the connection between the uterine tube and the ovary, as the surgery is always performed on the tubes, and these have to be observed very closely.[8]

The two most important characteristics of this new research were that "genitally healthy" women could be made the subjects of research and that these newly enforced sterilization procedures were performed on large numbers of women. At Königsberg University Women's Hospital, 199 of 216 women admitted for coercive sterilization were operated on before 1 July in 1935.[9] Drawing from this "material" (as he labeled his patients[10]), Mikulicz-Radecki presented observations on a series of twenty-six women (four of them fertility patients) to his colleagues of the Learned Society. He classified these patients according to his experimental design in always the same pattern, based on information from the individual patient files, which included the surgical protocols. All of these procedures were interventions aligned with the different stages of the menstrual cycle. The menstruation history of each woman was carefully recorded. Starting in 1935, every sterilization patient also had to submit herself to a curettage procedure of the uterus. The result of the study of the uterine lining—mucosa—removed during this procedure was matched with the patient's information on menstrual status. These data then were compared with the observed position of the uterine tubes "in situ" and recorded in the research notes.

The abdominal incisions during various phases of the menstrual cycle allowed the visualization of the positions of many tubes in many women on different days. Through these observations of their opened subjective bodies, the sterilization patients were unified and reduced to the same natural substance of woman. Their bodies were used as a matrix for studies of current scientific problems, for confirmation or rejection of contemporary doctrines, and for academic training. Moreover, pharmacological, surgical, and invasive diagnostic experiments in addition to the forced sterilization served the same purpose. Two young women from Mikulicz-Radecki's observation series were subjected to further experiments. One of them received two days before the planned sterilization and the other one three days before it several hormone injections of a very high dosage that was otherwise routinely used at the Königsberg hospital in fertility treatment, for which the hospital was well known.[11] These injections were aimed at bringing an ovarian follicle to early maturation so that ovulation would be artificially accelerated and the movements of the tubes could be explored under these conditions. Furthermore, these two women, as well as several other patients undergoing sterilization, were subjected to the invasive, complication-prone, and—in terms of the sterilization—unnecessary diagnostic procedure of hysterosalpingography. This procedure served the in vivo visualization of the uterus and tubes before and during the surgery. A contrast medium was injected transcervically into the uterus and its distribution to the uterine tubes documented with radiographs in surgery through direct observation. The situation of the hormonally stimulated women was then compared to that of women who had not received the hormone injections.

By performing research on women whom he forcibly robbed of the ability to give birth, Mikulicz-Radecki reached new results on what he called the "regularity of normal life": the evidence of a functional so-called *bursa-ovarica* position of the tubes during their extensive movements within the menstrual cycle before and after ovulation.[12] In October 1935, at the twenty-fourth convention of the Deutsche Gesellschaft für Gynäkologie (German Gynecological Society), he had presented his findings for the first time to the professional public.[13] He claimed for his results "not only a purely theoretical interest" but also their relevance "for the explanation of some causes of sterility," and he promised a practical application of his insights. He saw himself "entitled to establish special guidelines" for "helping women with a desperate wish for a child."[14]

The director of the Königsberg University Women's Hospital was not alone in his double assault on the female body in general and the bodies of a multitude of individual women specifically. In Nazi Germany, all university clinics conducted forced sterilizations.[15] In 1935, at the annual German gynecologists' convention, the hospital directors had a lively discussion on surgical sterilization methods, but not on how they dealt with coercion they deployed against their patients.[16] Most of the clinics intended "to exploit [their] own material scientifically."[17] Gynecologist Hans Albrecht from Munich, president of the society, presented a keynote lecture on "periodical fertility and infertility" and referred in his concluding sentences to the then just publicized theory of Hermann Knaus on cyclical fertility. Albrecht asked his colleagues "to note their findings at the ovaries for the question of ovulation in great detail, to study the extirpated tubes for spermatozoa and with reference to the patients' menstruation calendars, [and] to collaborate further on the definitive clarification of the question concerning the constancy of menstrual cycles."[18] At the Women's University Hospital in Halle, experiments involving the implantation of tissue and the transplantation of adnexa (tubes and ovaries) of two sterilization victims to sterility patients are documented. This meant for the victim whose ovaries were removed not only sterilization but also castration and precipitous menopause.[19] In Graz, pregnant women—most of them forced laborers—and their fetuses were experimented on by injections of radioactive contrast media into the uterus and multiple radiographs, before they had to undergo forced abortion.[20] In Königsberg, Mikulicz-Radecki performed fertility research on Nazi victims "only" in the first years of the regime when most of the forced sterilizations were conducted—different from Carl Clauberg, who worked as a resident in this hospital. After the beginning of the war, Clauberg transferred to the Miner's Hospital in Königshütte (Chorzòw today) in occupied Poland, intending to develop it into a "city of mothers"—a mecca for fertility treatments—whereas block 10 in the nearby concentration camp Auschwitz became Dept. II of his "Institute for the Biology of Reproduction." Here he conducted experiments on women prisoners of the camp that not only caused them excruciating pain but also killed many of them and rendered the majority of the survivors infertile.[21]

During the first years of Nazi rule, Mikulicz-Radecki was renowned for his work on forced sterilization.[22] He was an "expert" on the "physiology and pathology of the tubes" and author of a textbook on surgical techniques of the Stoeckel school, which was published in 1933 for the first time and in 1963 for the third.[23] Together with the Breslau (today's Wrocław in Poland) surgeon Karl Heinrich Bauer (1890–1978)[24] he wrote the book *Die Praxis der Sterilisierungsoperationen* (The practice of sterilization surgery), a guide for surgeons and gynecologists performing forced sterilizations according to the Nazi sterilization law.[25] Both authors had given talks on this topic at the Annual German Surgeon's Convention in 1935.[26] Mikulicz-Radecki also served as expert consultant on the topic in the Reich Ministry of the Interior.

The Interchangeability of Bodies and Medical Practices

The transition from "Miss N, admitted for sterilization for feeblemindedness" to the "patient with a burning wish for a child" took place seamlessly on the level of the female body perceived by the gynecologist as an object of medical science and the surgeon's skill. "The one who undertakes sterilization procedures on the woman," Mikulicz-Radecki wrote, "has . . . to be thoroughly aware of the anatomy and physiology of the female genital organs, especially of the processes of conception, which after all has to be prevented by the surgery."[27] The task was stylized as a challenge to the knowledge and prowess of his own profession:

> The sterilization of the woman does not only present a technical problem but encompasses questions of reproductive anatomy, physiology, and pathology; the complete mastery of the subject ultimately is the prerequisite of the true execution of the sterilization. Only the person in daily contact with these things and in posses-

sion of knowledge of their great diversity will be alive to the greatness of the task, but also of the responsibility.[28]

This enhancement of professional prestige of gynecologists can be explained partly by the competition between them and surgeons at smaller hospitals that did not have resident gynecologists—though Mikulicz-Radecki did not want to see this increase in professional standing as a matter of prestige but as concern for the best implementation of the law. However, his wording also uncovers an underlying attitude of violence against his patients: human beings are transformed into matter, into "material." The knowledge gained from individual bodies is generalized and becomes transferable from body to body. "Bilateral tube occlusion is the most frequent cause for sterility. . . . These occlusions represent the status we want to reach through surgical sterilization: the obstruction of the migration path of the ovum."[29]

The results of therapies, operations, examinations, and follow-up examinations of women who came to the hospital voluntarily seeking fertility treatment, on the one side, and, on the other side, research findings compiled from studies of women and girls who were forcibly sterilized "optimized" medical practices for the gynecologists' respective aims. The knowledge of "pathological states . . . that in all probability mean a 100 percent inability to conceive," gained through the study of sterile women, could save sterilization patients from surgery if they were diagnosed as infertile before the surgery. Conversely, the knowledge of their fertility led to medical justification for sterilization in all other women. In discussing these cases, the interchangeability of medical knowledge is made especially clear. A mentee of Mikulicz-Radecki investigated "the impact of prolonged amenorrhea on the generative functions of the female reproductive organs."[30] His results indicated that only after five years of absent menstruations was the probability for a pregnancy low, though he found exceptions. Mikulicz-Radecki concluded from this study "that a woman with normal or only slightly hypoplastic reproductive organs must be sterilized, even if she reports a longer period of amenorrhea or even one of several years."[31] Research on sterility patients with "infantile reproductive organs" led to the statement that "infantilism and hypoplasia if not accompanied by at least five years of amenorrhea" did not signify "a secure sterility" in cases of women younger than twenty-three years. Therefore, these girls and women had to be sterilized too.[32] Foreseeing a wave of eugenic sterilizations of children, Mikulicz-Radecki remarked that the sterilization of girls would take place in the "physiological state of infantilism" and warned, "It would be an illusion to believe that because of the genetic disease, for example debility, the reproductive function would not come to blossom, just because sometimes infantilism is found on the adult feeble-minded, and infantilism (albeit not always) might imply sterility. Therefore"—he concluded—"all those children will have to be operated on despite their infantile reproductive organs."[33]

It is important to look at the entirely different situations and intentions of the women concerned here. Sterility patients had invasive and quite often unpleasant and painful examinations to endure, such as hysterosalpingography, curettage, expensive hormone injections, and sometimes large operations. They did so voluntarily because they hoped to become pregnant after these treatments. Sterilization patients, however, were coerced into the surgical procedures—they came involuntarily; they were robbed of their fertility against their will by a forced operation and were further subjected to additional experiments for research purposes. At the Königsberg University Women's Hospital, not only living but also dead sterilization victims became research subjects, the latter to "ascertain . . . the success of the operation" even in the event of the patient's death. On suggestion by Mikulicz-Radecki, the governor of the Province of East Prussia ruled "to send to our hospital the reproductive organs removed by dissection of sterilized women deceased in mental hospitals."[34]

Surgical Skills "for the People"

Why did the surgeons and gynecologists accept the practice of coercive sterilization at all? Several points explain this phenomenon. First of all, historical research on "war and medical culture" stresses the great impact of World War I on the conservative-nationalistic mentality of the majority of German physicians, who were devastated and could not accept the lost war or the reality of the new Weimar Republic.[35] Healing the *Volkskörper* (people's body) from the losses of war became their foremost task. During World War I, doctors at the front had still taken care of their individual patients according to the medical ethos—in stark contrast to the merciless severity shown toward "shell-shocked" soldiers by the military medical advisors (most of them were university professors far away from the horrors of the front) to bring them back quickly to the trenches. Social differentiation in and debates on the medical treatment of soldiers and officers were based on Social Darwinist classifications of "fitness." These followed along class lines and extended beyond the end of war. In 1933, many physicians endorsed the eugenic aims behind the Law for the Prevention of Hereditarily Diseased Offspring. Furthermore, the state—through the public health office and the police—referred the patients to the hospital, and there was a division of labor concerning sterilization that may have contributed to the surgeons' ready acceptance of the situation. The Hereditary Health Court (Erbgesundheitsgericht), not the surgeon, decided if a person was to be classified under one of the genetic diseases stated in the law. His responsibility was to check the fitness for surgery and possible infertility of the patient, and then to perform the procedure. So the physician became only part of a scripted process, for which he never had to take on the overall responsibility.[36]

Considering the actual violence against the unwilling patients, Mikulicz-Radecki presented a bewildering self-concept: the person who performs "legally required sterilizations on women," he wrote, "always has to have the feeling of being engaged in the course of the law not only as a surgeon, but predominantly as a carefully attending physician."[37] The consent of the person was without legal relevance, and so it was of no concern for the gynecologist. This is reflected by the fact that only physical findings were recognized as contra-indications for a temporary postponement or abandonment of a planned forced sterilization, up to a uterine bleed "due to the shock of hospitalization."[38] However, the great risk to the patient through the forced operation itself was never considered.[39] Obviously, no discrepancy was perceived here to the professed "careful medical treatment."

Concerning the factual treatment in the hospital, however, the will of the patients and their potential resistance against the operation was taken into account and prepared for—mainly by using different applications of various narcotics.[40] In this context, "means of deception or surprise" to overcome the patient's resistance became so-called "medical aids," as spelled out by Mikulicz-Radecki in his book on sterilization procedures. Mikulicz-Radecki added here an extra chapter on "Special Care for Hereditarily Diseased Patients in a Women's Hospital." He advised, "Hereditarily diseased people are human beings, too, whom we will have to give all our medical care, of course," continuing with a remark that if it was "occasionally not possible to do the physical examination before surgery, an injection of morphine or an enema of Rectidon" could facilitate this exam.[41] Generally, the resistance of the sterilization victims was explained by the "mental illness" ascribed to them by the hereditary health court. "Mental illness" also was made responsible for their behavior against the instructions of the doctors after the forced operation. So they were to be blamed for their own death when resisting the inhalation anesthesia, going on a hunger strike, or jumping out of a window from great height. Contradictory to the emphasis on the "mental illness," it is striking how precisely the women—most of them convicted to sterilization because of "congenital debility"—knew to tell their menstrual history, and that Mikulicz-Radecki took it for granted that they were able to do so. He based his entire research design on the accuracy of these women's information! Only in a small number of cases was he unable to obtain "correct" details.[42]

Though contemporary doctoral dissertations described the days of sterilization surgeries in the hospitals as days of "chopping and stabbing,"[43] and despite their performance of acts of coercion, these gynecologists had no concept of themselves as violent perpetrators. The book *Die Praxis der Sterilisierungsoperationen* addresses two professional obligations: one toward the law and the state, and one toward the patients. Bringing both of them together was seen by the practitioners of gynecology at the time as practically difficult and demanding the full commitment of their skills and medical knowledge in any given case.

The obligation toward the state can be formulated in the common denominator of certainty. Firstly, the certainty that the sterilized woman was robbed completely of her generative ability; secondly, in the case of sterility the certainty that a pregnancy was indeed impossible; and thirdly, the question of the certainty of the safest date for sterilization after a delivery in cases where a pregnant woman had escaped an abortion despite a sterilization order. The central question of certainty was that of the most efficient sterilization method. Mikulicz-Radecki assumed most of them—there existed nearly one hundred different surgical techniques for sterilization—to be insecure or impractical. Often he emphasized the "great regeneration tendency of all parts of the female reproductive organs,"[44] and tying or dividing the tubes did not seem secure enough for him. His favorite method was the excision of the tube with wedges of some centimeters of the uterine wall—the removal of the intramural part of the tube. This technique also played a role in a special fertility surgery invented in the United States and included the grafting of an ovary into the walls of the uterus.[45] The second certainty aspect was the—forced—gynecologic examination before the intervention, to decide "if the surgery can be avoided because the patient is sterile already."[46] Here, hysterosalpingography was used as a diagnostic tool. Thus evading sterilization did not mean that women and girls were left alone. Some of them had "to undergo safety controls for several years because in some exceptional cases a conception has been observed at a later date."[47] The third certainty aspect concerned the question of pregnancy and forced sterilization: the linking of eugenic abortion with sterilization, and the sterilization after delivery in case the pregnant woman succeeded in giving birth to her child. Here Mikulicz-Radecki pleaded for a general delivery in hospital—which in the 1930s was not common practice—in coordination with the public health office. "To allow for the execution of the law," the sterilization should be performed "immediately after birth" to prevent another "escape into pregnancy."[48]

The traditional ethical obligation of a physician with respect to their patients can be seen as a special concept of protection, which primarily should minimize the operation risks. In the context of forced sterilization, "protection" only tangentially related to the victim-patient herself, but was much rather aimed at the statistics for minimizing the mortality rate. Mikulicz-Radecki urged his colleagues to be prudent and careful concerning both obligations of the surgeon: "the physician has to examine which approach to surgery—abdominal or vaginal—and which operation method would be most protective for the patient," but would concurrently "achieve sterility most securely."[49] To speak about the "protection of the patient" did not mean to respect the will of the actual woman or girl in front of the gynecologist. This is evident from the following sentence: "Under no circumstances must these examinations and decisions be interfered with through occasional resistance from the patient." Mikulicz-Radecki pleaded for individualization in choosing the surgical method for each woman, but he recommended wherever possible the "vaginal way" for opening the abdomen. This procedure provided the advantages "that no visible wounds remain, that the laparotomy incision will be avoided and with it the risk for a subsequent herniation, and that the patients often do not know at all that they were operated on. Thanks to its hidden position, the disturbance of the wound by the often unruly hereditarily diseased would not be possible."[50] Protection, individualization, and deception were linked in an inextricable bond. Also, the descriptions of the different surgical methods generally were not "neutral" but implicitly or explicitly related to the forced intervention. Monitoring of patients for the prevention of suicide and tranquilizing them through twilight sleep were the alternatives when the attempt to establish an emotional contact between the hospital staff and the patients and to meet their physical and spiritual pains during convalescence did not succeed. It is amazing though that the patients' pains were mentioned at all, and that doctors and nurses were admonished to try to develop empathy for their victims without canceling the intervention—and afterward to mitigate the sequelae.

Pondering both obligations of the surgeon, Mikulicz-Radecki decided clearly in which direction the scales should weigh: "Given the great relevance of the law for the *Volk*—our people—when in doubt, one will always decide against the patient and perform the operation."[51] With just a few words, these patients were quasi "surgically removed" from the body of the "people": they did not belong to this body and therefore were to be violated and separated from it.

After the war, from 1953 until his retirement in 1963, Felix von Mikulicz-Radecki served as the director of the Women´s Hospital of the Free University in Berlin. In an autobiography he declared his time in Königsberg (1932–45) as "thirteen very happy years—except for the end of war—during which one could clinically and scientifically draw from unlimited resources."[52]

Conclusion

Why could medical violence through forced sterilization coexist with the medical ethos of help toward women with sterility problems? As we have learned, the transition took place seamlessly on the level of the human body perceived as an object of medical science and the surgeon's skill. Human beings were transformed into matter, into "material." The knowledge gained from individual bodies was generalized and became transferable from body to body. However, despite their performance of acts of coercion, gynecologists and surgeons had no self-concept as violent perpetrators. After all, they felt more obliged to the state, to eugenics, and to a "*völkisch*" ethic of "common good for the German people" than to the traditional ethics of the doctor toward the individual patient.

For a long time after 1945, the sterilization surgeons exhibited no sense of guilt. Only in 1995 did the German Gynecological Society apologize to the sterilization victims,[53] and in 2013 the society initiated a research project on its history.[54]

Further empirical investigations are needed to understand how at university women's hospitals in Nazi Germany and its occupied territories victims of sterilization and others were made subjects of research, for which scientific topics they were misused, and how the results were utilized after the Nazi period. Historical research on victims and "normal" patients during National Socialism in academic institutions such as university hospitals is still a vast field of open questions.

Gabriele Czarnowski, is researcher at the Institute of Social Medicine and Epidemiology, Medical University Graz, Austria. She obtained her DPhil at the Otto-Suhr-Institute and the Institute for the History of Medicine, Free University, Berlin. Her main focuses are social history of gender relations, medicine, and public health in National Socialism, history of gynecology, and obstetrics.

Notes

1. Felix von Mikulicz-Radecki, son of the Breslau surgeon Johannes von Mikulicz-Radecki, was director of the Königsberg Women's University Hospital from 1932 to 1945. Fischer 1962, 1043.

2. Mikulicz-Radecki 1937, 185–214. Together with an appendix of sixteen reproductions—presumably slides shown during the session—the lecture was published in the series of the Society (Scientific Class), reviewed approvingly, e.g., by Bluhm 1937, 536–37. The author listed it in his publication index throughout his life. See Kürschners deutscher Gelehrtenkalender 1966, 1619.

3. Mikulicz-Radecki 1937, 185.

4. Mikulicz-Radecki 1926, 318–62.

5. Mikulicz-Radecki 1926, 322.

6. Mikulicz-Radecki 1937, 193.

7. The forced sterilizations in Nazi Germany had begun in 1934. See the pioneer study by Bock 1986.

8. Mikulicz-Radecki 1937, 194.

9. Horn 1936.

10. Mikulicz-Radecki 1937, 194, 196f, 209.

11. Since 1934, the chief resident Carl Clauberg was engaged in hormone therapy; Genzer 1937.

12. Mikulicz-Radecki 1937, 201ff.

13. Mikulicz-Radecki 1936b, 128–32.

14. Mikulicz-Radecki 1937, 209; see also Mikulicz-Radecki 1936c, 1037–43; Mikulicz-Radecki 1936d, 1441–57.

15. See, for example, Daum and Deppe 1991; Doetz 2011; Grimm 2004; Koch 1994; Link 1999; Rothmaler 1991.

16. In contrast, at the 1931 gynecologist's convention, Ludwig Fraenkel (1870–1951), director of the Breslau University Women's Hospital, in his main talk on "sterilization and contraception" had emphasized, "The sterilization of the feebleminded belongs to the surgeries on eugenic grounds.

One cannot be cautious enough with this. The feebleminded person particularly has a claim to legal protection... The refusal of sterilization by the feebleminded woman has to be considered, even in cases were the debility is very high" (Fraenkel 1932, 11). As a Jew, Fraenkel fell victim to the Gynecological Society's self-alignment with the Nazi regime in 1933 and was expelled from the university under pressure from students. Simmer 1986, 205; Kröner 1989, 9; Dross et al. 2016, 37–38, 76, 117–18.

17. For this reason at the Annual German Surgeon's Convention in the same year and in an article, Mikulicz-Radecki only presented his results of a survey on experiences with sterilization practices on 6,032 patients in 47 university and other large women's hospitals as cumulative statistics, but did not give details for each hospital. Mikulicz-Radecki 1935a, 632; Mikulicz-Radecki 1935b, 1749.

18. Albrecht 1936, 23–51, 157.
19. Grimm 2004, 44.
20. Czarnowski and Hildebrandt 2017.
21. See, e.g., Bock 1986, 453ff; Hildebrandt et al. 2017.
22. Mikulicz-Radecki, a Catholic, joined the NSDAP in May 1933 and was a SA member. Bundesarchiv (BA) Berlin (formerly Berlin Document Center), Felix von Mikulicz-Radecki 17.7.1892.
23. Mikulicz-Radecki 1933, 1962, 1963.
24. Karl Heinrich Bauer (1890–1978) was the director of the Breslau (now Wrocław, Poland) Surgical University Hospital; after the war he held the same position in Heidelberg, where in 1945 he was appointed as rector of the university (Laufs 1990, 237–41).
25. Bauer and Mikulicz-Radecki 1936.
26. Bauer 1935; Mikulicz-Radecki 1935a.
27. Mikulicz-Radecki 1936a, 63.
28. Mikulicz-Radecki 1936a, 62.
29. Mikulicz-Radecki 1936a, 74.
30. Hördt 1937.
31. Mikulicz-Radecki 1936a, 73.
32. Mikulicz-Radecki 1936a, 74.
33. Mikulicz-Radecki 1936a, 74.
34. Rolf Böhnke 1939, 2392 f.
35. See, also for the following: Prüll and Rauh 2014; Hofer, Prüll, and Eckart 2011.
36. Similarly, a *Oberstabsarzt* (senior military physician) in World War I especially welcomed that military physicians were exonerated by the *Sanitätsamt* (health authority) as the last decision maker for forced surgeries on soldiers (Michl 2007, 81–82).
37. Mikulicz-Radecki 1936a, 61.
38. Mikulicz-Radecki 1936a, 86.
39. August Mayer (1876–1968), director of the University Women's Hospital in Tübingen, proponent of eugenic sterilizations, had questioned in an unpublished article, "How and by whom will coercion be wielded if necessary? Are nurses and doctors who inwardly feel not justified to do this (because of fear of danger to life by anesthesia assault, for example) free to refuse their cooperation? Who will fill in for them?" (BA Berlin, R 1501/126244, Bl. 305).
40. Czarnowski 2019, 145–49.
41. Mikulicz-Radecki 1936a, 143.
42. See the operation records in Mikulicz-Radecki 1937 and Horn 1936.
43. See Bock 1986, 378; also to the disaster of the forced operations and the acquiescence of fatalities: Bock 1986, 372ff.
44. Mikulicz-Radecki 1936a, 99.
45. Mikulicz-Radecki 1936a, 122; Mikulicz-Radecki 1936d. In this paper he revised his notion on certain adhesions of the tube as certain signs for sterility and thus extended the indication for sterilization.

46. Mikulicz-Radecki 1936a, 61.
47. Mikulicz-Radecki 1936a, 72.
48. Mikulicz-Radecki 1936a, 149.
49. Mikulicz-Radecki 1936a, 62.
50. Mikulicz-Radecki 1936a, 112.
51. Mikulicz-Radecki 1936a, 71.
52. Mikulicz-Radecki 1963, 238. In January 1945 he evacuated the hospital (patients and personnel) to the west, and later he and his male assistants left Königsberg (now Kaliningrad) under hazardous conditions.
53. Stauber 1995.
54. See Dross et al. 2016.

References

Archives

Bundesarchiv (BA) Berlin:
Formerly Berlin Document Center, Felix von Mikulicz-Radecki 17.7.1892
Reichsministerium des Inneren R 1501 / 126244

Books and Articles

Albrecht, Hans. 1936. "Periodische Fruchtbarkeit und Unfruchtbarkeit." *Archiv für Gynäkologie* 161: 23–51, 156–57 (Schlußwort).
Bauer, Karl Heinrich, and Felix von Mikulicz-Radecki. 1935. "Über Technik und Methodik der Sterilisation beim Mann." *Archiv für Klinische Chirurgie* 183: 611–623.
———. 1936. *Die Praxis der Sterilisierungsoperationen.* Leipzig: Barth.
Bluhm, Agnes. 1937. "Rezension des Vortrags 'Der Eiauffangmechanismus bei der Frau und seine Bedeutung für die Sterilität' von Felix v. Mikulicz-Radecki." *Archiv für Rassen- und Gesellschaftsbiologie* 31: 536–37.
Bock, Gisela. 1986. *Zwangssterilisation im Nationalsozialismus: Studien zur Rassenpolitik und Frauenpolitik.* Opladen: Westdeutscher Verlag. Reprint 2010. Münster: Monsenstein und Vannerdat.
Böhnke, Rolf. 1939. "Mikroskopische Untersuchungen an Tuben, die aus eugenischen Gründen unwegsam gemacht wurden." *Zentralblatt für Gynäkologie* 63(44): 2392–99.
Czarnowski, Gabriele. 2008. "'Das unheilbar Erkrankte aus dem Volkswachstum ausschalten': Politische Gynäkologie an den Berliner Universitätsfrauenkliniken im Nationalsozialismus." In *Die Charité im Dritten Reich*, edited by Sabine Schleiermacher and Udo Schagen, 133–50. Paderborn: Ferdinand Schöningh. 2nd ed., 2019. Retrieved 30 July 2020 from https://charite.zeit-archiv.de/Inhalt__Onlinefassung/14__Politische_Gynaekologie_im_NS__Czarnowski/index.html.
Czarnowski, Gabriele, and Sabine Hildebrandt. 2017. "Research on the Boundary between Life and Death: Coercive Experiments on Pregnant Women and their Fetuses during National Socialism." In *From Clinic to Concentration Camp: Reassessing Nazi Medical and Racial Research, 1933–1945*, edited by Paul Weindling, 73–99. New York: Routledge.
Daum, Monika, and Hans-Ulrich Deppe. 1991. *Zwangssterilisation in Frankfurt am Main 1933–1945.* Frankfurt am Main: Campus.
Deutsche Gesellschaft für Gynäkologie. 1936. "Verhandlungen der Deutschen Gesellschaft für Gynäkologie: 24. Versammlung, München, 23. bis 26. Oktober 1935." *Archiv für Gynäkologie* 161.
Doetz, Susanne. 2011. *Alltag und Praxis der Zwangssterilisation: Die Berliner Universitätsfrauenklinik unter Walter Stöckel 1942–1944.* Berlin: be.bra wissenschaft.

Dross, Fritz, Wolfgang Frobenius, Andreas Thum, Alexander Bastian, with the cooperation of Ulrike Thoms. 2016. *"Ausführer und Vollstrecker des Gesetzeswillens"*: *Die Deutsche Gesellschaft für Gynäkologie im Nationalsozialismus.* Geburtshilfe und Frauenheilkunde. Supplement S01.
Fischer, Isidor (ed.). 1962. *Biographisches Lexikon der hervorragenden Ärzte der letzten fünfzig Jahre.* 2nd and 3rd ed. München, Berlin: Urban und Schwarzenberg.
Fraenkel, Ludwig. 1932. "Sterilisierung und Konzeptionsverhütung." *Archiv für Gynäkologie* 144: 86–132.
Genzer, Irmgard. 1937. *Erfolge der Hormonbehandlung bei hormonaler Sterilität.* Königsberg (Pr): Raabe.
Grimm, Jana. 2004. "Zwangssterilisation von Mädchen und Frauen während des Nationalsozialismus. Eine Analyse der Krankenakten der Universitäts-Frauenklinik Halle von 1934 bis 1945." Med. diss., Halle-Wittenberg. Retrieved 30 July 2020 from http://sundoc.bibliothek.uni-halle.de/diss-online/04/04H085/prom.pdf.
Hildebrandt, Sabine, Susan Benedict, Erin Miller, Michael Gaffney, Michael A. Grodin. 2017. "'Forgotten' Chapters in the History of Transcervical Sterilization: Carl Clauberg and Hans-Joachim Lindemann." *Journal of the History of Medicine and Allied Sciences* 72: 272–301.
Hofer, Hans-Georg, Cay-Rüdiger Prüll, and Wolfgang U. Eckart (eds.). 2011. *War, Trauma and Medicine in Germany and Central Europe (1914–1939).* Freiburg: Centaurus.
Hördt, Eduard. 1937. *Welchen Einfluß hat eine längerdauernde Amenorrhöe auf die generativen Funktionen der weiblichen Genitalorgane?* Berlin-Lichtenrade: Westkreuz-Druckerei.
Horn, Ruthardt. 1936. *Statistisches und Biologisches von 216 aus eugenischen Gründen sterilisierten Frauen.* Königsberg (Pr): Raabe.
Koch, Thomas. 1994. *Zwangssterilisation im Dritten Reich. Das Beispiel der Universitätsfrauenklinik Göttingen.* Frankfurt am Main: Mabuse.
Kröner Hans-Peter. 1989. *Die Emigration deutschsprachiger Mediziner im Nationalsozialismus: Berichte zur Wissenschaftsgeschichte, Sonderheft.* Weinheim.
Kürschners Deutscher Gelehrtenkalender. 1966. *Bio-bibliographisches Verzeichnis deutschsprachiger Wissenschaftler der Gegenwart.* 11th ed. München: Saur.
Laufs, Bernd. 1990. "Vom Umgang der Medizin mit ihrer Geschichte." In *Von der Heilkunde zur Massentötung: Medizin im Nationalsozialismus*, edited by Gerrit Hohendorf and AchimMagull-Seltenreich, 233–53. Heidelberg: Das Wunderhorn.
Link, Gunther. 1999. *Eugenische Zwangssterilisation und Schwangerschaftsabbrüche im Nationalsozialismus: Dargestellt am Beispiel der Universitätsfrauenklinik Freiburg.* Frankfurt am Main: Lang.
Michl, Susanne. 2007. *Im Dienste des "Volkskörpers": Deutsche und französische Ärzte im Ersten Weltkrieg.* Göttingen: Vandenhoeck & Ruprecht.
Mikulicz-Radecki, Felix von. 1926. "Experimentelle Untersuchungen über Tubenbewegungen." *Archiv für Gynäkologie* 127: 318–62.
———. 1933. *Gynäkologische Operationen.* Leipzig. 2nd completely new ed. Jena, 1962; 3rd reprint ed. Jena, 1963.
———. 1935a. "Indikation und Technik der Sterilisation bei der Frau." *Archiv für Klinische Chirurgie* 183: 624–35.
———. 1935b. "Sammelstatistik über eugenische Sterilisierungen bei der Frau und daraus sich ergebende Richtlinien." *Zentralblatt für Gynäkologie* 59(30): 1749–59.
———. 1936a. Die Sterilisierung bei der Frau. In *Die Praxis der Sterilisierungsoperationen*, Karl Heinrich Bauer and Felix von Mikulicz-Radecki, 61–149. Leipzig: Barth.
———. 1936b. "Der Eiauffangsmechanismus bei der Frau und die sich daraus ergebenden Schlussfolgerungen für die operative Behandlung der Sterilität." *Archiv für Gynäkologie* 161: 128–32.
———. 1936c. "Zur Sterilitätstherapie bei der Frau." *Deutsche medizinische Wochenschrift* 62(26): 1037–43.
———. 1936d. "Die Ovarienaufpfropfung auf den Uterus als Sterilitätsoperation." *Zentralblatt für Gynäkologie* 60: 1441–57.

———. 1937. *Der Eiauffangmechanismus bei der Frau und seine Bedeutung für die Sterilität*. Schriften der Königsberger Gelehrten Gesellschaft. Naturwissenschaftliche Klasse, vol. 13, no. 6. Halle (Saale): Max Niemeyer.

———. 1963. "Aus dem Leben und Wirken eines Frauenarztes und Hochschullehrers." *Hippokrates* 34(6): 235–40.

Prüll, Livia, and Philipp Rauh (eds.). 2014. *Krieg und medikale Kultur: Patientenschicksale und ärztliches Handeln in der Zeit der Weltkriege 1914–1945*. Göttingen: Wallstein.

Rothmaler, Christiane. 1991. *Sterilisationen nach dem "Gesetz zur Verhütung erbkranken Nachwuchses" vom 14. Juli 1933: Eine Untersuchung zur Tätigkeit des Erbgesundheitsgerichtes und zur Durchführung des Gesetzes in Hamburg in der Zeit zwischen 1933 und 1944*. Husum: Matthiesen.

Simmer, Hans H. 1986. "Gynäkologische Endokrinologie in den Verhandlungen der Deutschen Gesellschaft für Gynäkologie von 1886 bis 1935: Beiträge deutschsprachiger Frauenärzte." In *Zur Geschichte der Gynäkologie und Geburtshilfe*, edited by Beck Lutwin., 183–219. Berlin: Springer.

Stauber Manfred. 1995. "Gynäkologie im Nationalsozialismus—oder 'Die späte Entschuldigung': Verhandlungen der Deutschen Gesellschaft für Gynäkologie und Geburtshilfe, München, 23. bis 27. August 1994." *Arch Gynaecol Obstet* 257: 753–71.

CHAPTER 7

Deference, Pragmatism, Ideology
The Medical Student Kurt Gerstein and the Predicament of Ethical Conduct under National Socialism

Mathias Schütz

National Socialism (NS) is commonly understood as antithetical to morals and ethics. Still, the questions stand even if moral conduct was possible under the regime, and if the regime itself possessed and acted according to some kind of coherent ethical concept, however twisted it might appear. The question of ethics is almost naturally linked to medicine and the fact that healers easily became torturers and murderers under NS—often without acknowledging any contradiction between their professional ethos and their actions. The following remarks aim at contributing to a historical understanding of ethics during NS. They draw their inspiration from a recently discovered memorandum written by Kurt Gerstein (1905–45), during the time of his medical studies at Tübingen University, to the Reich's Ministry of the Interior. The memorandum addresses problems of anatomical procurement and treatment of human bodies. Although it only adds to the complicated and conflicting personality Kurt Gerstein has become famous for, it highlights a crucial fact about (medical) ethics under NS: that even an elaborate concept of deference, compliant to modern ethical standards, was compromised not only by pragmatic considerations but, eventually, by a punctual ideological conformity with NS.

Kurt Gerstein: Old Questions, New Sources

When, in 1967, Saul Friedländer coined the term "ambiguity of good" with regard to the life of Kurt Gerstein, it was not yet foreseeable that generations to come would be wondering about the motives behind Gerstein's actions.[1] Kurt Gerstein[2] was born into a conservative Prussian family in 1905 and grew up in northern Germany. He became a mining engineer, worked for the Prussian state, and joined the NSDAP together with his father and his brothers in 1933. At the same time, he was engaged in the Protestant Church's youth work, led a youth group and a Bible circle, and, through his activism, built a network of ties to the Bekennende Kirche (Confessing Church) opposition group. Gerstein was repulsed by the anti-Christian tendencies of some parts of the NS movement. When his youth group was slated to be absorbed into the Hitler Youth, he solemnly dissolved it, but kept in contact with his young followers. Instead of spreading God's word immediately—or his understanding thereof—he concentrated on editing and distributing brochures about sexual education and ethics. In the course of this engagement, he sometimes adopted the theory and rhetoric of anti-Semitism. Gerstein accused Jewish companies of wittingly weakening the youth's morals with blatant advertisement for condoms. Such claims connected his fight for austereness with the delusion of a Jewish conspiracy against the German people's community (*Volksgemeinschaft*). This apparent pro-regime rhetoric was in clear contrast to Gerstein's arrest for distribution of leaflets with disparaging and oppositional content, which led to his ouster from the NSDAP in 1936.

Torn between his father's demand to make peace with the regime and his own concepts of how to live a meaningful life, he decided to return to the university. After an initial leaning toward the Protestant ministry, he turned to the medical profession as a means of helping his fellow men. Gerstein studied medicine in Tübingen until he was, once again, arrested for contacts with oppositional activists and interned in the concentration camp of Welzheim for six weeks in 1938. Spiritually and financially on the verge of collapse, as well as responsible for his young family and constantly pressured by his father, he returned to the mining profession. In 1941, he suddenly joined the Waffen-SS, to the utter shock of his peers. He later claimed to have been motivated by the murder of one of his sisters-in-law in the *Aktion T4*, the mass killing of psychiatric and other patients—Gerstein said that he wanted to "look into those ovens and chambers to comprehend what is happening there."[3] Due to his education in engineering and in medicine, he joined the Waffen-SS's institute of hygiene and quickly became known internally as a specialist for all matters concerning disinfection. In 1942, he was assigned with the task of delivering a vast amount of prussic acid—the active component of the Zyklon B pesticide, which was later used for the mass murder of Jews in the gas chambers of German extermination camps—to an undisclosed location in occupied Poland. As he was suspicious of the ultimate potentially nefarious use of this chemical, he disposed of the load along the way under the pretense of safety concerns, as he claimed later. The journey led Gerstein to the extermination camps of the *Aktion Reinhard*,[4] where he witnessed the mass killing of deported Jews by carbon monoxide in Bełżec. Shocked by his gruesome discovery of what was actually going on "in those chambers and ovens," he returned to Germany and tried to alarm the Allies as well as the churches, and, allegedly, to sabotage the delivery of prussic acid to the extermination camps.

After the war, when he was in American and French custody, he wrote several versions of what has since become known as the *Gerstein Report* about his observations and actions. Gerstein committed suicide under unclear circumstances in a Paris prison for suspected war criminals.[5]

This short summary of Gerstein's life alone illustrates the difficulties of trying to understand his motives and actions. Indeed, Friedländer's first attempt to capture Gerstein's personality was followed by a great number of biographical research studies and theoretical explanations over the ensuing decades.[6] Despite all these efforts, certain important aspects of his life as well as basic questions about his character and motives have remained in dispute. Gerstein is still "a far greater mystery"[7] than any one narrative has given so far. Due to Gerstein's biography and actions, any research on him inevitably touches on concepts of good and evil, of justifiable and unjustifiable behavior. Thereby, it coincides with another, much younger field of research about the history of NS: A field that deals with the question of what morals and ethics meant for those who lived under the regime, as well as what they meant for actors within the regime. These rationales relate directly to philosophical concepts as well as to empirical practices, especially in medicine.[8] Based on insights from research into Gerstein's life as well as from a study of the question of morals and ethics under NS, this chapter attempts to understand and highlight Gerstein's actions: those that were owed to his personal moral concept as well as those in which he followed a National Socialist concept of ethical behavior. It will then be discussed in what way those concepts actually ran counter to or were consistent with each other. This attempt was made possible by the rather accidental discovery of an unknown document that Kurt Gerstein had written to the Reich's Ministry of the Interior on 18 April 1938.[9] The document, a memorandum dealing with the problems of anatomical body procurement, comprises seven typewritten pages and two pages of photographs from an anatomical burial ground with handwritten annotations. It thus represents one of the longest coherent texts produced by Gerstein other than the *Gerstein Report*. Additionally, it opens up a new perspective on the history of medicine and especially anatomy during NS: it highlights the fact that actual ethical considerations were possible and took place, the complacent claims of many contemporary anatomists notwithstanding.[10]

The memorandum does not only add to our knowledge about the period of his medical studies at Tübingen University. It also highlights Gerstein's ethical reflections in a time of soul searching. During this period, he turned away from the Protestant Church as a moral compass and toward the medical profession as a means of helping, advising, and evangelizing his fellow human beings.[11] Disillusioned by the demeanor of the church, the self-alignment of the pro-regime *Deutsche Christen* (German Christians) with the NS regime, and the toothless, theological opposition of the Bekennende Kirche, he was in dire need of a perspective for his career and his spiritual ambitions. And so he began to admire the "vital physicians, materialists, philistines," hoping that their "antithetical, but somehow endearing and pleasant companionship" would help to "grow and augment" the quality of his own inner being.[12] He expected that they would prepare him for the uniquely intimate situation between a doctor and his patient, a situation marked by need and trust. For this moral and spiritual task, which transcended the doctor's immediate, physical task, it was necessary to assure that the medical student's education and training met the highest standards—something Gerstein himself did not experience during the pivotal first contact with the human body, the anatomical dissection course. Gerstein's own experience with anatomical education in Tübingen led him to intervene with the Reich's Ministry of the Interior via his memorandum. The content of Gerstein's document will be presented here, put into its broader historical context and linked to the question of whether ethical conduct under NS was, after all, possible.

Critique and Reform: Gerstein's Memorandum on Anatomy

Long after Kurt Gerstein's death, his widow Elfriede recollected a scene from a visit at Tübingen's city cemetery and its separate burial ground "X." This area had been used by the anatomical institute for the burial of its dissected bodies for centuries and would continue to serve this purpose until the 1960s.[13] Elfriede Gerstein recalled that her husband was so outraged by what they saw at the anatomical burial field that he took pictures with his camera and filed a complaint with the university authorities.[14] It is not clear if the university reacted to this complaint or if the response was not deemed satisfactory by Gerstein. In either case, he decided to draft a memorandum on the conditions and the reform of the procurement and treatment of human bodies by anatomical institutes and sent it to the Reich's Ministry of the Interior. The missive was forwarded to the Reich's Ministry of Science and Education, which had the jurisdictional responsibility for this matter.[15] In the memorandum, Gerstein's concerns went far beyond a complaint about the conditions on the burial ground of Tübingen anatomy. Rather, those conditions seemed to have triggered his radical reexamination of the way human bodies were procured, treated, and disposed of by anatomical institutes. Although he acknowledged the imperative nature of anatomical work on the bodies of deceased persons, he wanted to change its conduct in a decisive manner.

Gerstein started his memorandum by reflecting on the history of anatomical body procurement and connecting it to the present situation. He detected a dialectic of stigmatization in the relationship between anatomical institutes and the corpses they procured. Since the early modern period, taboos surrounding anatomical dissection had been slowly removed, and bodies for anatomical use had been almost exclusively sourced from socially stigmatized persons. These included executed criminals, single mothers and illegitimate children, persons who had committed suicide, vagrants, the mentally ill—in short, anybody whose body was not claimed for burial or whose interment in sacred ground was refused by the religious authorities. Thus the work and workplace of the anatomist itself had become stigmatized. And exactly because anatomy was perceived as something unsavory, if not illegitimate, nobody wanted to end up on the dissection table. As a consequence, the enforced delivery of bodies stemming from the disenfranchised and marginalized remained the only source. Gerstein even believed to sense a veritable conspiracy of the churches and the relatives of suicidal persons to dispose of their bodies via anatomical institutes. However, this appeared to him as just an extreme version of the fundamental problem he detected: that the social stigmatization and exclusion of "the poorest of the poor of our people" extended beyond their death, a situation that he characterized as "brute and unbearable from a National Socialist point of view."[16] Instead of acknowledging the anatomical use of any body as a great—if involuntary—sacrifice and treating this body with the according respect, corpses were maltreated by cramming them into cheap coffins and hastily burying them in the anonymous common grave "X," without any ceremony whatsoever.

Gerstein then proposed six reform measures to end this mode of procurement and treatment of human bodies. Firstly, instead of placing all bodies and body parts in the same or a random coffin, each body would be assigned an individual coffin to transport it from the delivering institution to the anatomical institute and from the anatomy to the cemetery. Secondly, the acknowledgment of the body as an individual would have to replace its treatment as anonymous material and affect the way of storage at the anatomical institutes: instead of putting several bodies and body parts indiscriminately in the same bin, those bodies would be stored separately and the dissected parts collected in special containers. Hereby, all parts of one individual body would be placed back into its assigned coffin. Thirdly, the anatomical staff would be instructed according to those new rules and, fourthly, the students would receive a special explanatory note to raise their awareness and deference toward the human body during their work. Fifthly, while most of the bodies delivered to the anatomical institutes would receive such a deferent and individualized treatment, Gerstein saw the necessity as well as the moral legitimacy for one exemption from that strict rule: "The bodies of the executed—especially those executed for treason—could take an exceptional position, since they have placed themselves outside the people's community and, therefore, forfeited the right to be treated as members of this community. They could be used for the creation of anatomical specimens for teaching collections and the like."[17] And sixthly, disclosing his initial motive for writing the memorandum, Gerstein concluded that the anatomical burial needed to be completely reorganized, referring to the conditions he had witnessed on Tübingen's cemetery "X."

During his visit at burial ground "X," Gerstein had witnessed human bones spread across the soil, without any signs of maintenance or commemoration. These conditions, which he documented with several photographs, were the launching point for his criticism: "Humans are hastily buried here with less piety than a dog."[18] Such a treatment was not only unacceptable in itself, he argued, but appeared to be symptomatic for anatomists' general perception of the human body. Invoking National Socialist notions of honor, as well as the "law prohibiting cruelty against animals (lex Göring),"[19] Gerstein highlighted the necessity of acknowledging and expressly respecting what he understood as a difficult but necessary sacrifice for science and medical education. The only way out of the described vicious circle of social stigmatization surrounding anatomical body procurement would be a system of voluntary donation. To this end the highly negative image of anatomy needed to be overcome, and it would only be overcome by a transparent, dignified treatment of the human body. The measures he proposed culminated in his call for a ceremonial burial of the dissected bodies attended by faculty and students. The latter would also provide for the maintenance and care of the anatomical cemetery. The arranged burial ground would feature a huge boulder and an inscription in memory of those people who had "lent" their body to anatomy, to "honor their sacrifice."[20]

Gerstein's criticism and proposal for reform were intensively assessed at the Reich's Ministry of Science and Education but did not produce any immediate results. This was not only due to Gerstein's second internment in 1938, because of which his focus of attention shifted once again, away from medicine in general and anatomy in particular. Additionally, the reaction at the Ministry had been a mixture of bewilderment about the conditions documented by the memorandum and especially by the attached photographs, and even greater astonishment about the "extravagant"[21] reform measures Gerstein had proposed. Although the authorities acknowledged the obvious shortcomings at the undisclosed site,[22] they did not see the necessity for a fundamentally different approach toward the treatment of bodies in German anatomy. This position was further emphasized by Emil Abderhalden, professor of physiology and president of the academy of science Leopoldina in Halle, whom Gerstein himself had named as a possible reviewer of his proposals.[23] The fact that Abderhalden was also an early proponent of medical ethics, and even published and edited a journal called *Ethics*, highlights the complexity of ethical reasoning and conduct under NS—a problem that Gerstein also struggled with in his memorandum.

Gerstein's "Doubling": Ethics and Exclusion

In his famous attempt to illuminate the psyche of the Nazi doctors, Robert Lifton introduced the psychological concept of "doubling"[24]: He describes the physician's development of two autonomous selves, which are interconnected in a "Faustian bargain." Doubling allows the physician not only to function in an extreme environment but also to embrace this environment and the behavior it produces as legitimate and ethical. According to Lifton, doubling is not necessarily abnormal or immoral—it can be a necessary psychological reaction to counter and overcome an existential challenge. However, not everybody is similarly susceptible to doubling. Doctors, because of their training, almost immediately develop some variety of a professional self: "That doubling usually begins with the student's encounter with the corpse he or she must dissect, often enough on the first day of medical school. One feels it necessary to develop a 'medical self,' which enables one not only to be relatively inured to death but to function reasonably efficiently in relation to the many-sided demands of the work."[25] It needs to be stated that neither is Lifton's theory by any means the final word on the matter of the Nazi doctors' psyche, nor does his understanding of the effects of the dissection course on the development of the medical students still apply to current anatomical concepts.[26] Nonetheless, Lifton's concept of doubling might aid an understanding of the specific situation Gerstein was confronted with and reacted to. It was exactly the estranged and instrumental relationship of the medical student with the dead, naked human body that Gerstein understood as a problematic result from the dissection course—something he himself had experienced and described as utterly confusing: "Such experiences had in some way something liberating, in another way they did, for me, not suit the earnestness which is required when standing before a strange, defenseless body."[27] Gerstein explicitly reflected on the doubling he experienced, a process that obviously made him uncomfortable. It led him to see the root of this problematic experience in the way anatomy was organized.

Gerstein's criticism and his proposals for reform proclaimed the value of each individual person as a fundamental ethical principle: this value was not to be compromised by any scientific or medical consideration. This understanding and its application to the question of the procurement and treatment of human bodies by anatomical institutes went beyond anything even remotely under consideration at the time. Gerstein's critical analysis of the dialectic of stigmatization surrounding anatomical body procurement—social stigmatization as the reason for as well as the result of a body being procured by an anatomical institute—was a well-informed and clear-sighted assessment. It was the reason that, as Gerstein admitted in his memorandum, "the word anatomy has, in the vernacular, a gruesome and ... undignified connotation."[28] It was, in fact, one of the main reasons why anatomical institutes continuously had to complain about a shortage of bodies for teaching and research. It was also the reason why anatomical institutes could not imagine any other way of improving procurement than the strict enforcement of the delivery of those stigmatized bodies by the state.[29] Gerstein wanted to overcome this detrimental tradition by changing the way anatomy perceived and treated the human body: in procurement, in dissection, and in burial. Such an attitude was, as the reactions on the side of the Reich's Ministry of Science and Education as well as the "ethicist" Abderhalden indicate, way ahead of its time. It took another twenty-five years until anatomical body procurement began to transform into a system of individual body donations, putting an end to the social stigmatization associated with dissection. And it took even longer until the anatomical burial was turned into a ceremonial appreciation of the dead, organized and implemented by medical students.[30]

Considering such a progressive stance, it is all the more shocking how easily Gerstein excluded one particular group of persons—executed convicts—from his seemingly universal ethics. He designated them as objects not only of dissection but also of collection; he denied them the right not only to a dignified burial but to any burial at all. It appears that he was projecting all the social stigma associated with anatomy on those persons who, through their "treason," had forfeited being part of the German *Volksgemeinschaft*. It is striking that the historically informed Gerstein understood that anatomical dissection had always been an implicit punishment for a socially marginal way of life. Irrespective of this basic insight, he did not understand that his call for the indiscriminate dissection of executed persons was basically an explicit punishment. And he also did not comprehend that this concept of dissection as a postmortal penalty lay at the foundation of anatomical body procurement in early modern times and, therefore, at the very core of the inauspicious tradition he argued against.[31] In fact, just like his claim for the treatment as an individual of any body procured by anatomy was too progressive for his time, his claim for the postmortal punishment of executed convicts through dissection and collection was deemed as regressive even by NS.[32] Gerstein wanted to accommodate the anatomical need for collection and research through the bodies of the executed: the rule of a deferential treatment of the regular persons' bodies and their burial after having served the purpose of medical education would be based on the exception of executed convicts losing any self-determination and their bodies remaining in the anatomical institutes.

Gerstein could not anticipate the National Socialist execution machinery after the beginning of World War II, which produced thousands upon thousands of bodies for the German anatomies, delivered right after decapitation, willfully accepted by anatomists, and trivialized as "fresh material" in dozens of research papers.[33] Nevertheless, his general understanding of the bodies of executed persons as unreservedly disposable and their exclusion from his ethical concept raises the question of how he was able to integrate such contradictory positions. However, it is possible that he did not see them as contradictory. Rather, they might have appeared to him as conforming according to the generally accepted logic of the times, the society, and the regime Gerstein was a subject to no less than anybody else living under NS. Gerstein's memorandum is an example for the particular ethics that NS established, taught, and performed: an ethics that claimed to enforce natural law, which rewarded strength, courage, assertiveness, even brutality.[34] The social integration and cohesion, the National Socialist claim echoed by Gerstein that "Germany honored even the smallest member of its people's community,"[35] was built on exclusion; it was built on the "enormous dynamic of the process of withdrawing solidarity"[36] from those people identified as not belonging to or working against the community. Whether following an ideological and moral conviction or because of pragmatic and strategic considerations, Gerstein, time and again, tried to reconcile himself with National Socialist positions, not only by differentiating between good Germans and "traitors" unworthy of a respectful treatment but also by denouncing an alleged Jewish sexual conspiracy against the German youth.[37] Especially through his "entryism,"[38] his attempts to influence National Socialist organizations from within, Gerstein tried to implement his concepts of sexual education and abstinence. He concurred to cooperate even with the most sinister parts of the National Socialist movement, willfully renouncing his own confessional background.[39]

The National Socialist impregnation of Gerstein's moral considerations regarding the procurement and treatment of human bodies by anatomical institutes is highlighted by one of his undeniably progressive proposals. Himself a devout Christian, he harshly criticized the Christian tradition of refusing a proper burial for the socially stigmatized. He wanted the anatomical burial grounds to be transformed into dignified places of remembrance and reflection, especially for medical students who would also take care of the sites' maintenance. He promoted this proposal as a measure rendering "the highest value for people's education."[40] Gerstein combined his referral to such concepts with the notion of "sacrifice" for the community made by the deceased. In his imagination, the anatomical burial ground was an exact reflection of German military cemeteries, a place of national memory, resurrection, and revenge after the loss of World War I.[41] His claim for the appreciation of the individual could only be thought of as a service to the collective, the National Socialist *Volksgemeinschaft*. Gerstein could only argue for his views on the respectful and dignified procurement and treatment of human bodies in anatomy by being pragmatic enough to commit to some basic ideological convictions of NS. His ethics were, in the end, purchased by exclusion.

Conclusion: No Evasion

Gerstein's memorandum on the treatment of human bodies in anatomy, his commitment to sexual education and abstinence, and his entryism reveal that he was willing to engage in some kind of "Faustian Bargain," as Lifton has phrased it regarding the doubling of the Nazi doctor's self. Although neither a Nazi nor a doctor, Gerstein tried to enforce his ethical concepts by integrating parts of the National Socialist ideological and moral convictions: the framing of the Jews, the exclusion of "traitors," the denial of traditional religious beliefs, the search for compliance to the point of self-denial. He was willing to adapt to a certain extent to the ruling worldview in order to prevail with his personal worldview regarding those particular topics he held dear. Hereby, Gerstein—involuntarily as well as unconsciously—proved to be an integral part of the German *Volksgemeinschaft*, which, as has been noted, constituted itself as a "community of action,"[42] i.e. not exclusively through absolute ideological conformity but rather through the individual implementation of the social-Darwinist paradigm of assertiveness as the only valid and relevant ethics. By trying to maintain his influence and to live up to his morals, Gerstein confirmed what Hannah Arendt later analyzed as a flawed, if not doomed understanding of responsibility: "the almost universal breakdown, not of personal responsibility, but of personal *judgment*...."[43] This led sensible people like Gerstein to believe in the possibility of ethical conduct and positive influence—notwithstanding the overwhelming reality of the political regime, the *Volksgemeinschaft*'s social cohesion, and its everyday violence. "Whoever participates in public life at all, regardless of party membership or membership in the elite formations of the regime, is implicated in one way or another in the deeds of the regime as a whole.... For the simple truth of the matter is that only those who withdrew from public life altogether, who refused political responsibility of any sort, could avoid becoming implicated in crimes, that is, avoid legal and moral responsibility."[44] This was also Kurt Gerstein's ethical predicament.

Mathias Schütz is a historian who specializes in the development of German scientific medicine during the nineteenth and twentieth centuries. He received his PhD from the University of Hamburg and currently works at the Institute for Ethics, History and Theory of Medicine of Ludwig-Maximilians-University Munich.

Notes

1. Friedländer 1967. Cf. Hébert 2016.
2. For Gerstein's biography, cf. Friedländer 1967; Hey, Rickling, and Stockhecke 2003; Schäfer 1999.
3. The quote is taken from Rothfels 1953, 187. Translation from German by the author.
4. The *Aktion Reinhardt*, named after the infamous SS officer Reinhard Heydrich, who had been liquidated by Czechoslovakian agents in May 1942, was the first phase of the systematic murder of (Polish) Jews by means of gassing. It was executed with carbon monoxide in the three camps of Bełżec, Treblinka, and Sobibor, of which Gerstein claims to have visited the former two.
5. Until today, Gerstein's accounts remain an important source of documentation, especially regarding Bełżec. Cf. Kuwałek 2013, 298.
6. Brayard 2001; Brayard 2002; Brayard 2008; Dreßen 1997; E. Franz 1970; H. Franz 1964; Hébert 2006; Hébert 2016; Hey, Rickling, and Stockhecke 2003; Jersak 2004; Joffroy 1992; Schäfer 1999; Steinbach 1997.

7. Smith 1997, 367. Cf. Gross 2010, 144.
8. Bialas 2014; Bialas and Fritze 2014; Bruns 2009; Bruns 2014; Fasching 2001; Frewer 2000; Frewer and Bruns 2003; Gross 2010; Konitzer and Gross 2009; Konitzer and Palme 2016; Koonz 2003; Nickelsen 2018; Proctor 2000; Rütten 1996/97. The term "ethics," albeit without any conceptual elaboration, has also been adopted by Burleigh 1997 and Nicosia 2002.
9. Kurt Gerstein to Reich's Ministry of the Interior, 18 April 1938, Bundesarchiv-Berlin, R 4901/935, fol. 7–15. The discovery of the document by the author of this chapter occurred during research for a project regarding the history of the anatomical institute of Munich University during National Socialism. Cf. Schütz et al. 2017.
10. Cf. Hildebrandt 2013, 19f.
11. For Gerstein's relation to medicine and his memorandum's contextualization within the history of anatomy, cf. Schütz 2018.
12. Kurt Gerstein to Kurt Niedermeyer, 19 December 1937, Landeskirchliches Archiv der Evangelischen Kirche von Westfalen-Bielefeld, 5.2, 686. Translation from German by the author.
13. Mörike 1988, 99; Schönhagen 1987, 7–10.
14. Joffroy 1992, 104f.
15. Reich's Ministry of the Interior to Reich's Ministry of Science and Education, 2 May 1938, Bundesarchiv-Berlin, R 4901/935, fol. 6.
16. Kurt Gerstein to Reich's Ministry of the Interior, 18 April 1938, Bundesarchiv-Berlin, R 4901/935, fol. 9. Translation from German by the author.
17. Kurt Gerstein to Reich's Ministry of the Interior, 18 April 1938, Bundesarchiv-Berlin, R 4901/935, fol. 10. Translation from German by the author.
18. Kurt Gerstein to Reich's Ministry of the Interior, 18 April 1938, Bundesarchiv-Berlin, R 4901/935, fol. 11. Translation from German by the author.
19. Kurt Gerstein to Reich's Ministry of the Interior, 18 April 1938, Bundesarchiv-Berlin, R 4901/935, fol. 11. Translation from German by the author. The "German Reich's animal protection law" from 24 November 1933, named after then Prussian prime minister and NS's foremost hunter, Hermann Göring, forbade e.g. scientific experiments on living animals.
20. Kurt Gerstein to Reich's Ministry of the Interior, 18 April 1938, Bundesarchiv-Berlin, R 4901/935, fol. 11. Translation from German by the author.
21. Reich's Ministry of Science and Education, Bach to Scheer, 6 May 1938, Bundesarchiv-Berlin, R 4901/935, fol. 16. Translation from German by the author.
22. Gerstein was also in direct contact with the chair of Tübingen anatomy, Robert Wetzel, and did not want to jeopardize this relationship; only later did he reveal the location of the cemetery and the anatomical institute. Cf. Kurt Gerstein to Reich's Ministry of Science and Education, 23 June 1938; Reich's Ministry of Science and Education, Note by Scheer, 27 June 1939, Bundesarchiv-Berlin, R 4901/935, fol. 18, 33. For Robert Wetzel, a National Socialist activist, cf. Scharer 2014.
23. Emil Abderhalden to Reich's Ministry of Science and Education, 11 July 1938, Bundesarchiv-Berlin, R 4901/935, fol. 20 f. For Gerstein's relationship with Abderhalden, cf. Frewer 2000, 109f.
24. Lifton 1986, 418.
25. Lifton 1986, 426f.
26. Cf. Grodin 2010; Hildebrandt 2016a.
27. Joffroy 1992, 104. Translation from French by the author.
28. Kurt Gerstein to Reich's Ministry of the Interior, 18 April 1938, Bundesarchiv-Berlin, R 4901/935, fol. 12. Translation from German by the author.
29. Schütz 2018, 196f.
30. Schütz 2018, 200f. Cf. Schütz 2019.
31. Stukenbrock 2003, 230.
32. E.g. in discussions at the Reich's Ministry of Justice in 1935. Cf. Schütz 2018, 203.

33. For a comprehensive account of German anatomy during National Socialism, cf. Hildebrandt 2016b.
34. Cf. Bruns 2009: 44; Chapoutot 2016: 24f.; Konitzer 2009: 108; Proctor 2000: 343.
35. Kurt Gerstein to Reich's Ministry of the Interior, 18 April 1938, Bundesarchiv-Berlin, R 4901/935, fol. 11. Translation from German by the author.
36. Welzer 2005, 57. Translation from German by the author.
37. Schäfer 1999, 96.
38. The term relates to a Trotskyite concept of infiltrating reformist parties and transforming them into revolutionary organizations. Due to its historic failure, there exists the expression "entryism until self-denial," which could also be applied to Gerstein.
39. Kurt Gerstein to his closest associates and friend, 24 November 1939, Landeskirchliches Archiv der Evangelischen Kirche von Westfalen-Bielefeld, 5.2, 686. Cf. Schütz 2018, 206; Schäfer 1999, 139–41.
40. Kurt Gerstein to Reich's Ministry of the Interior, 18 April 1938, Bundesarchiv-Berlin, R 4901/935, fol. 13. Translation from German by the author.
41. Cf. Mosse 1990, 84–89.
42. Bajohr 2014.
43. Arendt 2003, 24 (emphasis in original).
44. Arendt 2003, 33f.

References

Arendt, Hannah. 2003. "Personal Responsibility under Dictatorship." In *Hannah Arendt: Responsibility and Judgement*, edited by Jerome Kohn, 17–48. New York: Schocken.
Bajohr, Frank. 2014. "'Community of Action' and Diversity of Attitudes: Reflections on Mechanisms of Social Integration in National Socialist Germany, 1933–45." In *Visions of Community in Nazi Germany: Social Engineering and Private Lives*, edited by Martina Steber and Bernhard Gotto, 187–99. Oxford: Oxford University Press.
Bialas, Wolfgang. 2014. *Moralische Ordnungen des Nationalsozialismus*. Bristol, CT: Vandenhoeck & Ruprecht.
Bialas, Wolfgang, and Lothar Fritze (eds.). 2014. *Nazi Ideology and Ethics*. Newcastle: Cambridge Scholars.
Brayard, Florent. 2001. "Humanitarian Concern versus Zyklon B." In *Remembering for the Future: The Holocaust in the Age of Genocide*. Vol. 2: *Ethics and Religion*, edited by John K. Roth and Elisabeth Maxwell, 54–65. New York: Palgrave.
———. 2002. "L'Humanité versus Zyklon B: L'ambiguïté du choix de Kurt Gerstein." *Vingtième Siècle: Revue d'Histoire* 73(1): 15–25.
———. 2008. "'Grasping the Spokes of the Wheel of History': Gerstein, Eichmann and the Genocide of the Jews." *History & Memory* 20(1): 48–88.
Bruns, Florian. 2009. *Medizinethik im Nationalsozialismus: Entwicklungen und Protagonisten in Berlin (1939–1945)*. Stuttgart: Franz Steiner.
———. 2014. "Medical Ethics and Medical Research on Human Beings in National Socialism." In *Human Subject Research after the Holocaust*, edited by Sheldon Rubenfeld and Susan Benedict, 39–50. Cham: Springer International.
Burleigh, Michael. 1997. *Ethics and Extermination: Reflections on the Nazi Genocide*. Cambridge: Cambridge University Press.
Chapoutot, Johann. 2016. "Eine nationalsozialistische Normativität? Über den Sinn und die Werte des Nationalsozialismus." In *"Arbeit," "Volk," "Gemeinschaft." Ethik und Ethiken im Nationalsozialismus*, edited by Werner Konitzer and David Palme, 13–25. Frankfurt am Main: Campus.

Dreßen, Willi. 1997. "Die Rolle eines Toten im sogenannten 'DEGESCH'-Prozeß: Kurt Gerstein und die Zyklon-B-Lieferungen." *Jahrbuch für Westfälische Kirchengeschichte* 91: 199–210.
Fasching, Darrell J. 2001. "Ethics without Choice: Lessons Learned from Rescuers and Perpetrators." In *Remembering for the Future: The Holocaust in the Age of Genocide*. Vol. 2: *Ethics and Religion*, edited by John K. Roth and Elisabeth Maxwell, 81–97. New York: Palgrave.
Franz, Egon. 1970. "Die sexualpädagogische Missionsarbeit Kurt Gersteins im Rahmen seines Widerstandes gegen die Machthaber des 3. Reiches." *Die Innere Mission* 60: 208–16.
Franz, Helmut. 1964. *Kurt Gerstein: Außenseiter des Widerstandes der Kirche gegen Hitler*. Zürich: EVZ.
Frewer, Andreas. 2000. *Medizin und Moral in der Weimarer Republik und im Nationalsozialismus: Die Zeitschrift "Ethik" unter Emil Abderhalden*. Frankfurt am Main: Campus.
Frewer, Andreas, and Florian Bruns. 2003. "'Ewiges Arzttum' oder 'neue Medizinethik' 1939–1945? Hippokrates und Historiker im Dienst des Krieges." *Medizinhistorisches Journal* 38(3–4): 313–35.
Friedländer, Saul. 1967. *Kurt Gerstein ou l'ambiguïté du bien*. Paris: Casterman.
Grodin, Michael A. 2010. "Mas, Bad, or Evil: How Physician Healers Turn to Torture and Murder." In *Medicine after the Holocaust: From the Master Race to the Human Genome and Beyond*, edited by Sheldon Rubenfeld, 49–65. New York: Palgrave Macmillan.
Gross, Raphael. 2010. *Anständig geblieben: Nationalsozialistische Moral*. Frankfurt am Main: S. Fischer.
Hébert, Valerie. 2006. "Disguised Resistance? The Story of Kurt Gerstein." *Holocaust and Genocide Studies* 20(1): 1–33.
———. 2016. "Hans Rothfels, Kurt Gerstein and the Report: A Retrospective." In *Holocaust and Memory in Europe*, edited by Thomas Schlemmer and Alan E. Steinweis, 85–105. Berlin: De Gruyter Oldenbourg.
Hey, Bernd, Matthias Rickling, and Kerstin Stockhecke. 2003. *Kurt Gerstein (1905–1945). Widerstand in SS-Uniform*. 2nd ed. Bielefeld: Verlag für Regionalgeschichte.
Hildebrandt, Sabine. 2013. "The Case of Robert Herrlinger: A Unique Postwar Controversy on the Ethics of the Anatomical Use of Bodies of the Executed during National Socialism." *Annals of Anatomy* 195: 11–24.
———. 2016a. "Practical Core Elements of an Ethical Anatomical Education." *Clinical Anatomy* 29(1): 37–45.
———. 2016b. *The Anatomy of Murder: Ethical Transgressions and Anatomical Science during the Third Reich*. New York: Berghahn Books.
Jersak, Tobias. 2004. "Die vermeintliche Ambivalenz des Bösen: Der SS-Offizier Kurt Gerstein." In *Karrieren im Nationalsozialismus: Funktionseliten zwischen Mitwirkung und Distanz*, edited by Gerhard Hirschfeld and Tobias Jersak, 255–62. Frankfurt am Main: Campus.
Joffroy, Pierre. 1992. *L'espion de Dieu: La passion de Kurt Gerstein*. Rev. ed. Paris: Seghers.
Konitzer, Werner. 2009. "Moral oder 'Moral'? Einige Überlegungen zum Thema 'Moral und Nationalsozialismus.'" In *Moralität des Bösen: Ethik und nationalsozialistische Verbrechen*, edited by Werner Konitzer and Raphael Gross, 97–115. Frankfurt am Main: Campus.
Konitzer, Werner, and Raphael Gross (eds.). 2009. *Moralität des Bösen: Ethik und nationalsozialistische Verbrechen*. Frankfurt am Main: Campus.
Konitzer, Werner, and David Palme (eds.). 2016. *"Arbeit," "Volk," "Gemeinschaft." Ethik und Ethiken im Nationalsozialismus*. Frankfurt am Main: Campus.
Koonz, Claudia. 2003. *The Nazi Conscience*. Cambridge, MA: Belknap Press.
Kuwałek, Robert. 2013. *Das Vernichtungslager BEŁEC*. Berlin: Metropol.
Lifton, Robert Jay. 1986. *The Nazi Doctors: Medical Killing and the Psychology of Genocide*. New York: Basic Books.
Mörike, Klaus D. 1988. *Geschichte der Tübinger Anatomie*. Tübingen: J. C. B. Mohr.
Mosse, George L. 1990. *Fallen Soldiers: Reshaping the Memory of the World Wars*. Oxford: Oxford University Press.

Nickelsen, Kärin. 2018. "On Otto Warburg, Nazi Bureaucracy and the Difficulties of Moral Judgment." *Photosynthetica* 56(1): 75–85.
Nicosia, Francis R. (ed.). 2002. *Medicine and Medical Ethics in Nazi Germany: Origins, Practices, Legacies*. New York: Berghahn Books.
Proctor, Robert N. 2000. "Nazi Science and Nazi Medical Ethics: Some Myths and Misconceptions." *Perspectives in Biology and Medicine* 43(3): 335–46.
Rothfels, Hans. 1953. "Augenzeugenbericht zu den Massenvergasungen." *Vierteljahreshefte für Zeitgeschichte* 1(2): 177–94.
Rütten, Thomas. 1996/97. "Hitler with—or without—Hippocrates? The Hippocratic Oath during the Third Reich." *Korot: The Israel Journal of the History of Medicine and Science* 12: 91–106.
Schäfer, Jürgen. 1999. *Kurt Gerstein—Zeuge des Holocaust: Ein Leben zwischen Bibelkreisen und SS*. Bielefeld: Luther-Verlag.
Scharer, Philip. 2014. *Robert Friedrich Wetzel (1898–1962): Anatom—Urgeschichtsforscher—Nationalsozialist*. Hamburg: Dr. Kovač.
Schönhagen, Benigna. 1987. *Das Gräberfeld X: Eine Dokumentation über NS-Opfer auf dem Tübinger Stadtfriedhof*. Tübingen: Kulturamt.
Schütz, Mathias. 2018. "Doppelte Moral: Der Medizinstudent Kurt Gerstein und die Geschichte des anatomischen Leichenwesens in Deutschland." *NTM Zeitschrift für Geschichte der Wissenschaften, Technik und Medizin* 26(2): 185–212.
———. 2019. "Erzwungener Wandel: Die Transformation der anatomischen Leichenbeschaffung in Bayern nach 1945." *Medizinhistorisches Journal* 54(1): 70–92.
Schütz, Mathias, Jens Waschke, Georg Marckmann, and Florian Steger. 2017. "Munich Anatomy and the Distribution of Bodies from the Stadelheim Execution Site during National Socialism." *Annals of Anatomy* 211: 2–12.
Smith, Lacey Baldwin. 1997. *Fools, Martyrs, Traitors. The Story of Martyrdom in the Western World*. New York: Knopf.
Steinbach, Peter. 1997. "Kurt Gerstein—Der Einzeltäter im Dilemma des exemplarischen Handelns." *Jahrbuch für Westfälische Kirchengeschichte* 91: 183–97.
Stukenbrock, Karin. 2003. "Unter dem Primat der Ökonomie? Soziale und wirtschaftliche Aspekte der Leichenbeschaffung für die Anatomie." In *Anatomie: Sektionen einer medizinischen Wissenschaft im 18. Jahrhundert*, edited by Jürgen Helm and Karin Stukenbrock, 227–39. Stuttgart: Franz Steiner.
Welzer, Harald. 2005. *Täter: Wie aus ganz normalen Menschen Massenmörder werden*. Frankfurt am Main: S. Fischer.

CHAPTER 8

LUDWIG STUMPFEGGER (1910–45)
A Career at the Interface of Hitler, Himmler,
and Ravensbrück Concentration Camp

Stephanie Kaiser and Mathias Schmidt

The role of medicine for the biopolitical nature of the Nazi ideology can be summarized in four key terms: health dictatorship, racial medicine, performance medicine, extermination medicine. These were characterized by anti-Semitic tendencies and "Nordic Aryan" superior notions with elements such as selection, perceptions of genetic value, artificial breeding (the "new man"), sterilization, "euthanasia" of a new quality ("annihilation of life unworthy of life"), and the fight against hereditary diseases.[1] For the rapid realization and implementation of this ideology, the cooperation with medicine was essential to the regime. The execution required the unconditional help of physicians, and many found themselves supporting these ideas, which is reflected in numbers: of all academic professions the physicians had the largest share of membership of the Nazi Party (NSDAP) with over 45 percent and also high membership rates for the Sturmabteilung (SA, paramilitary wing of the Nazi Party) or the Schutzstaffel (SS).[2] The purpose of the medical community had shifted. They were committed to the aims of Nazi state leadership: care for the *Volkskörper*, a collective body of racially pure Germans, became more important than the traditional care for the individual patient. A "race-ethical morality" was the supreme maxim of medical action, from which point of view even the systematic murder of care-dependent and sick people seemed morally correct and necessary for the sake of the German nation. Killing and healing became two inseparably linked but diametrically opposed strategies of action.

The work and support of the Nazi system by physicians led to the practical use of racial hygiene—the German version of eugenics—in human experiments, euthanasia, and unethical dealing with dead bodies, all in all to the moral downfall of the medical profession in Germany. Many questions regarding these physicians' character, intentions, career paths, networks, personal leeway, etc., have not yet been answered for all doctors involved. One of them is Ludwig Stumpfegger. Historians have long been aware of him, but his name was only noticed by the general public in the critically acclaimed movie *Der Untergang* (Downfall), which was nominated for the Academy Award for Best Foreign Language Film in 2004.[3] In one of the last scenes, which takes place one day after the suicide of Adolf Hitler on 30 April 1945, Magda Goebbels, the wife of Reich minister of propaganda Joseph Goebbels, entered the nursery of her six children accompanied by the physician Stumpfegger. First, the five girls and one boy were given morphine to fall asleep, then cyanide capsules were put in their mouths and crushed with their teeth. Although the exact circumstances of the children's deaths cannot be clarified in detail to date, testimonies and autopsies document this event. In those last days of the rapidly collapsing Third Reich, Stumpfegger and others who remained in the so-called *Führerbunker* (an air-raid shelter near the Reich Chancellery) tried to flee during the Battle of Berlin, but their traces were lost in the turmoil of war. Rumors of a successful flight to South America persisted, but in the year 1972—twenty-seven years later—two male skeletons were found in a construction pit near the area of the Lehrter Bahnhof in Berlin-Moabit (an inner-city train station that was heavily damaged during World War II and shut down in 1951). One body belonged to Martin Bormann, one of the most influential politicians in the Third Reich. He acted not only as chief of the Nazi Party Chancellery but also as Adolf Hitler's private secretary. The other body was identified as that of Ludwig Stumpfegger. An autopsy revealed that both men had committed suicide.[4]

To date, there is no comprehensive analysis of this German surgeon and SS leader's biography and actions available in English.[5] Although Stumpfegger is not an unknown protagonist of the Third Reich, there are still many gaps regarding his life story. Only a closer look explains what kind of person he was and how he ultimately gained a position in Adolf Hitler's inner circle, as his *Begleitarzt*[6] (escort physician). His is an exemplary character for a generation of young and ambitious physicians born at the beginning of the twentieth century—like Karl Brandt—who represent the ideological principles and political goals of National Socialism.

This study follows the rise of Stumpfegger in two areas. Firstly, the political and military area: Stumpfegger benefited from the relations of his superior Karl Gebhardt, the head physician of Hohenlychen Sanatorium. Through him, Stumpfegger became acquainted with Gebhardt's childhood friend Heinrich Himmler, the leader of the SS and chief of German police, and gained access to the highest political circles within the Nazi state. Through his personal contact with Himmler, Stumpfegger (whose physique corresponded to the ideal "racial image" of the SS[7]) was promoted quickly within the organization and thus utilized this relationship for a successful career advancement. Moreover, he was able to further strengthen his ties to Himmler, as he was appointed as his escort physician, which gave Stumpfegger access to the political and private environment of one of the most powerful men of the Nazi dictatorship.

Secondly, the medical area: as a very capable physician and a highly skilled surgeon, Stumpfegger worked at the Hohenlychen Sanatorium north of Berlin. Specializing in sports medicine, it had an excellent reputation far beyond the borders of the German Reich. During World War II, Stumpfegger was employed as a physician of the Waffen-SS (armed forces of the Nazi Party's SS) and was deployed both on the western and the eastern front. His medical focus changed accordingly from sports medicine to military medicine and war surgery. In order to make progress with his research in this area, he carried out medical crimes in the Ravensbrück concentration camp, which will be discussed here.

The main stations of Stumpfegger's life are used to illustrate the following central questions: How exactly did Stumpfegger enter the sphere of the most powerful men of the Third Reich? Was his successful career caused by coincidence or by his own calculation? What were the results of these interpersonal relationships in professional and social terms? And in which documented manner did Stumpfegger participate in the crimes of the Third Reich? These questions were investigated through examination of archival materials, especially from the Federal Archives in Berlin, the Archive of the Institute of Contemporary History in Munich, and military information from the Deutsche Dienststelle (WASt) für die Benachrichtigung der nächsten Angehörigen für Kriegsverluste und Kriegsgefangene.[8]

Stumpfegger's Connection to Gebhardt and Himmler and the Effects on His Career in the SS

Ludwig Stumpfegger was born on 11 July 1910 in Munich.[9] He grew up in a family of the social middle class in Landshut, a town in Lower Bavaria, and in this economically comfortable setting he was able to study medicine at the University of Munich from May 1930 until November 1935. Two years later he received his medical degree. He married in 1939 and had two children (born 1940 and 1944) with his wife Gertrud.

After Hitler's rise to power in January 1933, Stumpfegger joined the Allgemeine SS (General SS, the largest branch of the SS) with the membership number 83,668 in early June 1933. Two years later, on 1 May 1935, he became a member of the Nazi Party with the membership number 3,616,119. In joining the General SS first and at such an early stage of the Nazi regime, Stumpfegger revealed his political convictions. The General SS brought a certain prestige, and not everyone was able to become a member. However, Stumpfegger's choice is very interesting because before the so-called *Röhm-Putsch* (Night of the Long Knives) in summer 1934, the SS was actually subordinated to the SA and played a secondary role in the exterior view of National Socialism. Yet the SS styled itself to be more distinguished; from 1930 Himmler began to emphasize the differences between the SA and the SS, designating the SS as an "order" that was to be "racially more pure," "more faithful," and "tougher" than other organizations of the Nazi Party.[10] Stumpfegger appears to have shared these ideas.

During the 1936 Winter Olympic Games in Garmisch-Partenkirchen, a ski town in Bavaria, in February and the subsequent Summer Olympic Games that same year in Berlin, Stumpfegger worked in the medical center adjacent to the sports grounds under Karl Gebhardt (1897–1948).[11] It is possible that Stumpfegger's and Gebhardt's paths had already crossed long before in the Medical Faculty of the Ludwig-Maximilian-University in Munich. Both had completed their medical studies there, and Gebhardt had worked at the University as a private lecturer from the summer semester of 1933 onward. He was a pupil of Ferdinand Sauerbruch, one of the most important and influential surgeons of the twentieth century, as well as Erich Lexer, one of the founders of plastic surgery. Gebhardt led the internationally known and respected Hohenlychen Sanatorium in Brandenburg, which he had transformed into a flagship clinic of Nazi health policy and which was visited regularly by senior Nazi officials.[12] He was also a childhood friend of the *Reichsführer-SS* (literally Reich leader of the SS) Heinrich Himmler (1900–45) and, since March 1938, also his personal physician.[13]

At the beginning of the war, Hohenlychen, which used to be a sports medicine clinic, became a facility of the SS and changed its medical focus to the rehabilitation of war veterans.[14] Thus, part of Hohenlychen's SS staff was also involved in the crimes of the Nazi regime through involvement in human experiments (see below).

Stumpfegger was a talented and very capable surgeon, who had already entered the scientific field through numerous publications and had a special focus on sports medicine. Consequently, he was noticed by Gebhardt, who recruited the young physician to Hohenlychen in 1936. There Stumpfegger's career began as a surgical intern.[15] Gebhardt seemed to have valued Stumpfegger both professionally and personally, and appointed him to his adjutant in March 1940.[16] Thus

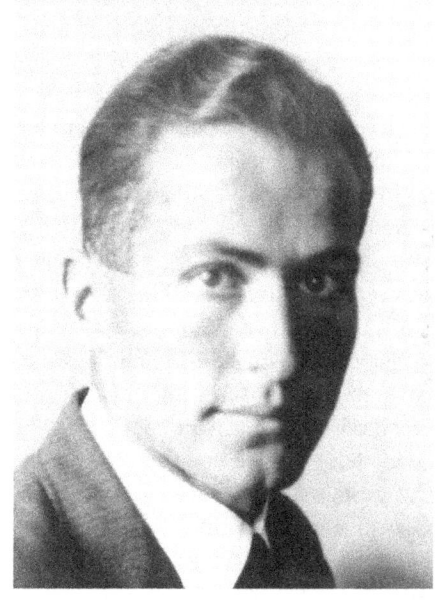

Figure 8.1. Portrait of Ludwig Stumpfegger, taken from a handwritten CV, undated. Courtesy Federal Archive Berlin, R 9361-III/559030, SSO-File Stumpfegger.

Gebhardt launched Stumpfegger on a successful career path and gave him access to the Nazi elite.

The exact date of Stumpfegger's first encounter with Himmler cannot be determined from the source material available.[17] It is highly likely that Gebhardt introduced him to Himmler at the Hohenlychen Sanatorium or during the Olympic Games. By 1938 at the latest, the relationship between Himmler and Stumpfegger was consolidated, and the latter profited from this: as SS-*Untersturmführer* (second lieutenant of the SS, the first commissioned SS officer rank) he was immediately awarded the *SS-Degen* (dress sword worn by the SS) on 26 August 1938 in accordance with a direct order of the *Reichsführer-SS*.[18] The sword served a priori as an indicator for those selected SS leaders who were in Himmler's personal favor. With the exception of the graduates of the *Waffen-SS-Junkerschulen* (SS leadership training facilities), who automatically received the sword, the conferring of the award did not follow any formal rule but was exclusively dependent on Himmler's personal decision and was accompanied by an increased status of the respective wearer.[19] The award of the *SS-Degen* proves Himmler's perception of and appreciation for Stumpfegger, whom he also addressed with the familiar "du" and the nickname "Stutz."

Stumpfegger first served in the German Wehrmacht. He completed a two-month basic training with the *15. Gebirgsjäger-Regiment 100* (mountain troops), most likely in 1937.[20] In the next year he took part in the annexation of the Sudetenland (northern, southern and western areas of former Czechoslovakia, which were inhabited primarily by German speaking inhabitants) to the German Reich and the occupation of Czechoslovakia. As Himmler's escort physician during that period, he would have spent a considerable amount of time in the direct vicinity of Himmler.[21]

In October 1939, after the German invasion of Poland, Stumpfegger volunteered for the later so-called Waffen-SS. This decision was clearly a political one, signifying Stumpfegger's ideological direction: he chose to perform his military service with the SS, Hitler's "political soldiers," and not with the traditional army, the German Wehrmacht. Initially not deployed with an SS unit, Stumpfegger soon belonged to Himmler's staff, for example when the latter inspected SS units in combat during the 1940 western campaign. The entourage included Gebhardt as well as Himmler's adjutant Joachim Peiper (1915–76), with whom Stumpfegger would later meet again on the eastern front.[22] In 1941 Stumpfegger was promoted to *SS-Sturmbannführer d. R.* (a major of the SS reserve) by the *Reichsführer-SS* himself.[23] In the same time period, Stumpfegger replaced Gebhardt as Himmler's physician, because the head of Hohenlychen became consulting surgeon of the Waffen-SS. Gebhardt himself described the tasks of Stumpfegger's new appointment as follows: "Whenever Himmler was in danger or went into a potential danger, he would always consult me [Gebhardt] or an assistant of mine or, from 1941 on, Dr. Stumpfegger in order to be provided with a surgeon."[24] However, Stumpfegger was most likely already aboard Himmler's private train as his physician from November 1939 onward,[25] a fact that demonstrates the increasingly trusting relationship between the men. In a postwar interrogation, Gebhardt explained that Stumpfegger, "as my substitute as Himmler's personal physician, had a particularly close relationship with him, as did I, because he was also from Landshut."[26]

At this point, Stumpfegger had become Gebhardt's "right hand" and been promoted to attending and deputy chief physician in Hohenlychen.[27] His surgical skills were also called for after a secret medical-statistical report by the Waffen-SS had shown that their units were particularly affected by the surgical supply crisis within the German Armed Forces.[28] The reason behind this was that those units operated at the focal points of the eastern front and were often poorly qualified, which had led to an extremely high number of casualties and deaths due to wound infection. In order to counter this and to achieve a reduction in the losses of so-called secondary dead (those who had died of their injuries and of wound infections), Gebhardt, by Himmler's command, created a *Chirurgensondergruppe beim Kommandostab des RfSS* (special surgeons' unit at the staff of the *Reichsführer-SS*) under Stumpfegger's leadership. This group's task was to actively intervene when the medical units were overloaded, or—in particularly severe individual cases—with a special consideration of members of the Waffen-SS.[29] A better training for the junior surgeons in the military hospitals of the Waffen-SS was to be introduced as well. And this was what Stumpfegger's *Chirurgengruppe* was sent out to do in 1941 in their deployment with the SS division Reich.[30]

Stumpfegger experienced World War II not only on the western but also on the eastern front, interrupted by a "research visit" at Ravensbrück concentration camp (see below). In spring 1943, he and the *Chirurgengruppe* "Hohenlychen" under his command were transferred to Peiper's 3rd Battalion, 2nd *Panzergrenadier Regiment* (armored infantry) of the restructured SS division *Leibstandarte SS Adolf Hitler*.[31] The two SS men knew each other from their time with Himmler. Stumpfegger most likely spent seven weeks with Peiper's battalion, receiving the Iron Cross 2nd Class for this service. In April 1943, the promotion to *SS-Obersturmbannführer* (lieutenant colonel of the SS) was granted following again an explicit request by Himmler. A few days later, Stumpfegger also received the Iron Cross 1st Class,[32] and in the early summer of 1944, Stumpfegger was awarded the coveted *SS-Ehrenring* (SS honor ring).[33] This was another personal honor bestowed by Himmler, similar to the *SS-Degen*. He was still assigned to the *Leibstandarte* in July 1944, which had been moved to France after the Allies landed in Normandy.

Medical Experiments in Ravensbrück Concentration Camp

Starting in late 1942 and throughout the first half of 1943, Stumpfegger worked on his *Habilitation* (senior thesis to become university lecturer) at the Medical

Faculty of the Friedrich Wilhelm University of Berlin. He did so in Hohenlychen as well as in Ravensbrück concentration camp, only fifteen kilometers away. In Hohenylchen as a staff member he had access to data from patients who were in care there, and in Ravensbrück he took part in medical experiments on female prisoners. These were designed to analyze the development of gas gangrene (clostridial myonecrosis) and to examine whether chemotherapeutic agents such as sulfonamides were superior to traditional surgical procedures for the treatment of wound infections.[34]

In the course of the Russian campaign, the German medical service had to face new challenges. The number of wounded and the type of injuries overwhelmed the organizationally and methodologically ill-prepared medical units and led to a high number of soldiers dying as a result of injuries and wound infections. Therefore, experiments were prepared to solve the dire situation. Recent research has shown that this experiments had already been designed when the assassination attempt on Reinhard Heydrich—chief of the *Reichssicherheitshauptamt* (SS Reich Main Security Office) and acting Reich protector of Bohemia and Moravia—on 27 May 1942 took place. His death by gangrene nine days later was by no means the reason for the experiments, only illustrating the problems.[35] In addition to experiments in Auschwitz, Sachsenhausen, and Dachau, Karl Gebhardt conducted experiments in the women's concentration camp Ravensbrück since June 1942. Bacteria, decay pathogens, wood splinters, and glass were introduced into specially inflicted wounds on the victims of the experiments, thus imitating injuries caused by bomb splinters. The course of the wound development and healing as well as the effect of the drugs tested were documented and analyzed.[36]

In November 1942 Stumpfegger and Fritz Fischer, an intern at the Hohenlychen Sanatorium who had carried out the experiments with sulfonamides under Gebhardt's supervision, started new experiments to further their own scientific careers.[37] Until February 1943 the two physicians carried out surgeries on at least twenty-five Polish female inmates in Ravensbrück, occasionally supported by other doctors from Hohenlychen. According to his own statements, Stumpfegger's goal was to check new research results from scientists from "enemy states" as he called it, which claimed that not only the periosteum but also the surrounding connective tissue could be bone-forming. Through his experiments, Stumpfegger wanted to develop new methods in the treatment of wounded or injured patients.[38] For this purpose, he and Fischer sawed out parts of both bones in the lower legs of the women, in some cases leaving the periosteum in situ, in others removing it. In addition, the shin-bones of at least two women were shattered to study new bone formation. These procedures led to severe lifelong suffering for the victims.[39] In these experiments, Stumpfegger had clearly exceeded his official tasks in the military surgical trial and had entered the field of reconstructive surgery, which was his personal scientific interest.

It is unclear if or to what extent the results of Stumpfegger's research were used. In 1944, he published his *Habilitation* with the title *Die freie autoplastische Knochentransplantation in der Wiederherstellungschirurgie: Erfahrungen und Ergebnisse* (Free autoplastic bone grafting in reconstructive surgery: Experiences and results). Here, Stumpfegger evaluated various documented cases from the therapeutic institutions of Hohenlychen, all of which were described in a standard scheme: the patient's personal information was followed by the patient's history, symptoms and diagnosis, the surgical procedures, and the course of the recovery period. In ten other cases, however, the information differed from this template. In these, only age, patient initials, and surgical procedure were documented.[40] Stumpfegger declared in his *Habilitation* that he had obtained his research results from material (medical records, X-ray images, histological preparations) of patients from Hohenlychen and "partly from my own experiments."[41] He received his license to lecture in 1944 at the Medical Faculty of the Friedrich Wilhelm University in Berlin. After comparing the testimonies of the victims during the Nuremberg Doctors Trial with the experiments described by Stumpfegger, medical historian Ulf Schmidt hypothesizes that the ten cases in Stumpfegger's habilitations are those of prisoners on whom he had experimented in Ravensbrück concentration camp.[42]

Stumpfegger was also involved in at least one human experiment, in which conditions for the success of heterologous bone grafts were tested. For this experiment, Fritz Fischer was sent to Ravensbrück to remove a shoulder blade from a living concentration camp inmate and bring it back to Hohenlychen immediately. There it was implanted in a patient whose shoulder girdle bones had been resected because of a bone tumor. The operation in Hohenlychen was either performed by Stumpfegger himself or at least with his assistance.[43] Although this case was discussed in detail at the Nuremberg Doctors Trial, it could not be conclusively determined who initiated this transplantation or who initiated Fischer's and Stumpfegger's experiments. On the one hand, during an interrogation in 1945, Fischer testified that Gebhardt had given him the order to carry out the surgery in Ravensbrück so that Stumpfegger could assist with the following operation in Hohenlychen. Gebhardt, on the other hand, stated at the Nuremberg court that the experiments were based on Stumpfegger's initiative and were approved by Himmler. Furthermore, so he claimed, he himself had had scientific objections at the time and agreed to the transplantation of the shoulder blade only under certain conditions.[44] Although the exact course of events can no longer be sufficiently clarified, it seems unlikely that Stumpfegger's experiments were approved by Himmler *against* Gebhardt's will. Also not credible is that Gebhardt had rejected Stumpfegger's experimental design and negotiated terms with his long-time colleague. These experiments corresponded with Gebhardt's own research interests, a fact to which Fritz Fischer also testified in 1945,[45] and Gebhard had served as reviewer of Stumpfegger's *Habilitation* as well.[46] Also, Fischer's line of defense was to deny all responsibility with the argument of command hierarchy, an argument that the Allied Powers had originally refused to accept as early as January 1942, instead holding every individual perpetrator personally accountable for his or her actions.[47] Fischer wanted to convince the court that the scientific and moral responsibility lay with the person in charge of the experiments, and this person had been Karl Gebhardt.[48] Therefore, it can either be assumed that the initiative came from Gebhardt, who gave Stumpfegger the opportunity to conduct medical experiments in a concentration camp, or that Stumpfegger specifically asked for it after he heard about this possibility. In either of these scenarios, Stumpfegger was not forced to do anything, but rather he initiated new experiments that furthered his own scientific interest and career, and which had been made possible within the framework of already existing experiments in Ravensbrück, where sulfonamides were tested for purposes of military medicine.

Stumpfegger as Hitler's Escort Physician and His Suicide in 1945

On 9 October 1944, Ludwig Stumpfegger ascended to the innermost circle of the crumbling Third Reich at the young age of thirty-four. In the wake of the dismissals of Karl Brandt, *Bevollmächtigter für das Sanitäts- und Gesundheitswesen* (Reich commissioner of sanitation and health), the surgeon Hans Karl von Hasselbach, and the otorhinolaryngologist Erwin Giesing, Stumpfegger became the new surgical attendant of Adolf Hitler—a position he had to thank Himmler for.[49] In this new role, Stumpfegger belonged to the personal staff of the Führer, and joined Hitler in the Berlin Bunker under the New Reich Chancellery from late February or early March 1945 on.[50] Himmler might have suggested Stumpfegger to Hitler for selfish purposes: Did the *Reichsführer-SS* want to consolidate his position with Hitler? Or did he want the surgeon to "spy" for him? Himmler's intention may not have been important for Stumpfegger; on the contrary, there are indications that he had transferred his loyalty completely to Hitler and that he was devoted toward his new task.[51] Martin Bormann commented on this situation:

> Yesterday Hasselbach was dismissed as the Führer's personal physician, and Dr. Stumpfegger, who until now was Uncle H.'s [Himmler's] doctor, is to replace him. The new man seems very pleasant. Brandt is no longer active as a personal physician either. There have been new quarrels between Morell on the one side and Hasselbach and Brandt on the other; but now this situation, which was so unpleasant for the Führer, is over![52]

To describe the relationship between Stumpfegger and Hitler is problematic. Three factors are responsible for this: (1) Their doctor-patient relationship lasted only a few months, and due to a lack of contemporary documents only a fragmentary image of the last months in the Berlin Bunker can be drawn. What is known is that the dictator initially had a fear of contact and reservations regarding treatment by his new escort physician.[53] (2) Theodor Morell was the physician treating Hitler since 1936. Morell, however, seemed to have trusted Stumpfegger and his medical skills. On several occasions he advised Hitler to let Stumpfegger perform injections during his absence. Later, the SS doctor was present at almost all treatments and examinations and was allowed to give Hitler injections.[54] He also assisted Carl Otto von Eicken—director of the ear, nose, and throat clinic at the Charité in Berlin—in November 1944 during the surgical removal of a polyp from Hitler's left vocal cord.[55] Joint walks with Bormann, Hitler, and his German shepherd Blondi in the garden of the Reich Chancellery complete the picture of the escort physician who permanently supervised the health of the Führer. Stumpfegger did not make the same mistake that Karl Brandt did. He never quarreled with Morell or contradicted him; rather, he dutifully fulfilled his medical assignments.[56] When he was on call, Stumpfegger lived in a room in the bunker; a second one served as a treatment and dressing room. (3) It is possible that Stumpfegger's close and long-standing association with Himmler had increasingly become a burden for the physician and his patient. In April 1945 Himmler had fallen out of favor with Hitler for his attempts to engineer a separate peace with the Western Allies. It may have been this event that caused Hitler to become suspicious of his physician Stumpfegger—who had been proposed to him by Himmler—and thus making the doctor-patient relationship, which had been established not long ago, more fragile. According to witness statements, Stumpfegger was very shaken by Hitler's suspicions and withdrew for the time being.[57]

Literature quoting witness testimonies suggests that Stumpfegger had renounced his former sponsor Himmler and that the dictator became his only point of reference.[58] The latter personally instructed his physician to obtain cyanide, which was to be distributed to the members of his closest circle in the bunker; the effectiveness was first tested on Hitler's dog Blondi.[59] In addition, Stumpfegger personally received his last promotion on the fifty-sixth birthday of the Führer by Hitler himself, being elevated to SS-Standartenführer (colonel of the SS).[60] One day later, on 21 April 1945, Stumpfegger was the only remaining physician in the Führerbunker. After Morell had been flown out of the besieged capital, he took over the role of Hitler's only physician.

Stumpfegger did not escape the collapse of the Third Reich. He remained in the bunker under the Reich Chancellery until the very end, and was somehow—the exact circumstances cannot be reconstructed—involved in the murder of the six children of Joseph and Magda Goebbels.[61] His last task as the physician of the Führer had been the determination of the death of Adolf Hitler and Eva Braun-Hitler on 30 April 1945.[62]

The downfall of the Third Reich went hand in hand with Stumpfegger's personal demise. The attempted escape of the bunker crew[63] from Berlin in the night from 1 to 2 May—one day after Hitler's suicide—failed, as the capital was surrounded by the Red Army. According to a postwar statement by *Reichsjugendführer* (Leader of the Hitler Youth) Arthur Axmann, Stumpfegger and Bormann were said to have been separated from the others. Later, Axmann claimed that he found the two of them lifeless on the Sandkrug Bridge near today's Berlin Central Station.[64] Stumpfegger was long considered missing. His fate could only be clarified in 1972, when two bodies were discovered during construction work in Berlin and Stumpfegger's bones were identified. An autopsy revealed splinters of glass between his teeth, suggesting that he had bitten down on a cyanide capsule to bring about his own death rather than getting captured by the Red Army.[65]

At the time of his death, Ludwig Stumpfegger was thirty-four years old. His remains were later buried in the Munich North Cemetery in the grave of his wife Gertrud (1915–2005).[66]

Discussion and Conclusion

Stumpfegger, born in 1910, belonged to the so-called "*Kriegsjugendgeneration*" (youth generation of World War I) or "*Generation des Unbedingten*" (uncompromising generation), which included the young men who were not old enough to have fought during World War I. From their point of view, they had missed the chance to fight at the front and thought they could have changed the course of the war. After the lost war, they witnessed the years of the Weimar Republic along with the reparations and hyperinflation as results of the Treaty of Versailles. This experience had led many to an ideological radicalization, especially the ambitious, academically educated young men. They became the young careerists and perpetrators of the Third Reich,[67] among them Ludwig Stumpfegger.

Stumpfegger was partly socialized during the time of the Third Reich (he was twenty-two years old when the Nazis came to power), and was a student during a period when the concepts of eugenics and racial hygiene were already a firm part of medical education and training and the practical implementation under state legitimation had already begun.[68] This means that measures of racial hygiene, starting with the *Gesetz zur Verhütung erbkranken Nachwuchses* (Law for the Prevention of Hereditarily Diseased Offspring), and the exclusion of Jews was legitimized by law and enforced. This, together with permanent indoctrination and thus internalization, may have shaped Stumpfegger's attitude and sense of responsibility, and may well have prepared him for the transgression of ethical boundaries in medical practice.

In the beginning, questions about the conditions of his career development and whether this was a product of chance or calculation had been raised. The latter must be answered with "both." His meeting with Gebhardt, and Stumpfegger's medical service at the Olympics, seem to have been a foreseeable coincidence—

foreseeable because he surely knew about the possibility of networking at such a highly anticipated event, and coincidence because he could not have calculated the chances for a lasting cooperation with Gebhardt. The connections to Himmler and finally to Hitler were a consistent development due to his political loyalty and networking ability, and were supported by his medical skills. He was an ambitious SS man who did not rest on his laurels. When a place at Hitler's side became available, he took it. However, these were patronage relationships, meaning Stumpfegger was the favorite or the sponsored. He also pushed his military and medical career by participating in war missions and scientific research. The latter led him toward the human experiments in Ravensbrück, which he used to fulfill his research interest and gain his *Habilitation*.

The research question about Stumpfegger's participation in the crimes of the Third Reich outlined above has definitively been answered: he was a perpetrator. Stumpfegger was clearly aware of the criminal nature of his research in Ravensbrück, as he omitted the origin of the data he collected there in his *Habilitation*. Furthermore, as a protégé of Gebhardt, Himmler, and later Hitler himself, he must have had insights into many of the crimes committed by Nazi Germany. This is also made clear by his suicide with the collapse of the Third Reich in 1945 at the age of nearly thirty-five years. The fact that he stayed by Hitler's side until the very end shows that he was a loyal and convinced supporter of the dictator and the Nazi ideology.

Parts of the medical profession were burdened with guilt in the Third Reich; physicians departed from the traditional doctor-patient relationship. Physicians followed "conscientiously" and unscrupulously the collective ethics, which culminated in a medical-biological and governmentally imposed state of terror during World War II and threatened and destroyed the existence of vulnerable population groups. Herein lies a constant danger, which medical historian Florian Bruns summed up in a nutshell: Medical care must never be subjugated to ideological dogmas that attribute people different values or rights to live,[69] and any expansion of doctors' societal power must be weighed carefully.

Acknowledgments

We thank our colleague Jens Westemeier for his constructive feedback on the manuscript. The project received funding by the START Program of the Medical Faculty of the RWTH Aachen University.

Stephanie Kaiser, PhD, is a research assistant at the Institute for History, Theory and Ethics of Medicine, Uniklinik RWTH Aachen. Her research interests include the history and ethics of anatomy and pathology in National Socialism, death and dead bodies in contemporary society, and regional history of World War I.

Mathias Schmidt, PhD, is research assistant at the Institute for History, Theory and Ethics of Medicine, Uniklinik RWTH Aachen. His main research focuses on the history of medicine during National Socialism, especially physicians in the Schutzstaffel.

Notes

1. Eckart 2012, 14; Mann 1989, 20.
2. Kater 1989.
3. Fest 2004, 374–77.
4. Anonymous 1998.
5. For a first analysis in German, see Kaiser 2018, on which this study is based.
6. The term *Begleitarzt* is not very common in German (used during the Third Reich) and has no counterpart in English. It describes a physician of the staff of high officers or political leaders who accompany them on travels.
7. He was 1.90 meters tall, had blue eyes and dark blond hair, was of slim stature, and was athletically active. See BArch B, R 9361-III/559030, Stumpfegger: Personalbericht.
8. A German government agency, which maintains records of members of the former German Wehrmacht and Waffen-SS who were killed, captured by Allied forces, or listed as missing in action, as well as other war-related records.
9. BArch B, R 9361-III/559030, Stumpfegger, passim.
10. Hein 2012, 11, 313, concludes that the General SS was in fact "more normal" than elitist in terms of its actual social structure but also in terms of its "racial," physical, and ideological selection criteria.
11. Hahn 2015, 189; Neumann and Eberle 2009, 106; Klee 2003, 613.
12. Helfen und Heilen 1943, 3; Cocks 2012, 98; Hahn 2018.
13. Hahn 2015, 345; Schulz and Wegmann 2003, 354. The acquaintance with Himmler and Gebhardt's medical work saw him rise quickly through the ranks within the SS. As an SS general, he was promoted to *Beratender Chirurg der Waffen-SS* (consulting surgeon of the armed SS) in 1940 and *Oberster Kliniker beim Reichsarzt SS und Polizei* (chief surgeon in the staff of the Reich physician SS and police), thus expanding his political influence within the SS considerably.
14. BA-MA, N 756-305/b: SS-Lazarett-Abteilung Hohenlychen/Kr. Templin (Uckermark).
15. Wedemeyer-Kolwe 2014, 96.
16. BArch B, R 9361-III/559030, Stumpfegger: Chef des Persönlichen Stabes RfSS to Chef des SS-Personal-Hauptamtes, 13 March 1940.
17. A search in surviving documents of Himmler and his staff in the Federal Archives Berlin, NS 19, provided no indication of the exact date.
18. BArch B, R 9361-III/559030, Stumpfegger: RfSS Persönlicher Stab an Personalkanzlei RfSS, 26 August 1938.
19. Ziegler 1989, 139.
20. IfZ, MA 293/1: Letter Gebhardt to Stumpfegger, 1 June 1939; Letter from unknown adjutant of Allgemeine Wehrmachtsangelegenheiten im Oberkommando der Wehrmacht to Wolff, 20 June 1939.
21. BArch B, R 9361-III/559030, Stumpfegger; IfZ, MA 293/1: Letter Gebhardt to Zöpfel, 1 June 1939.

22. Moors and Pfeiffer 2013, 256; BArch B, R 9361-III/559030, Stumpfegger; Longerich 2010, 509f.; Westemeier 2014: from 1939 to 1941, Peiper was Himmler's adjutant, a highly decorated *Standartenführer* of the Waffen-SS and responsible for war crimes of his unit in Italy in 1943 and Belgium in 1944.

23. WASt; BArch B, R 9361-III/559030, Stumpfegger: SS-Sanitätsamt to Kommandoamt der Waffen-SS, 9 September 1941.

24. Geheimes Staatsarchiv Preußischer Kulturbesitz (GStA PK), I. HA, Rep. 335 Fall 1, Protokoll Nr. 48, 3995f., quoted in Hahn 2015, 345 (translation by author).

25. Schulz and Wegmann 2003, 354; BArch B, R 9361-III/204053: Stumpfegger to SS-Rasse- und Siedlungshauptamt, 10 November 1939.

26. IfZ, Gebhardt 1946, 26 (translation by author).

27. IfZ, MA 293/1: Gebhardt to Wolff, 11 February 1940.

28. Ebbinghaus and Roth 2001, 192.

29. IfZ, Gebhardt 1946, 14; BArch B, R 9361-III/559030, Stumpfegger: Genzken to Kommandostab RfSS im SS-Führungshauptamt, 9 June 1941; IfZ, MA 293/1: Himmler to Schmitt, Grawitz, Jüttner, 21 May 1940, and Gebhardt to Prützmann, 15 October 1942.

30. IfZ, MA 293/1: Gebhardt to Stumpfegger, 14 September 1941.

31. IfZ, MA 293/1: Gebhardt to Himmler, 2 January 1943. In 1933 the *Leibstandarte* had been established as Hitler's personal bodyguard. With the murder of the SA leadership in the so-called *Röhm-Putsch*, it proved its unconditional loyalty to the Führer and is responsible for numerous war crimes committed on the western and eastern fronts. The unit was restructured several times, and by the end of the war it was known by the name 1st SS Panzer Division *Leibstandarte SS Adolf Hitler*.

32. BArch B, R 9361-III/559030, Stumpfegger: SS-Führungshauptamt Amtsgruppe D Sanitätswesen der Waffen-SS, 6 April 1943.

33. BArch B, R 9361-III/559030, Stumpfegger: Letter from Himmler, 20 June 1944.

34. Ebbinghaus and Roth 2002, 207–9; Baader 1986, 62–65; Hahn 2015, 458–62.

35. Testimony of Gebhardt during the Nuremberg Doctors Trial, Protokoll, 4040–46; Ebbinghaus and Roth 2002, 177–96; Roelcke 2014; Mitscherlich and Mielke 2012, 172; Hahn 2015, 458–62.

36. Ebbinghaus and Roth 2002, 207–9; Baader 1986, 62–65; Hahn 2015, 458–62.

37. Ebbinghaus and Roth 2002, 207–9.

38. Stumpfegger 1944, 496; Ebbinghaus and Roth 2002, 209.

39. Testimony of Gebhardt during the Nuremberg Doctors Trial, Protokoll, 4116–19; testimony of the witness Dr. Maczka during the Nuremberg Doctors Trial, Dok. No. 861, quoted in Mitscherlich and Mielke 2012, 200f.

40. Stumpfegger 1944.

41. Stumpfegger 1944, 498.

42. Schmidt 2009, 674.

43. Mitscherlich and Mielke 2012, 201f.; Ebbinghaus and Roth 2002, 211.

44. Testimony of Fischer in November 1945, Dok. No. 228; testimony of Gebhardt during the Nuremberg Doctors Trial, Protokoll, 4116–18, 4123f.; Mitscherlich and Mielke 2012, 201–3; Hahn 2015, 462f.

45. Testimony of Fischer in November 1945, Doc. No. 228; Hahn 2015, 463.

46. Hahn 2015, 463f.

47. Drinan 1992, 175.

48. Schmidt, Nebe, and Westemeier 2018, 191.

49. Katz 1982, 299; IfZ, Gebhardt 1946, 11; IfZ, von Hasselbach 1951, 34. The reason for the dismissals was that the three physicians had spoken out against Hitler's treatment with strychnine preparations by Morell. In this context, they were accused of breaching medical confidentiality.

50. Kellerhoff 2006, 71.

51. Schenck 1989, 476.

52. Genoud 1954, 137, quoted in Joachimsthaler 2004, 104f. (translation by author).
53. Irving 1983, 39; Katz 1982, 316.
54. Katz 1982, 325; Irving 1983, 39.
55. IfZ, Giesing 1945, 173; Schmidt 2009, 133–35; Klee 2003, 130.
56. Trevor-Roper 1965, 94.
57. Joachimsthaler 2004, 196.
58. Joachimsthaler 2004, 196; Trevor-Roper 1965, 93f.; Jochen von Lang 1979, 307.
59. Ryan 1966, 495; Joachimsthaler 2004, 251f., 258.
60. BArch B, R 9361-III/559030, Stumpfegger: Fegelein to SS-Personalhauptamt Berlin, 20 April 1945.
61. Joachimsthaler 2004, 197f., raises the question of the trustworthiness or even the existence of archival material concerning the actual course of the murders. Besymenski 1968, 79f.; Longerich 2010, 10; Liebrandt 2017, 286.
62. Sweeting 2000, 266.
63. Fest 2004, 173–75. Including, among others, General Wilhelm Mohnke, Hitler's personal adjutant Otto Günsche, Hitler's driver Erich Kempka, Hitler's pilot Hans Baur, Goebbel's adjutant Günther Schwägermann, diplomat Walter Hewel, Martin Bormann, and Artur Axmann.
64. Boldt 1973, 197; Joachimsthaler 2004, 86; Fest 2004, 175; Jochen von Lang 1979, 334f.
65. Janßen 1973; Anonymous 1998, 236. According to the WASt his death was recorded on 17 March 1949 at the registry office in Lychen/Templin.
66. World War II Graves.
67. Wild 2009.
68. Fiebrandt 2000, 510; Schmidt, Gutsul, and Kleinmanns 2017, 119.
69. Bruns 2009, 176–77.

References

Archival Sources

Documents NMT 1 (Medical Case)
Testimony in court of Karl Gebhardt during the Nuremberg Doctors Trial, protocol.
Testimony of Dr. Maczka during the Nuremberg Doctors Trial, Doc. No. 861.
Testimony of Fritz Fischer in November 1945, Doc. No. 228.
Archiv Institut für Zeitgeschichte München (IfZ)
Dr. med. Erwin Giesing, "Bericht über meine Behandlung bei Hitler," Wiesbaden, 12. Juni 1945.
MA 293/1: Reichsführer-SS, Persönlicher Stab—Professor Gebhardt.
Niederschrift der Unterredung des Herrn Prof. Dr. Hans-Karl von Hasselbach, geb. am 2. November 1903, wohnhaft Bielefeld, Anstalt Bethel, Tel. 63141, durchgeführt in Bielefeld am 27. und 28. Dezember 51, mit Dr. Frhr. von Siegler im Auftrag des Deutschen Instituts für Zeitgeschichte, München.
Vernehmung des Karl Gebhardt vom 17. Oktober 1946, 1000-1200 Uhr durch Mr. Rodell, im Auftrag von Dr. Hochwald. Index No. 201.
Bundesarchiv Berlin (BArch B)
R 9361-III/559030: Sammlung Berlin Document Center (BDC). Personenbezogene Unterlagen der SS und SA. SSO-File, Stumpfegger, Ludwig.
R 9361-III/204053: Sammlung Berlin Document Center (BDC). Personenbezogene Unterlagen der SS und SA.
Bundesarchiv-Militärarchiv Freiburg (BA-MA)
N 756: Nachlass Wolfgang Vopersal.

Deutsche Dienststelle für die Benachrichtigung der nächsten Angehörigen von Gefallenen der ehemaligen deutschen Wehrmacht, Berlin (WASt)
Auskunft zum militärischen Werdegang von Dr. Ludwig Stumpfegger.

Books and Articles

Anonymous. 1998. "Gentest: Bormanns Skelett eindeutig identifiziert." *Der Spiegel* 19: 230–39.
Baader, Gerhard. 1986. "Menschenversuche im Nationalsozialismus" In *Versuche mit Menschen in Medizin, Humanwissenschaft und Politik*, edited by Hanfried Helmchen and Rolf Winau, 41–82. New York: De Gruyter.
Besymenski, Lew. 1968. *Der Tod des Adolf Hitler: Unbekannte Dokumente aus Moskauer Archiven; Eingeleitet von Karl-Heinz Janßen.* Hamburg: Wegner Verlag.
Boldt, Gerhard. 1973. *Hitler—Die letzten zehn Tage.* Frankfurt am Main, Berlin: Ullstein Verlag.
Bruns, Florian. 2009. *Medizinethik im Nationalsozialismus: Entwicklungen und Protagonisten in Berlin (1939–1945).* Stuttgart: Franz Steiner Verlag.
Cocks, Geoffrey Campbell. 2012. *The State of Health: Illness in Nazi Germany.* New York: Oxford University Press.
Drinan, Robert F. 1992. "The Nuremberg Principles in International Law." In *The Nazi Doctors and the Nuremberg Code: Human Rights in Human Experimentation*, edited by George J. Annas and Michael Grodin, 174–82. New York: Oxford University Press.
Ebbinghaus, Angelika, and Roth Karl H. 2001. "Kriegswunden: Die kriegschirurgischen Experimente in den Konzentrationslagern und ihre Hintergründe." In *Der Nürnberger Ärzteprozeß und seine Folgen*, edited by Angelika Ebbinghaus and Klaus Dörner, 177–218. Berlin: Aufbau Verlag.
Eckart, Wolfgang Uwe. 2011. "Medizinische Forschung- Universitäten, Studierende, Medizinische Fakultäten." In *Medizin und Nationalsozialismus: Bilanz und Perspektiven der Forschung*, edited by Robert Jütte, Wolfgang Uwe Eckart, and Winfried Süß, 106–23. Göttingen: Wallstein Verlag.
———. 2012. *Medizin in der NS-Diktatur: Ideologie, Praxis, Folgen.* Wien, Köln, Weimar: Böhlau Verlag.
Fest, Joachim. 2004. "Der Untergang. Eine historische Skizze." In *Der Untergang: Das Filmbuch*, edited by Michael Töteberg, 7–208. Hamburg: Rowohlt Taschenbuch Verlag.
Fiebrandt, Maria. 2014. *Auslese für die Siedlergesellschaft: Die Einbeziehung Volksdeutscher in die NS-Erbgesundheitspolitik im Kontext der Umsiedlungen 1939–1945.* Göttingen: Vandenhoeck & Ruprecht.
Genoud, François. 1954. *The Bormann Letters.* London: Weidenfeld & Nicolsen.
Hahn, Judith. 2015. *Grawitz, Genzken, Gebhardt. Drei Karrieren im Sanitätsdienst der SS*, 2nd ed. Münster Ulm: Klemm & Oelschläger.
———. 2018. *Leibesübungen und Leistungsmedizin: Der Sportarzt Karl Gebhardt und die Heilanstalten Hohenlychen in der NS-Zeit.* Berlin: be.bra wissenschaft Verlag.
Hein, Bastian. 2012. *Elite für Volk und Führer? Die Allgemeine SS und ihre Mitglieder 1925–1945.* München: De Gruyter Oldenbourg.
Helfen und Heilen. 1943. "Helfen und Heilen: 10 Jahre Heilstätte und SS-Lazarett Hohenlychen." *Das Schwarze Korps* 9(45): 3–4.
Irving, David. 1983. *Die geheimen Tagebücher des Dr. Morell: Leibarzt Adolf Hitlers.* München: Wilhelm Goldmann Verlag.
Janßen, Karl-Heinz. 1973. "Der Fall Martin Bormann: Das Ende einer Phantom-Jagd." *Die Zeit* 17.
Joachimsthaler, Anton. 2004. *Hitlers Ende: Legenden und Dokumente.* 2nd ed. München: Herbig Verlag.
Kaiser, Stephanie. 2018. "Ludwig Stumpfegger—Eine Karriere im Nationalsozialismus" In *Die Ärzte der Nazi-Führer: Karriere und Netzwerke*, edited by Mathias Schmidt, Dominik Groß, and Jens Westemeier, 81–103. Münster: Lit.
Kater, Michael H. 1989. *Doctors under Hitler.* Chapel Hill: University of North Carolina Press.

Katz, Ottmar. 1982. *Prof. Dr. med. Theo Morell: Hitlers Leibarzt*. Bayreuth: Hestia.
Kellerhoff, Sven Felix. 2006. *Mythos Führerbunker: Hitlers letzter Unterschlupf*. 2nd ed. Berlin: Berlin Story Verlag.
Klee, Ernst. 2003. *Das Personenlexikon zum Dritten Reich: Wer war was vor und nach 1945*. Frankfurt am Main: S. Fischer Verlag.
Lang, Jochen von. 1979. *The Secretary: Martin Bormann; The Man Who Manipulated Hitler*. New York: Random House.
Liebrandt, Hannes. 2017. *"Das Recht mich zu richten, das spreche ich Ihnen ab!" Der Selbstmord der nationalsozialistischen Elite 1944/45*. Paderborn: Ferdinand Schöningh.
Longerich, Peter. 2010. *Heinrich Himmler: Biographie*. 3rd ed. München: Pantheon Verlag.
Mann, Gunter. 1989. "Biologismus—Vorstufen und Elemente einer Medizin im Nationalsozialismus." In *Medizin im Dritten Reich*, edited by Johanna Bleker and Norbert Jachertz, 11–21. Köln: Deutscher Ärzte-Verlag.
Moors, Markus, and Moritz Pfeiffer. 2013. *Heinrich Himmlers Taschenkalender 1940: Kommentierte Edition*. Paderborn: Ferdinand Schöningh.
Neumann, Hans-Joachim, and Henrik Eberle. 2009. *War Hitler krank? Ein abschließender Befund*. Bergisch Gladbach: Lübbe.
Roelcke, Volker. 2014. "Sulfonamide Experiments on Prisoners in Nazi Concentration Camps: Coherent Scientific Rationality Combined with Complete Disregard of Humanity." In *Human Subjects Research after the Holocaust*, edited by Sheldon Rubenfeld and Susan Benedict, 51–66. Cham: Springer.
Ryan, Cornelius. 1966. *The Last Battle: The Classic History of the Battle for Berlin*. New York: Simon & Schuster.
Schenck, Ernst G. 1989. *Patient Hitler: Eine medizinische Biographie*. Düsseldorf: Droste.
Schmidt, Ulf. 2009. *Hitlers Arzt Karl Brandt: Medizin und Macht im Dritten Reich*. Berlin: Aufbau Verlag.
Schmidt, Mathias, Nazarii Gutsul, and Jan Kleinmanns. 2017. "Medizin und Politik in der NS-Zeit am Beispiel der Ärzte des 'Sonderkommandos Künsberg' und des 'Einsatzstabs Reichsleiter Rosenberg.'" In *Neue Forschungen zur Medizingeschichte: Beiträge des "Rheinischen Kreises der Medizinhistoriker,"* edited by Mathias Schmidt, Dominik Groß, and Axel Karenberg, 103–28. Kassel: University Press.
Schmidt, Mathias, Julia Nebe, and Jens Westemeier. 2018. "Das Problem der Verantwortung in der Wissenschaft am Beispiel der Angeklagten im Nürnberger Ärzteprozess." In *Forschung zwischen Freiheit und Verantwortung: Die wissenschaftshistorische Perspektive*, edited by Dominik Groß and Julia Nebe, 187–98. Kassel: University Press.
Schulz, Andreas, and Günter Wegmann. 2003. *Die Generale der Waffen-SS und der Polizei: Die militärischen Werdegänge der Generale, sowie der Ärzte, Veterinäre, Intendanten, Richter und Ministerialbeamten im Generalsrang, Band 1*. Bissendorf: Biblio Verlag.
Stumpfegger, Ludwig. 1944. "Die freie autoplastische Knochentransplantation in der Wiederherstellungschirurgie: Erfahrungen und Ergebnisse." *Deutsche Zeitschrift für Chirurgie* 259: 496–746.
Sweeting, C. G. 2000. *Hitler's Personal Pilot: The Life and Times of Hans Baur*. Washington, DC: Brassey's.
Trevor-Roper, Hugh R. 1965. *Hitlers letzte Tage*. Frankfurt am Main: Ullstein.
von Lang, Joachim. 1985. *Der Adjutant: Karl Wolff: Der Mann zwischen Hitler und Himmler*. München/Berlin: Ullstein.
Wedemeyer-Kolwe, Bernd. 2014. "Die Sportheilstätte Hohenlychen: Reichssportsanatorium, SS-Reservelazarett, Versehrtensportzentrum." In *Rehabilitation und Prävention in Sport- und Medizingeschichte. Bericht der gemeinsamen Tagung des Niedersächsischen Instituts für Sportgeschichte e.V. Hannover (NISH) und des Instituts für Geschichte, Ethik und Philosophie der Medizin der Medizinischen Hochschule Hannover (MHH) vom 10. bis 11. November 2012, zugleich Tagungsbericht der 11.*

Tagung des NISH [Tagung "Prävention und Rehabilitation in der Sport- und Medizingeschichte" an der Medizinischen Hochschule Hannover], edited by Christine Wolters and Christian Becker, 89–108. Berlin: Lit.

Westemeier, Jens. 2014. *Himmlers Krieger: Joachim Peiper und die Waffen-SS in Krieg und Nachkriegszeit*. Paderborn: Ferdinand Schöningh.

Wild, Michael. 2009. *Uncompromising Generation: The Nazi Leadership of the Reich Security Main Office*. Translated by Tom Lampert. Madison: University of Wisconsin Press.

World War II Graves. Stumpfegger, Dr. Ludwig. Retrieved 5 August 2020 from https://ww2gravestone.com/people/stumpfegger-ludwig/.

Ziegler, Herbert F. 1989. *Nazi Germany's New Aristocracy: The SS Leadership 1925–1939*. Princeton, NJ: Princeton University Press.

CHAPTER 9

Between Participation in National Socialist Medicine and Everyday Administrative Action
On the Economic Argument of the Psychiatric Planning Commission (1941–45)

Felicitas Söhner

Approximately three hundred thousand mentally ill or mentally and physically disabled people were murdered between 1939 and 1945 as part of the National Socialist so-called "euthanasia" program.[1] The scientific investigation of these crimes, especially concerning the way in which postwar society dealt with the knowledge and the perpetrators of this patient murder, is underway and not yet complete.[2] So far, research into the crimes of Nazi medicine has focused intensively on the responsibility of politics, medicine, and science. However, research on the Holocaust in general shows that special attention should also be paid to the bureaucratic system and the role of the administration in order to investigate these "crimes against humanity."[3] Administrative staff of the T4 Headquarters (*Zentraldienststelle T4*) in Berlin led and supervised the systematic registration of patients by means of documents and forms, medical examination procedures, transport of patients to interim and killing institutions, organization of resources of personnel and space, bureaucratic management of deaths, and planning the future use of vacated properties. The bureaucratic structure of the "euthanasia" system fulfilled various functions. It not only served to effectively organize the program—as well as to impose secrecy—but also fulfilled economic goals such as the redistribution of estates and the reuse of buildings.[4]

The term "administrative mass murder," coined by Hannah Arendt with regard to the planned destruction of mentally disabled and mentally ill people in the context of National Socialist "euthanasia" crimes, is controversial.[5] But Arendt, as a political philosopher and observer of the Eichmann trial in Jerusalem (1961), directed her attention to the bureaucratic execution of the industrially organized Holocaust and thus described a criminal type of normality and banality deviating from the conventional understanding of the term "perpetrator" who has deliberately committed a criminal act. In this chapter, the role of the administration in the murder of patients will be examined using the example of administrative superintendent Ludwig Trieb,[6] who worked for the Berlin Nazi authorities. Trieb, who had previously worked as administrative manager at the psychiatric hospital in Günzburg, Bavaria (Heil- und Pflegeanstalt Günzburg), was temporarily transferred to Berlin in 1941 at the instigation of the Führer's office to handle special tasks. From 1941 to 1945 he worked as a member of the T4 Planning Commission of the Reich Working Group for Psychiatric Institutions (Reichsarbeitsgemeinschaft Heil- und Pflegeanstalten).[7] He played an essential role in his function as "economic expert" in the T4 Headquarters in Berlin, where he examined all German institutions and compiled "planning reports."[8] Trieb was regarded by the authorities as a very able administrator and in 1940 was appointed to the staff of the headquarters of the "T4 euthanasia operation" at Tiergartenstraße 4 in Berlin.[9] There, he was a member of a planning commission that prepared a national register of mental hospitals, focusing on buildings and bed capacities. The work of this commission was linked to the use of hospital facilities for the war effort, with the aim of planning inpatient mental healthcare for a postwar German Reich, and is also likely to have had (undocumented) links with the "euthanasia" program.

After the war and a brief interlude, from 1949 to the middle of the 1960s, Trieb was again the head of administration at the mental hospital in Günzburg.[10] Postwar proceedings at an Allied denazification tribunal and by the German Public Prosecution Office resulted in a ruling that Ludwig Trieb was a "fellow traveler" (Mitläufer). Some sources in the archival material suggest that Trieb was aware of the links between his work and the Nazi "euthanasia" program.[11]

With Ludwig Trieb as an example of an administrator's actions in Nazi Germany, this chapter endeavors to determine the mechanisms and objectives of administrative decision-making processes: first, by preparing a comprehensive inventory of the administrative processes in interactions between mental hospitals and T4 Headquarters in Berlin; second, by embedding the documented processes within the context of health and social policy. Specifically, administrative actions related to the management of real estate belonging to psychiatric institutions are reconstructed here.

The Current State of Research

Regarded as committed pioneers in the investigation of NS crimes are the publicists Götz Aly and Ernst Klee. Since the 1980s, Aly has been focusing on the connection between "euthanasia" and modernization in German psychiatry in

Nazi Germany.[12] Furthermore, the early work of Klee raised awareness of archival materials on the structures, dimensions, and course of medicine and "euthanasia" in the Third Reich, which had been largely unexplored until then.[13] Aly and other authors discussed and referred to the contribution of Heinz Faulstich, who analyzed the "economic acting and thinking of protagonists" in the "euthanasia" killings.[14]

Winfried Süß concluded a more comprehensive analysis with his sociohistorical study on health policy in the war.[15] Other relevant contributions to the history of medicine also address the role of nursing homes during the National Socialist era in general or in relation to what was known as Action T4—the deportation of the mentally ill to killing centers—in particular.[16]

Henry Friedlander's path-breaking *The Origins of Nazi Genocide* argues that "euthanasia was not simply a prologue but the first chapter of Nazi genocide."[17] The historian Yaacov Lozowick deals with the phenomenon of racial fanaticism among Nazi bureaucrats. To this end, the author analyzes precisely the Eichmann section with regard to personnel, tasks, structures, and working methods.[18]

The special role of Ludwig Trieb as outstanding organizer and agent of the T4 Planning Commission is examined by Heike Bernhardt. She describes the administrative director as "head of economics at the T4 Headquarters" and refers directly to his involvement in Action T4.[19] Florian Steger and Thomas Becker also mention Ludwig Trieb's activities as an employee of the psychiatric hospital in Günzburg.[20] They concentrate on the role of the Bavarian mental hospital in the programs of Nazi medicine. Hans-Walter Schmuhl refers to the planning reports written by Trieb and deals with the therapeutic idealism of psychiatry, with which he identified partly enthusiastic participation of psychiatrists in the National Socialist "euthanasia" program.[21] He ultimately follows a structural theory approach, seeing the "euthanasia" as the result of radicalization processes. Among other things, he attributes this radicalization to the polycratic structure of power (in National Socialist Germany) and its own momentum.[22] Bernd Walter also focuses his attention on those responsible for politics and administration. He sees racist ideological motivations increasingly superimposed on economic criteria.[23] Taking a decidedly materialistic approach, Roer and Henkel see the decisive explanation for the murder action in the economic conditions of psychiatry. First and foremost, that sick and disabled people lacked an ability to work was decisive for their murder.[24]

A number of further studies on the postwar epoch focus primarily on the attempt to reinterpret Nazi crimes[25] or consider them in relation to the attitude of the Postwar German public.[26] Thus, the political scientist Kerstin Freudiger examines differences in the punishment of these crimes and the related constructions of penalty mitigation.[27] Jurist Anika Burkhardt also analyzes the injustice of Nazi "euthanasia" from the point of view of criminal law.[28] However, any considerations of economic strategies and the role of lower- and middle-level managers in the administration of "euthanasia" processes have not yet been sufficiently investigated.

Sources and Methods

This chapter is based on a systematic collection of materials from various archives. The focus was on files from the Federal Archives in Berlin, particularly final reports on the journeys of the T4 Planning Commission in the German territories from April 1941 to December 1942, as well as reports and recommendations issued on the basis of these planning trips.

Another focus was on the public prosecutorial investigation files in the State Archive in Munich, in particular the arbitration board files of affected individuals. On the basis of these documents, it was possible to reconstruct processes and responsibilities. A further focus was on the records of the "euthanasia" witness statement collection in the central office of the State Justice Administration and court of appeal files in the State Archive, both in the Federal Archive Ludwigsburg. The witness documents of persons involved in the T4 Planning Commission constituted another resource. Testimonies by Ludwig Trieb, which are available in the State Archive in Wiesbaden and in the Federal Archives in Berlin, served as further sources. Documents with notes and reports on visits to the T4 Planning Commission, which are archived by church and private sponsors or their legal successors, were also included.[29]

The goal is to take a closer look at the economic acting and thinking of one of the co-organizers from different perspectives. The methodological approach of microhistory is followed. It is about portraying historical milieus both descriptively and analytically by the limitations of the object of investigation.[30] This analysis of activities of Ludwig Trieb focuses on the role of a typical administrator as an enabler of the functioning of the T4 "machine." Using this approach, this chapter aims to determine the extent to which political-ideological developments influenced the protagonist's administrative thinking and acting patterns.

Administration of "Euthanasia" in the Berlin Headquarters

In the years of the global economic crisis, social policy came under pressure several times. Economic arguments played an important role in fields such as unemployment benefits, welfare payments, pensions, or mental healthcare. The financial crisis of the state led to massive austerity measures for hospitals and to a reduction in social and health services.[31] The National Socialist hereditary and "racial" ideology was the basis for a new regulation of health administration: a law standardizing the health system was passed in 1934.[32] Relating thereto, the former municipal healthcare system was restructured and centralized.[33] There is a debate how far under National Socialism the state was able to enforce social and ideological "equality" of the social system by taking a radical political standpoint on public policy decisions.

At the same time, according to medical ethicists Dörries and Vollmann, under these political and economic conditions and with the further development of professional knowledge, psychiatrists agreed on a classification that even enabled statistical recording to promote cost-effective treatment, a system susceptible to abuse.[34] The *Würzburger Schlüssel*,[35] introduced in 1933, represented a pragmatic consensus based on scientific knowledge at the time, and this supported systematic routine documentation and administrative practices in mental healthcare.[36]

Apart from describing close cooperation between politics and psychiatry under National Socialism, medical historian Neuner observes that medical language became increasingly constricted, while at the same time politics and society became increasingly tolerant of repressive measures.[37] According to the historian Maren Richter, administrative staff welcomed some efforts of the National Socialist state with great approval, such as the project of centralizing the healthcare system and making it more efficient.[38] The fact that this centralization was intended to help enforce the criminal health policy of National Socialism was underestimated or not seen by many, but also deliberately supported by some.[39]

The systematic killing of patients in Action T4, as it was called, was implemented with strongly utilitarian motives. The term "Action T4" refers to the address of the administrative body set up to ensure implementation, the central office or T4 Headquarters (Tiergartenstraße 4 in Berlin). It stands for the targeted killing of more than seventy thousand people with mental and physical disabilities, as well as mental and neurological diseases, between 1939 and 1941.

All measures relating to the "euthanasia" action were the sole responsibility of the Führer's office. For reasons of secrecy, the administrative apparatus of the killing program was outsourced from the Führer's office and moved to its own address in April 1940. The central office, with more than four hundred employees, was divided into the following departments: the medical, administrative, main economic, transportation, human resources, and inspection departments.[40] This office directed and controlled the systematic registration of healthcare institutions and their inhabitants by means of registration forms, the organization of the evaluation procedure and filing of the data received, the preparation of hospital transfers, the procurement of premises and personnel, and the correspondence between the authorities and relatives after their family members were killed.[41]

In order to delegate responsibility and to disguise any connection between the state and the "euthanasia" program, five official front organizations were founded. All of these organizations were completely independent, but none had its own financial resources. The Reich Working Group for Psychiatric Institutions was the organ cited on paper for correspondence with medical institutions and nursing homes. The "Charitable Foundation for Institutional Care" (Gemeinnützige Stiftung für Anstaltspflege) took on the role of official employer of nonmedical personnel. The Reich Working Group for Psychiatric Institutions (Reichsarbeitsgemeinschaft Heil- und Pflegeanstalten) recorded as central office the mental hospitals and their inhabitants and ordered the transfer of the patients to the killing institutions. The "Charitable Ambulance" (Gemeinnützige Krankentransport GmbH) organized the transports of the residents. The "Central Clearing Center for Psychiatric Hospitals" (Zentralverrechnungsstelle Heil- und Pflegeanstalten) was responsible, for example, for offsetting the costs incurred in relocating the victims.

The historian Peter Sandner refers to the entanglement of the true structure of the T4 Headquarters and a "fictional structure"[42] of individual "non-profit" foundations whose boundaries are blurred and whose fields of activity are not always congruent. Both the confusion about the powers of the cover organization and a neutralizing nomenclature, using terms such as "treatment" or "disinfection" to describe murder, served to keep the proceedings secret.[43] In Burkhardt's terms, the institutional structure could be classified as a perfectly organized secret apparatus parallel to the state administration.[44] T4 employees used modern office equipment such as typewriters, forms, files, and folders in their work,[45] which standardized official business operations and thus increased regulatory capacity.[46]

All "euthanasia" officials working at the central office had joined the NSDAP in the early 1930s. Their routes into the authority were very different and, in many cases, based on old personal ties from previous involvement in the SA.[47] Information about a person's political reliability was always obtained before hiring that individual.[48]

Geographically, Action T4 began in the Polish territories and, over time, was gradually extended over East and South Germany to all parts of the Reich.[49] Within the scope of Action T4 and beyond it, medical commissions visited mental hospitals and nursing homes of the German Reich and recorded the patients there on registration forms.[50] By order of the Reich Ministry of the Interior (on 1 February 1943), every six months the nursing homes had to fill in a registration form for all patients admitted in the meantime.[51] These patient registrations were to be collated in a central registry of the entire inpatient population, to provide a reliable basis for reorganizing the asylum system.[52]

In addition to the residents, the real estate was recorded. All psychiatric facilities were registered on forms, including all associated building structures, along with their condition, size, construction, infrastructure links, capacity, hired staff, and economic conditions. This information was to serve as a basis for the planning of the continued use of vacant facilities.[53]

On 24 August 1941, Adolf Hitler gave the verbal order to discontinue Action T4. It can be assumed that this is due to popular disquiet and church protest.[54] Even after the official end of systematic patient killings in the spring of 1941, covert regional "actions" continued. In total, by 1945, up to three hundred thousand people fell victim to these crimes in the German Reich and its occupied territories.[55] However, even after Action T4 was discontinued, functionaries at the headquarters continued planning the utilization of future vacant real estate.

Activities of the Administrator Trieb in the Central Office

According to the business distribution plan of the central office dated August 1943, Department IIg: "Planning Hospitals and Nursing Homes," was directed by Herbert Becker (physician) and Ludwig Trieb (economic inspector) and was part of Department II: "Technical Handling."[56] This planning department was set up in the spring of 1941 under Becker; Trieb was appointed shortly thereafter as an organizer and business expert. Until then, he had been administrative director of the Günzburg mental hospital and was recommended for his excellent organizational skills. This department was verifiably active until the winter of 1943–44.[57]

The members of the department visited institutions from a comprehensive list of mental hospitals and nursing homes in the German Reich. From March 1941 onward, they traveled to psychiatric institutions in the various states and provinces. Visits were made by a planning commission, and from late autumn 1941 two commissions, each consisting of at least one doctor, one administrative expert, and one photographer.[58] The following commission inspections have been documented:[59]

In spring 1941, economic inspector Ludwig Trieb made his first visit as a member of a planning commission, with the physician Aquilin Ullrich, the administrative officer Wolfgang Grützner, the Bavarian upper governmental councilor Max Gaum, Willi Exner of the Reich Ministry of the Interior, and the photographer Franz Wagner. Continuing their work until the autumn of the same year, they inspected all Bavarian psychiatric institutions to determine their economic condition "with the same principles."[60] After this was completed for Bavaria, *Ministerialrat* Herbert Linden ordered that all other facilities in the German Reich be inspected in the same way.[61]

During their visits, the commission assessed mental health institutions, spoke with the institution directors, and prepared planning reports with proposals for using the facilities. The reports contain detailed information about people, treatment options, and financial resources, and all conclude with a recommendation or proposed use. For this purpose, the commission filled in questionnaires and took photographs, monitored site maps, farm maps, current balance sheets, patient and staff numbers, unit ratings, insurance policies, and farm production and income statements.[62] The heads of the institutes were aware of this inventory taking. Pastor von Bodelschwingh, director of the Bethel facility, noted on a visit there that Inspector Trieb was provided with information on economic and financial issues by the in-house economist.[63] The director of the Hephata

Table 9.1. Documented visits by the planning commission.

March–May 1941	Bavaria (excluding Palatinate)
June 1941	Mecklenburg
August 1941	Brandenburg, Saxony
September 1941	Schleswig
September–October 1941	Pomerania
September–October 1941	Silesia
October–December 1941	Former Rhine Province
October–November 1941	Thuringia
December 1941	Berlin-Rummelsburg
January 1942	Brunswick
February 1942	Hesse
March 1942	Hesse-Nassau
April 1942	Hamburg
April 1942	Bremen
April 1942	Oldenburg
May 1942	Westphalia
June 1942	Hannover
July 1942	Baden, partly Alsace
July 1942	Lippe
August 1942	Sudetenland
September 1942	Lippe
July–September 1942	Protectorate
September 1942	Warthegau
September 1942	Danzig-West Prussia
October 1942	East Prussia
October 1942	Bavaria
October–November 1942	Württemberg
October–November 1942	Westmark
November 1942	Alsace
November–December 1942	Saxony
December 1942	Pomerania

Institute in Bethel, Helmich, recorded in his files, "While Mr Trieb made statistical surveys, two other gentlemen went through the asylum and took outdoor and indoor shots. Mr Trieb also made an extensive visit of the economic facilities, such as the kitchen and laundry."[64]

A four-part questionnaire ("white, printed double sheet") was used for the survey, which was specially developed by Ludwig Trieb for the planning department.[65] On the basis of the data collected, the planning department of the T4

Headquarters set up a comprehensive index that provided—to a memorandum from the leading German psychiatrists Ernst Rüdin, Maximilian de Crinis, Carl Schneider, Hans Heinze, and Paul Nitzsche—a reliable basis for the envisaged reorganization of the mental hospital sector.[66] The specialist literature interprets this as a "legacy" of an initially realized goal of the NS psychiatry, whose further research and therapy activities are to be understood as the guise of further illness and disability killings.[67]

This file contained details of the year of construction, building system, area, supporters, businesses, infrastructure, and so on, and was to form the basis for the planning of psychiatric care for the entire Reich.[68] The aim of the surveys was to create a complete medical psychiatric, economic, and photographic documentation of psychiatric care in Germany, as well as to provide a basis for centralist planning for the future after the war. In addition to economizing the supply structure, another aim was deconfessionalization, thus eliminating the church's influence on the general population.[69]

Based on statistical data, psychiatric care was to be optimized across the Reich and plans were to be made for the postwar period, which was expected to be imminent.[70] After the initial investment, the index cards were updated regularly and occupancy figures entered.[71] Trieb remarked in his booklet "Thoughts and Suggestions Concerning the Future Development of Psychiatry" in May 1943, "The result of these findings is laid down in a file, which is constantly kept up to date through a duty imposed on the institutions to report all changes in the number of sick and institutionalized persons."[72] This fact alone shows that the commissioners must have been very well aware that the economically sensible use of real estate was not the only aim—the intention was also to keep track of patients' whereabouts.

Becker and Trieb also wrote a report for each planning trip. The economic inspector made suggestions as to which facilities residents could relocate to, so that residents could be put to military or administrative use.[73] One economization measure that Trieb recommended in the report on Rummelsburg in Berlin was that the residents be dealt with according to their work performance. After categorizing them by ability and willingness to work, he suggested that the nonworking patients in "Working Group 1 . . . should be reduced accordingly. . . . Working Group 2 . . . should be reduced to a limited extent,"[74] and the other groups should work more. This is a clear statement about the decimation of persons—and not of beds—by a few hundred.[75] Although the economic evaluation of the Rummelsburg facility had no direct consequences, there is a marked tendency here to propose how, in the case of a German victory, the "non-productive" members of the population would have been dealt with. It must have been clear to the administrative expert that attaining the guideline lower numbers of beds either meant the overcrowding of other healthcare facilities, the significant reduction in inpatient time, or indeed the displacement of psychiatric patients.[76]

In addition to business considerations, the commissioners also commented in their reports on the attitude of the managers in the facilities visited. Since some institutions were not very interested in achieving consensus, the planning reports contain critical comments, such as the "unauthorized action" of the administration in Pomerania. The decentralized, capricious evictions of the facilities and murders of the patients[77] were excoriated as "a reduction that can no longer be called planning because it has been done quite arbitrarily and wildly without any calculating foresight."[78] In some places, regional authorities clearly sought confrontation. For example, the senator for health of Hamburg refused any cooperation with the commission,[79] a medical officer in Rhine-Hesse refused to allow commissioners entry.[80] The Westphalian Provincial Administration threatened to "fight and resist" if the Commission "wanted to take away institutional space, make major interventions or orders . . . in its administration."[81] The commissioners noted these instances of actual or potential resistance in detail: in Westphalia they criticized a "most highly developed (and thus the most confident) central administration" of mental hospitals, compared to other regions.[82] The planning report on Bethel is also critical of the institution's self-confidence and lack of cooperation.[83] Inspector Trieb emphasized the atmosphere of suspicion in which the commission was received and noted that documents were withheld and only those the business administrator Kunze considered relevant were submitted.[84] For the most part, senior staff was described as being "at work" in Berlin, not least in determining which facilities could be expected to cooperate in restarting the so-called "e-measure."[85] In the postwar years, Ludwig Trieb never denied his commitment to the Reich Working Group for Psychiatric Institutions; however, he emphasized that the content of his tasks was far removed from the killing of patients. "The sense and purpose . . . was to bring together health and care institutions . . . this action had nothing to do with euthanasia."[86]

This statement is in discrepancy with the letter from psychiatrist Emil Gelny to Paul Nitsche (7 February 1944)[87] and to the regional official of the Lower Danube region Sepp Mayer (6 February 1944), concerning the unofficial continuation of the "euthanasia." The letter suggests that Trieb's benevolent perception is the reason behind declining patient numbers. In response to Gelny's concern about continuing his "previous activity [in the context of] the elimination of absolutely incurable and, in view of today's situation intolerable patients," Trieb reacted with "enthusiastic approval." Both had talked about plans to set up the mental hospital in Gugging (Austria) as an institution where "euthanasia" was possible. The fact that Trieb repeatedly asked his correspondents to "treat his advice as strictly confidential, since otherwise he would incur inconvenience," shows that he must have been aware of the explosiveness of the conversation content.[88]

The Reich Working Group took advantage of the state of limbo after the termination of Action T4 and the openness to possibly continuing the "action" through systematic future-oriented psychiatry planning. In order to accelerate progress on this issue, a meeting was to be held in the second half of January 1942 with the broadest possible involvement of institutional and supervisory bodies. Planned topics included information about bed supply, institute location, the functional orientation of the institutes toward the care of "Aryans," the use of vacant buildings, and future requirements in peacetime.[89] The concept of psychiatric care in the sense of "hospitals with a euthanasia option" was to remain secret until the end of the war and the publication of a "euthanasia" law.[90] Opinions differed among the planners about where this plan was to be carried out. The commission led by Ludwig Trieb preferred a combination of treatment-oriented psychiatric hospitals close to urban centers and less expensive "death asylums for expired cases."[91] Robert Müller, a member of the commission traveling at the same time in different commissions to Becker and Trieb, made significantly more concrete recommendations in his planning report on Baden: "One of the most important requirements in implementing euthanasia will be the most inconspicuous form possible. This includes, first, and foremost, the inconspicuous environment.... Thus, with few exceptions, the death of the euthanized will hardly differ from natural death. That is the goal to be achieved.... So for the future: no nursing home for incurable cases, but only hospitals with the most active therapy and scientific work and—with a euthanasia option."[92]

Classification of the Planning Department

The examination of the T4 Headquarters shows how an institution of the classic state administration could be created and became the instrument of the radical goals of the Nazi state without having to create special, regular administrative acts that would disrupt structures. The service considered here is an example of the fact that participation in crime did not require a particularly strong criminal effort. Only professional competence and a lack of commitment to the ethical principle of equal rights for all human beings were a prerequisite for the perpetration of atrocities.

The central office at Tiergartenstraße 4 in Berlin organized and controlled the systematic recording of patients, organization and operation of the killing facilities, transport of victims, financing and cost management, economic recording of the institutions, and bureaucratic handling of the deaths.[93] The bureaucratic activity of the department was organized by division of labor and split into a series of tasks, processes, and responsibilities. This necessarily entailed a limitation of individual roles to their own immediate tasks.[94]

The department "Planning Hospitals and Nursing Homes" had a significant role within the T4 Headquarters. In order to set this up, no previously used authority was instrumentalized or converted, but de novo structures were created to organize the "euthanasia." This means that employees of the T4 Headquarters can be seen as involved in "euthanasia," whether actively or not. They were active in the period of the highest radicalization of state action. The T4 Headquarters was an essential part of the economic aspect of "euthanasia": it served as a central instance in real estate management, more concretely in the conversion of an institution without a formal recruitment procedure. It was highly effective, especially as it had complete coverage of people and real estate. Measured by the number of victims, the entire central office with its front organizations can be classified as an effective system in which the working methods and decision-making processes of bureaucracy and party ideology were used.[95]

The rule-bound procedure and typically bureaucratic way of working must be seen in stark contrast to the content. Although the "euthanasia" officials repeatedly pointed out in later statements that the planning trips had nothing to do with Action T4,[96] or that the only connection was between planning commissions and the number of beds vacated by the medical commissions,[97] the establishment of the T4 Planning Commission changed the nature of the work. The final reports of the T4 Planning Commission were more far-reaching than a mere interim balance sheet; rather, they were to form the basis for plans to reorganize psychiatric care in the entire National Socialist state.

Another aspect of the planning reports is remarkable: they mark an important change of perspective in the organization of "euthanasia." When the operators had handed over the freed-up real estate to external users in the initial phase of the program (the Wehrmacht, the SS, and Nazi Party institutions were particular early profiteers of "euthanasia"[98]), the Planning Commission was established to utilize these buildings according to the recommendations of the Reich Working Group and the wishes of the hospital administrators.[99] The vacant buildings served as space buffers for sudden demand bottlenecks.[100] In this context, the murder of patients is no longer to be classified only as part of Nazi ideology; it must also be considered within the context of economizing measures in the psychiatric care system.[101] One of the most important tasks of the planning department was the creation of reliable data on the misappropriation of institutions as a basis for planning.[102] The sources confirm the suspicion that the agents of the mental healthcare accounting center were also planning to set up a card index and simplify the billing procedure based on a comprehensive reporting system.[103]

Administrative processes and methods played a major role in the planning and execution of the National Socialist policies of exclusion and extermination. In this context, bureaucratic methods fulfilled very different functions. They not only facilitated the organization and secrecy of the "euthanasia" program but also served economic interests, when those in the bureaucratic apparatus combined their ideological convictions with financial pragmatism—for example, in the systematic appropriation of estates.[104] The available archive material leads to the conclusion that the employees of the T4 organizations themselves developed National Socialist guidelines and radicalized existing administrative requirements.

Therefore, in the spirit of historian Hinz-Wessel, Hannah Arendt's notion of administrative mass murder, that is, the bureaucratic execution of industrially driven extermination of people, can also be accepted for the systematic murder of the mentally ill and mentally disabled as part of National Socialist "euthanasia." Action T4 was real.[105] Although there are no sequences in the written statements by administrative inspector Trieb that substantiate his clear support of "euthanasia," he played a major role as a member of the administrative authorities. He developed guidelines in the spirit of National Socialism and interpreted existing administrative guidelines according to the political zeitgeist. As an active agent who indirectly participated in the killing of mentally ill people with his deeds, he had a responsibility.[106] It was precisely his combination of organizational abilities and ideological motivation, along with instrumentalized administration, that ensured that the planned "euthanasia" in hospitals and nursing homes functioned and was economically beneficial to the Nazi state. So it was above all the structure that attained full effectiveness; the individual remained hidden behind it as an agent, but if he wanted to, he could be well aware of what he was doing.

Felicitas Söhner, DPhil, has held the position of assistant at the Department of History, Philosophy and Ethics of Medicine at the University of Düsseldorf since 2016. Her research focus is in medical and social history of the nineteenth and twentieth centuries, oral history, European memory culture, and biographical processes.

Notes

1. Faulstich 2000, 2003; Ebbinghaus and Dörner 2002, 297.
2. Hohendorf et al. 2002–6; Rotzoll et al. 2010.
3. Arendt 1986, 373–99.
4. Hinz-Wessels et al. 2005, 105–6.
5. Arendt 1964, 18.
6. 1899–1983; Member of the NSDAP 1.5.37, SA 1.11.33, Oberscharführer, NS-State Corps, Reichsbund of German Officials ab 1933, NS People's Welfare 1934, TV 1922, Reichskolonialbund 1938, NS-State Air Protection Corps 1933.
7. Cranach and Siemen 1999, 250.
8. Söhner et al. 2017.
9. Söhner et al. 2015.
10. Steger et al. 2010–12.
11. Söhner, Becker, and Fangerau 2016.
12. Aly 1985; Aly et al. 1985.

13. Klee 1986, 2010.
14. Faulstich 1993, 2000, 2003.
15. Süß 2003.
16. Schmuhl 1987; Frei 1991; Görgl 2008; Cording 2001.
17. Friedlander 1995, xii.
18. Lozowick 2003
19. Bernhardt 1994, 159, 80.
20. Steger et al. 2010–12.
21. Schmuhl 1987.
22. Schmuhl 1987 and 2016.
23. Walter 1996.
24. Roer and Henkel 1986, 13–24.
25. Loewy and Winter 1996.
26. Osterloh and Vollnhals 2011.
27. Freudinger 2002.
28. Burkhardt 2015.
29. These archives include the Archiv der Erzdiözese Salzburg, Archiv des Bezirksverbands Oldenburg, Archiv des Diakonischen Werks Rheinland, Archiv des Erzbistums München-Freising, Dokumentationsarchiv des österreichischen Widerstands, Landeswohlfahrtsverband Archiv Kassel, Hauptarchiv Bethel, and Hauptstaatsarchiv Bremen.
30. Medick 1994.
31. Grotjahn 1933.
32. Gesetz über die Vereinheitlichung des Gesundheitswesens, 3 July 1934.
33. Richter 2018, 536.
34. Dörries and Vollmann 1997, 553.
35. Classification introduced in Germany on the occasion of the annual meeting of the German Association for Psychiatry, held in Würzburg on 24 January 1933.
36. Agich 1994.
37. Neuner 2011, 255; Rotzoll et al. 2010, 32.
38. Richter 2018, 578.
39. Richter 2018, 578.
40. Burkhardt 2015, 93.
41. Burkhardt 2015, 96.
42. Sandner 2003, 374.
43. Pfeiffer 2005, 28.
44. Burkhardt 2015, 93–96.
45. HStAW 631a 887 W. Grützner (22.06.65).
46. Eichler 1995, 181.
47. Burkhardt 2015, 93.
48. Burkhardt 2015, 94.
49. Söhner 2018.
50. Hinz-Wessels et al. 2005, 33.
51. NAW, Film T-1021, Roll 11.
52. Hinz-Wessels et al. 2005, 99.
53. Burkhardt 2015, 99.
54. Burkhardt 2015, 104.
55. Faulstich 2000, 218–32.
56. BAB GStA DDR Best. DP 3 L. Trieb (16.12.65); HStAW 631a 890 L. Trieb (04.04.64), A. Ullrich (04.09.61).
57. BAB R96I/15 H. Becker/R. Müller (04.41–12.42).

58. Hinz-Wessels et al. 2005, 99.
59. BAB R96I/15 H. Becker/R. Müller (04.41–12.42).
60. BALu B162/18116 L. Trieb (03.04.62, 05.02.63, 04.04.63, 16.12.65).
61. BALu B162/18116 L. Trieb (03.04.62, 05.02.63, 04.04.63, 16.12.65).
62. ADWRh Ohl 86.2 Diakonissenanstalt Kaiserswerth (08.07.42).
63. HAB 2/39-198 F v Bodelschwingh (18.05.42).
64. ADWRh Ohl 86.2 Diakonissenanstalt Kaiserswerth (08.07.42); Kaminsky 1995, 415.
65. HStAW 631a 890 A. Ullrich (04.09.61), L. Trieb (04.04.64); HStAW 631a 887 W. Grützner (22.06.65).
66. Rüdin et al. 1943, Gedanken und Anregungen betr. die künftige Entwicklung der Psychiatrie BAB R96 I/9.
67. Sandner 2006, 138
68. Faulstich 1993, 291.
69. Walter 1996, 747; Sandner 2003, 237; BAB 96I/15 H. Becker/R. Müller (04.41–12.42).
70. HStAW 631a 1800 A. Ullrich (04.09.61), L. Trieb (06.06.61).
71. BALu B162/18116 L. Trieb (03.04.62, 05.02.63, 04.04.63, 16.12.65).
72. NAW, Film T-1021, Roll 12 L. Trieb (29.05.43).
73. Aly 1985, 108.
74. BAB R96I/15 L. Trieb (17.12.41).
75. Aly 1985, 47.
76. Baader 2009, 19.
77. Söhner 2018.
78. BAB R96I/15 H. Becker/R. Müller (04.41–12.42).
79. BAB R96I/15 H. Becker (17.04.42).
80. BAB R96I/15 H. Becker (14.03.42); Sandner 2003, 517.
81. BAB R96I/15 H. Becker (27.05.42).
82. BAB R96I/15 L. Trieb (20.05.42).
83. NAW, Film T-1021, Roll 11 L. Trieb (20.05.42).
84. NAW, Film T-1021, Roll 11 L. Trieb (20.05.42).
85. The so-called "e-measure" is a camouflage word for "euthanasia." ADWRh Ohl 86.2 Diakonissenanstalt Kaiserswerth (08.07.42); AAS 18/11/ Caritas -Anstalt.
86. HStAW 631a 890 L. Trieb (04.04.64), A. Ullrich (04.09.61).
87. Klee 1986, 82.
88. DOöW E 18.281LG Wien, Vg 8a Vr 455/46 E. Gelny (06.02.44)
89. Walter 1996: 745, BALu B 162, Ordner Nr. 132, Richtlinien des Reichsbeauftragten zur Planungsfrage.
90. Scheuing 2004, 360.
91. Aly et al. 1985, 25; Faulstich 1993, 292.
92. BAB R96I/15 H. Becker / R. Müller (04.41–12.42).
93. Hinz-Wessels et al. 2005, 105.
94. Schilde 2002, 212.
95. Sandner 2003, 368.
96. HStAW 631a 887 W. Grützner (22.06.65).
97. HStAW 631a 890 L. Trieb (04.04.64), A. Ullrich (04.09.61).
98. BAB R96I/15 H.Becker/R.Müller (04.41–12.42).
99. Sandner 2003, 517.
100. BAB R96I/15 H. Becker/R. Müller (04.41–12.42).
101. Baader 2009, 19.
102. Süß 2003, 318.
103. Hinz-Wessels et al. 2005, 100.

104. Hinz-Wessels et al. 2005, 106.
105. Hinz-Wessels et al. 2005, 105.
106. Volk 2005, 19.

References

Archival Sources

Archiv der Erzdiözese Salzburg (AES)
    18/11/Caritas-Anstalt St. Anton 1928–1945.
Archiv des Diakonischen Werks Rheinland (ADWRh)
    Ohl 86.1.1.4.
Bundesarchiv Berlin-Lichterfelde (BAB)
    GStA DDR Best. DP 3/1884.
    BAB R96 I/9.
    BAB R96 I/15.
Bundesarchiv Ludwigsburg (BaLu)
    B162/18116.
    B162/Heidelberger Dokumente, Ordner Nr. 132.
Dokumentationsarchiv des österreichischen Widerstands (DÖW)
    E 18.281LG Wien, Vg 8a Vr 455/46.
Hauptarchiv Bethel (HAB)
    HAB 2/39-198.
Hauptstaatsarchiv Wiesbaden (HStAW)
    HStAW 631a 887.
    HStAW 631a 890.
    HStAW 631a 1800.
National Archives Washington (NAW)
    Film T-1021, Roll 10, No. 126559-61.
    Film T-1021, Roll 11, No. 126867-928.
    Film T-1021, Roll 11, No. 127160-71.

Books and Articles

Agich, George J. 1994. "Evaluative Judgment and Personality Disorder." In *Philosophical Perspectives on Psychiatric Diagnostic Classification*, edited by J. Z Sadler, O. P. Wiggins, M. A. Schwartz, 233–45. Baltimore: Johns Hopkins.

Aly, Götz. 1985. *Aussonderung und Tod: Die klinische Hinrichtung des Unbrauchbaren*. Berlin: Rotbuch.

Aly, Götz, Karl Masuhr, Maria Lehmann, Karl-Heinz Roth, and Ulrich Schultz. 1985. *Reform und Gewissen: "Euthanasie" im Dienst des Fortschritts*. Berlin: Rotbuch.

Arendt, Hannah. 1964. *Eichmann in Jerusalem: Ein Bericht zur Banalität des Bösen*. Interview 9 November 1964. Stuttgart: SWR.

———. 1986. *Zur Zeit: Politische Essays*. Berlin: Rotbuch.

Baader, Gerhard. 2009. *Psychiatrie im Nationalsozialismus zwischen ökonomischer Rationalität und Patientenmord*. Speech 03.10.2009. Hall: UMIT.

Bernhardt, Heike. 1994. *Anstaltspsychiatrie und "Euthanasie" in Pommern 1933 bis 1945*. Frankfurt am Main: Mabuse.

Burkhardt, Anika. 2015. *Das NS-Euthanasie-Unrecht vor den Schranken der Justiz: Eine strafrechtliche Analyse*. Tübingen: Mohr-Siebeck.

Cording, Clemens. 2001. *Die Regensburger Heil- und Pflegeanstalt Karthaus-Prüll im "Dritten Reich."* Regensburg: DWV.
Dörries, Andrea, and Jochen Vollmann. 1997. "Medizinische und ethische Probleme der Klassifikation psychischer Störungen." *Fortschr Neur Psychiat* 65: 550–54.
Ebbinghaus, Angelika, and Klaus Dörner. 2002. *Vernichten und Heilen: Der Nürnberger Ärzteprozeß und seine Folgen.* Berlin: Aufbau.
Eichler, Volker. 1995. "Die Frankfurter Gestapo-Kartei." In *Die Gestapo: Mythos und Realität*, edited by P. Gerhard and K.-M. Mallmann, 178–99. Darmstadt: Primus.
Fangerau, Heiner, Sascha Topp, Klaus Schepker. 2017. *Kinder- und Jugendpsychiatrie im Nationalsozialismus und in der Nachkriegszeit.* Berlin: Springer.
Faulstich, Heinz. 1993. *Von der Irrenfürsorge zur Euthanasie.* Freiburg: Lambertus.
———. 2000. "Die Zahl der "Euthanasie"-Opfer." In *"Euthanasie" und die aktuelle Sterbehilfedebatte: Die historischen Hintergründe medizinischer Ethik*, edited by A. Frewer and C. Eickhoff, 218–33. Frankfurt am Main: Campus.
———. 2003. "Hungersterben in der Psychiatrie 1914–1949." *Sudhoffs Archiv* 87.
Frei, Norbert. 2003. "NS-Eliten nach 1945: Das Beispiel der Ärzteschaft." In *Nach der Diktatur*, edited by W. Woelk, F. Sparing, K. Bayer, and M. Esch, 57–69. Essen: Klartext.
———. 1991. *Medizin und Gesundheitspolitik in der NS-Zeit.* München: Oldenbourg.
Freudiger, Kerstin. 2002. *Die juristische Aufarbeitung von NS-Verbrechen.* Tübingen: Mohr-Siebeck.
Friedlander, Henry. 1995. *The Origins of Nazi Genocide: From Euthanasia to the Final Solution.* Chapel Hill: University of North Carolina Press.
Görgl, Andreas. 2008. "Die 'Aktion T4' und die Rolle der Heil- und Pflegeanstalt Günzburg." Dissertation, University Ulm.
Grotjahn, M. 1933. "Zur psychiatrischen Systematik und Statistik." *Allg Z Psychiat* 99: 464–80.
Hinz-Wessels, Annette, Petra Fuchs, Gerritt Hohendorf, Maike Rotzoll. 2005. "Zur bürokratischen Abwicklung eines Massenmords." *VfZ* 1: 79–107.
Hochmuth, Anneliese. 1997. *Spurensuche: Eugenik, Sterilisation, Patientenmorde und die von Bodelschwinghschen Anstalten Bethel 1929–1945.* Bielefeld: Bethel.
Hohendorf, Gerritt, Wolfgang Eckart, Christoph Mundt. 2002–6. DFG-Projekt: *Wissenschaftliche Erschliessung des Aktenbestandes R179 der NS-"Euthanasie."* University Heidelberg.
Kaminsky, Uwe. 1995. *Zwangssterilisation und "Euthanasie" im Rheinland.* Köln: Rheinland.
Klee, Ernst. 1986. *Was sie taten—was sie wurden.* Frankfurt am Main: Fischer.
———. 2010. *"Euthanasie" im Dritten Reich.* Frankfurt am Main: Fischer.
Loewy, Hanno, and Bettina Winter (eds.). 1996. *NS-"Euthanasie" vor Gericht.* Frankfurt am Main: Campus.
Lozowick, Yaacov. 2003. *Hitler's Bureaucrats: The Nazi Security Police and the Banality of Evil.* London: Continuum.
Medick, Hans. 1994. "Mikro-Historie." In *Sozialgeschichte, Alltagsgeschichte, Mikro-Historie. Eine Diskussion*, edited by W. Schulze, 40–53. Göttingen: V&R.
Neuner, Stephanie. 2011. *Politik und Psychiatrie.* Göttingen: V&R.
Osterloh, Jörg, and Clemens Vollnhals (eds.). 2011. *NS-Prozesse und deutsche Öffentlichkeit.* Göttingen: V&R.
Pfeiffer, Jürgen. 2005. "Wissenschaftliches Erkenntnisstreben als Tötungsmotiv?" In *Ergebnisse: Vorabdrucke aus dem Forschungsprogramm, Geschichte der Kaiser-Wilhelm-Gesellschaft im Nationalsozialismus*, edited by C. Sachse and S. Heim. Berlin: MPI.
Richter, M. 2018. "Von Seilschaften und Netzwerken: Die Abteilung Gesundheitswesen und die Gesundheitspolitik." In *Hüter der Ordnung*, edited by F. Bösch and A. Wirsching, 536–80. Göttingen: Wallstein.
Roer, Dorothee, and Dieter Henkel. 1986. "Funktion bürgerlicher Psychiatrie und ihre besondere Form im Faschismus." In *Psychiatrie im Faschismus*, edited by D. Roer and D. Henkel, 13–37. Bonn: Psychiatrie.

Rotzoll, Maike, Gerrit Hohendorf, Petra Fuchs, Christoph Mundt, and Wolfgang Eckart (eds.). 2010. *Die nationalsozialistische "Euthanasie"-Aktion "T 4" und ihre Opfer.* Göttingen: Schöningh.
Sandner, Peter. 2003. *Verwaltung des Krankenmordes.* Gießen: Psychosozial.
———. 2006. "Auf der Suche nach dem Zukunftsprojekt: Die NS-Leitwissenschaft Psychiatrie und ihre Legitimationskrise." In *"Moderne" Anstaltspsychiatrie im 19. und 20. Jahrhundert,* edited by H. Fangerau and K. Nolte, 117–42. Stuttgart: Steiner.
Schilde, Kurt. 2002. *Bürokratie des Todes.* Berlin: Metropol.
Scheuing, Hans-Werner. 2004. *". . . als Menschenleben gegen Sachwerte aufgewogen wurden."* Heidelberg: Winter.
Schmuhl, Hans-Walter. 1987. *Rassenhygiene, Nationalsozialismus, Euthanasie.* Göttingen: V&R.
———. 2016. *Die Gesellschaft Deutscher Neurologen und Psychiater im Nationalsozialismus.* Berlin: Springer.
Söhner, Felicitas. 2018. "Gedächtnis und Erinnerungskultur im deutsch-polnischen Grenzraum am Beispiel der Verbrechen der NS-Psychiatrie." In *Gedächtnistopographien im Grenzraum,* edited by M. Borzyszkowska-Szewczyk and M. Řezník. Warschau: DHI.
Söhner, Felicitas, Thomas Becker, and Heiner Fangerau. 2016. "Psychiatry at the Heil- und Pflegeanstalt Günzburg 1939–1945." *Neurology, Psychiatry and Brain Research* Special Issue: 46–55.
Söhner, Felicitas, Michael von Cranach, Heiner Fangerau, and Thomas Becker. 2016. "Nach der 'Aktion T4.'" *Nervenarzt* 88(9): 1065–73.
Söhner, Felicitas, Heiner Fangerau, and Thomas Becker. 2018. "Evakuierung psychiatrischer Patienten nach Kriegsbeginn." In *Der regionalvernetzte Krankenmord,* edited by M. Rotzoll et al. Köln: Psychiatrie: 104–19.
Söhner, Felicitas, Hans-Joachim Winckelmann, and Thomas Becker. 2015. Das Laboratorium der I.G. Farben an der Heil- und Pflegeanstalt Günzburg. *Medhist Journ* 2: 223–248.
Steger, Florian, Andreas Görgl, and Wolfgang Strube, Hans-Joachim Winckelmann, and Thomas Becker. 2010. "Die 'Aktion-T4' und die Rolle der Heil- und Pflegeanstalt Günzburg." *Psych Prax* 37(6): 300–305.
Steger, Florian, Andreas Görgl, Wolfgang Strube, Hans-Joachim Winckelmann, and Thomas Becker. 2011. "Die 'Aktion-T4': Erinnerung an Patientenopfer aus der Heil- und Pflegeanstalt Günzburg." *Nervenarzt* 82(11): 1476–82.
Steger, Florian, Andreas Görgl, Wolfgang Strube, Hans-Joachim Winckelmann, Thomas Becker. 2011. "'Transferred to Another Institution': Clinical Histories of Psychiatric Patients Murdered in the Nazi Euthanasia Killing Program." *Israel Journal of Psychiatry and Related Sciences* 48: 268–74.
Steger, Florian, Barbara Schmer, Wolfgang Strube, and Thomas Becker. 2012. "Zwangssterilisationen nach dem Gesetz zur Verhütung erbkranken Nachwuchses." *Nervenarzt* 83(3): 366–77.
Süß, Wolfgang. 2003. *Der "Volkskörper" im Krieg.* München: Oldenbourg.
Topp, Sascha. 2013. *Geschichte als Argument in der Nachkriegsmedizin.* Göttingen: V&R.
Volk, Christian. 2005. *Urteilen in Dunklen Zeiten.* Bamberg: Lukas.
von Cranach, Michael, and Hans-Ludwig Siemen. 1999. *Psychiatrie im Nationalsozialismus.* München: Oldenbourg.
Walter, Bernd. 1996. *Psychiatrie und Gesellschaft in der Moderne.* Paderborn: Schöningh.
Weise, Anton. 2017. *Nach dem Raub.* Göttingen: Wallstein.

CHAPTER 10

Dentists in National Socialist Germany
A Fragmented Profession

Matthis Krischel

Before 1933, the dental profession in Germany was fragmented in two main ways: First, it included university-educated dental surgeons as well as skilled dentists (dental technicians authorized to treat patients) who were educated outside universities. Members of both groups could be licensed to treat patients, and their treatment could be reimbursed by public health insurance. Second, it was divided along the political spectrum. Among dental surgeons in Germany were right-wing nationalists and early supporters of the National Socialist (Nazi) Party, but also social democrats, socialists, and communists. Skilled dentists were less sharply divided politically, with a majority taking a more moderate position. Some dentists' political affiliations also directly influenced their views of how dental care should be organized, either in individual private practice or in large clinics operated by the state or public health insurance agencies.

This chapter in part summarizes research on the history of dentistry in Nazi Germany previously published in German.[1] Much of the early research on the topic had been done by the Association for Democratic Dental Medicine (Vereinigung Demokratische Zahnmedizin, VDZM) and its members.[2] More recently, a monograph and an edited volume following a conference have been published.[3] The international literature is sparse. Significant contributions have been published in French, and the emigration of dental surgeons to Britain has been documented in English.[4] In addition to secondary sources, dental journals from the 1930s and 1940s have been analyzed as primary sources for this contribution.

The aim of this chapter is to present, for the first time in English, an overview of the history of the dental profession in Nazi Germany. It will shine a spotlight on aspects of political, institutional, and social history. Dental surgeons and skilled dentists will be compared with each other, and occasionally also with physicians, in order to highlight particularities. In part, the willingness of dental professionals to cooperate with the Nazi state will be understood as a conscious exchange of favors and resources between the domains of dental medicine and politics:[5] Dental surgeons and skilled dentists were prepared to comply with Nazi health policy and integrate into its system in part to gain professional advantages. In this way, this chapter contributes to the understanding of medicine and its institutions in Nazi Germany and their interaction with the National Socialist state and government.

This chapter will also sketch the parallel histories of dental surgeons and skilled dentists. Already before 1933, dental surgeons wanted to achieve a monopoly on dental care. This conflict continued under Nazi rule, but it was not resolved until 1952. Both groups went through similar phases of readjustment to the new political environment in 1933, the consolidation of power within their institutions, and the persecution of Jewish and "politically unreliable" members. They also found the spectrum of their practice potentially changed through Nazi health policies and under the conditions of World War II from 1939 on. Even though skilled dentists outnumbered dental surgeons until 1945, the smaller group was, as an academic profession, much more structured, had more and more differentiated institutions, and left more historical sources. Dental surgeons were also more involved in some of the fields with connections to Nazi health policy, such as eugenics. For these reasons, they will receive more attention in this chapter.

The contribution is part of an ongoing research project on the history of dentistry in Nazi Germany. The project was funded partially by the German Dental Assoication (Bundeszahnärztekammer), the German Society of Dentistry and Oral Medicine (Deutsche Gesellschaft für Zahn-, Mund- und Kieferheilkunde, DGZMK), and the National Association of Statutory Health Insurance Dentists (Kassenzahnärztliche Bundesvereinigung).[6]

Dental Surgeons

In 1933, 10,885 dental surgeons (Zahnärzte) worked in Germany.[7] Though the first German universities had started to train dental surgeons in the nineteenth century, they remained a small minority until after World War I. Between 1920 and 1925 their number had doubled from 4,459 to 9,137.[8] This was in part because the profession had become more attractive—as it was now part of the medical faculties at German universities, graduates could receive a doctorate in dental medicine (Dr. med. dent.)—and in part because men returning from World War I chose to go into this profession.[9]

Dental surgeons earned significantly less money than physicians. Like many professionals, they had suffered a dramatic setback from the financial crisis of 1929 and saw their overall income decrease by 20 percent. In 1933, dental surgeons on average earned 5,716 Reichsmark, while physicians on average earned 9,280 Reichsmark.[10] Skilled dentists, in turn, earned on average about 60 percent of dental surgeons' income. In the years after 1933, all groups saw their income rise around 10 percent per year. This can be understood as an economic recovery after the crisis of 1929, but it can also be explained by new positions being created in healthcare and healthcare bureaucracy, as well as the elimination of Jewish and "politically unreliable" healthcare professionals. This benefited some previously unemployed dental surgeons.

Dental surgeons blamed their inferior economic position in comparison to physicians on their rivalry with skilled dentists. In part, their efforts to fall in line with Nazi health policies can be understood as an effort to gain favors from the regime and eventually attain a monopoly in the profession. Subsequently, dental surgeons established Nazi organizations and positions similar to the ones in the medical profession. The most important of these positions was the Reich leader of dental surgeons (*Reichszahnärzteführer*), a position similar to that of the Reich leader of physicians (*Reichsärzteführer*).

The political alignment of the chief professional association of dental surgeons in Germany took less than a month. In March 1933, two weeks after the German people had elected the Nazi Party to power, Ernst Stuck (1893–1974), a dental surgeon from Leipzig, published an article titled "Nationale Revolution und Reichsverband" (National revolution and the Reich-association of dental surgeons)[11] in the association's journal. Stuck had been a member of the Nazi Party and the Nazi Physicians' League since 1931. In 1932 he also became an officer in the Nazi Party office for public health (*Hauptabteilung Volksgesundheit*) under his fellow dentist Bernhard Hörmann (1889–1977) of Munich.

In the article, Stuck pointed out the new directive of healthcare politics in Germany: "suprema lex salus publica," i.e. public health as the first and most important priority. Just after noting that "a blind politics of particular interests" would no longer be tenable, Stuck pointed out which measures would best serve public dental health: a solution of the "obvious legal uncertainty of German dental surgeons with regards to social security" and an end of "freedom of patient-care," i.e. the right to treat patients without holding a medical license or a university degree. In practice, Stuck wanted to shift power from public health insurances to dental surgeons and exclude skilled dentists from treating patients. With this, he addressed the two chief health political concerns of German dental surgeons and tried to align these particular interests with the new government's health policies.[12]

Stuck was elected president of the Reich Association of Dental Surgeons (Reichsverband der Zahnärzte) on 24 March. The published protocol notes that the meeting

> presented a different image from the usual. The gathering was under the exhilarating impression of the great national revolution. Many colleagues as delegates from the Reich had appeared in uniforms of the SA and the *Stahlhelm* [paramilitary

nationalist organization]. It is a proof of discipline and certainly a good omen for German politics on a large scale that despite an apparently belligerent image, no discord disturbed the negotiations and differences were settled in the politest collegial manner on stage and in the background.[13]

Delegates of the meeting also sent notes of loyalty to the new government and—after Stuck had been elected—a second note of loyalty to Chancellor Adolf Hitler personally.[14] A few weeks later, the board of the Reich Association turned over the power to make decisions in its name to Stuck. This completed the political alignment of the most important professional association of dental surgeons in Germany.

One year later, the most important scientific societies for dental medicine in Germany were united into the German Society of Dentistry and Oral Medicine (Deutsche Gesellschaft für Zahn-, Mund- und Kieferheilkunde, DGZMK). Its new president, Hermann Euler (1878–1961), had already been president of one of the constituent societies since 1929. He had become a member of the Nazi Teachers' League (NS-Lehrerbund) in 1933 and became member of the Nazi Party in 1937 and of the Nazi Physicians' League in 1938. Euler had studied first medicine and then dentistry in Heidelberg and later became professor of dentistry at the University of Breslau (today's Wrocław, Poland), where he was also dean of the medical school in 1930 and 1933–36. In this position he oversaw the persecution and expulsion of Jewish faculty from the medical school.[15] In 1940 he mentored a doctoral thesis "On the possibility of re-use of gold from the mouths of the dead."[16] In the context of the robbery of dental gold from murdered psychiatric patients and concentration camp prisoners, this work must be understood as supporting this aspect of Nazi "health policy." The author, dental surgeon Viktor Scholz, claims that the state could make a law allowing the removal of dental gold from the deceased. He claims that at the time of writing, for reasons of public opinion and professional ethics among dental surgeons, a law like this would not be tenable. But in his closing paragraph, Scholz states that his investigation does not mark the end of the question, but only its beginning.[17] Indeed, by September 1940, SS leader Heinrich Himmler had ordered SS doctors to collect gold teeth from the dead.[18]

When the German Society of Dentistry and Oral Medicine was re-formed in 1949, Euler was again elected as president and served in this role until 1954.

Like Euler, many German dental surgeons contributed rhetorically or practically to Nazi health policy. Some even sent patients with cleft lips or cleft palates to be sterilized, and some served as part of the SS in concentration camps, managing the robbery of prisoners' dental gold and selecting arriving prisoners to be murdered (see below). At the same time, numerous Jewish and politically opposing dentists were forced out of the profession, driven into exile, or murdered. Of the 10,885 dental surgeons who worked in Germany in 1933, 10 percent were considered Jewish by Nazi authorities. This included people of Jewish faith or with at least one Jewish grandparent. Their number is given between 1,050 and 1,150.[19] This means that their percentage was significantly higher than in the population as a whole, for which 1.5 percent was given, but smaller than among physicians, where it can be assumed that around 16 percent claimed Jewish religion of origin.[20] Jewish dental surgeons faced similar persecution as physicians[21]: Already in 1933 they were expelled from positions at universities and public hospitals, they were removed from the public health insurance system, they were only reimbursed by private insurance companies for treating Jewish patients, and quotas of 1.5 percent for Jewish students at medical faculties of universities were created. This quota affected medical and dental students and had especially strong repercussions in cities with high percentages of Jewish citizens and healthcare professionals, like Berlin and Frankfurt. By July 1938 the license to practice medicine was revoked for all Jewish physicians.[22] This law seems to have been applied to dental surgeons as well. Nonetheless, they, together with pharmacists and veterinarians, were explicitly targeted in January 1939.[23] Only a small number received licenses to treat the Jewish population as "dental treatment providers" (*Zahnbehandler*).[24] According to ongoing research, at least another fifty dental surgeons were terminated from jobs or removed from the public health insurance system for political reasons.

Jewish dental surgeons were unevenly distributed throughout Germany. More than a third of them practiced in Berlin.[25] Jewish dental surgeons were also more likely than average to work for the public health insurance system, in public health, or in school dentistry. The dismissal of these Jewish and/or politically opposed colleagues, of course, caused temporary shortages of dental surgeons. On the other hand, it made it easier for those not persecuted to find employment. This may help to explain why a relatively large number of dental surgeons were among the early supporters of Nazism.

Research is ongoing on the fates of persecuted dental surgeons. By January 1939, only 372 remained in Germany.[26] Taking into account that a number of persons died by suicide or natural causes between 1933 and 1939, it still seems likely that about two-thirds of dental surgeons were able to emigrate from Germany. This percentage would—again—be similar to physicians.[27] Dental surgeons could face problems similar to physicians when it came to licensing in their new host countries. In Berlin, more than three hundred Jewish dental surgeons participated in a course to train them as dental technicians before emigrating. This occupation might have been less prestigious and less economically attractive than dental surgery, but it was also much less strictly regulated.[28]

Two biographical sketches can illustrate the spectrum of fates of persecuted dental surgeons. Alfred Kantorowicz (1880–1962) was born in Posen, Prussia (todays Poznan, Poland), and studied dentistry and later medicine in Berlin.[29] Before World War I, this was still the usual career path for academic dentists.

After serving in the war, Kanzorowicz became a lecturer at the University of Bonn, where he was promoted to full professor in 1923. He distinguished himself in public dental health, establishing a system of dental screening and treatment of schoolchildren that was named the "Bonn model." In this model, dental surgeons employed by the municipality screened elementary school students' teeth and—when necessary—treated them immediately. Kantorowicz was also one of the pioneers of oro-maxillofacial surgery in Germany. After the National Socialists took power, Kantorowicz, as a Jew and member of the Social Democrat Party, was considered their obvious enemy. He was arrested in April and imprisoned in Bonn and the concentration camps Börgermoor and Lichtenburg. Kantorowicz had hoped for support from his university, but he received none. A condition of his release from concentration camp was emigration. He went to Istanbul, where he became professor of dentistry and a pioneer of pediatric dentistry in Turkey.[30] Kantorowicz was among the minority of Jewish German academics who wanted to return to Germany after the war. He intended to return to Bonn in spring 1947, but a heart attack suffered immediately beforehand caused him to retire. He eventually moved back to Bonn in 1950 and died there in 1962. As a highly qualified and world-famous academic dental surgeon, Alfred Kantorowicz was able to escape imprisonment to another academic position. In this regard, he represents the most successful class of emigrant dental surgeons from Germany.

The biography of the Düsseldorf dental surgeon Waldemar Spier (1889–1944) illustrates another outcome.[31] He was born in Düsseldorf into a Jewish family and studied dental surgery at the University of Würzburg. After serving in World War I, he settled in private practice in Düsseldorf, where he was active as a member and an elected official of Fortuna Düsseldorf soccer club. It is unclear if Spier, as a veteran of World War I, was subject to the anti-Semitic exclusion from working within the public healthcare system in 1933. After the pogrom of November 1938, he was arrested and sent to Dachau concentration camp, from which he was released after three weeks. Spier's wife was Catholic, which gave him some so-called "privileges." He received a license to practice as "dental treatment provider" (*Zahnbehandler*) for the remaining Jewish community in Düsseldorf in 1939. He continued to live there and became head of the Jewish community in 1943 by default—he was one of the few remaining Jewish citizens, and his three predecessors in this role had, respectively, either been driven to suicide, gone into hiding, or had been arrested. Spier was arrested in March 1944 and sent to Auschwitz concentration camp in September. There he survived the liberation of the camp by the Red Army, but he died subsequently of typhus and malnutrition. Spier had been well-integrated into German society. His wife supported him as much as possible, including visiting him during periods of imprisonment. It is unclear why Spier did not flee from Germany before 1939. His fate of deportation and subsequent death due to the murderous conditions of the camp must be assumed to be typical for the more than three hundred dental surgeons who had not emigrated at that point.

On the other end of the political spectrum, many dentists were among early supporters of Nazism. At least seventy-four of them received a golden party membership badge, signifying that they were among the first one hundred thousand party members. Around thirteen hundred dentists had joined the Nazi party before 1933, putting early party membership at 12 percent.[32] This is significantly higher than among physicians, were 7 percent were party members before 1933.[33]

The first two dental surgeons who were elected members of national parliament (Reichstag) were both members of the Nazi Party in 1933: Artur Kolb (1885–1945) of Amsberg and Bernhard Hörmann (1889–1977) of Munich.[34] Eighteen dental surgeons had joined the SS before 1933, and another 106 joined it that year, perhaps in part out of political opportunism after Hitler had been elected chancellor. Until 1945 around 1,500 dental surgeons joined the SS, and at least 251 joined the Waffen-SS.[35] The second number is significant, because it includes dental surgeons who were part of concentration camp personnel. Here they provided healthcare to SS soldiers and their families—and even to prisoners, in some cases—in camp dental stations. But they also participated in "selections" of prisoners to be murdered. In Auschwitz, Willi Schatz (1905–85)[36] and Willy Frank (1903–89)[37] "selected" prisoners on the ramp. Dental surgeons also oversaw the robbery of dental gold from the bodies of murdered prisoners.[38] In extermination camps, gold teeth and bridgework were broken out of the mouths by members of the *Sonderkommandos* before cremation. Accounts of surviving *Sonderkommando* prisoners describe the inhumane work they were forced to perform or observe.[39] In some cases, prisoners with dental training were selected for these tasks, and dental instruments brought to the camps by prisoners were used. In Auschwitz, more than ten kilograms of gold were robbed in this manner per week over many weeks. By the end of the war, at least two to three tons of dental gold had been taken in the concentration camps.[40] While a significant amount of the gold was traded inside the camps or stolen by SS guards, much of it was melted[41]—like precious metal acquired from other sources inside the camps—and send to Switzerland and other countries in order to pay for the German war efforts.[42]

In the area of eugenic sterilization, dentists were concerned with persons with cleft lip and cleft palate. The conditions were known in the German literature as "harelip" (*Hasenscharte*) and "wolf throat" (*Wolfsrachen*), terms that may have aided the dehumanization of persons with these conditions at the time. Dental surgeons were among the medical professionals required to notify public health offices about cases of hereditary diseases according to the Law for the Prevention of Hereditarily Diseased Offspring (Gesetz zur Verhütung erbkranken Nachwuchses). Cleft lip and cleft palate were included among the "severe physical deformities" that were, according to the law, indications for the usually forced sterilization of patients. At least two patients with cleft lip and sixty-nine patients with cleft palate were sterilized, and at least one patient's file was sent to be reviewed in the course of "euthanasia" patient murders.[43]

Dental surgeons were also involved in other aspects of Nazi health policy. Some of them supported "biological dentistry" (*biologische Zahnheilkunde*) as an aspect of naturalistic healthcare. Whole-grain rye bread was promoted as a natural way to preserve dental health and appropriate nourishment for racially German people. A research institute was founded and a journal published from 1934.[44]

Skilled Dentists

In 1933, 18,000 skilled dentists (*Dentisten*) worked in Germany, some of them in dental laboratories, but 11,648 were licensed to treat patients within the public health insurance system. They were trained for three years in an apprenticeship system and nonuniversity dental schools, and had to take a state exam before being allowed to treat patients. Their number rose to 20,885 in 1939, and 15,220 were licensed. Numbers on party membership and members of persecuted groups for skilled dentists are harder to find and not yet reliable: around 650 self-identified as Jewish, which would put the percentage around 3.6 percent.[45] Given that Nazi race laws tended to also target people of Jewish origin with other religious affiliations or none at all, the number of persecuted persons was likely higher than that. In 1933, Jewish and "politically unreliable" skilled dentists were excluded from working in the public health insurance system and their professional association, the Reich Association of German Dentists (Reichsverband Deutscher Dentisten, RDD). This included at least thirteen persons who were excluded for being active in communist or socialist parties without being considered Jewish.[46] When Jewish dental surgeons were stripped of their licenses to practice dental medicine in January 1939, the law also explicitly forbade all Jewish persons to practice dentistry.[47] In 1936, only two hundred Jewish skilled dentists remained in Germany.[48] This suggests that many of them had emigrated at this point.

Before 1933, around 12 percent of skilled dentists had been members of the Nazi Party. This number is comparable with dental surgeons.[49] Nevertheless, the political alignment of the RDD took until the autumn of 1933, significantly longer than that of the professional organization of dental surgeons. On 28 September 1933 the Reich leader of physicians Gerhard Wagner (1888–1938) informed the president of the RDD that the skilled dentist Karl Schaeffer (1898–?) would be named Reich leader of skilled dentists (*Reichsdentistenführer*) and take leadership of the RDD. Schaeffer had been a member of the Nazi Party and the SA since 1925 and was active in the party. After joining the SS in 1934, he advanced to the rank of *SS-Standartenführer* (similar to the rank of colonel in the army) within two years. Schaeffer had not been licensed to treat patients and had not been a member of the RDD before, indicating that he was chosen for his political allegiance and not his professional qualification. A letter by *Reichsärzteführer* Gerhard Wagner published in the journal of the RDD explicitly states that Schaeffer was not elected president of the association by its members but was chosen by the Reich minister of the interior to be Reich leader of all German skilled dentists after being proposed by Wagner. While the letter does not list any qualifications of Schaeffer as a skilled dentist, it praises him as an "old and tested party member and fighter."[50] Schaeffer was replaced in 1938 by Josef Schmid, who was subsequently replaced in 1939 by Fritz Blumenstein. The main reason for this seems to have been that members of the RDD feared that Schaeffer might be willing to agree to a monopoly of treating patients for dental surgeons. This had been an important point of contention between dental surgeons and skilled dentists, and both sides tried to use their influence and align themselves with Nazi health policy in part to maneuver into a favorable position in this conflict. It seemed that skilled dentists made some advances: in 1939 they were allowed to treat personnel of the armed forces and the police, a task that was previously performed exclusively by dental surgeons. Skilled dentists fit in well with some Nazi health policies, because their services were generally cheaper and considered of similar quality. Also, they proved that efficient healthcare did not require a university education, which may have been an attractive perspective within anti-intellectual circles among NS officials. The conflict was eventually resolved in 1952 when all licensed skilled dentists were given the status of dental surgeons, in turn agreeing to close all skilled dentist schools. Since then, the history of the profession of skilled dentists has received only limited attention by historians, in part because dental surgeons writing the history of their own profession have been more focused on the academic roots of their profession.[51]

Persons who actively opposed Nazism were rare in Germany, including those in the dental profession. Paul Rentsch (1898–1944) is an example of this minority.[52] In 1939, this dental technician from Berlin, together with his wife, joined the resistance group "European Union," which also included the socialist Berlin physician Georg Groscurth and the chemist Robert Havemann. The group provided shelter, food, medical treatment, and forged papers to persecuted people and helped men to avoid military service by providing drugs to them that would make it appear that they were unfit for service. Rentsch personally provided dental treatment to Jews who had gone into hiding. In 1943, Rentsch and his wife were arrested by the Gestapo. Subsequently, he was among the four main defendants who were tried at the peoples' court (*Volksgerichtshof*) for their activity in the European Union. A total of fourteen members of the group were sentenced to death. Rentsch was executed by guillotine on 8 May 1944. He was survived by his wife, who was released from prison after four months, and their two children.

Since 2006, Rentsch is remembered as a Righteous Among the Nations by Yad Vashem.

Conclusion

The dental profession in Germany in the 1930s and 1940s was twice fragmented. A duality between dental surgeons and skilled dentists persisted during this time period. The dental profession was also split along political lines. Dental surgeons were more politically active, and within this part of the profession a significant number of Jewish and politically left-leaning persons existed, but also many early supporters of Nazism. Comparing the two branches of the dental profession, it becomes obvious that dental surgeons fell in line with the new government more quickly, within weeks of Hitler being elected chancellor. The process of coordination took longer with skilled dentists.

Dental surgeons had fought for a strengthening of their profession in opposition to health insurers and for a unified dental profession, i.e. an integration of skilled dentists. Skilled dentists, on the other hand, were aware of the very real danger of their profession being absorbed and resolved to resist this. The two branches of the dental profession established rival bureaucracies centered on a Reich leader of dental surgeons and a Reich leader of skilled dentists. They can be described as a polycracy of competing bureaucracies, a typical feature of organization in Nazi Germany.[53] This led the two professions into a competition of radicalization in order to retain favor with the Nazi government and extend their power and competencies.[54] In this way, the radicalization can also be described as a competition for resources from the political regime.[55]

After 1945, German dental organizations, like so many others in the medical field, avoided critical research into their history for a long time. It was only in the 1980s that the first dentists started questioning the history of dentistry in Nazi Germany, but it took until the very recent past for the leading professional associations to establish and partially fund a research project on the topic. As research progresses, many aspects of dentistry in Nazi Germany are coming into focus, but much work remains to be done in the future. This includes a complete list of persecuted dental professionals; a fine-grain analysis of health policy conflicts between public health insurance agencies, dental surgeons, and skilled dentists; and a more detailed analysis of SS dentists in concentration camps, their role in the robbery of dental gold, and the forced involvement of prisoner dentists. A comparison of dental surgeons and skilled dentists during National Socialism with other medical disciplines and medical specialties has the potential to illustrate parallel developments and differences in different branches of medicine.

Matthis Krischel is lecturer of history of medicine and medical ethics at Heinrich Heine University in Düsseldorf, Germany. He received his PhD in history of medicine and medical ethics from Ulm University in Germany in 2013. His research interests include the history of Nazi medicine and its commemoration; the history of anthropology, eugenics, and human genetics; and the history of urology and sexology.

Notes

1. Schwanke, Krischel, and Groß 2016; Groß and Krischel 2020. Unless noted otherwise, translations from German to English in this chapter are by the author.
2. VDZM, Zahnmedizin im Faschismus; Kirchhoff 1987; Guggenbichler 1987.
3. Kirchhoff and Heidel 2016; Groß et al. 2018.
4. Riaud 2015a; Riaud 2003; Zamet 2006.
5. Ash 2002; Krischel 2014.
6. Krischel et al. 2017.
7. Maretzky and Venter 1974, 205.
8. Groß 2006.
9. Krischel 2017.
10. Maretzky and Venter 1974, 206; Möhrle 1996.
11. Stuck 1933.
12. Krischel 2017.
13. Hoffmann 1933.
14. Hoffmann 1933.
15. Groß, Schmidt, and Schwanke, 2016.
16. Staehle and Eckart 2005.
17. Scholz 1940.
18. Riaud 2015b.
19. Kirchhoff and Heidel 2016, 107–9.
20. Krischel 2014, 25.
21. Beddies, Doetz, and Kopke 2014.
22. Anonymous 1938.
23. Anonymous 1939.
24. Lutze 2006.
25. Köhn 1994.
26. Kirchhoff and Heidel 2016, 125.
27. Beddies, Doetz, and Kopke 2014.
28. Köhn 1994.
29. Forsbach 2018.
30. Doyum 1985.
31. Halling, Sparing, and Krischel 2018.
32. Schwanke, Krischel, and Groß 2016.
33. Kater 2000, 103
34. Anonymous 1933.
35. Westemeier, Groß, and Schmidt 2018.
36. Hördler, Kreutzmüller, and Bruttmann 2015.
37. Huber 2009.

38. Riaud 2003.
39. Greif 2005, 286–309; Nyiszli 2011.
40. Kirchhoff and Heidel 2006, 280–324.
41. Hayes 2007.
42. Ziegler 1998.
43. Thieme 2018.
44. Groß 2006, 173.
45. Schwanke and Groß 2016, 187.
46. Schwanke and Groß 2016, 189–90.
47. Anonymous 1939.
48. Schwanke and Groß 2016, 187.
49. Guggenbichler 1987, 269.
50. Wagner 1933.
51. Groß 2006.
52. Kirchhoff and Heidel 2016, 171–76.
53. Stone 2010, 133.
54. Groß and Krischel 2020, 28.
55. Krischel 2014.

References

Anonymous. 1933. "Zahnärzte im Deutschen Reichstag." *Zahnärztliche Mitteilungen* 12.
———. 1938. "Vierte Verordnung zum Reichsbürgergesetz." *Reichsgesetzblatt*, 969–70. Retrieved 6 December 2018 from http://www.ns-quellen.at/gesetz_anzeigen_detail.php?gesetz_id=26010&action=B_Read.
———. 1939. "Achte Verordnung zum Reichsbürgergesetz," *Reichsgesetzblatt* (1939): 47–48. Retrieved 6 December 2018 from http://www.nsquellen.at/gesetz_anzeigen_detail.php?gesetz_id=19110&action=B_Read.
Ash, Mitchell. 2002. "Wissenschaft und Politik als Ressourcen für einander." In *Wissenschaften und Wissenschaftspolitik: Bestandsaufnahmen zu Formationen, Brüchen und Kontinuitäten im Deutschland des 20. Jahrhunderts*, edited by Rüdiger Vom Bruch and Brigitte Kaderas, 32–51. Stuttgart: Steiner.
Beddies, Thomas, Susanne Doetz, and Christoph Kopke. 2014. *Jüdische Ärztinnen und Ärzte im Nationalsozialismus: Entrechtung, Vertreibung, Ermordung*. Berlin: De Gruyter.
Doyum, Ali Vicdani. 1985. *Alfred Kantorowicz unter besonderer Berücksichtigung seines Wirkens in Istanbul*. Diss. med. dent., Würzburg.
Forsbach, Ralf. 2018. "Verfolgt, vertrieben, rehabilitiert: Alfred Kantorowicz und seine Bonner Kollegen (1933–1962)." In *Zahnärzte und Zahnheilkunde im "Dritten Reich": Eine Bestandsaufnahme*, edited by D. Groß, J. Westemeier, M. Schmidt, T. Halling, and M. Krischel, 197–215. Berlin: Lit.
Greif, Gideon. 2005. *We Wept Without Tears: Testimonies of the Jewish Sonderkommando from Auschwitz*. New Haven, CT: Yale University Press.
Groß, Dominik. 2006. "Vom Gebissarbeiter zum staatlich geprüften Dentisten: Der Berufsbildungsprozess der nichtapprobierten Zahnbehandler (1869–1952)." In *Beiträge zur Geschichte und Ethik der Zahnheilkunde*, edited by Dominik Groß, 99–125. Würzburg: Königshausen & Neumann.
———. 2018. "Zahnärzte als Täter. Zwischenergebnisse zur Rolle der Zahnärzte im 'Dritten Reich.'" *Deutsche Zahnärztliche Zeitschrift* 73(3): 164–78.
Groß, Dominik, and Matthis Krischel. 2020. "Zahnärzte als Täter und Verfolgte im 'Dritten Reich.'" *Zahnärztliche Mitteilungen* 110(1–2): 26–29.
Groß, Dominik, Mathias Schmidt, and Enno Schwanke. 2016. "Zahnärztliche Standesvertreter im 'Dritten Reich' und nach 1945 im Spiegel der Lebenserinnerungen von Hermann Euler

(1878–1961) und Carl-Henz Fischer (1909–1997)." *Medizinische Fachgesellschaften im Nationalsozialismus: Bestandsaufnahme und Perspektiven*, edited by Matthis Krischel, Mathias Schmidt, and Dominik Groß, 129–72. Berlin: Lit.

Groß, Dominik, Jens Westemeier, Mathias Schmidt, Thorsten Halling, and Matthis Krischel (eds.). 2018. *Zahnärzte und Zahnheilkunde im "Dritten Reich": Eine Bestandsaufnahme*. Berlin: Lit.

Guggenbichler, Norbert. 1987. *Zahnmedizin unter dem Hakenkreuz*. Marburg: Mabuse.

Halling, Thorsten, Frank Sparing, and Matthis Krischel. 2018. "Erinnerungskulturen als Teil einer integrierten Geschichte des Holocausts: Der Düsseldorfer Zahnarzt Waldemar Spier (1889–1945)." *Zahnärzte und Zahnheilkunde im "Dritten Reich": Eine Bestandsaufnahme*, edited by D. Groß, J. Westemeier, M. Schmidt, T. Halling, and M. Krischel, 215–40. Berlin: Lit.

Hayes, Peter. 2007. *From Cooperation to Complicity: Degussa in the Third Reich*. Cambridge: Cambridge University Press.

Hoffmann, Lothar. 1933. "Die Hauptversammlung am 24. März 1933." *Zahnärztliche Mitteilungen* 11: 379–83.

Hördler, Stefan, Christoph Kreutzmüller, and Tal Bruttmann. 2015. "Auschwitz im Bild: Zur kritischen Analyse der Auschwitz-Alben." *Zeitschrift für Geschichtswissenschaft* 63(7–8): 609–32.

Huber, Barbara. 2009. *Der Regensburger SS-Zahnarzt Dr. Willy Frank*. Würzburg: Königshausen & Neumann.

Kater, Michael. 2000. *Ärzte als Hitlers Helfer*. Hamburg: Europa-Verlag.

Kirchhoff, Wolfgang. 1987. *Zahnmedizin und Faschismus: Arbeiterbewegung und Gesellschaftswissenschaften*. Marburg: Mabuse.

Kirchhoff, Wolfgang, and Caris-Petra Heidel. 2016. *". . . total fertig mit dem Nationalsozialismus"? Die unendliche Geschichte der Medizin im Nationalsozialismus*. Marburg: Mabuse.

Köhn, Michael. 1994. *Zahnärzte 1933–1945, Berufsverbot, Emigration, Verfolgung*. Berlin: Edition Hentrich.

Krischel, Matthis. 2014. *Urologie und Nationalsozialismus: Eine Studie zu Medizin und Politik als Ressourcen füreinander*. Stuttgart: Steiner.

———. 2017. "Zahnmedizin in Deutschland von der Mitte des 18. bis zur Mitte des 20. Jahrhunderts." In *100 Jahre Westdeutsche Kieferklinik: Festschrift zum Jubiläum*, edited by A. Hugger, 9–19. Düsseldorf: Universitätsklinikum Düsseldorf.

Krischel, Matthis, Enno Schwanke, Thorsten Halling, Jens Westemeier, and Dominik Groß. 2017. "Zum Stand der Aufarbeitung der Geschichte der Zahnmedizin im Nationalsozialismus." *Deutsche Zahnärztliche Zeitschrift* 72(6): 477–80.

Lutze, Kay. 2006. "Von Liegnitz nach New York: Die Lebensgeschichte des jüdischen Zahnarztes Fedor Bruck (1895–1982)." *Zahnärztliche Mitteilungen*, no. 10, 16 May: 124–27.

Maretzky, Kurt, and Robert Venter. 1974. *Geschichte des deutschen Zahnärzte-Standes*. Köln: Bundesverband Deutschen Zahnärzte.

Möhrle, Alfred. 1996. "Der Arzt im Nationalsozialismus: Der Weg zum Nürnberger Ärzteprozeß und die Folgerungen daraus." *Deutsches Ärzteblatt* 93(43): A-2766/B-2352/C-2089.

Nyiszli, Miklós. 2011. *Auschwitz: A Doctor's Eyewitness Account*. New York: Arcade Publishing.

Riaud, Xavier. 2003. *La pratique dentaire dans les camps du IIIe Reich*. Paris: Editions L'Harmattan.

———. 2015a. *Chirurgie dentaire et nazisme*. Paris: Editions L'Harmattan.

———. 2015b. "Nazi Dental Gold: From Dead Bodies till Swiss Bank." *Vesalius* 21: 32–53.

Scholz, Vikto. 1940. *Über die Möglichkeit der Wiederverwendung des Goldes im Munde der Toten*. Breslau: Paul Schwarzer's Buchdruckerei.

Schwanke, Enno, and Dominik Groß. 2016. "Der Reichsverband Deutscher Dentisten: Gleichschaltung—Ausschaltung—Standeskonsolidierung." In *Medizinische Fachgesellschaften im Nationalsozialismus: Bestandsaufnahme und Perspektiven*, edited by Matthis Krischel, Mathias Schmidt, and Dominik Groß, 173–96. Berlin: Lit.

Schwanke, Enno, Matthis Krischel, and Dominik Groß. 2016. "Zahnärzte und Dentisten im Nationalsozialismus: Forschungsstand und aktuelle Forschungsfragen." *Medizinhistorisches Journal* 51(1): 2–39.

Staehle, H. J., and Wolfgang Uwe Eckart. 2005. "Hermann Euler als Repräsentant der zahnärztlichen Wissenschaft während der NS-Zeit." *Deutsche Zahnärztliche Zeitschrift* 60: 677–94.

Stone, Dan. 2010. *Histories of the Holocaust*. Oxford: Oxford University Press.

Stuck, Ernst. 1933. "Nationale Revolution und Reichsverband." *Zahnärztliche Mitteilungen* 12: 314–15.

Thieme, V. 2018. "Das Fach Kieferchirurgie und die 'rassenhygienische Ausmerze' der Lippen-Kiefer-Gaumenspalte." In *Zahnärzte und Zahnheilkunde im "Dritten Reich": Eine Bestandsaufnahme*, edited by D. Groß, J. Westemeier, M. Schmidt, T. Halling, and M. Krischel, 169–86. Berlin: Lit.

Wagner, G. 1933. "An den Führer des Reichsverbands Deutscher Dentisten, Herrn Schaeffer." *Deutsche Dentistische Wochenschrift* 53: 646–47.

Westemeier, Jens, Dominik Groß, and Mathias Schmidt. 2018. "Der Zahnarzt in der Waffen-SS—Organisation und Arbeitsfeld." In *Zahnärzte und Zahnheilkunde im "Dritten Reich": Eine Bestandsaufnahme*, edited by D. Groß, J. Westemeier, M. Schmidt, T. Halling, and M. Krischel, 93–112. Berlin: Lit.

"Zahnmedizin im Faschismus." 1983. *Der Artikulator*, special issue.

Zamet, John S. 2006. "Aliens or Colleagues? Refugees from Nazi Oppression." *British Dental Journal* 201: 397–407.

Ziegler, Jean. 1998. *The Swiss, the Gold, and the Dead*. Boston: Houghton Mifflin Harcourt.

CHAPTER 11

Only Following Orders?
Aviation Medicine in Nazi Germany

Alexander von Lünen

Research on perpetrators of atrocities in Nazi Germany has evolved tremendously since the 1990s. Whereas the focus had previously been on the main culprits and their immediate minions, the books by Browning and Goldhagen—among others—marked a turning point not only in historiography but also in how the public in Germany and elsewhere would regard the notion of "perpetrator."[1] Recent court trials against John Demjanjuk (2009–11) or Oskar Gröning (2015) have shifted the goalposts even further, now regarding those who were comparably remotely involved in the killing during the Holocaust punishable by law.

This is a paradigm shift in more than one way. The standard excuse for many years—in fact, Gröning used it as part of his defense[2]—by Germans after World War II when confronted with their complicity in the crimes committed was that they had been "only following orders."[3] This statement became a token excuse, particularly after the trial against Adolf Eichmann in Jerusalem in 1961 and Hannah Arendt's controversial notion that Eichmann was a mere bureaucrat who embodied the "banality of evil."[4]

Arendt's discussion of Eichmann and the nature of evil regimes has drawn a plethora of criticism and is dismissed by many scholars, such as David Cesarani.[5] This makes it all the more interesting—and tantalizing—that Stanley Milgram's experiments on obedience seem to have lost nothing of their attractiveness for scholars, as Richard Overy outlines:

> Over the past decade Milgram's influence has if anything expanded as historians look for scientific corroboration of the argument that "normal" men can perform horrific acts without necessarily imbibing a hate-filled ideology or being driven by a visceral popular racism.[6]

Tantalizing indeed, as Milgram himself makes a direct reference to Arendt's *banality of evil*, which "comes closer to the truth than one might dare imagine," in his words.[7] Apparently, it does not seem to bother Richard Overy and other historians that what they are turning to is, after all, the attempt to scientifically corroborate Arendt's thesis.

Those tried for their involvement in the Dachau research in the Nuremberg Doctor Trials would argue exactly that; that they had to obey the chain of command and were in no position to stop the experiments, as much as they might have desired it.

This chapter considers Milgram's experiments, its critics, and recent reinterpretations of the experiments to discuss the culpability of aeromedical researchers in the unethical research in the Dachau concentration camp. One of the reinterpretations of Milgram's obedience experiments is the notion of "engaged followership," a theory that postulates that participants knew what they were doing was inhumane but accepted this to support the greater good of scientific research.

The Milgram Experiments

The experiments by Milgram, briefly, created a situation in which participants—the "teachers"—were recruited from the general public to supervise what they were told were learning and memory experiments. The "teacher" would ask a series of questions to a "learner," who was tied to a chair with electrodes attached to his body. At every wrong answer the "learner" would be punished by 15-volt electric shock, which would increase by increments of 15 volts at every subsequent wrong answer, ending at 450 volts. If the "teacher" hesitated to press the button at any time, an "experimenter" would use prods to encourage and eventually order the "teacher" to carry on. Milgram, in his first article on the experiments in 1961, demonstrated that 65 percent of his participants would apply the shocks, supposedly obeying the authority of the experimenter in his white lab coat, against the increasing protests of the "learner" who was at the receiving end of the shocks. Yet both "experimenter" and "learner" were actors hired to simulate the procedure and deceive the "teachers" into carrying out inhumane experiments. This, so ran Milgram's argument, would illustrate blind obedience among average Americans and their deference of responsibility to persons higher in authority.[8]

Milgram's *Obedience to Authority* experiments—commonly abbreviated as "OTA"—continue to draw their fascination from their apparent power to explain the behavior of perpetrators in atrocities—as alluded to in the above quote by Richard Overy.[9] Given Milgram's own arguments for cases of bureaucrats like Eichmann, other aspects seem to have been almost cast to the side, as can be seen by the phrasing of Laurent Bègue et al. who refer to Milgram's OTA study as "the Eichmann experiment."[10] As various authors (see below) have pointed out, Milgram would ignore or sideline results that would not align to his desired findings of OTA.

The OTA experiments drew sharp ethical criticism as soon as they were published, first and foremost because Milgram had deceived the participants, resulting in their traumatization.[11]

It was only in the last ten years or so that the methodological critique toward the OTA experiments gained traction. Jerry Burger, for example, initially supported Milgram's findings but developed doubts over time, and he revisited Milgram's own data with colleagues, coming to the conclusion: "Most striking is the fact that when participants heard the only prod that we might reasonably consider an order, not one individual 'obeyed.'"[12]

Other scholars had previously pointed to contradictions in Milgram's narrative and the actual conditions in the experiments.[13] Attention was now being paid to the fact that Milgram had conducted a whole series of experiments, all with different settings and participant groups; but prominent depictions—such as Milgram's film or his 1974 book—focused on a very few select experiments or, in the case of film, constrained themselves to one experiment and one participant. This led to debates over whether Milgram might have very selectively published his findings to further a certain narrative.[14]

Engaged Followership

Richard Griggs, for example, draws the conclusion from the above critiques that "obedience" was "motivated not by orders but appeals to science and that their behavior needs to be reconceptualized as an act of 'engaged followership.'"[15] This interpretation is further supported by the fact that Yale University, as the site of the experiments, played a role on participants' perception of the credibility of the experiments. Participants considered science a social good, and therefore their participation in experiments at one of the most prestigious scientific institutions made them proud—something further corroborated by Gina Perry in the interviews she did with former participants in the Milgram experiments.[16] Indeed, Milgram had pointed out to the participants that the experiments would help—among other things—in air traffic security and therefore would be to the immediate benefit to humanity.[17]

As this alternative analysis of Milgram's OTA experiments suggests, participants identified both with the experimenter and his goals. Apparently it was due to the pressure Milgram felt later—after the ethical criticism was leveled against him—that he focused on the OTA thesis in order to deflect the criticism by presenting more controversial findings.

The experiments of Milgram can thus be summarized as participants not blindly following orders but having a rather rational motive to bypass their ethical qualms and applying the shocks because they were convinced they served a greater purpose. Applied to the situation of the Holocaust in general, Brannigan and Perry point out that German officers carried out orders or served a system that they might not have aligned to morally, but they repressed these considerations in light of the feeling that it would be in the best interest of the German nation to carry them out.[18]

This, obviously, is an argument that Ian Kershaw had made earlier, one that represents the shift in Nazi historiography in the 1990s: a shift from the sociological models that explain the Holocaust and other atrocities, committed through a bureaucratic system that took individual agency away from perpetrators, to explanatory theories that highlight the choices that individuals had.[19]

The Dachau Experiments

In 1941, a young doctor named Sigmund Rascher (1909–45) proposed to the leader of the SS Heinrich Himmler an idea to conduct experiments on concentration camp inmates to investigate the effects of rapid decompression encountered in high-altitude flying.[20] Sigmund Rascher had no scientific credits and would certainly have remained an obscure figure, but he got engaged—and eventually married—to Karoline "Nini" Diehl, who was an acquaintance of Himmler.[21] This relationship paved the way for Rascher to pursue a scientific career, and Himmler took a personal interest in Rascher's research.

Medical experiments related to the human body at high altitude had been carried out in several countries since the late 1880s in mountaineering, ballooning, and then with aeroplanes, and always on animals or human volunteers. Rascher now claimed that the final details could only be revealed in experiments on humans. Because the participants might die, he suggested the use of "career criminals" incarcerated in concentration camps, who could be pardoned if they survived the experiments.[22] After the Battle of Britain had been lost by the Luftwaffe, its commander in chief Hermann Göring became increasingly obsessed with the idea of bombers and fighter planes attacking the Allies from superior height.[23] A proposal to study the physiology of stratospheric flying thus seemed attractive. While in previous experiments human volunteers had died accidentally, it was now Rascher's intention to deliberately kill experimentees to observe the final stages of high-altitude sickness.[24]

Much has been written on these experiments and about Rascher as their instigator.[25] He conducted the decompression experiments from May to August 1942, as well as the subsequent hypothermia experiments from August 1942 to May 1943; this was under the auspices of the general surgeon of the Luftwaffe Erich Hippke (1888–1969) and in cooperation with the SS-Ahnenerbe,[26] as Rascher had been drafted into the air force in 1939 despite his membership in the general

SS. The hypothermia experiments in particular have become the epitome of inhumane Nazi science and medicine for their cruelty. In the hypothermia experiments, inmates of Dachau concentration camp were forced to simulate the conditions of Luftwaffe pilots shot down over the North Sea, often having to endure exposure to cold water for hours before being rescued. The experiments thus tried to determine how long a pilot could be exposed to the cold before resuscitation was no longer possible, and what methods of resuscitation were the most effective. For this, inmates were put into basins with ice water or were forced to stand naked outside in freezing winter weather in order to gauge the stages of hypothermia—by monitoring their vital signs with ECG and thermometers— and to try different methods of revitalization. Around eighty to ninety inmates were killed in these experiments, many of them deliberately so, to study the final stages of hypothermia.[27]

Individual Culpability: The Doctors Trial

It is safe to say that the Nazi regime was an *enabler* of the human experiments by removing established legal, ethical, and institutional barriers to use "human material" in medical research. At the Doctors Trial in Nuremberg from October 1946 to August 1947, three of the defendants were tried specifically in regard to the decompression and hypothermia experiments: Siegfried Ruff (1907–89), director of the Institute for Aviation Medicine at the Deutsche Versuchsanstalt für Luftfahrt (DVL, German Experimental Flying Institute), and his assistant Hans-Wolfgang Romberg (1911–81). Also on trial in connection with Rascher's experiments was Georg Weltz (1889–1963), who joined the University of Munich in 1935 as lecturer in aviation medicine and set up an institute for aviation medicine there the following year. Sigmund Rascher had been transferred to Weltz's institute in April 1942. Rascher himself could not be tried, as he was shot by the SS in April 1945 at Dachau for fraud and child abduction; his wife Nini was executed in Ravensbrück for the same crime.[28]

All the defendants in Nuremberg accused of complicity in the Dachau aviation experiments would use a similar defense strategy: obedience to higher authority as excuse, and portraying Rascher as a psychopath with patronage from Himmler. This argumentation would very much align itself with the insights from Milgram's experiments. Yet, it has to be asked to what extent this notion of "obedience" was created during the Nuremberg trials by the defense lawyers. Several publications have pointed out that the lawyers across the Nuremberg trials had good communication networks and orchestrated their defense strategy.[29] The template was therefore quite similar for all defendants.

Ruff became involved with the Dachau decompression experiments because his institute at the DVL had a mobile decompression chamber that was used for high-altitude tests on pilot candidates. The mobile chamber had been developed to tour Luftwaffe airfields for screenings to avoid having candidates traveling across the country to the closest stationary chamber. During the war, the mobile chamber was also sent to field hospitals to be used in medical therapy.[30]

Ruff claimed that he was not aware of the murderous intentions of Rascher, i.e. that the latter had planned to willfully kill participants—yet, having the chamber transferred to Dachau concentration camp didn't seem to bother him. Furthermore, Ruff claimed, once Romberg—who was sent to Dachau as operator of the chamber—reported back to him what Rascher was up to, he recalled the chamber to Berlin at the earliest possible date, pointing out that he had to tread carefully in order to avoid upsetting Himmler.[31]

The only witnesses against Ruff were Walter Neff, a "Kapo" who was himself under investigation for his role at Dachau,[32] and the former inmate August Vieweg who was imprisoned at Dachau for being what the Nazis considered a "career criminal" (Berufsverbrecher). This led Ruff's attorney, Fritz Sauter, to say during the final plea at the Doctors Trial, "If anybody deserved to be sent to the concentration camp, it was this Vieweg."[33] All other witnesses were former Luftwaffe doctors who exonerated Ruff. The pattern was similar for the other defendants. It must therefore be noted that the myth of "only following orders" was first and foremost instigated by special interest groups as defense strategy and was communicated as such widely.

Romberg, as mentioned, was initialy sent with the decompression chamber to Dachau to operate it; however, he also used some of the results of the experiments for his own research on hypoxia, and requested data from Rascher after the experiments had ended.[34] Rascher, in turn, urged Romberg to publish their results of the decompression experiments jointly.[35] He also proposed Romberg for the *Kriegsverdienstkreuz* (War Merit Cross), the highest civilian award at the time, which Romberg received in September 1942.[36]

In the Doctors Trial, on the other hand, Romberg was adamant that he had no choice in the matter but to participate. Rascher had been an officer in the Luftwaffe, so Romberg argued, and he himself had only been a civilian employee in the service of an institute that was subordinated to the general surgeon of the Luftwaffe. However, Romberg also stressed that he did not endorse the lethal experiments. This assertion prompted the question of why Romberg did not interfere when he saw Rascher go beyond the tolerable threshold during the experiments on the prisoners. Romberg pointed to Rascher's higher rank, also refusing—upon further questioning—to call the experiments "murder," since they had been authorized by officers higher up in the chain of command.[37]

Georg Weltz, as mentioned, was Rascher's superior. Following Rascher's own account, however, the relationship was not harmonious. Rascher tried to stay independent and used his access to Himmler to maintain this independence from Weltz, a situation certainly to be considered untenable to the latter. The extent to which Weltz was thus informed of Rascher's experiments—let alone endorsed them—is up for speculation.[38] But given Rascher's and Weltz's disagreements, it was easy for the latter to get an aquittal from the court in Nuremberg.

Another interesting link was the initial involvement of Heinrich Kottenhoff, who had been Weltz's assistant from 1936 to 1939, as medical officer in the Luftwaffe.[39] Kottenhoff, however, remained in touch with Weltz and conducted joint experiments at the latter's institute after 1939. Kottenhoff was part of the original team with Weltz and Rascher in 1942; however, he was transferred to a military hospital in Romania before the experiments started.[40] On the other hand, Kottenhoff published a paper on aviation medicine in 1943 together with Marianne Stanislaus-Rühl, a zoologist who was assistant (since 1 August 1942) to Eduard May at the Institute for Entomology of the Ahnenerbe in Dachau.[41] A footnote in the publication indicates that the research was conducted at Weltz's institute at the University of Munich. While it is not quite clear to what degree Weltz was involved—the article does not indicate unethical research—his contact to the Ahnenerbe in Dachau may have been closer than he later admitted.

Networks

The hypothermia experiments were officially led by Ernst Holzlöhner (1899–1945) and assisted by Erich Finke (1905–45), both from the University of Kiel. Holzlöhner, however, committed suicide in June 1945, and Finke died in a field hospital in May 1945, and therefore neither could be tried. Gerhard Rose (also defendant at the Doctors Trial) and Georg Weltz testified that Holzlöhner was a decent person and only followed orders, suggesting that he might have committed suicide out of shame about his participation.

Generally speaking, the aeromedical community in Nazi Germany was closely knit. This was not least due to the specialized nature of the subject, its relatively low academic status as an "applied science" in the eyes of many academics, and that many of its protagonists knew each other from sports flying. This would also contribute to a closed network of researchers who would define their own habitus along both academic and aviator pedigrees.[42]

The war changed this. Now research for the Luftwaffe became increasingly important and attractive—not least as an argument for the researcher to be spared from frontline duty. While funding grew due to the war effort, those already established in aviation medicine were quite keen to guard their turf.[43] It is mainly because of this that Rascher's proposal was met with skepticism. Also, his academic performance so far, as pointed out above, was meager at best. Rascher needed a mentor for his habilitation thesis. His hypothermia experiments were specifically set up to produce results that no other researcher had ever achieved—not least because no one was willing to go as far as to purposely freeze someone to death to monitor the bodily functions. The first person considered as habilitation supervisor was Wilhelm Pfannenstiel (1890–1982), professor at the University of Marburg and well known for his role in the SS as advisor for hygiene. Also, Pfannenstiel lectured on aviation medicine at the university.[44] However, the habilitation did not come to pass in Marburg, apparently because the faculty did not agree to have it classified as "top secret," which is what Rascher and the SS wanted.[45] After the war, Pfannenstiel denied any agreement and claimed that he had never opened the envelope with Rascher's thesis draft.[46] Pfannenstiel furthermore maintained that he had little direct contact with Rascher and had not been particularly interested in supervising his thesis.[47] Later, in 1944, August Hirt from the University of Strasbourg was approached as supervisor. However, Hirt was not too interested, as there were serious doubts regarding Rascher's scientific qualification within the medical faculty.[48]

Rascher also won over Heinz von Diringshofen (1900–1967) as cosupervisor for the habilitation. Diringshofen had been medical officer in the armed forces since 1927; furthermore, he was associate professor at the University of Frankfurt and head of the Medical Research Laboratory of the German Air Force (Sanitätsversuchsstelle der Luftwaffe) at Jüterbog 1935–41, where Holzlöhner had been commanded to in 1942.[49] Diringshofen visited Rascher in Dachau on 18 July 1943, where the hypothermia experiments were demonstrated to him. According to Rascher, Diringshofen was keen to get involved in the research.[50] Equally interesting is the fact that Diringshofen was trained in aviation medicine by Hubertus Strughold from 1930 to 1932 at the University of Würzburg, when the latter was a lecturer in aviation physiology there. Strughold praised Diringshofen as "the medical adviser of the future air force" in a letter from 1931.[51]

Hans-Dietrich Craemer, head of research at the medical academy of the German mountain troops in Tyrol, on the other hand, corresponded with Rascher several times about a possible cooperation in hypothermia research after hearing him at the conference in 1942.[52] Craemer held seminars on hypothermia and high altitude at his institute quite regularly, where Luftwaffe researchers, such as Strughold, would present papers.[53]

It also seems that dissected brains from the victims of the decompression experiments made their way to the Kaiser-Wilhelm-Institute (KWI) for Brain Research in Berlin for further investigation (the institute became the branch for brain research of Strughold's institute in 1942). At least Rascher asked Romberg in January 1944 what had happened to the material sent to the institute.[54]

Furthermore, František Bláha, a Czechoslovakian doctor who was incarcerated at Dachau since 1941, stated that Rascher sent organs to the institute of pathology at the University of Munich for examination: "A number of visitors attended to these autopsies, members of the so-called scientific world, from Munich,

Berlin, Vienna, Bonn, Heidelberg and Cologne." Unfortunately, Bláha doesn't specify any names of these "visitors."[55] However, this sounds plausible, given that Maximilian Borst (1869–1946), professor of pathology and director of the institute of pathology at the University of Munich, provided Rascher with lab space in 1939 when the latter was doing his cancer research. Borst, a friend of Rascher's doctoral supervisor Joseph Trumpp, was also consultant for pathology for the Luftwaffe Munich district surgeon from 1939 to 1945.[56] The autopsies were conducted by Ludwig Singer (1896–1973), adjunct professor of pathology at Borst's institute and head of the department for pathology at the municipal hospital Munich-Schwabing, where Rascher had worked from 1936 to 1939. Singer claimed in November 1946 that he wasn't told that the bodies given to him for autopsy were from unethical experiments.[57]

After the war, several scientists claimed to have protested against Rascher's research when he presented at a conference in October 1942. As Rascher was not officially the lead on the hypothermia experiments, Holzlöhner presented some of his own research on hypothermia, and Rascher then added information about his work at the end of Holzlöhner's presentation.[58] Franz Büchner (1895–1991), professor of pathology at the University of Freiburg, also director of the Institute of Aviation Pathology there since 1940 and consultant for pathology to the general surgeon of the German air force, gave a public lecture against the "euthanasia" killing program on 18 November 1941.[59] This did not deter him from continuing his work for the Luftwaffe—and thus aiding in prolonging the war and consequently the "euthanasia" killings. He was also not too troubled about one of his habilitation students using the kidneys of executed deserters for his research.[60] Büchner claimed to have protested behind the scenes at the conference in October 1942, when Holzlöhner and Rascher presented their lethal hypothermia experiments.[61] There is little evidence to suggest that this actually happened, and it is somewhat strange that Büchner did not mention that he was on a panel together with Holzlöhner at a meeting of Wehrmacht doctors in December 1942, where the latter talked again about the resuscitation of persons who had spent time in cold water.[62] From the short synopsis of Holzlöhner's paper in the proceedings of the meeting, it seems rather obvious that he was talking about freezing humans to death to observe the development of hypothermia until the point of no return.[63] Büchner did not even mention this encounter, let alone claim that he had protested there or tried to cancel his participation in the meeting. Büchner also maintained that Hermann Rein and Strughold protested at the Nuremberg conference in 1942, but again, there is nothing on record that would confirm this.

Hermann Becker-Freyseng—research coordinator for aviation medicine in the Air Ministry—testified at the Doctors Trial that no one protested at the conference in 1942 at all.[64] Weltz claimed at the Doctors Trial that most people did not even notice Rascher's presentation, as they were too tired and overfed with information at the conference; others, however, had told him that they did not approve of Rascher's experiments, without complaining openly. He suggested that the only disagreement with Rascher's presentation was due to the latter's poor style and phrasing.[65]

Alternative Explanations: Layers of Perpetration

Consequently, as Weltz testified at the Doctor Trials, Rascher was regarded as an outsider. His presentation style was seen as unscholarly, the Ahnenerbe as a competitor, and his research as incompatible with established academic frameworks. This on the other hand, made him an attractive source of information. University researchers who would not ever have thought of doing these kinds of experiments at their own institutions saw the concentration camps as the scientific *heterotopia* where these things became possible.[66] It is thus no surprise that there was little—if any—protest or that a number of researchers would try to get data from Rascher.

In the past fifteen years or so, the dominant view on perpetrators developed that they were "ordinary people," either bigoted or compliant, and bureaucrats or careerists.[67] As commendable as this more nuanced view is, it seems to fall short of offering a view on those who were accessories to the murders, such as Ruff or Romberg. Neither of them committed murder—if we believe them that they did not know the experiments were going to be lethal—yet they enabled Rascher in conducting murderous experiments. What seems to be missing from research on perpetrators is a concept similar to what Kershaw has outlined for resistance in Nazi Germany: overlapping categories that are not mutually exclusive.[68]

Similarly, the accomplices in medical atrocities—and others—might have had overlapping interests with the "research" conducted on concentration camp inmates, in the sense of *engaged followership* outlined above. Neither Ruff, Romberg, nor Weltz resisted their participation in Rascher's experiments—not because they were "only following orders," not because of obedience to authority, but because they had some overlapping interest: scientific research and the war effort. Similarly, Franz Büchner protested publicly against the "euthanasia" murders, because this was an issue he cared about as a devout catholic; this did not translate into opposition to other areas of the regime.

Overall, however, there is little evidence of unethical research directly conducted by other scientists in aviation medicine.Some of them were card-carrying Nazis, but this usually was not reflected in their research.[69] The aeromedical scientists, while colluding with the regime in terms of support for the war effort, did not of their own volition initiate human experiments.

Conclusions

The experiments by Stanley Milgram in the 1960s have—inadvertently—provided corroboration to better understand participants in unethical research. The tragedy, as far as Milgram is concerned, is that he became the very thing he tried to research. His mission was to understand how humans can be made to engage in unethical behavior—in unethical experiments. His "the end justifies the means" defense is the very concept of "engaged followership" that the participants in his experiments have displayed.

The "engaged followship" paradigm does not claim that all scientists who participated in unethical research were "engaged" in the sense that they aligned themselves with all aspects of the Nazi regime, but that a partial overlap led them to engage in unethical research as long as the scientists felt that this served some greater purpose—if only to further their own careers. Even researchers who had no pronounced affection for the Nazis, such as Büchner, would support the war, and some found certain elements of the Nazi regime, e.g. authoritarianism, appealing.

While the war removed ethical barriers in scientific research, it did not remove the traditional hierarchies and "class" conceit in academia.[70] The Ahnenerbe and other nonacademic agencies were seen as turf invaders, and persons such as Rascher as usurpers who had no qualification—and thus no right—to be in academia. This tension is relevant when looking at the Dachau experiments. Carried out on behalf of the Luftwaffe on SS premises, they posed a major conflict within the polycratic nature of the Nazi regime. The SS with its Ahnenerbe encroached on many areas that were previously the monopoly of universities. As Kater points out, very few researchers of the Ahnenerbe managed to receive a habilitation, and none of them ever attained the rank of full professor (only a few managed to become nontenured associated professors)—unless they were already established professors by the time they joined the Ahnenerbe, like August Hirt was.[71] The rivalry between the Ahnenerbe and universities became thus quite stark.

Finding out how deep the involvement of other researchers in the Dachau experiment was proves to be difficult, not least because they covered for each other. However, there are ample clues that their rejection of the medical experiments was not as adamant as they portrayed it after the war.

Alexander von Lünen is senior lecturer in modern German history (with digital humanities) at the University of Huddersfield (UK). He has a doctorate in history of science and technology in 2008 from the Technische Universität Darmstadt, Germany, on aviator equipment in the interwar years in Europe. He is currently working on a monograph on aviation medicine in (Nazi) Germany and has created a bio-bibliographical database of all who published about aviation medicine in German journals during the Nazi era, as well as all who worked in that field: http://www.gaeromeddb.net (work-in-progress).

Notes

1. Browning 2001 [1992]; Goldhagen 1996. See Lawson 2013 for a good overview and discussion of the historiography of perpetrator research, and Hilberg 1995 for a more in-depth discussion.

2. Cf. "Auschwitz Guard Trial: Oskar Groening Admits Moral Guilt," BBC News, 21 April 2015, retrieved 24 September 2018 from https://www.bbc.co.uk/news/world-europe-32392594.

3. When the Allies discussed the statute for the International Military Tribunal in July 1945 in London, "superior orders" was explicitly prohibited as a defense argument, but some discretion was left to the judges to use it as mitigating circumstances. The subsequent Nuremberg trials—of which the Doctors Trial was the first—were held under Law No. 10 from 20 December 1945 by the Control Council of the four Occupying Powers. In this law the wording would allow more room to use "superior orders" as mitigating factor in the punishment. However, as Yoram Dinstein outlines, German defense lawyers ignored the prohibition in all these trials and tried to establish this narrative of "only following orders" as defense regardless. Dinstein 2012, 83ff., 114ff.

4. Cf. Arendt 2006 [1963].
5. Cesarani 2004.
6. Overy 2014, 520.
7. Milgram 1974, 6.
8. Blass 2004.
9. Overy 2014.
10. Bègue et al. 2015, 299.

11. As a matter of fact, the whole experiment was specifically designed to upset the participants, and Milgram had criticized other experiments for not putting their participants in moral dilemmas; Lunt 2009, 43–44. See Perry 2013, for the most comprehensive analysis of Milgram's experiments and the effects on participants.

12. Burger 2009; Burger et al. 2011, 464. Matthew Hollander, in a conversation analysis of the transcripts of the Milgram experiments, similarly found expressions of dissent without disobedience; i.e., participants obeyed the prod but clearly expressed that they did not approve of the experiment (Hollander 2015).

13. E.g. Packer 2008, 301–4.
14. Haslam et al. 2014, 8.
15. Griggs 2017, 34.
16. Perry 2013.
17. Russel 2011, 143. See also Haslam et al. 2015, 76–77.
18. Brannigan and Perry 2016, 299.
19. Kershaw 1993. See also Lawson 2013, 193.
20. Cf. Weindling 2004, chap. 6: "Aviation Atrocities."
21. Cf. Benz 1990.

22. Affadavit by Ruff at the Doctors Trial (NO-437). Transcripts of the trial can be found at http://nuremberg.law.harvard.edu (retrieved 1 December 2018). All statements from the Doctors Trial are taken from this source, unless otherwise noted.

23. Cf. Lünen, 2010.

24. According to Karl-Heinz Roth, decompression experiments were conducted on around two hundred inmates, of whom seventy were killed (Roth 2000, 49).

25. A good number of publications, such as Roth 2000, discuss the question how involved Hubertus Strughold (1898–1986) was in the Dachau experiments. Strughold was director of the Aeromedical Research Institute of the Air Ministry (Luftfahrtmedizinisches Forschungsinstitut des Reichsluftfahrtministeriums) from 1935 to 1945, subordinated to the general surgeon of the Luftwaffe.

26. The "Ahnenerbe" was founded in 1935 as a (legally) private scientific society with Heinrich Himmler as its "superintendent" and funded through the SS, although considerable funds also came from the DFG and German industry; it was incorporated into the SS in 1939. Its agenda was to research the prehistory of the "Aryan race" by conducting anthropologic, historic, and archaeological studies. Its managing director was Wolfram Sievers (1905–48), who also installed the Institut für wehrwissenschaftliche Zweckforschung (Institute for Military Scientific Research) of the Ahnenerbe at Dachau Concentration Camp in July 1942. This institute was set up to conduct medical experiments considered important for the war effort. It was the intention of Himmler and others to promote the Ahnenerbe to the status of a university or national academy. Cf. Kater 1997.

27. Roth 2000, 49.

28. Sigmund Rascher tried to make money off his work by industrially producing a hemostat that a Dachau inmate had invented. Initially this was accepted by the SS, but several irregularities in the finances of the enterprise led to him being arrested. His wife Nini had abducted children and pretended that they were hers; she was found out in 1944 but claimed Sigmund knew nothing of this. The Raschers were also investigated for the death of their housemaid, as they would have been the benefactors of her life insurance. See Benz 1990 for more details.

29. E.g. Seliger 2016.

30. Cf. Ruff and Strughold 1942, 1944.

31. Ruff's testimony on 28 April 1947.

32. "Kapo" (singl.) was a slang term used by the Germans for prisoner functionaries (Funktionshäftling, the official term). These were camp inmates put in charge as auxiliary guards to assist the SS in "keeping order" in the camps, turning inmate against inmate while minimizing SS staffing. Kapos had privileges and were known for their brutality in order to please their SS overseers; they were often recruited from criminals incarcerated in concentration camps, for it was believed that they had a lower threshold for brutality. Walter Neff was a political prisoner in Dachau. Cf. Zámečnik 2013.

33. Plea and Closing Brief for Ruff by Fritz Sauter at the Doctors Trial.

34. BArchB, NS 21/923.

35. On 3 January 1944, for example, Rascher wrote to Romberg about such joint publication, and mentions that he was still working in Dachau, "but not as blood-thirsty as I used to" (BArchB, NS 21/923, f120).

36. In a thank-you letter to Sievers from 2 October 1942, Romberg wrote, "I am convinced that the good cooperation [between Rascher and Romberg] will be an asset when continuing the experiments. . . ." BArchB, NS 21/914.

37. Testimony by Romberg on 1 May 1947. What worked in Romberg's favor in the Doctors Trial was Rascher's letter from April 1942 to Ahnenerbe boss Sievers, in which he claims that he conducted "extreme experiments" while Romberg was absent. BArchB, NS 21/922.

38. Leo Alexander, who had done the bulk of the investigations on the medical crimes committed by Luftwaffe doctors, remained convinced that Weltz supported Rascher to get permission to do the experiments. Wiener Library.

39. UA Munich: Habilitation Kottenhoff.

40. As Rudolf Brandt would testify for the Doctors Trial (NO 191). Weltz in his testimony from 6 May 1947 at the Doctors Trial mentions this too.

41. BArchB, NS 21/2177.

42. Katharina Trittel discusses this aspect in regard to Hermann Rein, one of the most prominent physiologists and aeromedical researchers in Germany (Trittel 2018).

43. Lünen 2009, 96–108.

44. UA Marburg, PA Pfannenstiel.
45. As Pfannenstiel wrote to Rascher on 2 December 1943; in this letter, he also mentions that he wants Rascher to do research in Dachau for him. BArchB, NS 21/918.
46. UA Marburg, PA Pfannenstiel.
47. IfZ, ZS-1952/2.
48. Letter from Hirt to Sievers, 27 March 1944; BArchB, NS 21/918.
49. UA Frankfurt, PA Diringshofen.
50. BArchB, NS 21/917.
51. Bayr. HStA, MK 35751.
52. BArchB, NS 21/922.
53. E.g. on 23/24 September 1943; BA-MA, RH 12-23/1893.
54. BArchB, NS 21/923. See also Schmuhl 2009, 108.
55. Archives Unbound.
56. Bayr. HStA, MK 43446.
57. Bayr. HStA, MK 44354. Nini Rascher wrote to Sievers on 16 June 1942 saying that Singer had been "not very nice" in a telephone call to Sigmund, and that Singer had insisted to involve Franz Büchner—on whom Nini commented as being "very very reactionary" ("stockstockschwarz"), and therefore his involvement would be out of the question. BArchB, NS 21/913.
58. BA-MA, RLD 15/90.
59. Leven 2002, 384–85.
60. UA Freiburg, PA Liebegott. Büchner, in his autobiography (1965, 72ff.), claimed that only Hippke's patronage protected him from prosecution. There had been investigations by the local Nazi Party office against Büchner, and his status as eminent scientist and his service for the Luftwaffe had indeed protected him from punishment (Leven 2000).
61. Büchner 1965, 72ff.
62. Franz Büchner filed for an injuction against Alexander Mitscherlich at the district court in Freiburg on 24 April 1947 to ban the publication of Mitscherlich's report on the Doctors Trial. Mitscherlich had stated that Büchner had not protested at the Nuremberg conference, and that he had also participated in unethical human experiments with Eugen Haagen in the context of research on hepatitis. The injunction was granted on 26 April 1947, but Mitscherlich was confident that the injunction would not be respected by the authorities in the American zone of occupation in Heidelberg, where he was living. It was Büchner then who sought a settlement, granted by the court on 3 June 1947, which stipulated that Büchner would no longer seek banning Mitscherlich's book, provided the latter would include a clarification that Büchner had nothing to do with Haagen's human experiments and that he had protested at the Nuremberg conference, albeit behind the scenes and not publicly. Mitscherlich and other intellectuals, such as Karl Jaspers, whom Mitscherlich had asked to comment, had their doubts about the last point, but were happy that the book could now be published and some light on medical crimes in Nazi Germany shed. When filing for the injunction, Büchner used an affadavit from Weltz to make his case, which stated that Büchner had told Weltz that he had protested (i.e., Weltz did not witness the protest himself). The evidence to support Büchner's position is thus somewhat inconclusive. The controversy and legal proceedings between Büchner and Mitscherlich is discussed in Peter 2013, 200ff.
63. BA-MA, RH 12-23/4552.
64. Testimony by Becker-Freyseng, 21 May 1947.
65. Testimony by Weltz, 7 May 1947.
66. Michel Foucault coined the term "heterotopia" to describe spaces of "otherness," spaces where the rules of normal life do not apply (Foucault 1994, 175–85). See also Roelke 2014, 66.
67. Cf. Mann 2000, 332–33.
68. As Ian Kershaw discussed, one can be a resister without being a full-scale opponent of the Nazi regime (Kershaw 2000, 183ff.). The members of the Stauffenberg group, for example, resisted

the regime by attempting to assassinate Hitler; but most of the members had much common ground with the Nazis, such as the war against the Soviet Union or an authoritarian form of government.

69. Pretty much all medical researchers at German universities were members of the Nazi Party or one (or more) of its subsidiaries, such as SA, SS, NSV, NSFK, etc. The aeromedical researchers were no exception to this. But I could find only a few examples where a genuine, wholehearted belief in the Nazi ideology was visible in their correspondence. The majority were German nationalists, however, and therefore shared some ideas with the Nazis. The research by aviation physiologists was usually carried out on themselves and volunteers (e.g. Luftwaffe soldiers); information was also gathered from the autopsies of pilots killed in accidents. By command of the general surgeon of the Luftwaffe, autopsies were carried out in order to gain an understanding of possible causes of accidents, even against the express wishes of the family of the deceased (BA-MA RL 6/178). Aviation medicine had a legacy of self-experimentation since its nestor Paul Bert started research in the 1870s. The French physiologist Bert, a former student of Claude Bernard, was asked in 1874 to help balloonists Sivel, Croce-Spinelli, and Tissandier beat the height record of British balloonists Coxwell and Glaisher by researching the supplemental oxygen required at high altitude. Due to some miscommunication, Sivel and Croce-Spinelli died from hypoxia (lack of oxygen) during the balloon ascent, and Tissandier was severly injured. Bert, although not at fault, took this very seriously, and committed himself to developing a general methodology of researching the organism at unusual ambient pressures, leading to his milestone publication *La Pression Barometrique* in 1878, which became the standard reference for both diving and aviation medicine for decades to come. In it, Bert advocated extensive research in controlled, indoor pressure chambers, carried out on animals and the researchers themselves to avoid ethical issues (cf. Lünen 2010, 34ff.). From this point of view, it could be argued that German aeromedical researchers indeed had reservations against human experiments, not necessarily because of ethical qualms but rather because these were seen as unscientific, given Bert's framework.

70. Cf. Herf 1984.
71. Kater 1997, 287.

References

Archival Sources

Bundesarchiv Berlin (BArchB; Federal Archives of Germany, Berlin branch)
    NS 21/913, NS 21/914, NS 21/917, NS 21/922, NS 21/923: Misc. Correspondence by and to Sigmund and Nini Rascher.
    NS 21/2177: Personnel file Ahnenerbe for Marianne Stanislaus-Rühl.
Bundesarchiv-Militärarchiv (BA-MA; Federal Archives of Germany, Military history branch in Freiburg im Breisgau)
    RLD 6/178: "Stellungnahme des Generalsanitätsinspekteurs zur Leichenöffnung nach Flugunfällen, 01.08.1941" [Statement from the General Surgeon of the Luftwaffe regarding autopsies after aviation accidents].
    RLD 15/90: Report of the conference: "Bericht über eine wissenschaftliche Besprechung am 26. und 27. Oktober 1942 in Nürnberg über Ärztliche Fragen bei Seenot und Winternot," published in 1943.
    RH 12-23/1893: "2. Gebirgsphysiologische Tagung" [2nd meeting on mountaineering physiology] in St. Johann, Tyrol, 23/24 September 1943 [Program, Manuscripts, List of participants].
    RH 12-23/4552: "Bericht über die 2. Arbeitstagung Ost der Beratenden Fachärzte in der Militärärztlichen Akademie in Berlin" [Report of the meeting of consultant doctors to the Academy of Military Medicine in Berlin, 30 Nov–03 Dec 1942].

Bayrisches Hauptstaatsarchiv (Bayr. HStA; Bavarian Main State Archive)
[MK files: Files of the Bavarian Ministry for Education]
MK 43446: PA [Personnel record] Maximilian Borst.
MK 44354: PA LudwigSinger.
MK 35751: PA Hubertus Strughold.
Misc. University Archives (UA)
UA Freiburg, B24/2104: PA Gerhard Liebegott.
UA Frankfurt, Abt 4, nr 388a+b, teil 1: PA Heinz von Diringshofen.
UA Marburg, Bestand 305a, Nr. 4377 & Bestand 307c, Nr. 5136: PA Pfannenstiel.
UA Munich, Sen-II-457: Files on the habilitation of Heinrich Kottenhoff.
Misc. Archives
Archives Unbound: Dachau And Subsidiary Camps: Case No. 000–50–2–103 (V): U.S. vs. Rudolf Brachtel et al., n.d. MS Holocaust and the Concentration Camp Trials: Prosecution of Nazi War Crimes: RG 153, Records of the Office of the JAG (Army), War Crimes Branch, Entry 149, Concentration Camp Trials. National Archives (United States). Archives Unbound, http://tinyurl.galegroup.com/tinyurl/4dfVZ1, accessed 03 April 2017.
Harvard University Law School Library. Transcripts of the doctors trial; retrieved 1 December 2018 from http://nuremberg.law.harvard.edu/nmt_1_intro#.
IfZ: Institut für Zeitgeschichte [Institute for Contemporary History], Munich; ZS-1952/2: Various post-war statements by Wilhelm Pfannenstiel.
Wiener Library, Document Collections, Ref 1943, Acc. No. 2014/29, f. 1943/1/7: Letter by Leo Alexander from 16 April 1959.

Books and Articles

Arendt, Hannah. 2006. *Eichmann in Jerusalem: A Report on the Banality of Evil*. London: Penguin Classics. First published in 1963.
Büchner, Franz. 1965. *Pläne und Fügungen: Lebenserinnerungen eines deutschen Hochschullehrers*. München and Berlin: Urban & Schwarzenberg.
Benz, Wolfgang. 1990. "Sigmund Rascher, M. D.: A Career." In *Dachau Review*, edited by Wolfgang Benz and Barbara Distel, 2:22–45. Dachau: Dachauer Hefte.
Bègue, Laurent, J.-L. Beauvois, Didier Courbet, D. Oberlé, J. Lepage, and Aaren A. Duke. 2015. "Personality Predicts Obedience in a Milgram Paradigm: Personality and Obedience." *Journal of Personality* 83(3): 299–306.
Blass, Thomas. 2004. *The Man Who Shocked the World: The Life and Legacy of Stanley Milgram*. New York: Basic Books.
Brannigan, Augustine, and Gina Perry. 2016. "Milgram, Genocide and Bureaucracy: A Post-Weberian Perspective." *State Crime Journal* 5(2): 287.
Browning, Christopher. 2001. *Ordinary Men: Reserve Battalion 101 and the Final Solution in Poland*. London: Penguin. First published in 1992 by HarperCollins.
Burger, Jerry M. 2009. "Replicating Milgram: Would People Still Obey Today?" *American Psychologist* 64(1): 1–11.
Burger, Jerry M., Zachary M. Girgis, and Caroline C. Manning. 2011. "In Their Own Words: Explaining Obedience to Authority through an Examination of Participants' Comments." *Social Psychological and Personality Science* 2(5): 460–66.
Cesarani, David. 2004. *Eichmann: His Life and Crimes*. London: Heinemann.
Dinstein, Yoram. 2012. *The Defence of "Obedience to Superior Orders" in International Law*. Oxford: Oxford University Press.
Foucault, Michel. 1994. "Different Spaces." In *Aesthetics, Method, and Epistemology*, edited by J. Faubion, 2:175–85. London: Penguin.

Goldhagen, Daniel. J. 1996. *Hitler's Willing Executioners: Ordinary Germans and the Holocaust.* London: Little, Brown and Co.
Griggs, Richard A. 2017. "Milgram's Obedience Study: A Contentious Classic Reinterpreted." *Teaching of Psychology* 44(1): 32.
Haslam, S. Alexander, Stephen D. Reicher, and Megan E. Birney. 2014. "Nothing by Mere Authority: Evidence That in an Experimental Analogue of the Milgram Paradigm Participants Are Motivated Not by Orders but by Appeals to Science." *Journal of Social Issues* 70(3): 473–88.
Haslam, S. Alexander, Stephen D. Reicher, Kathryn Millard, and Rachel McDonald. 2015. "'Happy to Have Been of Service': The Yale Archive as a Window into the Engaged Followership of Participants in Milgram's 'Obedience' Experiments." *British Journal of Social Psychology* 54(1): 55–83.
Herf, Jeffrey. 1984. *Reactionary Modernism: Technology, Culture, and Politics in Weimar and the Third Reich.* Cambridge: Cambridge University Press.
Hilberg, Raoul. 1995. *Perpetrators, Victims, Bystanders: The Jewish Catastrophe 1933–1945.* London: Secker & Warburg.
Hollander, Matthew M. 2015. "The Repertoire of Resistance: Non–compliance with Directives in Milgram's 'Obedience' Experiments." *British Journal of Social Psychology* 54(3): 425–44.
Kater, Michael H. 1997. *Das "Ahnenerbe" der SS 1935–1945: Ein Beitrag zur Kulturpolitik des Dritten Reiches.* 2. Aufl. München: Oldenbourg.
Kershaw, Ian. 1993. "'Working towards the Führer': Reflections on the Nature of the Hitler Dictatorship." *Contemporary European History* 2(2): 103–18.
———. 2000. *The Nazi Dictatorship: Problems and Perspectives of Interpretation.* 4th ed. London: Bloomsbury.
Lawson, Tom. 2013. *Debates on the Holocaust.* Manchester: Manchester University Press.
Leven, Karl-Heinz. 2002. "Der Freiburger Pathologe Franz Büchner 1941—Widerstand mit und ohne Hippokrates." In *Medizin und Nationalsozialismus: Die Freiburger Medizinische Fakultät und das Klinikum in der Weimarer Republik und im "Dritten Reich,"* edited by Peter Grün, Hans-Gorg Hofer, and Karl-Heinz Leven, 362–96. Frankfurt am Main: Peter Lang.
Lünen, Alexander. v. 2009. "'Splendid Isolation'? Aviation Medicine in World War II." In *Scientific Research in World War II,* edited by A. Maas and H. Hooijmaiers, 96–108. London: Routledge.
———. 2010. "Under the Waves, Above the Clouds: A History of the Pressure Suit." PhD thesis, TU Prints, Technische Universität, Darmstadt, http://tuprints.ulb.tu-darmstadt.de/2103.
Lunt, Peter. 2009. *Stanley Milgram: Understanding Obedience and Its Implications.* London: Palgrave Macmillan.
Mann, Michael. 2000. "Were the Perpetrators of Genocide Ordinary Men or Real Nazis—Results from Fifteen Hundred Biographies." *Holocaust and Genocide Studies* 14(3): 331–66.
Milgram, Stanley. 1974. *Obedience to Authority: An Experimental View.* London: Tavistock.
Overy, Richard. 2014. "'Ordinary Men,' Extraordinary Circumstances: Historians, Social Psychology, and the Holocaust." *Journal of Social Issues* 70(3): 515–30.
Packer, Dominic J. 2008. "Identifying Systematic Disobedience in Milgram's Obedience Experiments: A Meta-Analytic Review." *Perspectives on Psychological Science* 3(4): 301–4.
Perry, Gina. 2013. *Behind the Shock Machine: The Untold Story of the Notorious Milgram Psychology Experiments.* New York: New Press.
Peter, Jürgen. 2013. *Der Nürnberger Ärzteprozeß im Spiegel seiner Aufarbeitung anhand der drei Dokumentensammlungen von Alexander Mitscherlich und Fred Mielke.* Münster: LIT Verlag.
Roelcke, Volker. 2014. "Sulfonamide Experiments on Prisoners in Nazi Concentration Camps: Coherent Scientific Rationality Combined with Complete Disregard of Humanity." In *Human Subjects Research after the Holocaust,* edited by S. Rubenfeld and S. Benedict, 51–66. Cham: Springer.
Roth, Karl Heinz. 2000. "Strukturen, Paradigmen und Mentalitäten in der luftfahrtmedizinischen Forschung des 'Dritten Reichs' 1933 bis 1941: Der Weg ins Konzentrationslager Dachau." *Zeitschrift für Sozialgeschichte* 2(15): 49–77.

Ruff, Siegfried, and Hubertus Strughold. 1942. *Atlas der Luftfahrtmedizin*. Leipzig: Barth.
———. 1944. *Grundriß der Luftfahrtmedizin*. 2. Aufl. Leipzig: Barth.
Russell, Nestar. 2011. "Milgram's Obedience to Authority Experiments: Origins and Early Evolution; Obedience to Authority Experiments." *British Journal of Social Psychology* 50(1): 140–62.
Schmuhl, Hans-Walter. 2009. "Brain Research and the Murder of the Sick: The Kaiser Wilhelm Institute for Brain Research, 1937–1945." In *The Kaiser Wilhelm Society under National Socialism*, edited by S. Heim, C. Sachse, and M. Walker, 99–119. Cambridge: Cambridge University Press.
Seliger, Hubert. 2016. *Politische Anwälte? Die Verteidiger der Nürnberger Prozesse*. Baden-Baden: Nomos.
Trittel, Katharina. 2018. *Hermann Rein und die Flugmedizin: Erkenntnisstreben und Entgrenzung*. Paderborn: Schöningh.
Weindling, Paul J. 2004. *Nazi Medicine and the Nuremberg Trials. From Medical War Crimes to Informed Consent*. New York: Palgrave Macmillan.
Zámečnik, Stanislav. 2013. *Das war Dachau*. Frankfurt am Main: Fischer.

CHAPTER 12

BLOOD AND BONES FROM AUSCHWITZ
The Mengele Link

Paul J. Weindling

On 6 June 1985 there was international excitement when Josef Mengele's corpse was exhumed in a cemetery in Embu, a suburb of São Paolo, Brazil. The initial question was, could it be proved that the corpse was really that of Mengele, who had reputedly (and then proven as certainly) died of a stroke while swimming at Bertioga on 7 February 1979? His death was kept a secret by the Mengele family to protect intermediaries who had supported Mengele for over thirty years as a fugitive from justice. Proving Mengele's death would mean calling off international efforts to bring Mengele to justice, efforts which had ironically intensified in the years after his death. An international team of forensic pathologists analyzed Mengele's bones and teeth to prove the identity of the by now notorious figure in Nazi genocide. The identification meant that Mengele's corpse was subjected to forensic examination in some ways similar to what he had ordered in Auschwitz. Even though the identification confirmed without doubt that the corpse was that of Mengele, his demise left many questions unanswered concerning his Auschwitz period.[1] His skeleton has since been used at the São Paulo University Medical School to teach how to link physical remains with documents in forensic medicine.[2]

The revelation and forensic proof of Mengele's death coincided with an upswing in the study of the history of Nazi eugenics in the mid-1980s. Karl Heinz Roth linked Mengele's efforts to research twins in Auschwitz to innovative research in human genetics.[3] Robert J. Lifton's study of Nazi doctors as constituting a "biocracy" appeared in 1986, with Mengele as the apotheosis of the killer as "healer" of presumed racial ills. Lifton had dropped the idea of analyzing the medical experiments, so he analyzed Mengele on the ramp (conducting genocidal selections for slave labor or killing in the vast gas chambers) rather than Mengele the ambitious and opportunistic researcher.[4] Innovative research on ideology and social construction of genetics as eugenics was extended to Germany. At the time, I was engaged in studies of the formation of racial hygiene and its impact on public health and population policy.[5] Proctor's work on German racial hygiene was also in gestation.[6]

Importantly, the geneticist Benno Müller-Hill published in 1984 on how German geneticists were involved in the Holocaust. He showed how denial in his interviews with perpetrators was contradicted by records from the time. Müller-Hill documented collaborative research between the human geneticist Otmar von Verschuer and Mengele in Auschwitz using reports of the Deutsche Forschungsgemeinschaft (DFG, German Research Fund). Müller-Hill had used his understanding of how German genetic research was funded by requesting disclosure of the still not publicly archived DFG reports. The Reichsforschungsrat (Reich Research Council) and Berlin Document Center documents provided further details of Verschuer's funding.[7] Müller-Hill published critically on the geneticist Hans Nachtsheim and low-pressure experiments on epileptic children from the psychiatric hospital of Brandenburg-Görden.[8] Child "euthanasia" became an issue in 1984 when Götz Aly demonstrated that thirty-five children were killed on 28 October 1940 and their brain specimens transferred to the Kaiser Wilhelm Institute for Brain Research and retained after the war by the Max Planck Institute for Brain Research.[9] The Max Planck Society (MPS) researchers, notably Wilhelm Krücke and Gerd Peters, reacted with hostility and denial. In 1998, a new position of responsibility and historical scrutiny was demonstrated when the MPS president Hubert Markl initiated a historical commission and on 7 June 2001 delivered a momentous apology to a group of twins, who had been selected by Mengele at Auschwitz in 1944 for racial anthropological research.[10]

After the war, on 5 November 1946, Verschuer exculpated himself at a hearing held by senior figures in the still-existent Kaiser Wilhelm Society by declaring that he was the passive recipient of blood and eyes from Auschwitz, and that he was a scientist rather than a fanatical racist.[11] After some initial interest in prosecuting Verschuer by American war crimes investigators in late 1946, leading figures in the German research community settled that being a passive recipient of body parts from a concentration camp or "euthanasia" killing center was legitimate. This position defended the innocence of Verschuer and Julius Hallervorden, the recipient of brains from murdered psychiatric patients (and as we now know, also from Polish Jews who had died from infectious disease under the German occupation).[12] Many German medical institutes retained bodies from the murdered on the principle of being a passive recipient of research specimens rather than being actively involved in research on the persons when they were still alive.

The relations between Verschuer and Auschwitz have been described as close by the new generation of critical historians since the mid-1980s. Müller-Hill went so far as to call Auschwitz the "*Aussenstelle*" or external research station of the Kaiser-Wilhelm-Institut für Anthropologie, menschliche Erblehre und Eugenik (KWIA, Kaiser Wilhelm Institute for Anthropology).[13] The issue of the Auschwitz connection received close attention when the MPG's president, Hubert Markl, convened a Presidential Commission in 1998 for investigating the KWG under National Socialism. Other historians—notably Massin, Sachse, Schmuhl, Trunk, Weiss, and Richard Evans (in his very generalized introduction to his textually defective English edition of the 1946 memoir of the pathologist Miklós Nyiszli)—have seen the links between Mengele and the KWIA as tight. Mengele was Verschuer's former assistant at the Frankfurt Institute for Hereditary Biology and Racial Hygiene (established in 1935), as he had completed his MD dissertation there in 1938 where he was supervised by Verschuer. Mengele intended to complete a habilitation thesis (thesis to obtain license to lecture at German university) under Verschuer, but it is unclear when exactly the research for this commenced. It is certain, however, that Mengele considered Auschwitz as a source that could yield unique research "material" (for example in terms of numbers of twins available for research), and that scientific processing of his measurements, observations, and results from autopsies would establish his postwar career. What needs to be taken into account is that Mengele's dedicated service as an SS officer and *Lagerarzt* (camp physician) also meant that other duties shaped his priorities and filled his time.

In fact, Auschwitz did shape Mengele's postwar career, but in a way that he did not at first anticipate. Mengele became a fugitive from justice, but from judicial systems of the Federal Republic of Germany, Israel, and the United States, which had only a sporadic interest in locating him. The Federal Republic for many years turned a blind eye to the Mengele family from Günzburg bankrolling their fugitive scion.[14] However, a focus on Mengele's wide-ranging activities in Auschwitz and the evidence of the victims of forced research suggests that, rather than continuous research from the time of his arrival in Auschwitz in March 1943, Mengele intensified his research in Auschwitz only later, from the time of the destruction of the "gypsy camp" on 2 August 1944 until the end of November 1944. On 23 July 1944, the Majdanek concentration camp was liberated by the advancing Red Army, and it was clear to Mengele that he had only a limited time to perform his research on twins and others with growth anomalies, notably a large family of dwarves.

Twins were normally difficult to locate for human genetic research: Mengele began stockpiling Czech Jewish twins from the Theresienstadt ghetto from late 1943, and Jewish twins were primarily drawn from the Hungarians and Slovaks streaming into Auschwitz from May 1944. Finally, on fleeing Auschwitz on 17 January 1945, Mengele left the remaining Jewish twins and dwarves alive for reasons that are unclear. One can only speculate that this was either because the research was unfinished or because he hoped that if it came to a trial, any twins that survived could testify that Mengele's conduct was not gratuitously cruel or sadistic: incontrovertibly Mengele killed, but he did so for calculated "racial," scientific, or "sanitary" reasons.

There is irrefutable evidence of soft tissues—notably eye specimens and body fluids, especially blood—and skeletal bones being sent from Auschwitz to the KWIA. More open to debate is how extensive these tissue transfers were, the role of the DFG, and how close the links were between Auschwitz and the KWIA. The evidence for dispatches of body parts to the KWIA is fragmentary, made all the more challenging because Mengele's research notes from the Auschwitz period appear to have been dispersed. This chapter reviews the fragmentary evidence. Auschwitz was the largest center of coerced research under National Socialism, with at least 3,835 victims.[15] It was only with the arrival of male and then female Jews in 1942 in what had hitherto been a camp for non-Jewish Polish males that experiments began. Even so, the large-scale experiments by the gynecologist Carl Clauberg on chemical sterilization to seal the fallopian tubes—approved by Himmler on 7 July 1942—and Horst Schumann on X-ray sterilization were delayed until early 1943 by epidemic typhus (*Fleckfieber*). The victims of experiments can be documented from specimens of blood sent to the laboratory of the Hygiene Institute of the Waffen-SS at Raisko (outside of but close to Auschwitz-Birkenau), as well as from postwar testimonies, legal depositions in preparation of Mengele's trial, and compensation documents (when compensation was often refused on the basis that a "twin experiment" was not a damaging coerced experiment). Mengele's research victims were Jewish, Sinti, and Roma.

Eyes from Auschwitz

Three young dedicated Nazi medical scientists and SS officers have been identified as perpetrators, and all were close to Verschuer: Siegfried Liebau, Ernst Helmerstedt, and Josef Mengele. The physician and human geneticist Liebau was an informant of Verschuer concerning the research potential of Auschwitz. Massin stresses that Liebau was crucial in the supply of the heterochromic Sinti eyes. Between the start of December 1942 and October 1943, Liebau was *"wissenschaftlicher Assistent"* (scientific assistant) to Verschuer at the KWIA in Berlin-Dahlem.[16] In the early months of 1943, Liebau was also in Auschwitz-Birkenau. There he photographed for Karin Magnussen, assistant to geneticist Hans Nachtsheim, the members of the Mechau family of Sinti with heterochromic eyes. On 7 September 1943, the DFG noted research funding on eye color. This coincided with the scientific interest at the KWIA in the Mechau family.[17]

Karin Magnussen worked in Nachtsheim's Department for Experimental Hereditary Pathology. She combined hardline Nazi politics as an NSDAP member since 1931 with a "scientific appetite" for eyes. Nachtsheim had bred one thousand rabbits, and Magnussen collected over four hundred of their eyes and drew conclusions for the genetics of pigmentation in the human eye. Progressing from animal eyes to those of humans was a "logical" step.[18]

When Liebau was in Auschwitz, Mengele was stationed in Berlin for three months. In January 1943, Mengele was transferred from the SS division "Wiking" to the infantry battalion "Ost" and was stationed in Berlin.[19] This allowed him to reestablish contacts with Verschuer, who wrote with pride of Mengele's endurance on the eastern front.[20] After his arrival in Auschwitz on 30 May 1943, there was an interval when Mengele was absorbed in camp duties in the "gypsy family camp" and in epidemic control, suggesting that human research had to be postponed.

When Mengele came to Auschwitz, he was placed in charge of the medical supervision of the newly established *Zigeunerlager* (gypsy camp)—in Birkenau. He was joined by Erwin von Helmersen, a physician who obtained an MD from the KWIA, in this case working under Fritz Lenz (who in contrast to Verschuer withdrew from any links with concentration camps).[21] (Helmersen was handed over to Poland for trial and executed in 1949.) Mengele was also assisted by a staff of around thirty prisoner doctors, notably Berthold Epstein and Bruno Weisskopf from Prague, and Lucie Adelsberger, dismissed from the Robert Koch Institute Berlin, as well as sixty prisoner nursing orderlies.[22] The pathologist Nyiszli wrote of his autopsies on Sinti with heterochromic eyes.and his discovery that all eight bodies had Dubois tumors.[23]

Mengele became interested in the medically specific condition noma (orofacial gangrene) in malnourished Roma children.[24] Apart from his work on noma, there is no evidence of Mengele being engaged in research until later in 1943 or indeed early in 1944. Mengele then became interested in a small group of twelve Sinti and Roma twins. Although Mengele showed a wish to retain them, they did not survive the genocidal destruction of the gypsy camp in early August 1944, as part of genocidal policies against Sinti and Roma.

Verschuer's report to the DFG indicated that between October 1943 and March 1944 Mengele became involved in the KWIA director's DFG project on hereditary pathology. Verschuer stated that anthropological investigations were being carried out and that blood specimens were sent to his laboratory. In a further report to the DFG of October 1944, Verschuer reported that over two hundred blood samples of different races were being analyzed in conjunction with Dr. Günther Hillman of the Kaiser Wilhelm Institute for Biochemistry.[25] The Reichforschungsrat's (Reich Research Council) funding cards indicate a grant for comparative hereditary pathology on 20 March 1944. The motives for the blood research have been differently interpreted notably by Müller-Hill, who attributed an interest to Mengele and Verschuer in the Abderhalden Ferment Reaction, and Achim Trunk, who attributed an interest to Verschuer in racial susceptibility, tuberculosis, or serological racial diagnosis.[26]

Mengele as *Lagerarzt* was engaged in genocide on a colossal scale at the Auschwitz "ramp" in deciding on which newly arrived prisoners were fit for work and could fulfill forced labor quotas and who were to be immediately killed with the cyanide salt Zyklon B. Mengele also selected prisoners for the gas chambers among those in the camp and ordered killings to control epidemic infections. He took advantage of his position to conduct research: he could select twins, dwarves, and those with genetic anomalies from the new arrivals at Auschwitz, especially from the Hungarian transports, which coincided with Mengele's decision to retain and research twins. He had research opportunities in the so-called *Zigeunerlager*. Indeed, the chief camp physician Eduard Wirths rewarded Mengele with resources, because Mengele was punctilious in carrying out his sanitary and medical duties, not the least in selections for the gas chambers. Wirths's assessment was that "he has used every free moment to educate himself further as an anthropologist."[27]

Mengele improvised an extensive research infrastructure during June 1944. He found prisoner assistants, notably the pathologist Nyiszli and his three assistants who commenced work from 27 June 1944, and the prisoner anthropologists Erzsebet Fleischmann and the Polish princess Martina Puzyna.[28] Mengele was convinced that artists could render skin color better than color photography, so he employed Dina Gottliebová, "Mausi" Hermann, and Maria Zombirt in such capacity.[29] Mengele organized barracks for often very young male and female twins and arranged for their care, notably by Zwi Spiegel, who was an older Slovak twin. In short, an elaborate research infrastructure arose between June and late November 1944 to sustain several hundred Jewish twins. Occasionally Mengele would accept two or three generations from the same family. There were also some "fake" pairs of twins (notably the Kun and Reichenberg brothers, and the Bucci sisters), as being recognized as twin meant survival; these were in fact merely brothers or sisters who looked similar and were born a year or so apart. There is no record of payments by the DFG or by the SS for this research. That Mengele did not appear in SS records concerning human experiments meant that he was not noticed at first as a war criminal by the Americans who worked from captured German documents.[30]

Many twins who survived Auschwitz confirm that large amounts of blood were taken—as often as twice weekly. In addition, the twins underwent constant anthropological measurements and detailed uncomfortable examinations of eye color, at times with eye drops.[31] Researchers like Verschuer and Butenandt, or Hallervorden in the case of brains from "euthanasia" victims, showed indifference to having obtained body parts and fluids supplied from concentration camps or killing institutions. This postwar position detached the science from genocidal killings, although in the case of Verschuer he was a convinced anti-Semite.

Prisoners and twins speculated much on Mengele and the status of his research. Was it part of a wider plan for Germans to have twins who should be blond and blue-eyed, and that having twins would promote racial expansion? Again, evidence is lacking that Mengele formed part of an SS-sponsored research plan. The killing of Jews and Roma were major SS priorities. Mengele served genocidal aims of the SS by making selections at the ramp. But his research on twins was not embedded in SS racial policies of organizations such as the Lebensborn, Ahnenerbe, or the Rasse und Siedlungs-Hauptamt (Race and Settlement Office).[32] Mengele's research is not mentioned in the Himmler papers, and there is no record of any special finance being made available—Mengele thus seemed a low priority to war crime investigators until prisoners reported on his role in selections for the gas chambers, as well as the twin research. For although twins were killed for research, it appears that the majority of the twins did survive and later provided a steadily growing set of testimonies on Mengele's research and what it involved.

The Mechau family of Sinto origin from Bremen had attracted the attention of Karin Magnussen before their deportation. The family included one pair of twins, who were photographed by Magnussen at the KWIA in March 1943. They were therefore marked prior to their deportation as scientific specimens. Magnussen, in an interrogation of 25 May 1949, referred to photographing heterochromic eyes of twins. This leaves open whether they were Sinti and Roma or Jewish twins.[33] Magnussen explained that she met Mengele at the KWIA. When the Mechau family was interned in Auschwitz, Liebau kept them under observation and then Mengele facilitated the transmittal of the eyes to Magnussen.[34] Magnussen was guarded in the interrogation and did not admit to having requested the killing of the Mechau family for their eyes. Magnussen worked with the doctoral student Georg Wagner, whose PhD dissertation was based on physical measurements of 209 Sinti and Roma including 74 twins, some of whom had eye anomalies.[35] Magnussen and Wagner allegedly received forty pairs of eyes from Auschwitz through the agency of Liebau and Mengele.[36]

The Prisoner-Pathologist's Testimony

Miklós Nyiszli, Auschwitz number A 8450, arrived on a Hungarian transport with his wife and daughter, along with twenty-six district physicians on 29 May 1944, and was transferred to Monowitz.[37] After twelve days at the IG-Farben Buna Factory at Monowitz, Mengele ascertained that Nyiszli had trained in pathology in the German university of Breslau (today's Wrocław in Poland).[38] There were three additional assistants: Denis Görög from Szombathely, Adolph Fischer from Prague, and Joseph Kolner from Nice, and there was originally a fourth, a pathologist from Strasbourg, possibly Jonas Silber.[39] At the end of June 1944, Nyiszli transferred from Monowitz to an improvised pathology room in Crematorium 3 in Birkenau. This transfer is indicative of Mengele's upscaling of his Auschwitz research, using improvised resources of prisoners as research staff in makeshift accommodations.

Nyiszli is the origin of three sources about Mengele's Auschwitz research: first, a 1945 deposition that found its way to Yad Vashem; second, a series of

Hungarian newspaper articles that Nyiszli developed into his memoir, *I Was Mengele's Autopsy Doctor in Auschwitz: A Hungarian Doctor's Diary from Hell*, first published between 16 February 1947 and 5 April 1947; third, a deposition that became the Nuremberg document NI-11710, dated 8 October 1947, when "Dr Nikolai Nyiszli" was summoned to Nuremberg to give evidence for the IG Farben Trial, when he testified about the use of Zyklon gas in the crematoria.[40] Franciszek Piper's translated edition represents an effort to return to Nyiszli's original text, as it reinstates an additional chapter concerning lethal research in Auschwitz on digestion. The short chapter outlines pathological observations as recollected by Nyiszli, showing how Nyiszli worked not only for Mengele but also for other experimentally minded doctors in Auschwitz. The original Hungarian edition, a German typescript translation, and the edition edited by Piper in 2010 incorporated this additional chapter. The first published German edition in 1991 similarly contains the additional chapter. The edition introduced by Richard Evans omits the chapter without comment and contains minor inaccuracies, such as the correct name of the controversial Polish physician Roman (not Zenon) Zenkteller.[41]

In his 1945 deposition, Nyiszli referred to how he, along with a French colleague, had to take measurements of persons with anomalies. The SS officer in charge of the crematoria, Erich Muhsfeldt, would then shoot them, and the corpses were returned for pathological autopsy. The bones were cleansed with chlorinated lime and then sent to the KWIA. Nyiszli described Mengele's killing of fourteen Roma twins.[42]

Nyiszli's memoir has been a standard source of information on Mengele's sending blood and bones from Auschwitz. The memoir uniquely records a series of killings and dispatches of specimens. Nyiszli cites Mengele as demanding, "I require top-quality documentation, because it is going to the Institute of Anthropological, Biological and Racial Research in Berlin-Dahlem." On another occasion the institute was referred to as: "Berlin-Dahlem Institut für Rassenbiologische und Anthropologische Forschungen."[43] Indeed, Nyiszli felt that his life was dependent on the Berlin-Dahlem institute.

Nyiszli did not exhaustively list every instance in which he dispatched specimens for the KWIA, but he provided select examples. He conducted autopsies of twelve sets of Roma twins with great care. The twins were killed at the liquidation of the *Zigeunerlager* on 2–3 August 1944.[44] When conducting autopsies on four sets of the twins, Nyiszli recorded, "I also discovered that three of the four pairs of twins had different colored eyes: one brown, the other blue. . . . I took out the eyeballs and placed each in separate jars containing a formaldehyde solution."[45] In his work Nyiszli found Dubois tumors—arising from congenital syphilis— and evidence of tuberculosis, which were of interest to Verschuer.[46]

An indication of scale is provided by Mengele's demands for seven dissections a day, whereas Nyiszli restricted Mengele to a maximum of three dissections a day. In the 1945 testimony, Nyiszli said four dissections a day when referring to the doomed Roma twins. He gave instances of body parts being sent to Berlin: "4 pairs of twins from the Gypsy Camp." The victims were killed with lethal chloroform injections, and their organs were extracted. Nyiszli describes the shipping process: "They were then appropriately packed and sent off through the post. In order to make them reach the Institute faster, the parcels were stamped: 'Urgent, contents important for the war effort.'"[47]

Nyiszli described with dismay pre- and postmortal clinical examinations of a Jewish father who had a hunchback and his son who had a leg deformity from the liquidated Litzmannstadt/Łódź Ghetto. Transports from the ghetto arrived in Auschwitz from mid-August 1944. By then Mengele had more time to pursue his research interests.[48] Exactly when Mengele began researching children other than Sinti and Roma is of interest. The sisters Liliana and Tatiana arrived in Auschwitz on 23 April 1944. They were an anomaly in that they were baptized and had a non-Jewish father. They were held with other children, including their cousin Sergio de Simone, who had similar Christian-Jewish parentage. Sergio was one of the twenty children transported to Neuengamme for a tuberculosis immunization experiment and then killed in the cellar of a Hamburg school.[49] Liliana and Tatiana Bucci were measured and had blood taken from them, and they were held with the twins—they may have been regarded as such. Soon other twins began to be added to what soon became a collection of several hundred, as well as dwarves.[50]

Mengele initially "stockpiled" Jewish twins from the Theresienstadt family camp in Auschwitz, which came into existence 8 September 1943. These eleven "earmarked" pairs of twins survived two gruesome mass liquidations on 8–9 March and 11 July 1944 when the majority of the family camp inmates were sent to the gas chambers. From 17 May 1944, Mengele began retaining Hungarian Jewish twins and twins from former Slovak territory.[51] The interest in developmental abnormalities was evident with Mengele's excitement about the Ovitz family of dwarves, who arrived in Auschwitz on 19 May 1944. A possible correlation is with the geneticist Hans Grebe at the KWIA. Grebe studied the genetics of growth variations, with dwarfism as a topic of special interest, and it is conjectured that he was interested in the specimens sent by Mengele.[52]

Mengele stated regarding the hunchback father and the son with the leg deformity, "These bodies cannot be burnt. Their skeletons must be conserved and sent to the Anthropological Museum in Berlin." Nyiszli recollected that "he next asked me what I knew about cleaning skeletons. . . ." Nyiszli then advised, "You simply boiled the corpse in water until the flesh came easily off the bone. Next you bathed the skeleton in petrol. . . . An improvised stove was built . . . the two barrels with their macabre contents and the process of cooking the corpses began. . . . The skeletons and accompanying documentation were packed in tough paper sacks and posted to Berlin."[53]

Nyiszli thus gives detailed insight into the sending of body fluids, soft tissues, and bones (and associated documents) from Auschwitz-Birkenau to the KWIA in Berlin. Nyiszli believed that the KWIA's wider aim was a museum presenting the degeneracy of the Jewish race.[54]

Postwar Developments

Testimonies provide some further evidence of the consignments. Puzyna testified that Mengele consigned a wooden case to her, which she was to take to the camp post office. She secretly opened the case and found specimen jars with human eyes. This taught her Mengele's capacity as a killer. On 1 May 1946, *Die Neue Zeitung* in Munich reported that Mengele sent Verschuer eyes and blood samples from *Zigeunern* (Sinti and Roma). On 10 May 1946, Verschuer in an affidavit defended Mengele as physician and helper of the sick.[55] President of the rump KWG, chemist, and resistance activist Robert Havemann wrote on 15 August 1946 to An die Betreuungsstelle für Sonderfälle, Frankfurt am Main (welfare office for special cases, American Military Forces Frankfurt, Main), providing a detailed analysis of Liebau and Mengele in Auschwitz as scientific assistants to Verschuer, who they supplied with body parts and fluids for research. Havemann characterized Verschuer as a Nazi fanatic and activist.[56]

Havemann's report reached the attention of US war crime document analysts. The result was a memorandum to the neurologist Leo Alexander who was advising the US prosecution at the Nuremberg Doctors Trial which had just commenced.

> 12 Dec 1946
> Memo: To: Dr. Leo Alexander
> Please advise me of your opinion of the attached report which I wrote in Berlin. What action, and along what lines, do you propose
> M. Wolfson
> Room 223[57]

The response:

> 13-12-46 [At foot of same page in blue ink]
> I think that Mengele, Verschuer and Magnussen should be arrested, interrogated and tried. I suggest that you let Gen. Taylor and Mr. MacHaney see this.
> Thanks,
> Leo Alexander

These consignments were dated from early 1944 until late November 1944. There is an explanatory note:

> Verschuer tries to create the impression that Dr Mengele went to Auschwitz against his will and frequently tried to effect a transfer but was unsuccessful in leaving his Auschwitz environment. This statement of von Verschuer is easily disproven by quoting a personal evaluation entered into the SS personnel record of Mengele by SS-Hauptsturmführer MATTES, dated 19 August 1944. This evaluation states in part:
> "Mengele has always proven to be an excellent officer, respected and well-liked. His ideological views show maturity and strength. Because of his particular merits he was awarded the German War Merit Cross 2nd Class. He thoroughly commands the field of anthropology. And, therefore, he is particularly suited for a higher position. Mengele has not displayed any weakness in character (inhibition). As a camp physician he has always displayed great anthropological abilities."
> Dr von Verschuer admits, both in his reply to the "Neue Zeitung" article as well as to Professor Dr GOTTSCHALDT that Mengele was one of his assistants while von Verschuer was director of the Kaiser Wilhelm Institute. He further admits that in order to carry on medical research on Aberhald [sic]'s Ferment reaction he received 20 to 30 shipments of blood at regular intervals. He admits that this blood was derived from Auschwitz and was obtained through the help of Dr. Mengele. It goes without saying, that this blood was not derived from any blood donors, in fact the Auschwitz inmates were forced to submit to Dr. Mengele who then syphoned their blood. Three affidavits, submitted to me by Professor Havemann show how Mengele would syphon blood from people until they would die.
> Dr. Verschuer further admits that in his Dahlem Institute, research had been carried on regarding the development of the pigments of the human eye. It was with von Verschuer's knowledge but most likely through his direct intervening efforts that one of his assistants, Dr. Karin MAGNUSSEN obtained the eyes of inmates of Concentration Camp Auschwitz, which were used for studies in the pathological, anatomical section of the Kaiser Wilhelm Institute. Von Verschuer's admission establishes that at least 4 pairs of eyes were delivered to the Dahlem Institute in this manner, while it might be claimed that these inmates died a natural death, one cannot fail to overlook the fact that von Verschuer and Dr. Magnussen were interested in eyes of inmates who had heterochromic eyes, i.e. eyes whose respective color differed. In view of the fact that this occurrence of different coloring is rare and since Dr. Mengele knew of the request of von Verschuer's Institute and since his character evaluation showed him to have been highly cooperative in fact labels him as having contributed to anthropological research, it goes without saying that to gas these inmates after they had been carefully selected was not impossible. In fact, inmates state in affidavits that it was Dr. Mengele himself who was charged with the selection of inmates to be dispatched to the gas chambers at Auschwitz. When questioned by Professor Dr. Gottschaldt (head of the Kaiser Wilhelm Gesellschaft, Institute for psychological research), von Verschuer admitted having been informed of the detailed setup as it existed in Auschwitz. Since it is established

that Dr. Mengele rarely visited the Kaiser Wilhelm Institute in Berlin-Dahlem it is likely that von Verschuer's first-hand information stems either from a personal visit to the Auschwitz laboratories or from detailed reports supplied by Mengele.[58]

The lack of prosecution meant that Mengele was able to leave Germany through incompetence. The Mengele family at Günzburg informed a US search team that Mengele was dead. This evidence suggests that, from late 1946, there was compelling evidence against Verschuer and Mengele but that efforts had been made to conceal Mengele along with evidence of the supportive KWIA. The reconstructions of the mid-1980s only resurrected what had been well documented.

What evidence is there of Mengele's notes and specimens? In his biography of Simon Wiesenthal, Alan Levy alleged that in 1948 the Mengele family's go-between, Hans Sedlmeier, delivered to Mengele in Bolzano in the South Tyrol (a favored area for Nazis on the run) "a small suitcase with scientific specimens, including two glass slides with a blood sample between them, plus his precious notes from Auschwitz."[59] This is likely to have been part of a larger collection of specimens, notes, and documents that the Mengele family were engaged in dispersing to their fugitive scion. No record exists of the police ever searching thoroughly in Günzburg for incriminating documentation. (It is regrettable that the family has dispersed items like Mengele's South American diary for profit rather than making them available for scholarship.)

In 1964 Fritz Bauer, the Hessen chief prosecutor, prepared evidence for an eventual trial against Mengele, collecting many victim testimonies. In 1989 Yad Vashem asked whether the archives of the Kaiser Wilhelm Society had transferred documentation on Mengele's victims to the University of Frankfurt.[60] The human genetics department of the university wrote on 19 October 1989 to the dean of the medical faculty that it had no idea where the Verschuer collections of bones and soft tissue could be.[61]

In 1987 there were efforts to draw attention to the former KWIA as a site of atrocity. Götz Aly described how he, along with a group of historian colleagues including Anna Bergmann, Gabriele Czarnowski, and Susanne Heim, attached a plaque to the Otto Suhr Institute in Dahlem. The plaque accused Eugen Fischer and Verschuer of laying the fundamental principles of the race and population policy of the Nazi state. Moreover, it accused Mengele, as SS camp physician in Auschwitz, of conducting twin research and sending blood and organs to the KWIA. In 1988 the plaque was replaced with a bronze memorial plaque by the Free University, which omitted the wider role of Fischer and Verschuer in the Nazi state. The core issue of Mengele's dispatching of organs was allowed to stand.[62]

By this time I was engaged in researching the post-1945 efforts of Verschuer, Nachtsheim, and Lenz, as well as a resurfaced Pater Hermann Muckermann, to sustain their jobs and their institutional positions. The plaque was (and still is) in error that the KWIA ceased in 1945. In fact, the KWIA did not cease to operate after Germany's liberation by the Allies, as Hans Nachtsheim remained as acting director, and the KWIA sustained itself into the postwar period until 1948. At the installation of the new plaque I wrote on 20 June 1988 to *Der Tagespiegel* and to Dieter Heckelmann, the president of the Free University at the time, hoping that the crucial error could be corrected. Needless to say, this was unwelcome information, and I received no reply from the Free University, and the letter was not published. When I contacted President Peter-André Alt of the Free University on behalf of the Center for Medicine after the Holocaust (CMATH) in 2015 about preventing bones found in a scientific collection from Auschwitz from being incinerated, President Alt undertook to keep CMATH informed but failed in this commitment.[63] Having escaped the cremation furnaces of Auschwitz, President Alt's inactivity meant that the bones were in fact incinerated.[64] Continuities from the Nazi past are unwelcome news and remain unresolved as long as victims remain incidental and marginal.

Paul J. Weindling, MA, PhD, ML, is research professor in the history of medicine, Oxford Brookes University. His research covers medical refugees from 1930 to 1945, eugenics, international health organizations, and the victims of Nazi coerced experimentation. He is a trustee of CARA, the Council for At-Risk Academics. He was awarded the Anneliese Maier Prize, which he holds at the German National Academy of Sciences, Leopoldina in Halle, Germany, and was elected an honorary member of the German Association of Psychiatry (DPGNN) for investigating its role under Nazism. His books include *Health, Race and German Politics* (1989), *Epidemics and Genocide in Eastern Europe* (2000), *Victims and Survivors of Nazi Human Experiments* (2014), and *From Clinic to Concentration Camp* (2017).

Notes

1. Ralph Blumenthal, "U.S. Report on Mengele Reaffirms His Death," *New York Times*, 9 October 1992.
2. Associated Press in São Paulo, "Nazi Doctor Josef Mengele's Bones Used in Brazil's Forensic Medicine Courses," *The Guardian*, 11 January 2017, retrieved 18 September 2019 from https://www.theguardian.com/science/2017/jan/11/josef-mengele-bones-brazil-forensic-medicine.
3. Roth 1985.
4. Lifton 1986.
5. Weindling 1985a, 1985b, 1989.
6. Proctor 1988.
7. Müller-Hill 1984.
8. Müller-Hill 1987.
9. Aly to MPG president Heinz Staab, 17 September 1984, letter and report; in MPG E-II-1a 1963; Aly 2015.

10. Max Planck Society 2001.
11. Weindling 1989, 568–69; Schmuhl 2005, 530; Kröner 1998.
12. Palacz and Weindling 2020.
13. Müller-Hill 1999/2000.
14. Keller 2003.
15. Weindling 2014, 226. The figure aggregates the entries in Victims of Biomedical Research under NS. Collaborative Database of Medical Victims.
16. Sachse 2003, 256.
17. Weindling 1989, 560; Weindling 2014.
18. K. Magnussen, "Die Einwirkung der Farbgene auf die Pigmententwirkung in Kaninchenaugen," unpublished paper sent to author by Widukind Lenz on 12 October 1987; Weindling 2003.
19. Berlin Document Center, SS file for Josef Mengele.
20. Weindling 1989, 562; Trunk 2003, 13–14.
21. Massin and Sachse 2000, 26–27.
22. Völklein 2000, 120–21; Adelsberger 2001.
23. Nyiszli 1946/2010, 47–48.
24. Szymański 1962.
25. Trunk 2003, 8.
26. Müller-Hill 1999; Trunk 2003, 23–48.
27. Cited by Czech 1990, 690–91.
28. HHStA Wiesbaden, 631a, deposition of Martina Puzyna.
29. Nyiszli 1946/2010, 22, 42. This Piper edition is more accurate than the defective Evans edition.
30. Weindling 2004.
31. Cf. Weindling 1989, 563
32. Weindling 2014, 157–65.
33. Schmuhl 2005, 492–93; Hesse 2001.
34. AMPG Abt I, rep. 3, nr. 26.
35. Wagner 1943; Schmuhl 2005, 494–502.
36. Hesse 2001.
37. Czech 1990, 636, 690–92.
38. Nyiszli 1930.
39. My thanks to Georges Hauptmann for this identification.
40. NI-11710—affidavit sworn by the Hungarian medical doctor Nyiszli Nikolae on 8 October 1947 at Nuremberg, regarding the use of Zyklon B at Auschwitz. Dr. Nyiszli was transported to Mauthausen in January 1945 and eventually liberated at the Ebensee subcamp by the U.S. Army. German- and Hungarian-language signed original documents.
41. Uzarczyk 2018.
42. Nyiszli 1946/2010, 46–48. Nyiszli, testimony 28 July 1945, Yad Vashem 015/21-2. C, copy at Landgericht Frankfurt, 6 Dec 1972.
43. Nyiszli 1946/2010, 45.
44. Nyiszli 1973, 100.
45. Nyiszli 1946/2010, 47.
46. Nyiszli 1946/2010, 47–48. Note: the Penguin translation with an introduction by Richard Evans mistranslates "congenital syphilis" as "hereditary syphilis."
47. Nyiszli 1946/2010, 47.
48. Nyiszli 1946/2010, 136
49. Groschek and Vagt 2012
50. Bucci 2018.
51. Czech 1990, 628, entry for 17 May 1944.
52. Schmuhl 2005, 374–379.

53. Czech 1990, 138–41. The Piper edition has the correct spelling of "Muhsfeldt," incorrect in the Panther edition. The Oswiecim edition includes an additional chapter (chapter 17) on autopsy findings of prisoners who died from dysentery. The chapter is missing from the Penguin edition without explanation by Evans as editor.
54. Nyiszli 1946/2010, 85.
55. MPGA Abt II Rep. 1A Personalia Verschuer, Nr. 5 Verschuer affidavit.
56. Cf. Weindling 2003, 274. Archives de France BB/35/260 Havemann memorandum to Betreuungsstelle für Sonderfälle, 15 August1946.
57. Leo Alexander Papers, Medical Archives Durham NC, 4/35 M. Wolfson to Leo Alexander, 7 January 1947. Archives de France BB/35/269 memorandum of Wolfson to B.B. Ferencz Summary Report on an Investigation, 7 November 1946. Wolfson to Alexander 12 December 1946, reply Alexander 13 December 1946. Weindling 2004, 246–247.
58. Archives de France BB/35/269 Wolfson, Summary Report of an Investigation.
59. Levy 1993, 263.
60. University Archive Frankfurt, fax from Tel Aviv to German Foreign Office 6 January 1989, Az 2.49.00 f. 47.
61. University Archive Frankfurt, fax from Tel Aviv to German Foreign Office 6 January 1989, Az 2.49.00 f. 47.
62. Aly 2015, 219–20.
63. Cf. communication from Aly to Weindling 1 February 2015.
64. See Hildebrandt et al., "The History of the Vienna Protocol," in this volume.

References

Archival Sources

Alexander, Leo, Papers, Medical Records Center, Durham NC.
Archive of the Max Planck Society (AMPG) Abt I, Rep 3 Nr 26.
Berlin Document Center, Josef Mengele SS file, consulted in Berlin1985.
Hessen Hauptstaatsarchiv (HHSTA) Wiesbaden, Abt 631a Ermittlungsakten Mengele.
Max Planck Society Archives (MPSA).
University Archive (UA) Frankfurt am Main.

Books and Articles

Adelsberger, Lucie. 2001. Ein Tatsachenbericht. *Das Vermächtnis der Opfer für uns Juden und für alle Menschen*. Bonn: Bouvier.
Aly, Götz. 2015. *Volk ohne Mitte: Die Deutschen zwischen Freiheitsangst und Kollektivismus*. Frankfurt am Main: S. Fischer.
Bucci, Andra, and Tatiana Bucci (eds.). 2018. Umberto Gentiloni and Marcello Pezzetti, *Noi, Bambine ad Auschwitz*. Rome: Mondadori
Czech, Danuta. 1990. *Auschwitz Chronicle 1939–1945*. New York: Henry Holt.
Groschek, Iris, and Christina Vagt. 2012. ". . . dass du weißt, was hier passiert ist." *Medizinische Experimente im KZ Neuengamme und die Morde am Bullenhuser Damm*. Bremen: Edition Temmen.
Hesse, Hans. 2001. *Augen aus Auschwitz: Ein Lehrstück über nationalsozialistischen Rassenwahn und medizinische Forschungen; Der Fall Dr. Karin Magnussen*. Essen: Klartext.
Keller, Sven. 2003. *Günzburg und der Fall Josef Mengele: Die Heimatstadt und die Jagd nach dem NS-Verbrecher*. München: Oldenbourg Wissenschaftsverlag.
Kröner, Hans-Peter. 1998. *Von der Rassenhygiene zur Humangenetik: Das Kaiser-Wilhelm-Institut für Anthropologie, menschliche Erblehre und Eugenik nach dem Kriege*. Stuttgart: Gustav Fischer

Levy, Alan. 1993, *Nazi Hunter: The Wiesenthal File*. London: Robinson
Lifton, Robert J. 1986. *The Nazi Doctors: Medical Killing and the Psychology of Genocide*. New York: Basic Books.
Markl, Hubert. 2003. "Die ehrlichste Art der Entschuldigung ist die Offenlegung der Schuld." In *Die Verbindung nach Auschwitz. Biowissenschaften und Menschenversuche an Kaiser-Wilhelm-Instituten: Dokumentation eines Symposiums*, edited by Carola Sachse, 41–51. Göttingen: Wallstein.
Massin, Benoît. 2003. "Mengele, die Zwillingsforschung und die 'Auschwitz-Dahlem Connection.'" In *Die Verbindung nach Auschwitz. Biowissenschaften und Menschenversuche an Kaiser-Wilhelm-Instituten. Dokumentation eines Symposiums*, edited by Carola Sachse, 201–54. Göttingen: Wallstein.
Massin, Benoit, and Carola Sachse. 2000. "Biowissenschaftliche Forschung in Kaiser-Wilhelm-Instituten und die Verbrechen des NS-Regimes." *Ergebnisse* 3.
Max Planck Society. 2001. *Symposium in Berlin: Biomedical Sciences and Human Experimentation at Kaiser Wilhelm Institutes—The Auschwitz Connection*. Munich: Max Planck Society.
Müller-Hill, Benno. 1984. *Tödliche Wissenschaft*. Hamburg: Rowohlt.
———. 1987. "Genetics after Auschwitz." *Holocaust and Genocide Studies* 2: 3–20.
———. 1999. "The Blood from Auschwitz and the Silence of the Scholars." *History and Philosophy of the Life Sciences* 21: 331–65. A German version of this article has appeared in *Geschichte der KWG im Nationalsozialismus*, vol. 1, ed. D. Kaufmann (Göttingen: Wallstein Verlag, 2000), 189–227.
Nyiszli, Miklós. N.d. "Ich war Prosektor bei Dr. Mengele im Krematorium Auschwitz." Typescript in Instituut voor Oorlogs-, Holocaust- en Genocidestudies (NIOD).
———. 1992. *Im Jenseits der Menschlichkeit: Ein Gerichtsmediziner in Auschwitz*. Berlin: Dietz Verlag.
Nyiszli, Nicolaus. N.d. "Ich war Prosektor bei Dr. Mengele im Krematorium Auschwitz." Typescript. Translated by Thaddeus R. Gébert.
———. 1930. "Selbstmordarten auf Grund des Sektionsmaterials des Breslauer gerichtsärztlichen Instituts von Juni 1927–Mai 1930." MD diss., Breslau.
Nyiszli, Miklós. 1946/2010. *I Was Doctor Mengele's Assistant: The Memoirs of an Auschwitz Physician*. Edited by Franciszek Piper. Oświęcim: Frap-Books. [Translated from the Polish edition, 2000, and this from the Hungarian edition.]
———. 1973. *Auschwitz: Dr Miklos Nyiszli's Eye-Witness Account*. London: Panther.
———. 1992. *Im Jenseits der Menschlichkeit: Ein Gerichtsmediziner in Auschwitz*. Berlin: Dietz Verlag.
———. 2012. *Auschwitz: A Doctor's Eyewitness Account*. Introduction by Richard J. Evans. London: Penguin Books.
Proctor, Robert. 1988. *Racial Hygiene: Medicine under the Nazis*. Cambridge, MA: Harvard University Press.
Roth, Karl-Heinz. 1985. "Die wissenschaftliche Normalität des Schlächters. Josef Mengeleals Anthropologe. Eine Dokumentation." *Mitteilungen der Dokumentationsstelle zur NS-Sozialpolitik Hamburg* 1(2): i–ix.
Sachse, Carola. 2003. "Menschenversuche in Auschwitz überleben, erinnern, verantworten." In *Die Verbindung nach Auschwitz—Biowissenschaften und Menschenversuche an Kaiser-Wilhelm-Instituten*, edited by Carola Sachse, 7–34. Göttingen: Wallstein Verlag.
Schmuhl, Hans-Walter. 2005. *Grenzüberschreitungen: Das Kaiser-Wilhelm-Institut für Anthropologie, menschliche Erblehre und Eugenik 1927–1945*. Göttingen: Wallstein.
Szymański, Tadeusz. 1962. "Noma cases among the Roma in Auschwitz-Birkenau." Translated by M. Kantor. Medical Review—Auschwitz. Retrieved 10 June 2019 from https://www.mp.pl/auschwitz/. Originally published as "Noma (rak wodny) w obozie cygańskim Oświęcim-Brzezinka," Przegląd Lekarski—Oświęcim, 68–70.
Trunk, Achim. 2003. *Zweihundert Blutproben aus Auschwitz: Ein Forschungsvorhaben zwischen Anthropologie und Biochemie (1943–1945)*. Berlin: Research Program "History of the Kaiser Wilhelm Gesellschaft in the National Socialist Era."

Uzarczyk, Kamila. 2018. "Auschwitz Doctors on Trial: The Cases of Hans Münch, Johann Paul Kremer and Roman Zenkteller." Special Issue, *Wiener klinische Wochenschrift* (June): 8202–6.

Völklein, Ulrich. 1999. *Josef Mengele der Arzt von Auschwitz*. Göttingen: Steidl.

Wagner, Georg. 1943. "Rassenbiologische Beobachtungen an Zigeunern und Zigeunerzwillingen." Math.-naturwiss. F., diss., Berlin.

Weindling, Paul J. 1985a. "Blood, Race and Politics." *The Times Higher Education Supplement* (19 July): 13.

———. 1985b. "Weimar Eugenics in Social Context: The Founding of the Kaiser Wilhelm Institute for Anthropology, Human Heredity and Eugenics." *Annals of Science* 42: 303–18.

———. 1989. *Health, Race and German Politics from National Unification to Nazism*. Cambridge: Cambridge University Press.

———. 2003. "Genetik und Menschenversuche in Deutschland 1940–1960: Hans Nachtsheim, die Kaninchen von Dahlem und die Kinder vom Bullenhuser Damm." In *Rassenforschung an Kaiser-Wilhelm-Instituten vor und nach 1933*, edited by Hans-Walter Schmuhl, 245–74. Göttingen: Wallstein Verlag.

———. 2004. *Nazi Medicine and the Nuremberg Trials: From Medical War Crimes to Informed Consent*. Basingstoke. Palgrave Macmillan.

———. 2014. *Victims and Survivors of Nazi Human Experiments: Science and Suffering in the Holocaust*. London: Bloomsbury.

Weindling, Paul J., Gerrit Hohendorf, Axel C. Hüntelmann, Jasmin Kindel, Annemarie Kinzelbach, Aleksandra Loewenau, Stephanie Neuner, Michał Adam Palacz, Marion Zingler, and Herwig Czech. 2020. "The Problematic Legacy of Victim Specimens from the Nazi Era: Identifying the Persons behind the Specimens at the Max Planck Institutes for Brain Research and Psychiatry." *Journal of the History of the Neurosciences* 29(4).

Part II

THE PRESENT
Postwar Continuities, Legacies, and Reflections

CHAPTER 13

Renewed Trauma
Abraham de la Penha's Testimony against Dr. Franz Lucas in the Frankfurt Auschwitz Trial

Andrew Wisely

In immediate postwar Nazi trials in Nuremberg, Allied courts drew upon a deep reservoir of incriminatory documents to bring high-ranking SS defendants to speedy justice. As the responsibility for trials was passed to courts in the Federal Republic of Germany following its founding in 1949, survivor testimonies became critical for reinforcing the stated murder indictments against lesser-known war criminals. In courtrooms dominated by remorseless defendants with skilled defense lawyers, survivor witnesses encountered hostile environments for telling about their harrowing experiences. Anomalies that arose during cross-examination were cause for the court to doubt the truthfulness of their accounts.

Such skepticism met one Auschwitz survivor whose testimony against an SS doctor was ultimately dismissed. Abraham de la Penha, a Jewish plumber from Amsterdam, traveled to Frankfurt in March 1965 to testify against Dr. Franz Lucas in the Frankfurt Auschwitz Trial (1963–65), which brought to light for the first time the scope of extermination in Auschwitz-Birkenau. De la Penha's failure stemmed from his difficulty to encapsulate the functions of *Kläger* and *Ankläger*[1]—that is, to bear witness while being a witness, as Devin Pendas has put it.[2] Much more, his failure to win a hearing also reflects the slowness of many German legal and medical circles to deal with past in a way that honored its victims instead of continuing to traumatize them. I thus propose that de la Penha's confusion of forensic details does not lessen the value of his lament. The evidence wielded by defense lawyers to shred the testimony of prosecution witnesses was enough *then*, but should not be allowed the last word *now*. De la Penha's plight becomes clearer after a brief discussion of Nazi medical crimes, the role of witnesses in postwar trials, and the ritual of medical evaluation required for camp survivors such as de la Penha who sought compensation from the FRG.

There is no question that the Nazi regime was intentional about inflicting suffering on racial prisoners. The *Gesetz zur Verhütung erbkranken Nachwuchses* (Law for the Prevention of Hereditarily Diseased Offspring) passed in July 1933 was a warning of the harm, especially sterilization, awaiting the feeble-minded, Jews, Sinti, and Roma on the "inner front." In the camps, SS doctors were empowered to inflict damage in the form of experiments justified as benefiting the German ethnic community. While Carl Clauberg and Josef Mengele have long been associated with merciless experimentation, treachery for most prisoners came at the hands of lesser-known doctors. Alexander Mitscherlich estimated that some 350 members of 90,000 active German doctors chose to use "Menschenmaterial" for medical crimes.[3]

Doctors transplanted tissue and injected prisoners with disease to determine reactions, tolerance thresholds, and pace of death. They operated without anesthesia, administered drug overdoses, and injected lethal phenol dosages to the heart. They sterilized children under ten years old. They falsified death certificates and presided at executions, or left patients to starve and freeze to death. When it came time to answer for such crimes, however, SS camp doctors claimed that their efforts to improve sanitary and dietary conditions had been resisted by their superiors. Eduard Wirths, chief doctor at Auschwitz, for example, claimed that his "Christian and doctoral" conscience motivated him to help sick prisoners while rendering him suspicious to his superiors in Berlin and to the Political Division within Auschwitz.[4]

Under Wirths's leadership, SS doctors at the ramp at Auschwitz-Birkenau shared the duty of signaling mothers with children along with elderly and fragile prisoners toward the line that ended with suffocation in the gas chamber. Able-bodied or simply lucky prisoners, rarely more than 25 percent of a transport, were motioned toward another line that exploited them as laborers.[5] After monitoring the safety of orderlies who fed Zyklon B granules through the gas chamber roof, doctors confirmed the suffocation of the deportees. Surviving a ramp selection did not guarantee immunity from later selections in hospitals and barracks, held by often volatile doctors for the sake of controlling disease and making room for additional prisoners. Hence, selections strengthened the disorientation already produced by a harrowing train journey. Involvement in selections was a common charge leveled against camp doctors in postwar trials. The twenty-year statute of limitations for murder was extended in 1965, but no extension came after the 1955 deadline passed for prosecuting beatings, sterilizations, and other harm done to prisoners. SS laws emphasized the opposite of civil laws: they prohibited excess brutality but rewarded the following of orders that ensured an efficient killing machine. Doctors could count on extra rations following selection stints.

In the aftermath of war, racial prisoners especially were understandably more concerned about finding family members and convalescing than about testifying against their captors. Still, whether volunteered or requested, their affidavits and depositions were among the documents available as evidence against the twenty-four Nazi officers tried by the International Military Tribunal in Nuremberg in 1946. Donald Bloxham has pointed out that Robert H. Jackson, chief prosecutor for the United States, privileged documentary evidence over the testimony of racial victim groups that he worried would detract attention from political or religious "victims of fascism" and endanger impartiality.[6] While it is easy to agree with Bloxham's negative assessment of Jackson's view of victim testimony, one must also remember that urgent deadlines for fashioning indictments affected the choice of which documents to present as evidence from the vast body available to the Allies.

In the 1946 Doctors Trial, one of the American-hosted subsequent trials, thirty-two witnesses appeared for the prosecution, although documentary evidence sufficed to easily hang a third of the twenty doctors while bringing to light the decisions that paved the way for euthanasia inflicted on both German and non-German citizens, as well as for experimentation on prisoners considered unworthy of life.[7] Another important subsequent trial was the Einsatzgruppen Trial against Otto Ohlendorf and others in 1947. Ohlendorf and his defense lawyer Rudolf Aschenauer, a former Nazi Party member whose scores of Nazi clients later included Franz Lucas, justified the murder of ninety thousand Jewish noncombatants by Ohlendorf's *Einsatzgruppe D* as the result of superior orders issued in the context of preventing Soviet expansionism.[8]

For trials of mobile killing units whose goal was racial annihilation, it was harder for prosecutors to find witnesses alive to testify. Three major British trials benefited from witness affidavits and court appearances, however. The Belsen Trial of "Josef Kramer and 44 Others" that began in Lüneburg in September 1945 featured the commandant of Birkenau who supervised the extermination of Hungarian deportees beginning in May 1944 and later earned the title "Beast of Belsen" as commandant of Bergen-Belsen from December 1944 to April 1945. In this trial, the military court adjudicated war crimes against British citizens, not crimes against humanity. Because only thirty-one witnesses were available to testify—twenty of them Jewish survivors—the court allowed affidavits to be submitted as evidence. Despite the defense's focus on inconsistencies between affidavits and cross-examinations, defendants were overwhelmingly identified as having instigated and participated in selection parades.[9]

Hamburg's Curio-Haus hosted two other important British trials. In the "Zyklon-B Trial against Tesch & Stabenow" in March 1946, defendants were called to account for promoting inhumane camp objectives. The prosecution relied on the firm's employees to testify how the pesticide was multiplied for use in genocide.[10] Half a year later, in the first Ravensbrück Trial of December 1946, five camp doctors among the sixteen defendants were forced to answer for their selections, sterilizations, and other experiments on inmates. Survivor testimonies reflected their subpopulations: Dutch political prisoners petitioned the court to have mercy on Dr. Percy Treite, for example, but medical prisoners testified about his tissue transplants on racial prisoners. One doctor who all witnesses agreed deserved no mercy was Adolf Winkelmann, who came from Sachsenhausen to change places with Lucas at Ravensbrück. As women shuffled past him during selections in March 1945, Winkelmann glanced at their legs to determine their fitness for life or death.[11]

Bonn's parliament outlawed the death penalty in 1949, shortly before West Germany began to prosecute Nazi crimes whose victims were citizens of countries invaded by Hitler's forces.[12] In 1951, "Article 131" pardoned or diminished the sentences of former Nazis while restoring their privileges and positions.[13] The number of trials in West German courts thus dropped in the 1950s due to a lack of any organized effort to hunt down criminals. Ambitious state attorneys lacked support, while witnesses resided in countries lacking diplomatic ties with West Germany. In the climate of amnesty, defendants rarely received life in prison, the highest possible sentence for murder with malicious intent. Instead, by denying charges, shifting blame, and insisting on being forced to carry out superior orders, most defendants received prison sentences as *Gehilfen* (accomplices), ranging from three to fifteen years. The landmark Ulm Einsatzkommando Trial of 1958 set the precedent by ruling that the defendants could only be punished for carrying out the orders of the main perpetrators Hitler, Himmler, and Heydrich.[14]

Two events from the 1950s illustrate the struggle of working through the past, both for victim and perpetrator. The first was the *Bundesentschädigungsgesetz* (Federal Compensation Law, BEG) of 1956, concerned with restitution of victim damages. The second event (examined here first) was the aforementioned Ulm Einsatzkommando Trial of 1958, which showed a renewed effort to prosecute war criminals integrated into West German society. Against formidable odds, chief prosecutor Erwin Schüle broke through the collusion and networking among the ten defendants and the former Nazi judges and physicians (i.e. those who declared defendants fit or unfit for trial) involved in the evidentiary phase.[15] Schüle's two evidence streams included "non-perpetrator, non-German witnesses to the shootings" and "scholarship, which led to the discovery of wartime records and documentation."[16] Schüle was the first West German state attorney to request and receive documents from places such as Nuremberg, Berlin Document Center, and the Deutsche Dienststelle (WASt).[17] With the help of Göttingen historian Hans-Günther Seraphim as an expert witness, Schüle identified areas of responsibility, hierarchies of command, and possibilities of individual agency.[18] If Ohlendorf's trial at Nuremberg had shown the numbers of Jews murdered by mobile killing units, the Ulm trial was the first major focus in German courts on the mass executions of Jews. With no help from the judge, who hoped for a cathartic and didactic effect from the trial,

Schüle's ten-hour-long closing argument featured the testimony of the Lithuanian eyewitness Ona Rudaitis, the only known witness to a mass shooting of Jewish women and children in a meadow outside her village.[19] The trial's conclusion brought calls for a system no longer dependent on chance to discover crimes and recognize criminals.[20] The *Zentrale Stelle der Landesjustizverwaltungen zur Aufklärung nationalsozialistischer Verbrechen* (Central Office of the State Justice Administrations for the Investigation of National Socialist Crimes) that opened in Ludwigsburg in 1958 began coordinating investigations of Nazi murders of civilians in camps outside German borders.[21]

Preceding the Ulm trial by two years was the passing of the BEG in 1956, in which the expert witnesses were psychiatrists who evaluated injuries of claimants to determine whether a loss of 25 percent in productivity was present, thereby qualifying claimants for a pension. It is worth noting, to use José Brunner's terms, the parallels involving claimants as medicalized survivor witnesses, in which they testified for themselves, and as juridical witnesses, in which they testified against war criminals.[22] Whether as subjects of a health court or as witnesses in a criminal court, they had to work doubly hard to reinforce their juridical or compensatory claims.

Most claims were rejected, in Svenja Goltermann's view, because psychiatrists still believed that severe malnourishment (dystrophy) was responsible for psychological suffering.[23] Absent an organic cause, symptoms either derived from preexisting pathologies or were faked by a claimant to draw a pension.[24] Nothing else explained such a late appearance of disturbances, since the psyche was resilient enough for "normal" persons to recover from the effects of stress, whether they were racial victims or German war returnees.[25] Against Goltermann, Dagmar Herzog contends that the German psychiatrists who rejected claims "used every rhetorical strategy at their disposal to refute their critics and justify their decisions."[26] For example, Ernst Kretschmer, the lead researcher on neuroses in West Germany in the 1950s, maintained that most neuroses "had nothing to do with past experiences, but rather with future hopes (for money) or with a 'hypochondriacal' inability to master one's present."[27]

Collusion among evaluators matched the collusion among the doctors who rejected Mitscherlich's efforts in the Doctors Trial in 1947 and the jurists who sabotaged Erwin Schüle's efforts during the Ulm trial. Against reluctance to compensate racial victims, sympathetic assessors made slow inroads. After Hans Strauss requested in 1957 that *Entwurzelungsdepression* (depression caused by being uprooted) be considered a legitimate factor in compensation claims, German legal and medical circles discussed whether psychic damages with no visible organic origin manifested preexisting symptoms or were the delayed result of Nazi persecution.[28] Ulrich Venzlaff, resident physician at the university clinic in Göttingen, suggested that persons overcome by their persecution became psychologically ill beyond the hope of healing, producing a change in personality that was not the result of brain damage.[29]

Sympathizers writing dissenting opinions against initial "rejecters" included such psychiatrists as William Niederland, Kurt Eissler, Klaus Hoppe, and Henry Krystal in the United States, and (besides Strauss and Venzlaff) Walter von Baeyer, Kurt Kolle, and Ernst Kluge in West Germany. Niederland insisted that beatings were not the only abuses that left permanent marks. There was no checkbox—i.e. beyond the formulaic *kein Krankheitswert* (no measurable illness), *nicht verfolgungsbedingt* (not caused by persecution), or *Krankheitswert nicht feststellbar* (indeterminable illness value)—to quantify the humiliation and brushes with death posed by selections, for example.[30] He noted that persecution damaged a survivor's sense of time, accounting for confusion about when events occurred, even what year they were deported to a camp, and such puzzlement hurt one's chances for compensation.[31]

Hundreds of evaluations informed Niederland's compilation of symptoms. What later became ubiquitously referred to as trauma, Niederland first designated as "soul murder" or "survivor syndrome": the loss of initiative, energy, concentration, performance, creativity, and emotional stability, appearing with irritability and restlessness, paranoia, moodiness, dizziness, chronic pain, and sleep disturbances.[32] It was imperative that compensation authorities not view an anxiety disorder as a disposition that predated acute stress. Such "survivor syndromes" anticipated the description of "post-traumatic stress disorder" (PTSD) that entered the *Diagnostic and Statistical Manual of Mental Disorders* in 1980. The symptoms adhered to a schedule of "belated temporality,"[33] as the past frequently intruded into the present years after the survivor had achieved outward normalcy in community, career, and family.

The literary critic Cathy Caruth suggests that pathology consists of the inability to assimilate or experience fully the traumatic event and therefore to be possessed by it: "Central to the very immediacy of this experience . . . is a gap that carries the force of the event . . . at the price of simple knowledge and memory."[34] Insisting on clarity, sociologist Kai Erikson notes that the center of gravity has shifted from the classical medical usage of trauma—as the blow that provoked the injury and which informs the usage "post-traumatic" in PTSD—to the understanding of "trauma" as the disordered state of mind brought about by the event. In this second meaning, how people react to events gives them their traumatic quality, not the events themselves. Hence trauma results "from a *persisting condition* as well as from an acute event . . . from a sustained exposure to battle as well as from a moment of numbing shock, from a continuing pattern of abuse as well as from a single searing assault."[35] Beatings and selections at Auschwitz exemplify the acute and extended trauma endured by Abraham de la Penha. His story is an apt example of the title chosen by neurobiologist Bessel van der Kolk for his bestselling 2015 book, *The Body Keeps the Score*.[36]

Abraham de la Penha's Grievances in the Frankfurt Auschwitz Trial (1963–65)

When magistrate Heinz Düx began his pretrial investigations in October 1962 for the Frankfurt Auschwitz Trial, he was thwarted by his colleagues in much the way that Erwin Schüle was in Ulm.[37] The public *Schlußstrich* mentality wanted the preoccupation with the past to end. A public opinion poll taken in 1966, a year after the trial, showed 69 percent in favor of ending all trials against war criminals, half the percentage determined at the beginning of the Ulm trial.[38] Nearly 1,500 witnesses gave statements. Of the 356 witnesses heard during the trial itself, 220 were survivors of Auschwitz and other camps; of these, 188 resided outside of Germany.[39] Some had waited for years to face their captors, while others dreaded hearing the language of their captors again. The memory of their own transports was still with them when they disembarked in Frankfurt.[40] But when they revealed the crimes that the defendants had committed, they were met with denial and ridicule, while defense lawyers accused them of revenge motives and accepting bribes.[41] A venue such as the Eichmann Trial in Jerusalem in 1961 for telling stories was not possible in Frankfurt.[42]

Abraham de la Penha was thirty-four years old when he arrived at Auschwitz-Birkenau on 19 May 1944 in a transport of Dutch Jews from Westerbork, an SS-controlled transit camp in the Netherlands. When Auschwitz closed in January 1945, he was transferred to Ravensbrück, then to Sachsenhausen in March 1945. When the camp closed the next month, he was forced to march toward Lübeck and was liberated on or about 24 April 1945. He returned to Holland in June 1945 and emigrated to Haifa in February 1950, but returned to Amsterdam in the mid-1950s.[43]

On 26 March 1965, de la Penha testified in Frankfurt that Dr. Lucas had selected him for hard labor upon his arrival. He had recognized Lucas's name from a television special in Amsterdam on 19 December 1964 showing the Auschwitz inspection by the court from 14 to 16 December 1964.[44] A month later, he gave a statement to the Amsterdam police, and two months after that he was in Frankfurt.[45] Lucas, brought into custody only two days before de la Penha's arrival, had finally admitted on 11 March 1965—following fifteen months of denial—to having selected prisoners "three to four times."[46] Instead of supporting the indictment during his forty-four-minute appearance, de la Penha failed to identify Lucas from among the defendants.

De la Penha's first grievance consisted of two beatings suffered at the hands of SS guards. The first beating came during his twelve-hour shift in the munition factory, when a broken machine produced only ten grenade heads instead of two hundred. Twenty lashes from an electric cable made it impossible for him to lie on his back for three months. The second beating came in July or August 1944 after he stumbled and fell against an SS guard, who kicked him and forced him to roll on the ground for over two hundred meters. De la Penha entered the barrack hospital black and blue: "Understand that when you've been beaten, you feel the pain everywhere."[47]

The second grievance involved a selection of de la Penha and fellow prisoners in the hospital. Two SS guards, beaten for poaching lumber in Riga, somehow knew that Lucas would be the selecting doctor in the barrack hospital. When Lucas did arrive, de la Penha recognized him from the ramp selection. He fought his way to the back of the barrack and stood with arms raised in a group of five while numbers from selected prisoners were recorded. Two days later, two trucks arrived to take 150 prisoners to the gas chamber.[48]

When asked to identify his victimizer, de la Penha pointed to the defendant standing next to Lucas. He acknowledged not recognizing Lucas from Dutch newspaper or television footage either, due to the civilian clothes Lucas wore and the span of twenty years that had passed since Auschwitz.[49] He had recognized only the name, not the face, from television footage.[50] As for why he had waited so long to testify, de la Penha averred that he had not followed trial coverage— "I've gone through so much misery, I don't want to read about it"—and that on 19 December 1964 he had happened to watch the news only at a guest's request. Now that his testimony had harmed him more than it had helped the court, he regretted coming forward.[51] Although de la Penha also became flustered having to defend his Dutch mispronunciation ("Lücas"),[52] it was the failure of the visual test that sealed his fate.

Rudolf Aschenauer, Lucas's defense lawyer, asked whether de la Penha was even the prisoner he claimed to be. The deportation date of April 1944 that de la Penha claimed did not match the tattoo A-2744. Aschenauer declared that this number was given to a Belgian Jew who arrived on a transport from Malines on 21 May 1944, and that tattoos beginning with A only went into effect after 13 May 1944 anyway. To believe Aschenauer, if de la Penha could neither identify Lucas nor substantiate his own camp identity, his motive for appearing in court must have been to seek revenge, a natural step after receiving damages from the government. Aschenauer, who with fellow defense lawyer Hans Laternser posed cynical questions to undermine the motives of witnesses for testifying, asked whether de la Penha had applied for compensation. The witness confirmed that he had received "not quite 3,000 Marks" from an office in Amsterdam.

The audio recording of Abraham de la Penha's court performance leaves no doubt that interrogative pressure caught him by surprise and unraveled him after about twenty minutes. Near the end of his forty-four minutes, he blamed his blurred responses on nervousness, and his inability to orient himself on a court map on a poor memory for details. Agitated, he complained, "I've already explained that" and "I won't take that back." He himself had not traveled to Frankfurt to lie, but to explain what he knew: "And what I know I've told, and I can tell you no more than that."[53] His deposition of 25 January 1965 was similarly emphatic: "If this man claims during the trial that he never carried out selections autonomously, then he's lying, because I experienced it twice."[54] Skepticism from both accuser and accused created a stalemate. If the prosecution could not trust Lucas because of his fifteen months of denial, the judges and defense lawyers could scarcely trust de la Penha after his inability to identify his victimizer or to prove himself to be the victim he claimed.

De la Penha's Return to Amsterdam

Christian Raabe, who co-represented fifteen plaintiffs in the trial, resisted Aschenauer's discrediting strategy. Because de la Penha attributed his anxiety to two calamities in the week leading up to 18 December 1964—he witnessed the death of his son from his first marriage and had a kidney removed—Raabe asked the court to accept that de la Penha had recognized Lucas only by name, and that stress accounted for his modifying in court that aspect of his earlier deposition.[55] Translating the experience of Auschwitz to an audience was difficult enough, even when witness and interlocutors spoke the same language.[56] When literal translation was required, interpreters had to settle on terms, convey emotional content, and edit minor mistakes of the witness. When the Red Cross finally found a Belgian translator for de la Penha, he found her incompetent because she spoke softly and translated with difficulty, and this led him to begin his testimony in halting German.[57] The situation improved after Raabe encouraged him to speak Dutch instead, and the interpreter to translate directly instead of indirectly in the third person.[58] Although agitation had created imprecision in de la Penha's deposition and court remarks, Raabe argued that minor errors conveyed more authenticity than testimony that sounded rehearsed: "If he had really wanted to falsely incriminate the defendant, he could have done it much more simply."[59] The court disagreed: "Neither did he recognize Dr Lucas in the main hearing, nor could he give a corresponding description of him. This statement was thus not fruitful for the court."[60]

Even though Lucas had admitted to ramp selections, de la Penha was unable to crack the veneer of Lucas's good behavior that dominated the accounts of mostly prisoner doctors.[61] When he returned to Amsterdam, he told reporters that he had been treated like trash. He had been summoned to appear in Frankfurt, but no one met him when he arrived. At the courthouse, a doorman had ushered him to a room with ten former SS members waiting to give testimony. After two hours, a representative from the Red Cross apologized and brought him to another waiting room. These factors contributed to his perception that he was treated more poorly than the defendants on trial.[62] Abraham de la Penha died on 6 September 1965, less than a half year after testifying. Cancer finished what Auschwitz injuries to his kidneys and other organs had started. Joseph Slagter, director of the Dutch Auschwitz Committee, commented, "There are only a few that have suffered so much as Abraham de la Penha. For him the suffering did not end after a year and a half of KZ-Lager, but it continued for another twenty years."[63]

Conclusion and Implications

Revisiting the account that required so much of de la Penha's fading stamina to convey takes a step toward restoring the integrity stolen from him not just in the camps and in the courtroom but from the very beginning of his racial persecution. The choices that Jewish victims such as de la Penha had between bad and worse aligns with their accidental survival of a war meant to eliminate them.[64] De la Penha's recovery in a barrack hospital with its threat of selections was no less traumatic than receiving the beatings that sent him there. Until Auschwitz, de la Penha had likely never seen doctors trade caregiving for torture, a volatile infliction of pain based on consensus. As Jean Améry pointed out on the basis of his own torture, trust disappeared with the first struck blow: "Whoever was tortured, stays tortured. Torture is ineradicably burned into him, even when no clinically objective traces can be detected."[65] Améry's description of invisible yet burned-in memories overlaps with medical assessments of "survivor syndrome." How were applicants for compensation supposed to quantify such an "invisible" psychological ravage that included selections? The Heidelberg psychiatrist Walter von Baeyer found that witnesses balked when forced to relive traumatic memories in the courtroom: "They became uncertain, hesitated, stuttered, broke into tears, got a rapid heartbeat, could go no further, and the hearing had to be interrupted." They forgot details, especially the sequence of events, partly because the fear and surprise of the initial trauma intake narrowed their level of consciousness. Referring to the *Wahrheitsliebe* (love of truth) of witnesses free of revenge or exaggeration, Baeyer found that minor imprecisions spoke in their favor.[66]

Hearing Lucas's name by accident triggered de la Penha's memories associated with eight months of abuse in Auschwitz. The forensic details were not sharp enough nor the courtroom parameters accommodating enough for de la Penha to communicate his experience to a critical audience. His *Klage* entered an arena of *Anklage* less hospitable to lament.[67] From the standpoint of the court, his testimony was unnecessary to prove that Lucas had performed ramp selections, and Rudolf Aschenauer was eager to point out its flaws.[68] Nevertheless, de la Penha had the courage to express indignation toward former perpetrators who ignored uncomfortable memories by denying responsibility.[69]

Victim testimony is not by nature obliged to concede the victory in the domain of facts to the "hard" evidence generated by the perpetrator. It too contributes to the history, not just the memory, of National Socialism.[70] Renewed investigations may thus deliver the proof for claims made by witnesses whose memories were earlier considered too fragile and unreliable, so long as one follows Christopher Browning's advice to subject survivor testimony "to the same critical analysis and rules of evidence as other sources."[71] Examining de la Penha's attempt to turn lament into accusation—his insistence in the courtroom that he didn't "come here to lie"—points the way for research into earlier discredited victim testimony. The Frankfurt Auschwitz Trial provides over six hundred interrogation protocols from the preliminary investigation alone as a foundation to retrace stories.[72] The International Tracing Service contains Red Cross certificates of incarceration, applications for compensation, and transport lists of deportations. Moreover, the German Federal Archives has recently promised improved access to compensation records by digitizing hundreds of thousands of restitution files that "reflect the unique perspective of the persecuted who described their stories of suffering in compensation hearings."[73]

Abraham de la Penha's failure to have his story acknowledged illustrates the gap between justice and law from the victim's point of view. No such gap adheres in the perspective of the perpetrator. Dr. Lucas's acquittal in 1970, as that retrial transcript shows, came as a foregone legal conclusion, based on his putative fear of Josef Kramer's retaliation if he refused to perform selections on the Birkenau ramp. Lucas's self-depiction as fearful victim was enhanced by character references from predominantly defense witnesses and resulted in a verdict that restored his civil rights and allowed him to return to medical practice. While serving all but three months of his sentence of three years and three months, Lucas had time to fashion a narrative that effectively retracted the confession he gave under pressure in March 1965. In 1970, his defense lawyers went on the offensive, criticizing the Frankfurt court in 1965 for putting behind bars a meek man long since punished beyond measure.[74] Rather than conceding an inevitable triumph of law over justice—comparable to the "learning by doing" that may account for the slow acknowledgment of victim-compensation claims—the historian needs to be the first to shatter resignation. Devoting thoughtful attention to victims robbed of dignity through trauma and retraumatization contributes to the ongoing labor of justice that overturns disorder with order, as Hannah Arendt insisted shortly after witnessing a day of the Frankfurt Auschwitz Trial.[75]

Andrew Wisely, PhD, is associate professor of German in the Department of Modern Languages and Cultures at Baylor University (Waco, Texas). He is the author of *Arthur Schnitzler and Twentieth-Century Criticism* (2004). He is currently completing the book *Between Auschwitz and Frankfurt: The Exception and Deception of SS-Doctor Franz Lucas (1911–1994)*.

Notes

1. Weigel 2000, 128.
2. For a summary of witness participation, see Pendas 2006, esp. 161–68.
3. Mitscherlich and Mielke 1960, 17. See note 7 below.
4. See Wirths 1945/2005, 38–57, esp. 39.
5. "Straftaten des Angeklagten Dr. Lucas," *Der Auschwitz-Prozess: Tonbandmitschnitte, Protokolle, Dokumente*, ed. Fritz Bauer Institut Frankfurt am Main and Staatliches Museum Auschwitz-Birkenau (Zeno.org: Berlin, 2007), DVD-ROM, AP 37,878–79. Subsequent source references appear as AP followed by page numbers.
6. Bloxham 2008, 541–42.
7. Appointed as trial observers for the Chamber of West German Physicians, Alexander Mitscherlich and his student Fred Mielke printed a compilation of the trial evidence and protocols as "Das Diktat der Menschenverachtung" in 1947 and in 1949 as "Wissenschaftlichkeit ohne Menschlichkeit." A year after Mielke died, Mitscherlich published the documentation as *Medizin ohne Menschlichkeit: Dokumente des Nürnberger Ärzteprozesses* (Mitscherlich and Mielke 1960). For a summary of the resistance from German physicians to Mitscherlich's documentation, see Pross 1991, 13–16.
8. For a full account of the trial's origins and outcomes, see Earl 2009.
9. *Law Reports of Trials of War Criminals*, vol. 2: *The Belsen Trial* (London: United Nations War Crimes Commission, 1947), 9–23, 132, 138.
10. Ebbinghaus 1998, 19.
11. Testimony of Marie Claude Vaillant-Couturier, 28 January 1946, *Nuremberg Trial Proceedings*, vol. 6, IMT Day 44, p. 224, Yale Law School, Lillian Goldman Law Library, *The Avalon Project: Documents in Law, History and Diplomacy*, retrieved 24 December 2019 from https://avalon.law.yale.edu/imt/01-28-46.asp.
12. The GDR executed former Auschwitz doctor Horst Fischer in 1966. See Dirks 2005.
13. Frei 1996 [repr. Munich: DTV, 2003], 19.
14. Langbein 1963, 79–83. Langbein also showed that the number of German trials concluded between 1958 and 1963 for mass murder (42) almost doubled the number of similar trials completed before 1958 (23). The number of defendants rose almost 500 percent from 28 before 1958 to 136 thereafter. Of those 136 defendants, 9 were convicted of murder, 77 were convicted as accomplices to murder, and 36 were acquitted. Of the 77 accomplices—i.e. they did not "will" the murders or carry them out with "bloodlust"—43 received three to five years in prison. Of those 43, 30 were charged with assisting in the murders of between 100 and 15,000 victims (Langbein 1963, 117–18). See also Miquel 2004, 158–59. Also helpful for an overview are Rückerl 1979 and Reichel 2000.
15. See Tobin 2013 and Weinke 2008.
16. Tobin 2013, 192.
17. Tobin 2013, 187–206; Weinke 2008, 15.
18. Tobin 2013, 217.
19. Miquel 2004, 156–57.
20. Miquel 2004, 160–61.
21. Rückerl 1979, 50–53.
22. Brunner 2012, 93–110, esp. 94–97.
23. Goltermann 2009, 431.
24. Goltermann 2009, 430–31.
25. Goltermann 2009, 435–36.
26. Herzog 2014, 132.
27. Herzog 2014, 140.

28. Goltermann 2009, 437–40.
29. Goltermann 2009, 444–45.
30. Niederland 1980, 7.
31. Niederland 1980, 230–31.
32. Niederland 1980, 233–34.
33. LaCapra 2001, 89.
34. Caruth 1995, 4–5, 7.
35. Erikson 1995, 184–85 (emphasis in original).
36. Kolk 2015.
37. Düx 2003.
38. Wojak 2001, 25.
39. Renz 2000, 41.
40. Wagner 2010, 349–50.
41. See Ritz 2007, 57; and Wagner 2010, 349–50.
42. For a discussion of testimony in the Eichmann Trial, see part 2 of Douglas 2001.
43. Douglas 2001, AP 31,026. Yad Vashem, scan of International Tracing Service file, Abraham de la Penha (1909–1965), "Antrag d. Compensation Treuhand GmbH. Frankfurt/Main, Az: CP/9802 SD," 23 October 1962.
44. De la Penha 1965b, AP 30,998. See also Nina Burkhardt, *Rückblende: NS-Prozesse und die mediale Repräsentation der Vergangenheit in Belgien und den Niederlanden* (Münster: Waxmann, 2009), 170–71. The twenty defendants consisted of three administrators, four Political Division officers, five guards, a doctor, two dentists, a pharmacist, three medical orderlies, and a former prisoner. Lucas was also the only free defendant who elected to make the fact-finding trip to Auschwitz along with prosecutors, judges, and journalists.
45. De la Penha 1965b, AP 30,987–91.
46. Lucas served thirty-six months of the thirty-nine-month sentence levied on 19 August 1965 for four counts of accessory to genocide of at least a thousand Jews in each of the transports he selected. Lucas was the only one of the eventual twenty defendants to be granted a trial on appeal in 1970 that ended in his acquittal.
47. De la Penha 1965b, AP 30,992–94; 31,007–8.
48. De la Penha 1965b, AP 30,995–98.
49. De la Penha 1965b, AP 31,012–13.
50. De la Penha 1965b, AP 31,005–6; 30,098.
51. De la Penha 1965b, AP 31,001–2.
52. De la Penha 1965b, AP 31,009–10.
53. De la Penha 1965b, AP 31,019–27; 31,033.
54. De la Penha 1965a.
55. De la Penha 1965b, AP 31,020–23.
56. Insana 2009, 17.
57. *Het Parool* 1965a.
58. De la Penha 1965b, AP 31,022.
59. "Plädoyer des Nebenklagevertreters Raabe zu Lucas, Frank, Schatz, Breitwieser, Stark, Boger, Baretzki, Scherpe, Hantl, Mulka u. Höcker," 21 May 1965, AP 33,874.
60. "Fortsetzung der mündlichen Urteilsbegründung des Vorsitzenden Richters," 20 August 1965, AP 36,966.
61. Some examples are the prisoner doctors Tadeusz Sniesko, Tadeusz Szymanski, and Aron Bejlin from Auschwitz-Birkenau, and the prisoners Margareta Armbruster, Johanna Dyer, Karl Gerber, Louise le Porz, Cäcilie Neideck, and Helene Schwesig from Ravensbrück.
62. "Nederlandse ooggetuige in een hoek gedreven," *Trouw*, 30 March 1965.
63. *Het Parool* 1965b.

64. Langer 1991, 71.
65. Améry 1980, 34. Améry's description of his experiences emerged as he observed the Frankfurt Auschwitz Trial (xii).
66. Von Baeyer 1970, 85, 87–89.
67. Weigel 2000, 128.
68. Calling de la Penha the most unreliable witness for the prosecution, Aschenauer maintained that Auschwitz was never used as a prison for SS members and that in 1944 no Aryan prisoners were subject to *Aktion 14f13*—that is, to selections (Rudolf Aschenauer, "Plädoyer für Lucas, 21 June 1965," 11).
69. LaCapra 1998, 10.
70. Weigel 2000, 124.
71. Browning 2003, 40, 43.
72. Renz 2002, 637.
73. See 12 November 2019 report on Bundesarchiv conference of 14–15 October 2019 in Bayreuth: "Kriegsfolgenarchivgut: Entschädigung, Lastenausgleich und Wiedergutmachung in Archivierung und Forschung," retrieved 13 January 2020 from https://www.bundesarchiv.de/DE/Content/Meldungen/2019-11-12_kriegsfolgenarchivgut.html.
74. "Revisionsverfahren Dr. Franz Lucas," Öffentliche Sitzung des Schurgerichts 4 Ks 2/63, Frankfurt am Main, 20 August to 8 October 1970, Hessisches Hauptstaatsarchiv Wiesbaden, 461/37638.
75. Arendt and Fest 2011, 57.

References

Améry, Jean. 1980. *At the Mind's Limit: Contemplations by a Survivor of Auschwitz and its Realities*. Translated by Sidney Rosenfeld and Stella P. Rosenfeld. Bloomington: Indiana University Press.
Arendt, Hannah, and Joachim Fest. 2011. "'Eichmann war von empörender Dummheit': Hannah Arendt—Joachim Fest: Die Rundfunksendung vom 9. November 1964." In *Eichmann war von empörender Dummheit: Gespräche und Briefe*, edited by Ursula Ludz and Thomas Wild, 362–60. Munich: Piper.
Aschenauer, Rudolf. "Plädoyer für Lucas, 21 June 1965." Fritz Bauer Institut Archiv (Frankfurt), FAP 1, V-23.
Auschwitz-Prozess, Der. Tonbandmitschnitte, Protokolle, Dokumente. 2007. Edited by Fritz Bauer Institut Frankfurt am Main and Staatliches Museum Auschwitz-Birkenau. Berlin: Zeno.org. DVD-ROM. Referenced as *AP*.
Bloxham, Donald. 2008. "Jewish Witnesses in War Crimes Trials of the Postwar Era." In *Holocaust Historiography in Context: Emergence, Challenges, Polemics and Achievements*, edited by David Bankier and Dan Michman, 539–53. Jerusalem: Berghahn Books.
Brunner, José. 2012. "Medikalisierte Zeugenschaft: Trauma, Institutionen, Nachträglichkeit." In *Die Geburt des Zeitzeugen nach 1945*, edited by Martin Sabrow and Norbert Frei, 93–110. Göttingen: Wallstein.
Burkhardt, Nina. 2009. *Rückblende: NS-Prozesse und die mediale Repräsentation der Vergangenheit in Belgien und den Niederlanden*. Münster: Waxmann.
de la Penha, Abraham. 1962. Yad Vashem, scan of International Tracing Service file, Abraham de la Penha (1909–1965). Antrag d. Compensation Treuhand GmbH. Frankfurt am Main. Az: CP/9802 SD, 23 October.
———. 1965a. "Deposition of 25 January 1965 to Reiner Scherer, Reichsfahndungsdienst Amsterdam." Fritz Bauer Institut (Frankfurt). Lucas file.
———. 1965b. "Vernehmung des Zeugen Abraham de la Penha." 26 March. AP 30,987–31,035.

Dirks, Christian. 2005. *Die Verbrechen der anderen: Auschwitz und der Auschwitz-Prozess der DDR. Das Verfahren gegen den KZ-Arzt Dr. Horst Fischer*. Paderborn: Schöningh.
Douglas, Lawrence. 2001. *The Memory of Judgment: Making Law and History in the Trials of the Holocaust*. New Haven, CT: Yale University Press.
Düx, Heinz. 2003. "Der Auschwitz Prozess: Ein unerwünschtes Strafverfahren in den Zeiten der Verbrechensleugnung und des Kalten Krieges." In *Im Labyrinth der Schuld: Täter—Opfer—Ankläger*, edited by Irmtrud Wojak and Susanne Meinl, 267–84. Frankfurt am Main: Campus.
Ebbinghaus, Angelika. 1998. "Der Prozeß gegen Tesch & Stabenow: Von der Schädlingsbekämpfung zum Holocaust." *1999: Zeitschrift für Sozialgeschichte des 20. und 21. Jahrhunderts* 13(2): 16–71.
"Fortsetzung der mündlichen Urteilsbegründung des Vorsitzenden Richters [Hans Hofmeyer], 20 August 1965." AP 36,875–37,081.
Frei, Norbert. 1996. *Vergangenheitspolitik. Die Anfänge der Bundesrepublik und die NS-Vergangenheit*. Munich: Beck [repr. Munich: DTV, 2003].
Goltermann, Svenja. 2009. "Kausalitätsfragen: Psychisches Leid und psychisches Wissen in der Entschädigung." In *Die Praxis der Wiedergutmachung: Geschichte, Erfahrung, und Wirkung in Deutschland und Israel*, edited by Norbert Frei, José Brunner, and Constantin Goschler, 427–51. Göttingen: Wallstein.
Herzog, Dagmar. 2014. "The Obscenity of Objectivity: Post-Holocaust Anti-Semitism and the Invention-Discovery of Post-Traumatic Stress Disorder." In *Catastrophes: A History and Theory of an Operative Concept*, edited by Nitzan Lebovic and Andreas Killen, 128–55. Oldenbourg: De Gruyter.
Het Parool (Amsterdam). 1965a. "A. de la Penha, die in Auschwitzproces ex-kamparts dr. Lucas moest aanwijzen: 'Getuigen was ellendig.' Amsterdammer zat twee uur tussen Duitse SS'ers te wachten en kreeg slechte tolk." 29 March.
———. 1965b. "Na-oorlogse jaren brachten niets." 7 September.
Insana, Lina. 2009. *Arduous Tasks: Primo Levi, Translation, and Transmission of Holocaust Testimony*. Toronto: University of Toronto Press.
LaCapra, Dominick. 1998. *History and Memory after Auschwitz*. Ithaca: Cornell University Press.
———. 2001. *Writing History, Writing Trauma*. Baltimore: Johns Hopkins University Press.
Langbein, Hermann. 1963. *Im Namen des deutschen Volkes: Zwischenbilanz der Prozesse wegen nationalsozialistischer Verbrechen*. Vienna: Europa Verlag.
Langer, Lawrence. 1991. *Holocaust Testimonies: The Ruins of Memory*. New Haven, CT: Yale University Press.
Mitscherlich, Alexander, and Fred Mielke. 1960. *Medizin ohne Menschlichkeit: Dokumente des Nürnberger Ärzteprozesses*. Frankfurt am Main: Fischer.
Miquel, Marc von. 2004. *Ahnden oder amnestieren? Westdeutsche Justiz und Vergangenheitspolitik in den sechziger Jahren*. Göttingen: Wallstein.
Nuremberg Trial Proceedings. 1945. Testimony of Marie Claude Vaillant-Couturier, 28 January 1945. Vol. 6, Day 44. Yale Law School, Lillian Goldman Law Library, *The Avalon Project: Documents in Law, History and Diplomacy*. Retrieved 24 December 2019 https://avalon.law.yale.edu/imt/01-28-46.asp.
Pendas, Devin. 2006. *The Frankfurt Auschwitz Trial, 1963–1965: Genocide, History, and the Limits of the Law*. New York: Cambridge University Press.
Pross, Christian. 1991. "Breaking through the Postwar Coverup of Nazi doctors in Germany." *Journal of Medical Ethics* 17 (supplement): 13–16.
Raabe, Christian. 1965. "Plädoyer des Nebenklagevertreters Raabe zu Lucas, Frank, Schatz, Breitwieser, Stark, Boger, Baretzki, Schere, Hantl, Mulka u. Höcker." 21 May. AP 33,854–976.
Reichel, Peter. 2000. *Vergangenheitsbewältigung in Deutschland: Die Auseinandersetzung mit der NS-Diktatur in Politik und Justiz*. Munich: Beck.
Renz, Werner. 2000. "Der erste Frankfurter Auschwitz-Prozeß: Völkermord als Strafsache." *Zeitschrift für Sozialgeschichte des 20. und 21. Jahrhunderts* 15(2): 11–48.

———. 2002. "Der 1. Frankfurter Auschwitz-Prozess: Zwei Vorgeschichten." *Zeitschrift für Geschichtswissenschaft* 50(7) (July): 622–41.

Ritz, Christian. 2007. "Die westdeutsche Nebenklagevertretung in den Frankfurter Auschwitz-Prozessen und im Verfahrenskomplex Krumey/Hunsche." *Kritische Justiz* 1: 51–72.

Rückerl, Adalbert. 1979. *Die Strafverfolgung von NS-Verbrechen 1945–1978: Eine Dokumentation*. Heidelberg: C. F. Müller Juristischer Verlag, 1979.

Tobin, Patrick. 2013 "Crossroads at Ulm: Postwar West Germany and the 1958 Ulm EKO Trial." PhD thesis, University of North Carolina, Chapel Hill.

Trouw (Amsterdam). 1965. "Nederlandse ooggetuige in een hoek gedreven." 30 March.

van der Kolk, Bessel. 2015. *The Body Keeps the Score: Brain, Mind, and Body in the Healing of Trauma*. London: Penguin.

von Baeyer, Walter. 1970. "Gutachten über Fragen der Glaubwürdigkeit und Erinnerungszuverlässigkeit bei der Beurteilung von Zeugenaussagen rassisch Verfolgter, die weit zurückliegenden Extrembelastungen ausgesetzt waren." *Nervenarzt* 41: 83–89.

Wagner, Julie. 2010. "The Truth about Auschwitz: Prosecuting Auschwitz Crimes with the Help of Survivor Testimony." *German History* 28(3): 343–57.

Weigel, Sigrid. 2000. "Zeugnis und Zeugenschaft, Klage und Anklage: Die Geste des Bezeugens in der Differenz von 'identity politics,' juristischem und historiographischem Diskurs." In *Einstein Forum Jahrbuch 1999: Zeugnis und Zeugenschaft*, edited by Rüdiger Zill, 111–35. Berlin: Akad. Verlag.

Weinke, Annette. 2008. *Eine Gesellschaft ermittelt gegen sich selbst: Die Geschichte der Zentralen Stelle Ludwigsburg 1958–2008*. Darmstadt: WBG.

Wirths, Eduard. 1945/2005. "Verteidigungsschrift." In *Dr. med. Eduard Wirths: Ein Arzt in Auschwitz. Eine Quelleneditiion*, edited by Ulrich Völklein, 38–57. Norderstedt: Books on Demand.

Wojak, Irmtrud. 2001. "'Die Mauer des Schweigens durchbrochen': Der erste Frankfurter Auschwitz-Prozess 1963–1965." In *"Gerichtstag halten über uns selbst . . .": Geschichte und Wirkung des ersten Frankfurter Auschwitz-Prozesses*, edited by Irmtrud Wojak, 21–42. Frankfurt am Main: Campus.

Wojak, Irmtrud, and Susanne Meinl (eds.). 2003. *Im Labyrinth der Schuld: Täter—Opfer—Ankläger*. Frankfurt am Main: Campus.

CHAPTER 14

"SCHLUSS MIT DER RASSENSCHANDE!" FROM SEPARATION TO EXTERMINATION

The Fate of Jewish Mentally Ill Patients in Germany and Occupied Poland, 1939–42

Kamila Uzarczyk

The history of National Socialist (NS) "euthanasia" has been a subject of much research over the last decades. However, the stories and fates of victims and survivors of this medical crime need further exploration, especially when it comes to atrocities that were committed in the occupied territories. This study aims to contribute to this narrative by investigating the larger history of German medical atrocities in Poland through the detailed study of the activities at one psychiatric hospital for Jewish patients, the sanatorium Zofiówka in Otwock Ghetto. Based on archival materials and eyewitness statements, this chapter presents an insight into the machinations of the destruction of Jewish psychiatric patients. This subject is placed here also in the background of the wider plans by the National Socialist regime for the destruction of not only of the Jewish mentally ill but of all of European Jewry.

"The Branches of the Acacia Tree"

... In the morning of 19. August I woke up because of shooting. Shots were discharged isolated and in salvoes, and then again more powerful explosions—dull, like a hammer's blow against a wooden panel—hand grenades. I approached the window. Perfectly clear sky, sun, motion-less branches in the trees. Another day was about to start, hot and sultry. ... I went back to bed and I was trying to read. *Lord Jim* by Conrad. However, the continuous shooting was quite disturbing. I put the book aside. Many quarter hours went past while I was smoking one cigarette after another and thinking what was happening there, in the ghetto, Jewish orphanage and the sanatorium. . . . Knocking on the door, Mary, our maid, brought breakfast. She was pale and agitated. In short, interrupted, sentences she reported the events of this night. At 3 a.m. the Gestapo began clearing the ghetto. Jews had been thrown out of the sanatorium and rushed to the main ghetto. Some of them ran away looking for hiding places in the surrounding forest and the bushes. They are now hunting for them. Those who were more severely sick, not able to walk on their own, were shot on the premises. The doctors committed suicide. The mentally ill were killed with grenades.[1]

This excerpt from the 1942 essay "Gałązki akacji" (The branches of the acacia tree) by the theater director Edmund Wierciński (1899–1955) is a rare example of Polish literature referring specifically to the killings of mentally ill Jewish patients in the occupied territory, General Government. These few lines have been "inserted" into the main narrative on the liquidation of ghetto in Otwock, near Warsaw, on 19 August 1942. "Jewish patients were not distinguished as a group because of their illness. They were killed because they were Jews and the way the other Jews were killed."[2]

The author did not personally witness the events of that night; however, he did have a firsthand impression of the town as the scene of annihilation, since at the time he was a patient at the clinic for pulmonary diseases, located in the immediate vicinity of the Hospital for Nervous and Mentally Ill Jews—Zofiówka in Otwock.

"Isolation Colony for Distorted Human Souls"— Sanatorium Zofiówka

The Asylum for Nervous and Mentally Ill Jews in Otwock was founded on the initiative of the Society for Care of Nervous and Mentally Ill Poor Jews, established in Warsaw in 1906. In 1907, the society acquired a piece of land in Otwock, near Warsaw, and thanks to a generous donation from Zofia Endelman, two pavilions with the capacity for forty male and forty female patients began to operate in 1908 and 1910 respectively. The third pavilion, opened in 1926, completed the asylum complex surrounded by pine forest and commonly known as "Zofiówka." Apart from the pavilions for the poor patients, scattered comfortable villas for wealthier convalescents complemented the picturesque, hilly landscape.[3]

The choice of location for Zofiówka Sanatorium, as it was often referred to, was not an accidental one. For a long time Otwock had enjoyed a high reputation for its beneficial climatic conditions and had become increasingly famous as a health resort for pulmonary diseases, mostly tuberculosis. Here, in 1893, Dr. Józef Marian Geisler (1859–1924) opened the first lowland sanatorium specializing in the treatment of tuberculosis, followed soon by the initiative of Dr. Władysław Przygoda (1880–1937) and his sanatorium for Jewish patients, which opened in 1895. The rising popularity of Otwock as a health resort among the Jewish middle classes went hand in hand with an increase of the Jewish population in the town. Thus, in turn, Otwock may have been seen as an obvious location for further similar institutions, to mention only the Martów Sanatorium (1908), the Abram Górewicz rest home (1906–1921) or famous Brijus Sanatorium (1914). Additionally, the specific microclimate of the region was also believed to have a soothing influence on patients suffering from nervous disorders and general apathy, who "thanks to the particular working of the Otwock air regain appetite, willingness to work and sexual desire."[4]

The majority of the patients admitted to Zofiówka suffered from milder nervous dysfunctions and were usually put on work therapy, the concept first introduced in 1905 in Gütersloh by Hermann Simon (1867–1947). In Zofiówka it was initiated by the eminent neurologist Samuel Goldflam (1852–1932), director of the hospital from 1910 to 1926, and remained a method of choice even when more expensive shock therapies such as insulin therapy or cardiazol convulsive therapy became available in 1930. Cezary Jellenta vel Napoleon Hirszband (1861–1935), a writer and poet who spent the last months of his life on a rest cure in Otwock, described the miraculous efficacy of work therapy, which was supposed to ensure serenity and a feeling of belonging:

> This aspect of Inferno [sic] has an immediate soothing effect on the visitors. . . . It's now work-time. All patients—or almost all—and there are around 200 of both men and women, do something, all the quiet ones let themselves be brought under control, put in order and rhyme, experience some kind of social bonding, social rhythm.[5]

In the course of time, the asylum developed into a well-organized hospital with a farm and workshops, and on the eve of the war around 120 staff members and 9 full-time physicians were employed on contracts.[6] Directed by distinguished scientists and practitioners, such as Goldflam, Rafał Becker (1891–1939?) and Jakub Frostig (1896–1959),[7] Zofiówka became a widely recognized center of psychiatric care and in 1938 provided the most recent methods of treatment for nearly 400 patients. The outbreak of the war radically changed this situation. Zofiówka was designated as the only hospital for Jewish patients in the General Government; inevitably, overcrowding and staggering financial troubles resulted in a dramatically increased mortality rate, which preceded the final liquidation of the hospital on 19 August 1942.

"Schluss mit der Rassenschande!"[8] From Separation to Extermination

First NS German demands to separate Jewish from non-Jewish patients in designated institutions were formulated a few years before the war. As early as 1936, during a meeting of the directors of mental care institutions in Brandenburg on 15 January 1936, concerns were raised over various incidents that had occurred when Jewish and non-Jewish patients shared lodgings in the clinics, and therefore the practice should be discontinued. Jewish patients—it was suggested—should be housed separately in Jewish institutions.[9] Shortly afterward, in a letter to provincial authorities, Hans Pfundtner, German secretary of state from 1933 to 1943, pointed out that this fundamental shortcoming of the health service system posed a threat of *Rassenschande* and recommended that, in order to minimize the danger of race defilement, Jewish patients should be physically isolated in separate wards or institutions. Referring to the ministerial decree of 22 June 1938, he also ordered the provincial administration to prepare a detailed survey of the conditions in local medical and social care institutions, including the number of Jewish patients and their distribution according to sex.[10] Historian Henry Friedlander commented,

> This bureaucratic order, designed to apply the Nürnberg racial laws with utmost stringency, caused consternation in government agencies that administered state hospitals. Although the administrators agreed with the goal of the order, they argued that race defilement was impossible because male and female patients were housed in separate wards. They also objected to the financial burden physical separation would impose on their hospitals. . . . Nevertheless, local agencies moved to comply.[11]

By the end of August 1938, the various institutions submitted their required data; however, interesting arguments were voiced by provincial authorities of Saxony:

> On the one hand—it was argued—putting into practice ministerial instructions could mean better conditions for Jewish patients in the hospitals; on the other, however, medical personnel in the hospitals might have reservations to attend exclusively Jewish patients.[12]

Therefore the concentration of Jewish patients in one designated Jewish hospital, managed by Jewish personnel, was suggested as the best way to deal with the problem. The wheel had been set in motion and efficiently nurtured a race defilement panic. "In May 1939 the state hospital in Weinsberg notified the Ministry that it feared the relatives of German patients would protest if they [the patients] continued to share quarters with Jews."[13] Also, medical personnel were said to have complained that they had to attend Jewish patients.[14] These claims, however, have never been documented.

On 4 July 1939 the tenth directive to the Reich Citizenship Law (*Reichsbürgergesetz*) ordered the Reich Association of Jews in Germany (Reichsvereinigung der Juden in Deutschland—RdJ) to take over the cost of treatment for Jewish patients and to place all mentally ill Jews—estimated between twenty-five hundred and three thousand—exclusively in Jewish institutions. The only Jewish psychiatric hospital near Koblenz, founded in 1870 by Meier Jacoby (1818–1890),[15] had a capacity for only around two hundred patients; therefore the RdJ suggested a concentration of Jewish patients in separate wards in public mental care institutions. In Silesia, for example, female patients were to be transferred to Branitz (Branice) and male patients to Leubus (Lubiąż), and the first steps to organize the transfers were taken in August 1939. The outbreak of the war put a stop to this initiative.[16] Soon Jewish patients were targeted within the T4 and "euthanasia" special action (*Euthanasie-Sonderaktion*).

During the first months of the T4 program, Jewish patients were included in the "euthanasia" program as individuals. In summer 1940 they were targeted as a group and selected for the transports without any of the medical examination afforded to non-Jewish patients.[17] On 15 April 1940 Herbert Linden of the Reichsministerium des Innern (RMdI) demanded detailed information as to the number of Jewish patients in provincial psychiatric clinics. Shortly afterward, a ministerial directive instructed that all Jewish patients should be transferred to one of the designated assembly clinics: Berlin-Buch, Egfling-Haar, Hamburg-Langenhorn, Wunsdorf, Am Steinhof in Wien, Leubus, Giessen, Heppenheim, Grafenberg, and Andernach.[18] According to the official version, from there the patients were to be deported to psychiatric hospitals in General Government. In fact they were transported to "euthanasia" killing centers in Brandenburg, Hadamar, and Hartheim.[19] Group transports to the killing facilities took place from July 1940 (Berlin-Buch) to December 1940 (Leubus), and in autumn 1940 Jewish communities in various provinces began to receive death notifications from the psychiatric clinic Cholm/Chelm near Lublin in the General Government.[20] An estimated 1,794 patients,[21] identified by name, perished during the "euthanasia" *Euthanasie-Sonderaktion* in the summer of 1940. Despite intensive research, it remains unknown how many Jewish patients were included in T4[22] transports or killed during the liquidation of psychiatric hospitals in occupied territories. In Poland, Jewish patients in prewar years were frequently admitted to hospitals other than Zofiówka, but witness statements only occasionally refer the deportations of Jewish inmates as a distinguished group.[23] Historians approximate that altogether up to five thousand mentally ill Jews fell victim to the deportations and "euthanasia" operations.[24]

To avoid future admissions of Jewish patients to German clinics, Herbert Linden of RMdI decreed on 12 December 1940 that Jewish patients, apart from those admitted before 1 October 1940, should be admitted exclusively to Bendorf-Sayn near Koblenz. Due to the wave of new arrivals, conditions in the hospital deteriorated dramatically, and many patients had to be placed in ad hoc barracks built in the garden. According to the report filed by medical director Wilhelm Rosenau (1898–1968) in response to a demand by the Gestapo, as many as 422 patients (167 men and 255 women) were treated in Bendorf-Sayn in February 1942.[25] This report served as a basis for transport lists to the east: from March to November 1942, an estimated 512 patients[26] were deported to the death camps, where they perished. On 10 November 1942 Bendorf-Sayn ceased to exist as a Jewish psychiatric hospital, and after a period of discussions it was used as an alternate hospital facility for Koblenz. Henceforth, all remaining Jewish patients were to be sent to the psychiatric ward of the Jewish hospital in Berlin in Iranische Strasse. From there, within a year, all patients were deported to the death camps, and on 22 November 1943 the ward was dissolved.[27]

As Bendorf-Sayn served as a central psychiatric hospital for Jewish patients in Germany, the corresponding institution in the occupied Polish territory—General Government—was Zofiówka.

"Spa District" in the Ghetto

The outbreak of the war radically changed the situation in Zofiówka in many aspects. Some members of the medical personnel decided to leave and look for safety in Soviet-occupied eastern territories, in psychiatric hospitals in Kulparków and Choroszcz. Even though several were replaced by Jewish physicians who had been evicted or fled from Kraj Warty (Warthegau),[28] the number of physicians and nursing assistants was insufficient in relation to the increasing number of patients.[29] Moreover, from the very beginning the hospital's administration had to face great financial problems. A majority of the patients could not cover the cost of treatment and had to rely on Jewish welfare agencies, which were also lacking funds; payments were often much delayed, and the hospital was drowning in debts, to the point that in December 1940 the hospital's existence was threatened through a seizure of its assets by the courts.[30]

The situation worsened when in January 1941 Zofiówka was incorporated into the Otwock Ghetto as part of a so-called "spa district." In May 1941, due to the alleged threat of an epidemic, the Jewish district was sealed off, and conditions in the hospital deteriorated drastically. Extreme shortages of food and other supplies inevitably resulted in an increased mortality rate,[31] and within few months, from May to November 1941, about 210 out of a total of 406 patients died of starvation and cold.[32] Stanisław Nissenszal, who had been a steward in Zofiówka from 1939 until his dismissal toward the end of 1941 due to the financial difficulties, recollected,

> In October 1939 there were 450 patients and around 120 members of personnel. . . . Due to the ban on leaving the ghetto, formed at the end of 1940, the financial

situation and food supplies worsened catastrophically. Insufficient food ratios and epidemics (dysentery and typhus) resulted in increased mortality rate that reached 50 percent of the hospital population.[33]

Despite the dramatic financial situation, admissions of patients continued, including transfers from other psychiatric hospitals. On 18 March 1941 the administration of Zofiówka was notified of the upcoming transfer of 150 Jewish patients from Kobierzyn, near Kraków. Within a few months, the number of patients in the announced transport was reduced to 110,[34] and eventually 91 arrived at Zofiówka on 8 and 9 September 1941.[35] The fate of the missing 59 patients remains unclear: most likely, however, is that the majority of them died of starvation and exhaustion within these few months.[36]

In such financial circumstances, the management of Zofiówka sought to find additional sources of income to contribute to the extremely limited budget of the hospital. One such attempt was a rest home for wealthy Jews, and a coffeehouse, "Café Variete," opened in December 1941. Both were frequently visited by Jewish elites, mostly from Radom and Warsaw, and these two initiatives enjoyed a rather ill reputation among the impoverished inhabitants of the ghetto. Nissenszal reported,

> On the premises of "Zofiówka" doctor Miller, back then the head of the hospital,[37] set up a so-called rest home for wealthy Jewish people. All kinds of wealthy Jews from the Warsaw ghetto and from Radom would come there and give parties and orgies. Supposedly, the income was to financially support the hospital budget and improve living conditions for the patients; in fact, however, it served the ringleaders of those revelries, including Dr. Miller himself. There would come Jewish Gestapo men, recruited from *Ordnungspolizei* in Warsaw and Radom, namely: Kohn, Heller, Wejsberg, some of the commanders of *Ordnungsdienst* from Radom and other nouveau riche, who thrived on the poverty of Jewish people in the ghettos. This part of the ghetto has been visited by Professor Bałaban, the editor Einhorn and a few physicians from Warsaw, who came with the Warsaw Ambulance.[38]

"Warsaw Diary of Adam Czerniaków"

On a few occasions also Adam Czerniaków (1880–1942), the chairman of Warsaw Ghetto Jewish Council (Judenrat), visited Otwock spas for a few hours of rest or for inspection. Glimpses of everyday life in Zofiówka survived in his famous diary:

> May 31, 1940 . . . "Zofiówka" threatened to discharge their mentally ill patients because of the lack of funds.

July 20, 1940 . . . Today, at 7 in the morning I gave myself a 24-hour holiday after all these months—I'm leaving for Otwock. We are having beautiful weather; at 5 a.m. it is 61F; an inspection of the Brijus TB sanitarium and later of Zofiówka. I notice in Zofiówka the woman troublemaker who cost us 100000 zlotys, adult lunatics and children. One child in a straitjacket to prevent self-injury, the face covered with flies. Another one is scratching wounds on his head. A female singer in bed executes some operatic arias: she used to perform in Italy. Other women by the piano were playing and singing; I joined them. Somebody built himself a tombstone in a cemetery with his name carved on it. It is to this address that he would direct his creditors.

September 25, 1940 . . . In Otwock the Polish authorities are to take over Brijus. Zofiówka is threatened, etc.

September 27, 1940 . . . Brijus and Zofiówka have been saved for the time being, although they are forbidden to register new patients.

December 10, 1941 . . . In the "Zofiowka" in Otwock a coffeehouse [Café Variete] was set up to provide additional income.

January 29, 1942 . . . Disturbing news from "Zofiowka"[39]

Czerniaków did not say what exactly troubled him in regard to Zofówka at the beginning of 1942. Most likely, in the months to come starvation and cold further decimated the hospital's patients until it ceased to function during the liquidation of Otwock Ghetto.

"The Action"

At dawn on 19 August 1942 the Jewish district in Otwock was surrounded by troops, and "the Action"—liquidation of the ghetto—began. Even though there were rumors circulating about similar actions in other towns and cities, the people of Otwock did not expect it to happen this particular night, and, not being warned, many were taken by surprise. As Calel Perechodnik (1916–44) reported,

> In other towns policemen felt that it was their obligation to inform the local Jews about the impending deportation. The Otwock police did not consider it their obligation and did nothing. . . . Yes, there were a few instances when the policemen warned close friends of expected deportations. They made them promise, however, on their word of honor, that they would not reveal this any further. I know for example, that officer Pietras warned the administration of the hospital Zofiówka. Thanks to that, several people were saved; some others, not having the means or energy to save themselves, committed suicide that same night.[40]

Indeed, the administration of Zofiówka had been informed about the planned action and almost all guests staying at the rest home and a few members of the personnel managed to leave. Three doctors[41] and several patients committed suicide.[42] Dramatic scenes were seen in the sanitaria district as the Ukrainian troops rushed the personnel and the patients from Zofiówka and Brijus to the courtyard and the first pavilion in Zofiówka. The doctors assisted the patients on their way, and, as Adela Rejmanowa recollected,

> ... They walked dressed in much too long hospital robes and were rushed by the Germans. They marched to their "slaughter" exclaiming all sorts of bizarre phrases such as "green pigeons on the heads" or "where is grandmother?"—Some of them escaped. Some were forced to dig graves and started fighting. One of them crushed a German soldier's skull with a shovel. 300 mentally ill Jews were killed. While digging graves they covered themselves with sand, they did not want to dig and threw their arms onto German soldiers' necks and did not want to dig. Germans killed them one by one.[43]

Whereas this might be a rather dramatized description, an estimated 140 people were killed on the hospital premises,[44] among them 108 mentally ill patients. Around noon a unit of Jewish ghetto police was sent to Zofiówka to clean up the hospital site.[45] Stanisław Nissenszal, who had served as ghetto policeman from 1 December 1941 on, remembered, "24 people, some members of *Ordnungspolizei*, were sent to the hospital to tidy up 'Zofiówka' and 'Brijus' [and] threatened with capital punishment, were forced to bury 108 still warm corpses, including those of three physicians."[46] Those who survived this massacre were deported to Treblinka on the same day. The unit of ghetto policemen remained stationed at the hospital's premises until 1 December 1942, when they were ordered to leave. Zofiówka was to become a home for German orphans of the war.[47]

News about the liquidation of Zofiówka, albeit not entirely accurate, traveled across the Atlantic. The authors of *The Black Book of Polish Jewry*, first published in 1943, alarmed,

> "We hear about many mentally deranged persons in the streets of the Ghettos. Some of them are former inmates of asylums in Tworki, Choroszcze and Wadowice outside the Ghettos who were deported by the Nazis into the Ghettos of Warsaw, Krakow and Lwow. The only Jewish psychiatric hospital, Zofiowka in Otwock, near Warsaw, was already overcrowded and could not admit additional patients from other institutions. That institution is reported to have been liquidated at the end of 1942 and the insane were driven into Ghettos to mix with the sane"[48]

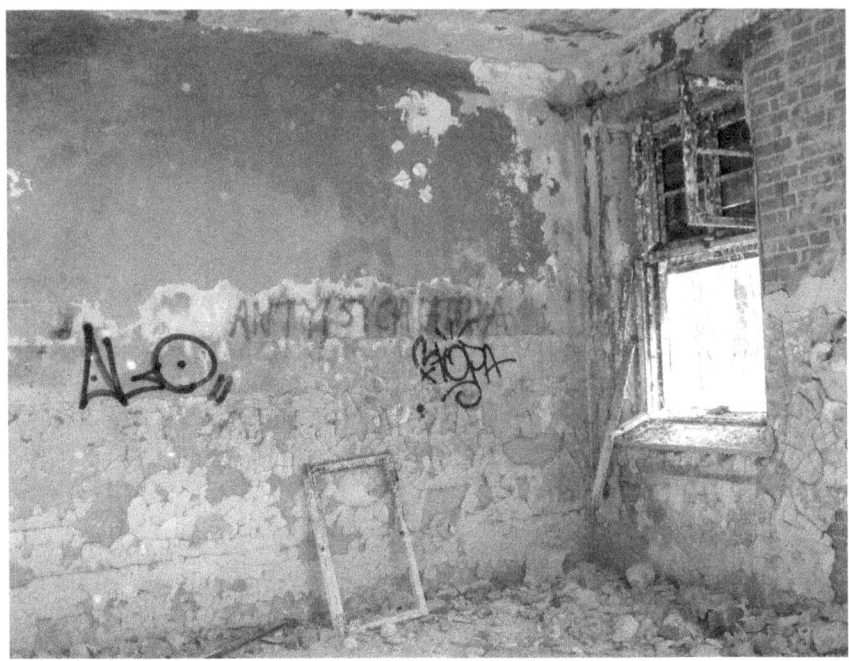

Figure 14.1. View of the former Jewish psychiatric hospital Zofiówka, 2019, interior (1002). Photo by the author.

"1.071.563 *Aufrufe*"

In the postwar years Otwock continued to enjoy a reputation as a health resort for pulmonary diseases, and in the whole complex of state-run local sanatoria Zofiówka has become a home for male youth diagnosed with tuberculosis. In 1985 its former name and field of expertise were resumed, as the hospital began to specialize in treating neuropsychiatric disorders in children and youth.

In 1998 Zofiówka ceased to exist, and the abandoned pavilions began to deteriorate. Over time, the remains of the former psychiatric hospital, where "moans and shrieks are heard among the ruins after dark" and "ghosts—the souls of the dead—are reputed to roam the corridors,"[49] became a rather rewarding object for thrilling stories and one more playground for urban exploration teams. An amateur short motion picture titled *Noc w nawiedzonym szpitalu psychiatrycznym "Zofiówka"/Opuszczony szpital psychiatryczny "Zofiówka" w Otwocku* (A night in haunted psychiatric hospital "Zofiówka"/Deserted psychiatric hospital "Zofiówka" in Otwock) attracted the attention of thousands of viewers. The camera captures remnants of the hospital buildings while the narrator keeps asking about the events buried in the remote past, which remains unknown to most of a broader audience.

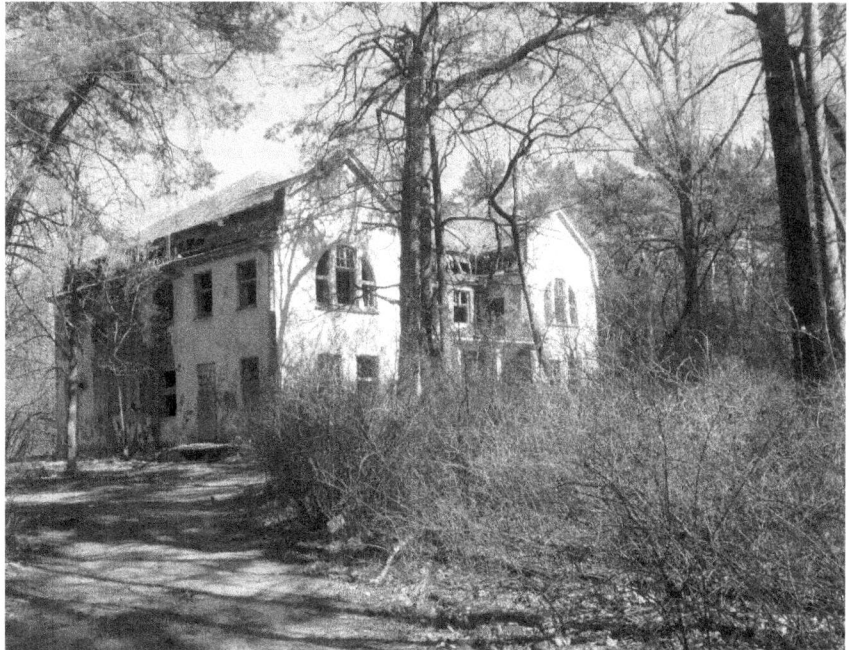

Figure 14.2. View of the former Jewish psychiatric hospital Zofiówka, 2019, exterior (1033). Photo by the author.

The Politics of "No Memory"

For decades, historians did very little to pursue systematic research on the fate of thousands of patients that perished in institutions of psychiatric care in occupied Poland during World War II. The first news referring to the brutal liquidation of psychiatric institutions, published as early as 1942 and 1943,[50] did not alert authorities in exile or spur thorough investigation in the immediate postwar years. Admittedly, the Main Commission for Investigation of German Crimes against the Polish Nation collected volumes of data on Nazi atrocities, but—as one of its members remarked—"extermination of the mentally ill in Poland by the Germans might seem to be—in comparison with all other German crimes committed in Polish territory—not important enough to be dealt with in any special way."[51] Indeed, historians of medicine focused on other, perhaps also more heroic aspects of medicine and the medical profession during the Holocaust; providing healthcare in turbulent war conditions, martyrdom and losses of medical personnel, long-term health consequences for the survivors of concentration camps and victims of medical experiments, etc., dominated the postwar array of publications on the topic. With the exception of a collection of reports published in *Psychiatry Yearbook*,[52] a series of articles in *Medical Review: Auschwitz*,[53] and the collected volume edited by Zdzisław Jaroszewski in 1993,[54] scholarly work on the subject has been scarce until recently.

By and large, the systematic annihilation of psychiatric patients has been a matter of marginal importance also in literature. Little is known about this crime, and "if the writers mentioned it at all, they would usually put it in a broader context, as an element of some other, and perhaps more severe crime, or used it as a pretext to discuss more fundamental problems."[55] Moreover, shortly after the war, artists in Poland became a target of increasing ideological pressure and were encouraged to produce art that would strengthen enthusiasm rather than fatalism and brooding over the war trauma. The new cultural politics, vaguely sketched by President Bolesław Bierut (1892–1956) already in 1947, soon became a reality. From 1949, artists preoccupied with traumatic war experiences were often silenced by censorship and their work excluded from circulation.[56] This was also the fate of *Szpital Przemienienia* (*Hospital of the Transfiguration*) by Stanisław Lem (1921–2006); the manuscript was completed in 1948 but published only in 1955, on the wave of a political thaw. In 1978 this popular novel lent itself to a film adaptation under the same title, directed by Edward Żebrowski (1935–2014). Final scenes, portraying the massacre of mentally ill patients by SS troops, clearly indicate that the artist(s) knew well what had happened in psychiatric hospitals during German occupation. Ten years later, the same motive was used in the famous film *Gdzieśkolwiek jest, jeśliś jest* (*Wherever You Are*) by Krzysztof Zanussi. However, in both productions, extermination of the mentally ill is a motive but not the leitmotiv of the plot.

Forgotten by historians, artists, and often by their families, thousands of murdered patients have been pushed into a space of nonbeing as if "'life not worth living' found continuity in 'life not worth mourning.' Those murdered, those who died of exhaustion, starvation, and negligence 're-died' after the war, this time falling into oblivion and social insensibility."[57] Cenotaphs and commemorating plaques installed on the premises of various psychiatric hospitals in postwar decades did not commemorate the patients but medical personnel or, broadly speaking, "the victims of fascism." The only exception, in Kobierzyn, nowadays a district of Kraków, deserves a few words.

As early as 1967, a gravestone devoted specifically to the memory of the patients killed at the hospital site in June 1942 was placed at the communal cemetery, formerly adjacent to the hospital. Additionally, a monument dedicated to Polish and Jewish patients from Kobierzyn has been installed on the hospital premises. The composition, created by Professor Józef Sękowski, consists of two parts and was erected and unveiled in two stages. First, two plaques, united by the impressive figure of Pieta, were unveiled in 2002 to commemorate 535 Polish patients killed in Auschwitz on 23 June 1942. The names of 91 Jewish patients transferred from Kobierzyn to Zofiówka in 1941 and killed on 19 August 1942 have not been included. In 2005 the names of these patients were identified on the list of 1,200 Jewish "euthanasia" victims held at Yad Vashem[58] and another two plaques, visually resembling *matzevah*, were unveiled in 2007 to preserve the memory of Jewish victims.[59]

> "Thus" —commented Tadeusz Nasierowski—"we have eventually two monuments. This situation is a falsification of reality, as it materializes the idea, supported by some Jewish circles, to separate what is Jewish from non-Jewish, creating the misleading impression that the fate of Jewish patients was somehow different."[60]

In fact it was. Jewish patients in Kobierzyn were put on a lower-calorie diet (see endnote 36), and those in the psychiatric hospital in Gostynin, taken over on 6 March 1940 by the German administration, were segregated in the dining room. Dr. Anna Kulikowska, at that time employed in one of the wards, remembered how,

> within few days of his tenure, German director W. ordered that all patients of Jewish origin should be seated separately during the meals. They received the same meals and portions, but they were seated separately. The Poles and Germans were not separated. The treatment and behavior towards the patients remained generally normal and unchanged. A few weeks later it was ordered that all patients of Jewish origin should be assembled and transported away with lorries covered with a black tarpaulin. It was not known in the clinic where these patients were murdered.[61]

Jewish mentally ill were doubly excluded: as mentally ill and as Jews, they were killed regardless of their health condition or ability to work. On 9 June 1941 a group of fifty-nine patients, thirty-seven Poles and twenty-two Jews, was deported from Gostynin to the home for elderly people in Śrem. The official version claimed that the patients would remain there. In all likelihood the patients were murdered.[62] Dr. Eugeniusz Wilczkowski, the last director of the facility before the war, stated, "These were the last Jewish patients that were still in the hospital. For this transport only the patients not able to work were selected, but in the case of Jewish patients all of them were qualified as not able to work."[63] According to director Wilczkowski, "the Germans demonstrated different approach to the patients, depending on their nationality. Jews experienced the worst treatment and they were all annihilated; the next were Poles—partly annihilated."[64]

Collective experience, most often traumatic, passed on to the next generation unites those who identify with this experience. In each country there are many "commonwealths of memory"[65] nursed and nurtured by those who survived and/or their families, but the memory of annihilation of people with mental disabilities has been marginalized for decades. The victims remained enveloped in overwhelming silence, as they did not leave any letters or memoires and have been erased from family annals and sagas due to the pervading embarrassment of mental illness; often the only trace of their life is a piece of official documentation—the case history from the hospital. In words of Paul Ricoeur,

> A devious form of forgetting is at work here resulting from stripping the social actors of their original power to recount their actions themselves. But this dispossession is not without a secret complicity, which makes forgetting a semi-passive, semi-active behavior, as is seen in forgetting by avoidance (*fuite*), the expression of bad faith and its strategy of evasion motivated by an obscure will not to inform oneself, not to investigate the harm done by the citizen's environment, in short by a wanting-not-to-know. Western Europe and indeed all of Europe, after the dismal years of the middle of the twentieth century, has furnished the painful spectacle of this stubborn will. Too little memory . . . can be classified as a passive forgetting, inasmuch as it can appear as a deficit in the work of memory. But, as a strategy of avoidance, of evasion, of flight, it is an ambiguous form of forgetting, active as much as passive. As active, this forgetting entails the same sort of responsibility as that imputed to acts of negligence, omission, imprudence, lack of foresight, in all of the situations of inaction, in which it appears after-the-fact to an enlightened and honest consciousness that one should have and could have known, or at least have tried to know, that one should have and could have intervened.[66]

Conclusion

The only psychiatric hospital for Jewish patients in General Government ceased to exist in summer 1942, and the patients, shot on the premises or deported to the death camp Treblinka, shared the fate of thousands of Jews from Otwock Jewish district. The killing was not hidden behind any camouflage operations. Jewish psychiatric patients in the occupied Polish territory were not included in NS "euthanasia operations": the T4 program and "euthanasia special action." Additionally, an unknown number perished during the liquidation of Polish psychiatric hospitals by SS troops and due to starvation and exhausting conditions in the hospitals during the war. Extremely fragmented contemporary sources do not allow for final conclusions; however, there are indications that Jewish patients were doubly stigmatized: as mentally ill and as Jews.

Kamila Uzarczyk is assistant professor in the Department of Medical Humanities and Social Sciences in Medicine at the Medical University of Wrocław, Poland. She received her PhD in history from the University of Wrocław in 2001 with a dissertation titled *The Concept of Race Hygiene and Implementation of Race Hygiene Legislation in German Province of Lower Silesia* (Toruń: Marszałek, 2002).

Notes

1. Wierciński 1991, 147.
2. Morawiec 2017, 276.
3. Wierciński 1991, 148.
4. Jellenta 1935, 109.
5. Jellenta 1935, 91.
6. Szymańska 2002, 39. Due to financial difficulties, until 1927 only volunteer-consulting physicians attended the patients.
7. Directors of Zofiówka: Aleksander Tumpowski (1870–1910) in the years 1908–10, Samuel Goldflam 1910–26, Rafał Becker 1927–32, Jakub Frostig 1932–38, Włodzimierz Kaufman 1938–42. Frostig was best known for pioneering the insulin shock therapy for schizophrenia in Poland—in 1936 he opened an insulin therapy ward in Zofiówka.
8. Translation: "End this race defilement!"
9. Hinz-Wessels 2002, 261–62.
10. Konieczny 1995, 236.
11. Friedlander 1995, 268.
12. Konieczny 1995, 237–38.
13. Friedlander 1995, 269.
14. Friedlander 1989, 39; Hinz-Wessels 2002, 263.
15. Rosenau 2012, 212. The hospital provided care for "Jews suffering from slight mental disorders, paralysis, epilepsy, mental retardation and idiotism." In 1937 non-Jewish medical personnel were dismissed and replaced by Jewish staff. In spring 1940 Dr. Wilhelm Rosenau (1898–1968) was appointed as "the main medical curator." The only non-Jewish member of administration was Paul Kochanek, managing director of the institution.
16. Konieczny 1995, 241; Hinz-Wessels 2013, 69.
17. Friedlander 1989, 40; Lilienthal 2009, 5; Hinz-Wessels 2010, 143.
18. Hinz-Wessels 2010, 143.
19. Lilienthal 2009, 8. It is not clear which of the "euthanasia" centers was the destination for Silesian Jewish patients.
20. Bardzik 1949, 77; Ossendowski 1949, 74. The choice of Chełm made the operation all the more plausible, because the facility did exist until 12 January 1940 when SS troops shot between 330 and 440 patients and personnel and the hospital was turned into a German military hospital.
21. Lilienthal 2009, 8; the author calculated 1,645, but this number does not include 149 patients (96 women and 53 men) taken in two transports from the assembly center in Leubus, in Silesia, on 17 and 18 December 1940. Konieczny 1995, 246.
22. Hinz-Wessels 2010, 143; Hinz-Wessels 2013, 66.
23. Witness statements only occasionally specify the number of Jewish patients deported from the hospital; one such example is report from psychiatric hospital in Gostynin: "In a series of seven transports from 3 February 1940 to 9 June 1940 altogether 48 patients, including 11 Jews, were taken from the hospital and in all likelihood killed—the transports were supervised by Gestapo and on two occasions shovels were seen in the lorry." Wilczkowski 1949, 55–56.
24. Friedlander 1995, 270; Hinz-Wessels 2010, 143.
25. Roseanu 2012, 216.
26. Hinz-Wessels 2002, 282.
27. Hinz-Wessels 2002, 284.
28. Nasierowski 2008, 201 and 205. Włodzimierz Kaufman, Stefan Miller, and Irena Miller-Themerson, as well as Kenda [Lewin] Adler, remained in Zofiówka. Jan Wolański (Izaak Bueckner), Helena and Marian Kisterowie, Stanisław Sierpiński (Wiktor Margulies), and Marian

Strumień (Mendel Strumwasser) fled to Kulparków, and Izaak Frydman escaped to Choroszcz. New members of the staff included: Maks Maślanka, Jadwiga Goldman, Zbigniew Rom, and Miriam Szmuszkiewicz-Włosko.

29. From 20 February to 31 May 1940 as many as 994 patients were consulted in the facility (Nasierowski 1993, 151).

30. Korespondencja ŻSS z Radą Żydowską i Zakładem dla Umysłowo Chorych "Zofiówka" w Otwocku, ŻIH, JUS, 769, p. 14.

31. Recorded mortality rates in 1941: May—10.1 percent; June—16.1 percent; July—12.1 percent; August—9.5 percent; September—7 percent; October—14.8 percent; November—18.2. ŻIH, JUS, 772, p. 10.

32. Szymańska 2002, 39; Nasierowski 2008, 207.

33. ŻIH, Relacje, 301/4064.

34. ŻIH, JUS, 210/541, p. 3 and 5.

35. According to Roman Kiełkowski 41 female patients were transported on 8 September 1941 and 50 patients, both male and female, on 11 September 1941, and only 3 or 4 Jews in terminal health condition remained in the hospital. Salvaged hospital documentation allows one to conclude that in 1940 an estimated 109 Jewish patients died in Kobierzyn (Kiełkowski 1967, 70).

36. From October 1940, daily food ratio for the patients in Kobierzyn was systematically reduced, and Jewish patients received lower calorie input than non-Jewish patients (50 grams of bread per day, whereas non-Jewish patients received 75 grams) ŻIH, Relacje, 301/1006.

37. Stefan Miller (1903–42), often incorrectly referred to as the director, was in fact the head of one of the wards (Seeman 2014, 5n1).

38. ŻIH, Relacje 301/4064.

39. Hilberg et al. 1979, 156, 176, 201, 202, 306, 320.

40. Perechodnik 1996, 30–31.

41. Szymańska 2002, 39; Dr. Lewin, Dr. Maślanko, and Director Kaufman committed suicide; Dr. Miller and his wife left for Mińsk Mazowiecki, where on 21 August 1942—the day of liquidation of Mińsk Ghetto—they also committed suicide.

42. Nasierowski 1993, 155.

43. ŻIH, Relacje, 301/1980.

44. Szymańska 2002, 84.

45. Perechodnik 1996, 38.

46. ŻIH, Relacje, 301/4064.

47. Nasierowski 1993, 155.

48. Lustiger 1995, 189.

49. Seeman 2014, 5.

50. German Order 1942, 70–71; Pospieszalski 1943, 78–80.

51. Quoted in Morawiec 2018, 93.

52. *Rocznik Psychiatryczny* 1 (1949), printed also as *Zbrodnie niemieckie wobec umysłowo chorych w Polsce*. Praca zbiorowa, Warszawa: PZWL 1949.

53. Kiełkowski 1967; Milczarek 1979; Monkiewicz and Krętowski 1984; Moska 1975.

54. Jaroszewski 1993.

55. Morawiec 2017, 276.

56. Brodzka-Wald et al. 2000, 22.

57. Gajewska 2016, 13.

58. Strous 2010, 208.

59. Taborska 2012, 487.

60. Nasierowski 2012, 525; quoted in Taborska 2012, 488.

61. Kulikowska 1989, 46.

62. The nurses that accompanied the patients reported "in the evening a steward of the home, a German who could speak Polish, revealed, while being drunk, that the facility saw horrifying scenes and this was not the first and not the last of the transports; that they murdered not only sick people but also healthy priests, doctors and young girls who had just graduated from a lyceum." Wilczkowski 1949, 58.
63. Wilczkowski 1949, 58.
64. ŻIH, Relacje, 301/1008.
65. Wolf-Powęska 2011, 34.
66. Ricoeur 2006, 448–49.

References

Archives

Archive of Jewish Historical Institute in Warsaw:
Jüdische Soziale Selbsthilfe [JUS]
    Sign: 769-772; 210/410; 210/54
Testimonies [Relacje]—Testimonies of Jewish Survivors of the Holocaust
    Nissenszal Stanisław 301/4064
    Goldin Zalman 301/1980
    Władysław Issajewicz 301/1006
    Eugeniusz Wilczkowski 301/1008

Books and Articles

Bardzik, Franciszek. 1949. "Zbrodnie niemieckie w szpitalu psychiatrycznym w Chełmie Lubelskim." In *Zbrodnie niemieckie wobec umysłowo chorych w Polsce*, 76–77. Praca zbiorowa, Warszawa: PZWL.

Batawia, Stanisław. 1947. "Zagłada chorych psychicznie." *Biuletyn Głównej Komisji Badania Zbrodni Niemieckich w Polsce* 3: 104–6

Brodzka-Wald Alina, Dorota Krawczyńska, and Jacek Leociak (eds.). 2000. *Literatura polska wobec zagłady*. Warszawa: ŻIH.

Friedlander, Henry. 1989. "Jüdische Anstaltspatienten in NS-Deutschland." In *Aktion T 4 1939–1945. Die "Euthanasie"-Zentrale in der Tiergartenstrasse 4*, edited by Götz Aly, 34–44. Berlin: Edition Hentrich.

———. 1995. *The Origins of Nazi Genocide: From Euthanasia to the Final Solution*. Chapel Hill: University of North Carolina Press.

Gajewska, Grażyna. 2016. *Bezużyteczni: Studia nad losami chorych i upośledzonych psychicznie w okresie rządów nazistowskich*. Gniezno: UAM.

German New Order in Poland. 1942. London: Hutchinson for Polish Ministry of Information.

Herczyńska, Grażyna. 2014. "Zofiówka." *Psychiatra: Pismo dla Praktyków* 5(7): 40–41.

Hilberg, Raul, Stanisław Staron, and Josef Kermisz (eds.). 1979. *The Warsaw Diary of Adam Czerniakow, Prelude to Doom*. Jerusalem: Yad Vashem, 1979

Hinz-Wessels, Anette. 2002. "Das Schicksal Jüdischer Patienten in brandenburgischen Heil- und Pflegeanstalten im Nationalsozialismus." In *Brandenburgische Heil- und Pflegeanstalten in der NS-Zeit*, edited by Kristina Hübner and Martin Heinze, 259–86. be.bra wissenschaft Verlag.

———. 2010. "Jüdische Opfer der Aktion T4 im Spiegel der überlieferten Euthanasie Krankenakten im Bundesarchiv." In *Die nationalsozialistische"Euthanasie"-Aktion T4 und ihre Opfer: Geschichte und ethische Konsequenzen für die Gegenwart*, edited by Maike Rotzoll, Gerrit Hohedorf, Petra Fuchs, Christoph Mundt, and Wolfgang Eckart, 143–46. Paderborn: Ferdinand Schöningh.

———. 2013. "Antisemitismus und Krankenmord. Zum Umgang mit jüdischen Anstaltspatienten im Nationalsozialismus." *Vierteljahreshefte für Zeitgeschichte* 61: 65–93

Jaroszewski, Zdzisław (ed.). 1993. *Zagłada chorych psychicznie w Polsce 1939–1945. Die Ermordung der Geisteskranken in Polen 1939–1945*. Warszawa: PWN.

Jellenta, Cezary. 1935. *Sosny Otwockie*. Warszawa: Wydawnictwo Współczesne.

Kiełkowski, Roman. 1967. "Zagłada chorych szpitala psychiatrycznego w Kobierzynie." *Przegląd Lekarski* 1: 68–78.

Konieczny, Alfred. 1995. "Rozwiązanie kwestii umysłowo chorych Żydów na Śląsku w latach 1938–1943." *Acta Universitatis Wratislaviensis* no. 1715, *Studia nad Faszyzmem i Zbrodniami Hitlerowskimi* 18: 235–60.

Kulikowska, Anna. 1989. "Erinnerungen an das psychiatrische Krankenhaus in Gostynin während der Okkupationszeit." In *Aktion T-4 1939–1945: Die "Euthanasie"-Zentrale in der Tiergartenstrasse 4*, edited by Götz Aly, 45–46. Berlin: Edition Hentrich.

Lilienthal, Georg. 2009. "Jüdische Patienten als Opfer der NS-'Euthanasie-Verbrechen.'" *MEDAON: Magazin für Jüdisches Leben in Forschung und Bildung* 5: 1–16.

Lustiger, Arno (ed.). 1995. *The Black Book of Polish Jewry: An Account of the Martyrdom of Polish Jewry under the Nazi Occupation*. Bodenheim: Syndikat Buchgesellschaft.

Marcinkowski, Filip, and Tadeusz Nasierowski. 2016. "Rafał Becker: psychiatra, eugenik, syjonista." *Psychiatria Polska* 50(1): 261–68. DOI: http://dx.doi.org/10.12740/PP/38918.

Milczarek, Jan. 1979. "Wymordowanie chorych psychicznie w Warcie." *Przegląd Lekarski* 1: 115–19.

Monkiewicz, Waldemar, and Józef Krętowski. 1984. "Los chorych psychicznie, kalek i starców w okupowanym białostockiem." *Przegląd Lekarski* 1: 80–84.

Morawiec, Arkadiusz. 2009. *Literatura w łagrze, łagier w literaturze. Fakt-temat-metafora*, Łódź: WSHE.

———. 2017. "'Dezynfekcja': Literatura polska wobec eksterminacji osób psychicznie chorych." *Przestrzenie Teorii* 27: 261–95

———. 2018. *Literatura polska wobec ludobójstwa*. Łódź: Wydawnictwo Uniwersytetu Łódzkiego.

Moska, Dionizy. 1975. "Eksterminacja w zakładzie'Loben." *Przegląd Lekarski* 1: 112–14.

Nasierowski, Tadeusz. 1993. "Zofiówka-Otwock: Szpital dla Umysłowo i Nerwowo Chorych." In *Zagłada chorych psychicznie w Polsce: Die Ermordung der Geisteskranken in Polen 1939-1945*, edited by Zdzisław Jaroszewski, 150–53. Warszawa: PWN.

———. 2008. *Zagłada osób z zaburzeniami psychicznymi: Początek ludobójstwa*, Warszawa: Neriton.

———. 2012. "Trzeba nieść tę noc . . . Dlaczego i jak upamiętniać ofiary tanazji przewrotnie zwanej eutanazją." In *Zagłada chorych psychicznie. Pamięć i historia*, edited by Tadeusz Nasierowski, Grażyna Herczyńska, and Dariusz Myszka, 523–29. Warszawa: Eneteia.

———. 2014. "Zofiówka." *Psychiatra: Pismo dla Praktyków* 5(7): 37–39

Ossendowski, Aleksander. 1949. "Zbrodnie niemieckie w stosunku do umysłowo chorych w szpitalu psychiatrycznym w Chełmie Lubelskim." In *Zbrodnie niemieckie wobec umysłowo chorych w Polsce*, 72–75. Praca zbiorowa, Warszawa: PZWL.

Perechodnik, Calel. 1996. *Am I a Murderer? Testament of a Jewish Ghetto Policeman*. Translated and edited by Frank Fox. Boulder, CO: Westview Press.

Pospieszalski, Karol Marian. 1943. *Z pierwszej linii frontu*. Glasgow: Książnica Polska.

Rosenau, Renate. 2012. "Wilhelm Rosenau—ostatni dyrektor medyczny żydowskiego zakładu psychiatrycznego w Sayn." In *Zagłada chorych psychicznie. Pamięć i historia*, edited by Tadeusz Nasierowski, Grażyna Herczyńska, and Dariusz Myszka, 209–22. Warszawa: Eneteia.

Ricoeur, Paul. 2006. *Memory, History, Forgetting*. Translated by Kathleen Blamey and David Pellauer. Chicago: University Chicago Press.

Seeman, Mary. 2014. "The Jewish Psychiatric Hospital 'Zofiówka' in Otwock, Poland." *History of Psychiatry* 15: 1–7. DOI: 10.1177/0957154X14542570.

Strous, Rael D. 2010. "Psychiatric Genocide: Reflections and Responsibilities." *Schizophrenia Bulletin* 36(2): 208–10. DOI: 10.1093/schbul/sbq003.

Szymańska, Sylwia. 2002. *Ludność żydowska w Otwocku podczas drugiej wojny światowej*. Warszawa: ŻIH.

Taborska, Halina. 2012. "Dokąd nas zabieracie: Dzieła sztuki publicznej upamiętniające chorych psychicznie zgładzonych w czasie II wojny światowej." In *Zagłada chorych psychicznie: Pamięć i historia*, edited by Tadeusz Nasierowski, Grażyna Herczyńska, and Dariusz Myszka, 273–91. Warszawa: Eneteia.

Wierciński, Edmund. 1991. "Gałązki akacji." In *Edmund Wierciński: Notatki i teksty z lat 1921–55*, edited by Anna Chojnacka, 147–64. (Wrocław: Wiedza o Kulturze.

Wilczkowski, Eugeniusz. 1949. "Los chorych psychicznie w szpitalu dla psychicznie i nerwowo chorych w latach okupacji niemieckiej." In *Zbrodnie niemieckie wobec umysłowo chorych w Polsce: Praca zbiorowa*, 54–62. Warszawa: PZWL.

Wolf-Powęska, Anna. 2011. *Pamięć: Brzemię i uwolnienie; Niemcy wobec nazistowskiej przeszłości (1945–2010)*. Poznań: ZYSK I S-KA.

Zabłotniak, Ryszard. 1992. "Sanatoria żydowskie w Otwocku (1939–1942) w pięćdziesiątą rocznicę Zagłady." *Zdrowie Publiczne* 103(10): 551–55.

Zbrodnie niemieckie wobec umysłowo chorych w Polsce: Praca zbiorowa. 1949. Warszawa: PZWL.

CHAPTER 15

"SINCE SHE WAS IN AUSCHWITZ, THE PATIENT FEELS THAT SHE IS BEING PERSECUTED"
Holocaust Survivors and Austrian Psychiatry after World War II

Herwig Czech

By the end of World War II and following the murder of approximately two hundred thousand patients,[1] psychiatry in Germany and Austria was deeply discredited, both in the eyes of the public and of its practitioners. In Austria, the National Socialist "euthanasia" campaigns had taken a massive toll, with victim numbers often proportionally higher than in Germany itself.[2] The "euthanasia" murders had also played a role in the Holocaust, with Action T4 providing personnel, experience, and the killing technology for the extermination camps installed in occupied Poland.[3] In Vienna, approximately four hundred Jewish psychiatric patients had been concentrated at Steinhof, the city's largest mental institution, from where they were sent to the gas chamber in Hartheim near Linz.[4] After Austria's liberation from Nazi rule and despite an official policy of denazification imposed by the victorious Allied powers and reluctantly implemented by Austrian authorities, many of the perpetrators were able to evade prosecution and—after a first wave of anti-Nazi measures had subsided—often resumed their careers.[5]

Against this backdrop, the present chapter explores how psychiatry dealt with the mental consequences of trauma and loss suffered on an unimaginable scale and how survivors of persecution by the Nazi regime influenced postwar psychiatry, either as psychiatrists or as patients. Most prominent in Austria's postwar psychiatric landscape was its undisputed academic and intellectual center, Vienna University's Department of Psychiatry and Neurology, which was home to many former victims of Nazi persecution. In 1945, its first director Otto Kauders (1893–1949) published an analysis of what he called the psychological effects of terror, one of the first attempts to describe the impact of persecution on victims' mental health.⁶ His successor Hans Hoff (1897–1969) had been forced into exile and spent the war years in Baghdad and New York. Hoff also published discussions of clinical questions related to persecution, but much later, in 1971.⁷ Viktor Frankl, the most influential of these psychiatrists, was a survivor of Auschwitz and other camps and soon rose to worldwide fame as the author of the bestselling book *Man's Search for Meaning* and as the creator of existential analysis and logotherapy.⁸

After the Shock: Holocaust Survivors in Post–World War II Vienna

In 1945, Vienna's once-thriving Jewish community, which had comprised nearly a tenth of the city's population before 1938, had been reduced to a small fraction of its former size.⁹ Jonny Moser, who was the first to provide detailed demographic data on the destruction of Vienna's Jews, put the number of those who had survived in Vienna at 989.¹⁰ A list dated 30 November 1945 compiled by the American Jewish Joint Distribution Committee of "Austrian Jews residing in Vienna during the occupation" gives a higher number of 1,365 persons.¹¹ Another list from the same source contains 2,229 names of "Austrian Jews returned from various concentration camps to Vienna."¹² Apart from this core group of Holocaust survivors, Austria's postwar Jewish population comprised those who returned from various countries of exile and successive waves of refugees from Eastern Europe. In 1948, Vienna's official Jewish community organization had 6,000 registered members. Additionally, 6,000 to 7,000 officially registered Jewish Displaced Persons (DPs) resided outside Vienna, primarily in the American zone of occupation.¹³ In the Vienna region, the most important camp for Jewish DPs was the Rothschild Hospital in the eighteenth district, which from 1873 until its takeover by the SS in the summer of 1943 had served the medical needs of Vienna's Jewish community. Between 1945 and 1952, approximately 250,000 Jewish refugees passed through the camp on their way to Palestine/Israel, the United States, and other destinations.¹⁴

The presidium of the reconstituted Vienna Jewish Community reported in 1948 that, despite their poor physical and mental health, the survivors returning from the camps or from emigration in the aftermath of liberation were mostly left to their own devices, with temporary housing in overcrowded refugee shelters the only help they could count on. In order to assess the health damages suffered, the community organized serial examinations for its six thousand registered members, three thousand of whom followed the invitation. The results were dire: "These records reflect the sad picture of the overall state of Vienna's Jews. Not one Jewish family was spared the barbarism of the recent years. They [the records] testify to the suffering, hardship, fear, and pain Vienna's Jews experienced during those years."¹⁵ An examination of 1,060 survivors of Nazi persecution organized in the summer of 1945 by Austrian health authorities in cooperation with a welfare organization dedicated to helping Nazi victims (Verein Volkssolidarität) painted a similarly bleak picture. Despite the fact that the screening did not include those hospitalized, most of the examined survivors showed clear signs of damage to their health. Around 10 percent required treatment for tuberculosis, while others suffered from heart problems, emphysema, malnutrition, and ulcers. The report does not mention mental health problems, reflecting both the immediate necessity of addressing the acute pathologies resulting from physical violence, malnutrition, and the abysmal conditions in the camps, as well as the widespread ignorance of the medical profession and beyond concerning the impacts of traumatic experiences.

A Discredited Discipline: Austrian Psychiatry, National Socialism, and "Euthanasia"

In September 1947, a scandal over alleged medical experiments on Jewish refugee children shook Vienna's DP community and the wider public. The fresh memory of Nazi medical atrocities (the previous month had seen the sentences passed in the Nuremberg Doctors Trial) loomed large when the director of the Rothschild DP hospital convened the press in order to denounce medical abuses committed against the children of Jewish refugees from Romania, who had been quarantined because of measles—of all places, in pavilion 15 of the Steinhof psychiatric hospital, the former killing pavilion of the Spiegelgrund "child euthanasia" center. A mother had discovered a fresh scar on her eighteen-month-old son, where without her consent a piece of skin had been removed. Subsequently, a doctor from the Rothschild hospital found out that a total of twelve children had been subjected to similar interventions. Additionally, the head physician at pavilion 15 had taken lung biopsies from six children. In the presence of journalists, the director compared these incidents with human experiments in Auschwitz, citing them as proof that the spirit of Nazism was still alive in Austria.[16] The DPs successfully mobilized the Allied authorities, who demanded an immediate investigation into the issue. Ultimately, a commission hastily convened by the mayor concluded that some of the interventions could be justified on diagnostic grounds, but remaining doubts about the skin biopsies and the failure to obtain the parents' consent led to a recommendation to inform the public prosecutor. The social democratic *Arbeiter-Zeitung* took a clear stance in the affair, defending the involved physicians and accusing the leadership of the Rothschild hospital of intentionally damaging Austria's international reputation.[17]

This incident not only sheds light on the precarious existence of Jewish DPs on the margins of Austrian postwar society, it also shows to what extent the trust of survivors in medical institutions had been shattered. The fact that the children of Jewish Holocaust survivors were quarantined in the former Spiegelgrund killing pavilion shows a blatant lack of sensibility toward their recent traumatic experiences. The involved Austrian parties—including the *Arbeiter-Zeitung*—were primarily concerned with defending the reputation of the involved physicians and medical institutions. During the preceding years, the Vienna institutions Steinhof and Spiegelgrund had been at the center of medical crimes committed against psychiatric patients—a fact that had become widely known among the population and even led to public protests during the war.[18]

Throughout the twentieth century, psychiatric patients in Austria were placed in a relatively small number of large, public institutions. During the T4 program in 1940–41, this concentration of patients facilitated their selection for the gas chamber at Hartheim near Linz. In all, the ratio of patients murdered during T4 on formerly Austrian territory was 2.6 times higher than in Germany proper. Vienna's Steinhof mental hospital, one of the largest institutions of its kind in Europe, lost two-thirds of its 4,280 patients (as of 1 July 1940), among them approximately 400 Jews, many of whom had been transferred there from other psychiatric institutions throughout Austria.[19] Among the Steinhof patients was Margarethe Trude Neumann née Herzl, the daughter of Theodor Herzl. Thanks to her father's prominence, she survived the T4 transports, only to be deported to Theresienstadt in September 1942, where she died six months later.[20] A number of the *Steinhof* pavilions that had been emptied of patients by the T4 killings were used in July 1940 to set up a new facility under the name of Spiegelgrund, which was dedicated to the implementation of the "child euthanasia" program. Over the following years, 789 children, most of whom suffered from mental disabilities, died at the institution, many of them by poisoning with barbiturates. Heinrich Gross, one of the Spiegelgrund doctors, built his postwar career in neuropathology on the systematic scientific exploitation of specimens from these victims' brains and other body parts.[21] After widespread protests, the gassing of patients through the T4 program was suspended on Hitler's order in August 1941, while the "child euthanasia" program continued. During the following phase, patients in psychiatric hospitals were exposed to increasingly inhumane and deadly conditions, leading to ever-increasing mortality rates. In some institutions, patients died not only due to hunger, infections, neglect, and cold; many were also actively killed by physicians and nurses in what is now commonly referred to as "decentralized euthanasia."[22]

Against this backdrop, the case of Leo Moses Aschkenasy stands out as highly unusual. In August 1944, at age thirty-six, he was diagnosed with schizophrenia first at the Vienna Jewish hospital and then by the University Department of Psychiatry and Neurology, which had him transferred to Steinhof. By this time, the vast majority of Austrian Jews had already been deported and murdered; only those precariously protected by factors such as a non-Jewish spouse or a position at the Council of Elders of the Jews in Vienna remained.[23] The authorities continued to deport Jews, often in smaller groups, on pretexts such as failure to wear the yellow star or other infractions against the numerous restrictions imposed on "racial" grounds. On admission to the hospital, Aschkenasy claimed to have lived in Vienna for thirty years; his patient file contains no indication of any of the abovementioned protective factors. As a Jew diagnosed with mental illness, he must have been in considerable danger of being reported to the Gestapo and then deported. However, he appears to have been treated like any other patient; treatment included rest and repeated electroshocks. While many hundreds of (mostly non-Jewish) patients died at Steinhof, he survived the Nazi period, to be released on 23 May 1945, six weeks after Vienna's liberation from Nazi rule.

Another unusual aspect of this case is that the diagnosis established by the court that ordered his commitment to a mental hospital, despite the biologistic doctrines prevailing at the time, came very close to recognizing Aschkenasy's experiences as a Jew in Nazi-dominated Austria as the root cause of his illness. Aschkenasy had shown up at an acquaintance's home pretending to be Adolf Hitler and asked for shelter because he had nowhere to go. His medical evaluation stated that he suffered from "psychogenically triggered stupor with loss of contact." He had reported earlier hallucinations—clearly based on fears linked both to air raids and anti-Jewish persecution—involving airplanes circling above his workplace and shouting at him "Jew! Jew! Jew!"[24] Despite losing over 10 percent of his body mass during his hospitalization, he survived because apparently nobody reported him to the Gestapo and due to his otherwise good physical health and relatively young age.

Leo Aschkenasy's survival is all the more astonishing given the fact that in Steinhof alone, although there is no evidence for active killings, an estimated thirty-five hundred people died under circumstances that were intentionally designed to increase mortality rates and reduce the hospital's population of patients who were deemed incurable. Crucially, the high mortality rate at Steinhof continued after liberation, peaking as late as October 1945.[25] On the one hand, it is to be assumed that the effects of years of indoctrination regarding "lives unworthy to live" on the attitudes of nurses and other staff did not change overnight. On the other hand, many psychiatric patients were weakened by years of neglect and were thus especially vulnerable to the general food crisis in postwar Vienna.

Despite the officially mandated secrecy surrounding the Nazi "euthanasia" program, knowledge about the killings of psychiatric patients spread quickly among the population and discredited psychiatry as a whole.[26] Further details emerged after liberation, for example when Ernst Illing, the first director of Spiegelgrund, was put on trial and sentenced to death in 1946.[27] Other perpetrators, however, never had to pay for their crimes. The most prominent case of those evading judgment is Heinrich Gross, who has received widespread attention since a murder trial against him in the year 2000 failed because of his alleged dementia. While Gross ultimately did not achieve his goal of pursuing a university career, Hans Bertha (1901–64) did so, despite the fact that as a T4 "expert" he had helped decide which patients should be gassed. As director of Steinhof in the years 1944–45, he was also responsible for the exorbitant death rates among patients. After a short professional hiatus due to postwar denazification, he became chair of psychiatry at Graz University and, in 1963, was even elected dean of the Graz Medical School.[28] Against this background, it is hardly surprising that Wolfgang Holzer, an assistant at the Graz Department of Psychiatry, still insisted as late as 1948 that his field had "passed a severe test during the last war" without as much as mentioning the "euthanasia" killings.[29]

At Rosenhügel, Vienna's largest neurological hospital, Holocaust survivors clearly were not welcome. Rosenhügel had become a municipal hospital only in 1938 after the liquidation of the Rothschild Foundation, and the hospital was then occupied by the German military until March 1945.[30] In May 1945, Erwin Stransky (1877–1962) became the first postwar director of the institution, which developed into a hideout for former National Socialists mentally shaken by Nazi Germany's defeat. In July 1945, Stransky tried to obtain an exemption for his patients from the obligation of registering as former Nazi Party members, claiming that "several cases have shown that the mere thought of it compromises the recovery of the patients." On another occasion, Stransky—who was himself of Jewish descent—asked his superiors to remove a survivor of the Theresienstadt concentration camp because of the "depressing impression" he made on the other patients.[31]

A Precarious Break with the Past: Vienna University's Department of Psychiatry

After the liberation, Austrian psychiatry was confronted with its legacy of forced sterilizations, mass murder of psychiatric patients, and the continued presence of many of the perpetrators. Prompted by the Allied powers' denazification policies, a clean break with the past was attempted in the academic field, at least initially in 1945. The directors of Austria's three psychiatric university departments in Graz, Innsbruck, and Vienna were dismissed on political grounds and replaced with candidates who had no compromising ties to the Nazi regime. These appointments followed the general pattern of academic denazification. Immediately after liberation, former National Socialists, especially those who had joined the Nazi Party as so-called "illegals" before 1938, usually lost their positions. However, it usually took only a few years before nearly all of them managed to put their careers back on track, including those directly involved in crimes.[32] Generally, the positions made available by the denazification program were not awarded to Jewish scholars expelled in 1938, but to representatives of the

Christian social political camp. Before the *Anschluss*, these academics had often sympathized with the Austrofascist dictatorship that ruled from 1933/34 to 1938 and as a result had suffered political repression under the Nazis, but after the war were able to reconstitute their dominant influence over Austrian academia.[33]

The first postwar appointee to the Vienna chair of psychiatry was Otto Kauders, who had been dismissed by the Nazis from his position in Graz in 1938 and spent the following years first in exile in Washington, D.C., and from 1939 onward in private praxis in Vienna.[34] As early as July 1945, in a lecture that was published the following year, he called for the creation of a new medical diagnosis to cover a broad range of symptoms apparently arising from a dysfunction of the autonomic nervous system observed by him in a great number of his patients. As the most characteristic and common of these symptoms, Kauders mentioned a state of pathological fatigue, which in some cases reached a state of complete physical and mental exhaustion. As the root cause of this apparently new disorder, Kauders identified the "severe traumatic pressure" to which the population was exposed during the war. Although Kauders suggested that he had personally experienced some of the described symptoms, he did not explicitly draw a connection to political or racist persecution. Rather, he opened the way to a medical version of collective victimhood, where everyone had suffered under the conditions created by the Nazi regime and the war. Nevertheless, Kauders broke with psychiatric orthodoxy in one important respect, stating that the symptoms he described could be caused by traumatic experiences in previously healthy individuals rather than requiring previous constitutional defects.[35] It took many years before this idea would be accepted by mainstream psychiatry, paving the way for what is today called post-traumatic stress disorder (PTSD). Before this was the case, thousands of victims of Nazi persecution saw their claims for compensation rejected because they could not prove that their health problems were a direct result of their traumatic experiences. Another of Kauder's articles from the same period, titled "On the Psychological Effects of Terror," is one of the first attempts in the psychiatric literature to reflect on the profound and lasting effects of Nazi persecution on the victims' mental health.[36] According to this text, states of "vegetative exhaustion," including complete breakdowns, were common among victims of "political terror" (anti-Jewish persecution is not mentioned explicitly). Kauders also described a forced regression of the organism to the level of biological survival, leading to the intended effect behind the use of terror as a political weapon: the "annihilation of human beings in their mental-moral sphere." In his inaugural lecture, Kauders called for a renewal of the entire psychiatric discipline in order to overcome earlier aberrations such as the concept of "life unworthy of living."[37]

The staff at the Vienna psychiatric clinic were confronted firsthand with the impact of imprisonment in a concentration camp when on 10 June 1945 a group of eleven former prisoners were transferred from Mauthausen, two of whom were

Jewish. Bernhard Kellner, sixteen years old, came from Zenta (Vojvodina) and had spent two years in the Mauthausen concentration camp. When admitted to the clinic, he weighed forty-four kilograms, his body was covered with scars from furuncles and edema, and he felt tired and weak. The overall diagnosis was "starvation" and "state of exhaustion." Martin Fischer, forty years old, had been imprisoned in Mauthausen for fourteen months and presented a similar picture. Both men were transferred to a rest home for former concentration camp prisoners after a few days; they were not diagnosed in psychiatric terms, but the clinical descriptions in their files point toward the idea of "vegetative exhaustion" put forward by Otto Kauders shortly afterward.[38]

Another Holocaust survivor admitted early on to the Vienna Psychiatric University Clinic was Tibor Guttmann, age sixteen, originally from Mukachevo in Ukraine. He had been imprisoned in several labor and concentration camps during the Nazi period and was transferred from the Jewish hospital because he had been aggressive to other patients. He was declared mentally ill by the court and transferred to Steinhof on the basis of the diagnosis of "abnormal reaction during adolescence with inhibition of speech, negativism, and state of excitement." His fate is unknown; what is clear, however, is that neither the Jewish hospital nor the Psychiatric University Clinic had found a way to deal with his state of severe traumatization. Instead, by pathologizing his reaction to years of traumatization as "abnormal," he was once again deprived of his freedom, this time by forced hospitalization.[39]

A similar failure can be observed in the case of a thirty-two-year-old woman who was admitted in March 1946. Classed as a *"Mischling* of the first degree" by the Nazis because of her father's Jewish descent, she had lost her job as a graphic designer, had been prohibited from marrying, and had suffered other harassments. After liberation, she was raped by a Soviet soldier while her mother was forced to watch. These facts were dutifully documented in her case file, but she was diagnosed with schizophrenia without consideration for a potential traumatic etiology. Over the following months and despite a lack of response to treatment, she received thirty insulin shock treatments and more than forty courses of electroshock.[40]

Otto Kauders's tentative steps to reflect on the experiences of National Socialism and to draw conclusions for psychiatric thought were cut short by his sudden death in 1949. His successor, Hans Hoff, had been forced to leave Austria in 1938 because of his Jewish background and survived the Holocaust in Baghdad and New York. He developed a strong interest in mental hygiene, especially with regards to former prisoners of war. Paradoxically, he was also one of the early proponents of the most invasive of the somatic psychiatric therapies, namely leucotomy (also known as lobotomy).[41] Under Hoff's leadership, the official orientation of Viennese psychiatry rested on the assumption of a multifactorial causation of mental illnesses; therapeutic methods were therefore eclectic and covered a range of procedures from psychosurgery to psychoanalysis. This self-professed pluralism allowed for individually tailored therapies for each patient, but it also meant that decisions were not so much evidence-based as they were a result of intuition and experience. Consequently, until the 1960s the hospital relied on somatic therapies which in other places had long been discredited, such as insulin shock and malariotherapy.[42]

In 1949, Walter Spiel und Karl Heinz Boysen reported high numbers of patients diagnosed with vegetative neuroses or states of vegetative exhaustion, comparable to Otto Kauders's findings a few years earlier. In response, the Vienna University Clinic introduced group therapy sessions in 1948, which were meant to facilitate a "spiritual unloading" within a "community of kindred spirits." The authors explicitly mentioned refugees, war invalids, and war widows as traumatized groups, but only obliquely referred to victims of Nazi persecution as "individuals, whose . . . existence has been shattered to the extreme in its entire uncertainty and has become wholly unpredictable."[43]

In what terms could the mental health consequences of extreme traumatization through persecution be articulated within psychiatric terminology after 1945? A study of psychiatric doctrine on psychological traumatization as reflected in German-language textbooks concluded that specific findings on Holocaust survivors did not begin to enter textbooks before the mid-1970s. Until the late 1960s, the dominating concept applied to survivors with mental health complaints was that of "traumatic neurosis," which had been introduced at the turn of the twentieth century.[44] According to this view, traumatic experiences could trigger lasting effects only in individuals with a corresponding predisposition but could never be considered the root cause of the symptoms. Furthermore, it was believed that the patients were driven by the unconscious wish to obtain benefits such as pensions ("pension neurosis" or "pension-seeking"), which provided additional arguments to deny compensation.[45] Hoff's own textbook, published in two volumes in 1956, echoes these views while never explicitly mentioning the effects of persecution suffered under National Socialism. Concerning the question of compensation after (post-)traumatic neuroses, however, he supported what he called the "modern view" that such claims could not be summarily denied based on the assumption of simulation or the implication of a "pension neurosis," a position that was at least in principle more favorable to survivors than the classical view on "traumatic neuroses" as invariably caused by (conscious or unconscious) pension-seeking. At the same time, he also maintained the detrimental view that only those individuals would suffer from longer-lasting effects who were already burdened with preexisting conditions of a genetic or other nature.[46] In a 1953 paper on evaluations for purposes of compensation in cases of neuroses, psychopathy, and vegetative dystonia (traumatic neuroses and vegetative dystonia being two of the few officially recognized psychiatric diagnoses that were applied to survivors), Hoff strongly argued against awarding victim's pensions, lest the neurotic, pension-seeking symptomatology become fixated.[47]

Hoff's first and only explicit examination of clinical questions concerning Nazi persecution was published two years after his death and was based on a paper he presented to a 1969 conference dedicated to the long-term effects of "extreme stress" in the context of National Socialist persecution. In this paper, which he presented as the consensus standpoint of the "Vienna School," he discussed, as possible consequences of persecution, the older concepts of vegetative dystonia and neurosis, but also, indicating an important development, chronic depression and the possibility of traumatic causation of psychosis. While he dismissed vegetative dystonia as a mere veil disguising the real origin of the symptoms and, in keeping with Freudian doctrine, insisted that neuroses had their roots in early childhood and could only be triggered but not caused by later trauma, he put forward chronic depression as the most important direct consequence of severe psychological trauma. What is more, he argued that it was the historical experience of National Socialist persecution that had led psychiatry to fully understand chronic depression. His paper contains a drastic description of the suffering of considerable numbers of his patients. They were "joyless, with very little zest for life, they cannot bring themselves to do anything, even the tendency to suicide is relatively low. They are actually the living dead." Hoff considered the clinical picture these survivors presented as a clearly defined syndrome with causal roots in the patients' experiences. In his view, the decisive moment often happened after liberation, when the survivors found out that all their family members had been murdered. The irreversibility of immense loss was also the main reason why Hoff had very little hope in helping such patients: they would sometimes be able to "function" again, but never fully recover.[48]

The reception of this paper within the Vienna School seems to have been limited. A textbook on "Systematic Psychiatry" published in 1977 by Peter Berner, Hans Hoff's disciple and successor, contains no reference to political persecution as possible etiological factor. In the context of a discussion of *"abnorme Erlebnisreaktionen"* (abnormal experiential reactions), however, Berner conceded that in some cases it is not the reactions that have to be considered "abnormal" but the stress that triggered them.[49]

Viktor Frankl, Auschwitz, and the Third Viennese School of Psychotherapy

Tellingly, neither Hans Hoff nor Peter Berner mentioned Viktor Frankl in their respective psychiatry textbooks, who was one of the first and also one of the most influential authors to reflect on the meaning of suffering and persecution for the mental health of former victims. Frankl based his existential analysis and logotherapy on his experiences in concentration camps, founding what came to be known as the "Third Viennese School of Psychotherapy" after Freud's psychoanalysis and Adler's individual psychology. The book that would bring him worldwide fame, *Man's Search for Meaning*, was based on lectures he gave in Vienna during the immediate postwar period.[50] Over the years, Frankl published a number of papers on his experiences, including some of the earliest chapters on the consequences of persecution to appear in psychiatry textbooks.[51]

An important factor in Frankl's popularity—at least in Germany and his home country Austria—was his willingness to accept a community of victims including both Holocaust survivors such as himself and those traumatized by the war, both as civilians and as members of the German armed forces. A paper from 1951 illustrates his specific brand of collective victimhood: "The new psychotherapy and the conception of man that underlies it was not concocted at the green table or the desk in the doctor's practice; rather, it formed itself in the hard school of the bomb craters and air-raid shelters, of the prisoner-of-war camps and the concentration camps."[52]

The Vienna Psychiatric Department, the American Joint, and the Assessment of "Hard Core Cases"

In 1954, the Vienna Psychiatric Department prepared a report for the American Jewish Joint Distribution Committee on a number of displaced persons who "had become conspicuous by their behavior or by their lack of social adjustment." The document provides a unique insight into how a representative of the "Vienna School" of psychiatry approached a group of Holocaust survivors with mental health issues, almost all of whom either had spent years in concentration camps or had been deported to Siberia and among whom there was "not a single patient who had not lost at least a part of his family during the war or in postwar times." In all, thirty-eight individuals had been designated for a psychiatric examination, six of them living in a DP camp in Hallein (Salzburg), twenty-one in camp Asten (Upper Austria), and nine in private care in Bad Ischl (Upper Austria). The author of the report was Raoul Schmiedek, a psychiatrist working under Hans Hoff. From the outset, Schmiedek emphasized that he was dealing "with human beings having gone through immeasurable sufferings and where judgment certainly requires all possible consideration." At the same time, he made clear that he felt justified in applying the usual diagnostic standards with regards to the line "between healthy and pathological," since so many other survivors had gone through similarly traumatic experiences without "becoming conspicuous." In line with the established view at the time (the 1953 paper by Hans Hoff quoted above is one typical example), Schmiedek found that "most of them have run into a kind of 'pension mentality,' a condition which makes them feel eligible for compassion because of the suffering they have gone through, and like children—at times even quite demanding—they expect that their wishes are complied with by the organization which for them replaces the father." Fulfilling these expectations was neither possible nor desirable, since this would only aggravate the supposed neurotic symptoms. This denial of "unrealistic, infantile wishes" should explain, in Schmiedek's view, why so many of the refugees he examined showed strong feelings of frustration and even aggression toward the American Jewish Joint Distribution Committee, and why so many of them tried to avoid being examined by a psychiatrist, whom they perceived as an agent of the aid organization—by feigning language difficulties, hiding, or outright refusing the examination. This attitude also colored Schmiedek's recommendations. While he considered psychotherapy time-consuming and not very promising because of the mentioned "pension mentality," he also stressed that a lack of opportunities to work and the uncertain future had a considerable influence on the examined individuals' conditions, recommending as a remedy vocational courses, creating opportunities for regular occupation, and ameliorating the living conditions in the camps.[53]

Toba Grosskind, born in 1927, survived Auschwitz as an adolescent. Following her liberation, as Raoul Schmiedek put it, "the patient [felt] that she [was] being persecuted." She spent several years in psychiatric institutions, mostly at Haus Bauer in Bad Ischl, where she received insulin and Cardiazol shocks and a leucotomy (lobotomy) was performed.[54] At the time of her examination, she lived in foster care, but Schmiedek diagnosed her with schizophrenia and insisted on her institutionalization.[55] Her later fate is unknown. Moische Friedmann, born in Poland in 1919, lost his parents and two siblings in 1942, apparently all shot at the same time. He fled to Austria after the war and lived in various DP camps, where he developed symptoms that Schmiedek qualified as a "neurotic reaction" to his experiences and "conversion hysteria." In this case, Schmiedek recommended two possible methods of psychotherapy: suggestive psychotherapy under Pentothal (popularly known as a "truth serum") or hypnosis therapy (a classic method first developed in the nineteenth century and a precursor to psychoanalysis).[56]

Some of the most difficult cases the American Jewish Joint Distribution Committee had to deal with concerned families who could not emigrate because they had children with mental disabilities who would not be allowed into their desired destination countries. The fourteen-year-old Martha Oesterreichischer from Hungary, who suffered from post-meningitis brain damage, had to be left behind by her family when they received an "excellent resettlement opportunity" (probably to the United States) that the parents felt "should not be denied their other children who could profit so much by it."[57] Similarly, Sabine Klapper had to leave behind her adult son Moses, born in Poland, when she received a visa for the United States under the DP act, but he was excluded by the US Public Health Service on grounds of mental disability.[58]

Youth Psychiatry and *Heilpädagogik*

In postwar Austria, two distinct if related disciplines competed for the responsibility to deal with mentally troubled or difficult children: child or adolescent psychiatry, which had gained ground during National Socialism, and the older *Heilpädagogik* (curative pedagogy), which had been institutionalized since the beginning of the century as a branch of pediatrics. The following case study stems from the work of Hans Asperger, the dominant figure in *Heilpädagogik*, and illustrates the impact of the belief that constitutionally healthy children could not suffer consequences from war-related trauma. Any observable symptoms, in this view, were attributed to some inborn constitutional defect or arose from the desire to gain material advantages, such as pensions.[59] Max G. was six years old in 1938 when his family was torn apart by the Nazis' anti-Jewish policies. His father, who was Jewish, was forced into a divorce and spent five years in a concentration camp. With his mother, Max then moved to Znojmo, a town annexed from Czechoslovakia after the Munich Agreement of 1938, from where the two were expelled along with the German-speaking population after Germany's defeat in 1945. At fourteen years of age, Max lived with his father in war-ravaged Vienna. In August 1946, Asperger wrote an expert opinion for the Juvenile Criminal Court on Max, who was accused of a series of thefts. Not a single word in Asperger's assessment of the boy referred to the fate of Max's father or to the fact that as a "half-Jew" Max had been in danger of persecution himself during half of his lifetime. While other documents in the file stressed that the boy had finished school with good grades despite his difficult situation, Asperger described him as "intellectually clearly reduced." Based on the boy's apparent "overfamiliarity" and "unreliability," he diagnosed him as an "epileptoid psychopath." In November 1946, after Max was fired from an apprenticeship that was seen as his last chance to prove his worth, and based on Asperger's diagnosis and recommendation, the boy was sent to the Eggenburg reformatory.[60]

Austria's Victim Welfare Law and the Quantification of Suffering

Barely three months after liberation, on 17 July 1945, the Austrian Provisional State Government enacted the first "Victim Welfare Law" ("Law on the Care for the Victims of the Fight for a Free and Democratic Austria"). Those officially recognized as victims on the basis of this law would be accorded certain benefits in terms of social insurance, access to housing, pensions, healthcare, and other things. From the outset, the criteria were narrowly defined. Only those who were deemed to have fought National Socialism "without reserve," "with weapon in hand," or at least "in words or deed" qualified for this welfare. Those who had survived would only be recognized if they had either been imprisoned for at least a year or, and this is particularly relevant in our context, if they suffered from severe health damages as a direct consequence of these same circumstances, namely combat, imprisonment, or mistreatment. With this first law, important parameters for the treatment of Nazi survivors were established early on. Most importantly, the law introduced an official hierarchy of victimhood, with the top of the symbolic pyramid being occupied by active fighters against National Socialism, especially those who had lost their lives because of their commitment to Austria's liberation.[61]

In 1947, a new version of the law was promulgated that extended the circle of those who could hope to be officially recognized as Nazi victims by introducing a new category, one that would also have significant repercussions on later medical debates. Henceforth, there would be a distinction between the "active" participants in the fight for Austria's freedom and the "passive" victims of political or "racial" persecution. A two-tier system was introduced, with two different types of identity cards and a graduated system of privileges and benefits according to the two different categories. Even this extended two-tier system continued to deny recognition to large numbers of survivors.[62]

The law also cemented the central position that medical experts would occupy for decades to come in the assignation of victim status and the symbolic, material, and medical benefits that came with it. At the same time, the scientific debates surrounding health effects of persecution became an important arena in the struggle for recognition and compensation, in which many different actors took part: medical experts, legislators, lawyers, and survivors along with their various organizations. Together with the role of medical experts, the law also laid the foundations for an important segment of the Second Austrian Republic's welfare state. Over the decades, a total of approximately one hundred thousand persons filed applications for benefits under the Victim Welfare Law.[63] To put this into perspective: this number is significantly lower than the two hundred thousand victims of anti-Jewish persecution alone. Under the provisions of the first version of the Victim Welfare Law, persecution for so-called "racial" or other reasons was not taken into account at all. Jews, Roma and Sinti, homosexuals, so-called antisocials, victims of medical crimes, and other groups remained excluded. Victims of forced sterilization were routinely told that there was no reason to believe that the surgeries had been ordered for other than purely medical reasons.[64] Those who had been forced into exile were excluded by a clause that demanded residency in Austria at the time of the benefit application.

The distinction between "active" fighters and "passive" victims shaped the perception of physicians dealing with survivors of persecution. In 1954, an Austrian physician told an international conference on healthcare for Nazi survivors that the state of the "passive" victims of "racial" persecution, who had often lost their whole families, was dominated by symptoms of depression, which had barely changed with liberation. In contrast to these passive victims, the author invoked the character of the heroic resistance fighter, whose morale and consciousness allowed him to overcome the adverse effects of persecution and imprisonment, even if his body might be affected. This polarization was also organized according to a clear gender dichotomy. While the male resistance fighters might suffer from well-defined physical health effects, female victims were pictured as more prone to psychosomatic reactions, echoing much older discourses on female hysteria.[65]

According to a study by the Austrian Historical Commission, health damages were invoked by 24.4 percent of victims; in the applications contained within the sample, 7.3 percent of survivors named neurological conditions and 7.3 percent mental illness. Put together, psychiatric and neurological complaints constituted the most frequently named group of conditions, before cardiovascular diseases.[66] In those cases in which a leading illness could be identified, psychiatric and neurological conditions were accepted as causally linked to persecution at a proportion of 70 percent, much higher than the group with the lowest acceptance rate—gynecological complaints—which was recognized in only 25 percent of cases.[67] While the diagnoses applied early after the war (such as "vegetative dystonia" or "traumatic neurosis") left survivors hardly any possibility of having their symptoms recognized as a consequence of what they had gone through, the chances of a positive outcome of an application improved after 1965, when two specific new diagnoses were introduced, namely "bionegative personality change" and "uprooting depression" (*Entwurzelungsdepression*).[68] Even so, the process of obtaining benefits on the grounds of the Victim Welfare Law remained riddled with bureaucratic hurdles. Survivors had to convince medical experts that their suffering was genuine and a direct consequence of persecution. The proceedings could take years and were humiliating and often re-traumatizing. Although some of the medical experts were sympathetic to their cause, in other cases they were confronted with experts who had been National Socialists prior to 1945.[69]

Although a number of survivors of Nazi persecution rose to positions of influence in Austrian psychiatry after 1945, for a long time attempts to integrate the traumatic experiences of the recent past into psychiatric thought remained limited to isolated episodes without much discernible impact on the mainstream. Until decades after the war, based on doctrines established since long before World War II, psychiatry—not only in Austria—failed to recognize the devastation wrought on the human mind by experiences of persecution, loss, and fear.

Herwig Czech studied history at the Universities of Graz, Vienna, Paris VII, and Duke (North Carolina). In 2007, he obtained his PhD from Vienna University with a thesis on medicine in National Socialist Vienna. He has widely published on topics related to the history of medicine and National Socialism in Austria. In 2020 he was appointed professor of the history of medicine at the Medical University of Vienna.

Notes

This chapter is an outcome of the research project "Physical and Psychological Consequences Suffered by Survivors of Nazi Persecution in Post-WWII Austria." It was carried out from 2014 to 2017 under the direction of the author, first at the Documentation Center of the Austrian Resistance (DÖW) and then at the Medical University of Vienna, and generously financed by the National Fund of the Republic of Austria for Victims of National Socialism and the Future Fund of the Republic of Austria.

1. Jütte et al. 2011, 214.
2. Czech 2012b.
3. Friedlander 1995.
4. Neugebauer 2002.
5. Czech 2017.
6. Kauders 1945.
7. Hoff 1971.
8. Frankl 1946b.
9. On the difficulties of establishing how many Jews lived in Vienna before the war, how many survived, and how many lost their lives, see Kranebitter 2018.
10. Moser 1999, 76–86.
11. JDC Archives Jerusalem, Geneva Office, Countries/Austria, AU.139. Remarkably, of these, 890 were men and only 468 were women. (I thank Marion Zingler for extracting this data.)
12. JDC Archives Jerusalem, Geneva Office, Countries/Austria, AU.140. In this group, there was a majority of women (1,207) over men (1,012).
13. Präsidium der Israelitischen Kultusgemeinde Wien 1948; JDC Archives Jerusalem, Geneva Office, Countries/Austria, AU.132, Memorandum by J. Benson Saks, 30 July 1946. Benson Saks, the American Jewish Joint Distribution Committee's representative in Vienna, estimated that an additional twenty thousand Jewish "infiltrees" [sic] were present in Austria. On Jewish DPs in postwar Germany, see, for example, Grossmann 2002.
14. Patka 2001; Jewish Museum Vienna, Wartesaal der Hoffnung. Das Rothschild-Spital im November 1947—Fotos von Henry Ries. Retrieved 12 May 2019 from http://www.jmw.at/en/node/3074.
15. Präsidium der Israelitischen Kultusgemeinde Wien 1948, 28, 35.
16. Archives des Affaires étrangères (La Courneuve), AUT-0201, Sécurité Publique, Renseignements Généraux, Note d'information Nr. 692, 22 September 1947.
17. "Die angeblichen Experimente im Infektionskrankenhaus," in Arbeiter-Zeitung Nr. 220, 21 September 1947, 3.
18. Czech 2018, 23.
19. Czech 2012b, 52–59.
20. Neugebauer 2002, 108.
21. Czech 2014; Czech 2019a.
22. Faulstich 1998. On Austria, see Czech 2012a.
23. Central Archives for the History of the Jewish People Jerusalem (CAHJP), Archiv der Israelitischen Kultusgemeinde Wien, A/W 415, Aufgliederung der in Wien und Niederdonau lebenden Juden, January to December 1944.
24. WStLA, 1.3.2.209.2.A12.3, Krankengeschichte Leo Aschkenasy.
25. Schwarz 2002.
26. Czech 2018, 23.
27. Czech 2019a.
28. Watzka 2016.
29. Holzer 1948, 41.

30. Czech 2003, 22.
31. WStLA, 1.3.2.209.A1. Nervenheilanstalt Rosenhügel, Stransky an Wiener Magistrat, Abt. II/3 Anstaltenverwaltung, 9 June, 7 July, and 28 December 1945.
32. On the denazification of the Austrian medical profession, see Czech 2017.
33. Arias 2009.
34. Hubenstorf 1987, 382–83; Gabriel 2016.
35. Kauders 1946b.
36. Kauders 1945.
37. Kauders 1946a, 711.
38. WStLA, 1.3.2.209.1.A57/222, Krankengeschichten Bernhard Kellner and Martin Fischer (with thanks to Tobias Röck for his help with archival research).
39. WStLA, 1.3.2.209.1.A57/224, Krankengeschichte Tibor Guttmann.
40. WStLA, 1.3.2.209.1.A56.1947, Journal-Nr. 7871.
41. Hoff et al. 1955; Hoff 1951.
42. Heiss 2015.
43. Boysen et al. 1949. ("Aber auch bei Menschen, bei denen, um mit *Kauders* zu sprechen, 'das eigene Dasein in seiner ganzen Fragwürdigkeit aufs äußerste erschüttert und völlig unberechenbar wird,' trifft das vorher Gesagte zu.")
44. Kloocke et al. 2005, e1; see also Priebe et al. 2002, and Söhner et al. 2018.
45. The concept of "pension neurosis" was introduced by German psychiatrists after World War I. Its history is inextricably linked to the denial of benefits to war veterans who suffered from what today would be called PTSD by denying a direct causal link between traumatic experiences and long-term effects on mental health (Baumann 2006, 166). A more flexible use of the term "trauma" can be found in Erwin Ringel's (1921–94) pioneering study on suicide, which explicitly mentions concentration camp survivors in the context of what he calls "political traumatization" (Ringel 1953).
46. Hoff 1956, 578–83, 666–75.
47. Hoff 1953.
48. Hoff 1971. In the paper, Hoff furthermore argued that experiences of persecution could play a role in triggering psychoses, provided there was a genetic or "constitutional" predisposition. Overall, Hoff's approach meant that expert evaluators (such as himself) had almost unlimited powers to define the conditions that would be recognized as caused (or at least triggered) by trauma linked to persecution and that would be attributed to some unrelated childhood trauma or a preexisting constitutional defect. Concerning the external causation of psychoses, Nagy (1959, 705) already argued along similar lines, albeit without any direct reference to National Socialist persecution.
49. Berner 1977, 57.
50. Frankl 1946b; Frankl 1946a; Frankl 1946c.
51. Frankl 1959; Frankl 1961.
52. Frankl 1951, 472. ("Nicht am grünen Tisch, nicht am Ordinationsschreibtisch wurde die neue Psychotherapie und das Menschenbild, das ihr zu grunde gelegt ist, ausgeheckt; sondern es hat sich geformt in der harten Schule der Bombentrichter und Bombenkeller, der Kriegsgefangenen- und Konzentrationslager"). After the war, Frankl claimed that he and Pötzl had worked together to transfer Jewish patients from Pötzl's Psychiatric University Clinic to the Jewish hospital in order to save them from "euthanasia." See Czech 2018, 35. For the controversy around Frankl's life in Vienna before his deportation, see Pytell 2000; Pytell 2005 (translated as Pytell 2015); Biller et al. 2002; Batthyany 2007.
53. JDC Archives Jerusalem, Geneva Office, Countries/Austria, AU.114, Mental Hygiene 1949, 1951, 1954. Report by the Psychiatric-Neurologic Clinic of the University of Vienna to American Jewish Joint Distribution Committee, Vienna, 27 February 1954. Signed Dr. Raoul Schmiedek and Professor Hans Hoff. A similar approach occurred when the committee in Austria concluded an agreement with August Aichhorn, one of the few psychoanalysts who had remained in Vienna during

the Nazi period, to offer therapy to survivors, starting with "mild cases." An important goal of these therapies was to liberate patients from "infantilistic, father-bound tendencies" and to bring them to a point where they would contribute financially to their treatment, echoing familiar concerns about "pension neurosis": JDC Archives Jerusalem, Geneva Office, Countries/Austria, AU.114, Mental Hygiene 1949, 1951, 1954. P. Robinson, AJDC Austria to William Schmidt, AJDC Paris, 22 March 1949. On August Aichhorn, see Aichhorn et al. 2012; Aichhorn 2005.

54. Haus Bauer was a hotel in Bad Ischl that served during the war as a neurological hospital for the German Luftwaffe and after 1945 became a civilian neurological hospital (Schaller 2000, 14). Several of Schmiedek's case histories mention lobotomies performed at Haus Bauer, sometimes more than once on the same patient.

55. JDC Archives Jerusalem, Geneva Office, Countries/Austria, AU.114, Mental Hygiene 1949, 1951, 1954. Psychiatric report on Toba Grosskind, 24 January 1954.

56. JDC Archives Jerusalem, Geneva Office, Countries/Austria, AU.114, Mental Hygiene 1949, 1951, 1954. Psychiatric report on Moische Friedmann, 24 January 1954.

57. JDC Archives Jerusalem, Geneva Office, Countries/Austria, AU.114, Mental Hygiene 1949, 1951, 1954. AJDC Geneva to AJDC Amsterdam, 12 June 1951.

58. JDC Archives Jerusalem, Geneva Office, Countries/Austria, AU.114, Mental Hygiene 1949, 1951, 1954. American Joint Distribution Committee, US Zone Headquarters, Salzburg to ADJC Geneva, 19 July 1951.

59. Asperger 1952, 141, 194.

60. Czech 2018, 29–30. I thank Gertrude Czipke for these documents. On the concept of the "epileptoid personality," see Asperger 1952, 132–34. There is no indication that Max actually suffered from epilepsy; Asperger's diagnosis was based purely on personality traits he observed during his interaction with the boy, which he considered typical for epileptics. On Asperger's role during National Socialism, see Czech 2015; Czech 2018; Sheffer 2018; Czech 2019b.

61. Gesetz vom 17. Juli 1945 über die Fürsorge für die Opfer des Kampfes um ein freies, demokratisches Österreich (Opfer-Fürsorgegesetz), Staatsgesetzblatt Nr. 90, 22. Stück, 27 July 1945, 111–13. See also Bailer-Galanda 1993; Berger et al. 2004.

62. Bundesgesetz vom 4. Juli 1947 über die Fürsorge für die Opfer des Kampfes um ein freies, demokratisches Österreich und die Opfer politischer Verfolgung (Opferfürsorgegesetz), Bundesgesetzblatt, 39. Stück, 1 September 1947, 821–24.

63. Berger et al. 2004, 34–36.

64. Neugebauer 1989; Bailer-Galanda 1992; Spring 2002.

65. Huk 1955.

66. Berger et al. 2004, 53, 193. The most frequent category, "loss of freedom," was mentioned by 89.6 percent; it was possible to name more than one category.

67. Berger et al. 2004, 204.

68. Berger et al. 2004, 189. The official guidelines for awarding pensions to war veterans and survivors of Nazi persecution stipulated that a diagnosis of neurosis, psychopathy, or vegetative dystonia would not be recognized as grounds for compensation, except in cases in which neurotic or psychopathic symptoms were so severe as to be comparable to a psychosis: Birti 1958, 394–95.

69. As was the case of SS member Dr. Kurt Zemann, see Neugebauer et al. 2005, 261.

References

Aichhorn, Thomas. 2005. "Blicke zurück und nach vorne: Aus der Korrespondenz August Aichhorn—Anna Freud nach 1945." In *Trauma der Psychoanalyse? Die Vertreibung der Psychoanalyse aus Wien 1938 und die Folgen*, edited by Wiener Psychoanalytische Vereinigung, 249–73. Wien: Psychosozial-Verlag.

Aichhorn, Thomas, and Christiane Rothländer. 2012. "Zur Errichtung der 'Wiener Arbeitsgemeinschaft' des 'Göring-Instituts' und der Arbeits- und Ausbildungsgruppe von August Aichhorn." In *Materialien zur Geschichte der Psychoanalyse in Wien 1938–1945*, edited by Mitchell G. Ash, 347–373. Frankfurt am Main: Brandes & Apsel.

Arias, Ingrid. 2009. "Die Wiener Medizinische Fakultät 1945: Zwischen Entnazifizierung und katholischer Elitenrestauration." In *Wissenschaft macht Politik. Hochschule in den politischen Systembrüchen 1933 und 1945*, edited by Sabine Schleiermacher and Udo Schagen, 247–62. Stuttgart: Franz Steiner Verlag.

Asperger, Hans. 1952. *Heilpädagogik. Einführung in die Psychopathologie des Kindes für Ärzte, Lehrer, Psychologen und Fürsorgerinnen*. Wien: Springer-Verlag.

Bailer-Galanda, Brigitte, 1992. "Verfolgt und Vergessen: Die Diskriminierung einzelner Opfergruppen durch die Opferfürsorgegesetzgebung." *Jahrbuch des Dokumentationsarchivs des österreichischen Widerstandes*: 13–25.

Bailer-Galanda, Brigitte. 1993. *Wiedergutmachung kein Thema: Österreich und die Opfer des Nationalsozialismus*. Wien: Löcker.

Batthyany, Alexander, and Mythos Frankl. 2007. *Geschichte der Logotherapie und Existenzanalyse 1925–1945: Entgegnung auf Timothy Pytell*. Wien/Berlin/Münster: LIT.

Baumann, Stefanie. 2006. "Opfer von Menschenversuchen als Sonderfall." In *Grenzen der Wiedergutmachung: Die Entschädigung für NS-Verfolgte in West- und Osteuropa 1945-2000*, edited by Hans-Günther Hockerts, Claudia Moisel, Tobias Winstel, 147–86. Göttingen: Wallstein.

Berger, Karin, Nikolaus Dimmel, David Forster, u.a., 2004. *Vollzugspraxis des "Opferfürsorgegesetzes." Analyse der praktischen Vollziehung des einschlägigen Sozialrechts. Entschädigung im Sozialrecht nach 1945 in Österreich 2. Veröffentlichungen der Österreichischen Historikerkommission. Vermögensentzug während der NS-Zeit sowie Rückstellungen und Entschädigungen seit 1945 in Österreich, Band 29/2*. Wien/München: Oldenbourg Verlag.

Berner, Peter. 1977. *Psychiatrische Systematik: Ein Lehrbuch*. Bern/Stuttgart/Wien: Verlag Hans Huber.

Biller, Karlheinz, Jay I. Levinson, and Timothy Pytell. 2002. "Viktor Frankl—Opposing Views." *Journal of Contemporary History* 37(1): 105–13.

Birti, Burkhart (ed.). 1958. *Das Opferfürsorgegesetz in seiner derzeitigen Fassung und sonstige Vorschriften des Fürsorgerechtes für die Opfer des Kampfes für ein freies, demokratisches Österreich und die Opfer der politischen Verfolgung unter besonderer Berücksichtigung der Rechtsprechung des Verwaltungsgerichtshofes, erläutert von Dr. Burkhart Birti, Sektionsrat im Bundesministerium für soziale Verwaltung*. Wien: Verlag der Österreichischen Staatsdruckerei.

Boysen, K.-H., and W. Spiel. 1949. "Vorläufiger Bericht über Gruppenbehandlung vegetativer Erschöpfungszustände." *Wiener Zeitschrift für Nervenheilkunde und deren Grenzgebiete* 2(3): 270–79.

Czech, Herwig. 2003. *Erfassung, Selektion und "Ausmerze": Das Wiener Gesundheitsamt und die Umsetzung der nationalsozialistischen "Erbgesundheitspolitik" 1938 bis 1945*. Wien: Deuticke.

———. 2012a. "Jenseits von Hartheim: Dezentrale Krankenmorde in Österreich während der NS-Zeit." In *NS-Euthanasie in der "Ostmark." Fachtagung vom 17. bis 19. April 2009 im Lern- und Gedenkort Schloss Hartheim*, edited by Arbeitskreis zur Erforschung der nationalsozialistischen Euthanasie und Zwangssterilisation, 37–60. Münster: Klemm&Oelschläger.

———. 2012b. "Nazi 'Euthanasia' Crimes in World War II Austria." *Holocaust in History and Memory* 5: 51–73.

———. 2014. "Abusive Medical Practices on 'Euthanasia' Victims in Austria during and after World War II." In *Human Subjects Research after the Holocaust*, edited by Sheldon Rubenfeld and Susan Benedict, 109–25. Cham/Heidelberg/New York u.a.: Springer.

———. 2015. "Dr. Hans Asperger und die 'Kindereuthanasie' in Wien—mögliche Verbindungen." In *Auf den Spuren Hans Aspergers. Fokus Asperger-Syndrom: Gestern, Heute, Morgen*, edited by Arnold Pollak, 24–29. Stuttgart: Schattauer.

———. 2017. "Braune Westen, weiße Mäntel: Die Versuche einer Entnazifizierung der Medizin in Österreich." In *Österreichische Ärzte und Ärztinnen im Nationalsozialismus*, edited by Herwig Czech and Paul Weindling (im Auftrag des Dokumentationsarchivs des österreichischen Widerstandes), 179–201. Wien: Dokumentationsarchiv des österreichischen Widerstandes.

———. 2018. "Hans Asperger, National Socialism and 'Race Hygiene' in Nazi-Era Vienna." *Molecular Autism* 9(29): 1–43.

———. 2019a. "Der Spiegelgrund-Komplex. Kinderheilkunde, Heilpädagogik, Psychiatrie und Jugendfürsorge im Nationalsozialismus." In *Behinderung und Gesellschaft. Ein universitärer Beitrag zum Gedenkjahr 2018*, edited by Gottfried Biewer and Michelle Proyer, 85–106. Wien: Universität Wien/ÖH Uni Wien (Open-Access Publikation).

———. 2019b. "Response to 'Non-complicit: Revisiting Hans Asperger's Career in Nazi-era Vienna.'" *Journal of Autism and Developmental Disorders* 49: 3883–87.

Faulstich, Heinz. *Hungersterben in der Psychiatrie 1914–1949: Mit einer Topographie der NS-Psychiatrie*. Freiburg: Lambertus.

Frankl, V. E. 1946a. *. . . trotzdem ja zum Leben sagen. Drei Vorträge gehalten an der Volkshochschule Wien-Ottakring*. Wien: Franz Deuticke.

———. 1959. "Psychohygienische Erfahrungen im Konzentrationslager." In *Handbuch der Neurosenlehre und Psychotherapie. 4. Band: Spezielle Psychotherapie II und Neurosenprophylaxe*, edited by Viktor E. Frankl, Victor E. Freiherr von Gebsattel, and J. H. Schultz, 735–47. München/Berlin: Urban & Schwarzenberg.

Frankl, Viktor E. 1946b. *Ein Psycholog erlebt das Konzentrationslager*. Wien: Verlag für Jugend und Volk.

———. 1946c. *Man's Search for Meaning*. New York: Washington Square Press.

———. 1951. "Zweites Referat über 'Psychotherapie.'" *Wiener Zeitschrift für Nervenheilkunde und deren Grenzgebiete* 3: 461–74.

———. 1961. "Psychologie und Psychiatrie des Konzentrationslagers." In *Psychiatrie der Gegenwart: Forschung und Praxis. Band III: Soziale und angewandte Psychiatrie*, edited by H. W. Gruhle, R. Jung, W. Mayer-Gross, and Max Müller, 743–59. Berlin/Göttingen/Heidelberg: Springer Verlag.

Friedlander, Henry. 1995. *The Origins of Nazi Genocide: From Euthanasia to the Final Solution*. Chapel Hill: University of North Carolina Press.

Gabriel, Eberhard. 2016. "Zum Wiederaufbau des akademischen Lehrkörpers in der Psychiatrie in Wien nach 1945." *Virus—Beiträge zur Sozialgeschichte der Medizin* 14: 35–77.

Grossmann, Atina. 2002. "Victims, Villains, and Survivors: Gendered Perceptions and Self-Perceptions of Jewish Displaced Persons in Occupied Postwar Germany." *Journal of the History of Sexuality* 11(1/2): 291–318.

Heiss, Gernot. 2015. *Die Malariatherapie und weitere diagnosekorrelierte Therapien: Ihre Anwendung an der Wiener Universitätsklinik für Psychiatrie und Neurologie in den 1950er und 1960er Jahren und ihre Diskussion in der zeitgenössischen Forschung* (unveröffentlichter Endbericht für den Jubiläumsfonds der Österreichischen Nationalbank). Wien.

Hoff, H., and W. Spiel. 1955. "Der Stand der psychischen Hygiene." *Wiener Archiv für Psychologie, Psychiatrie und Neurologie* 5: 1–8.

Hoff, Hans. 1951. "Psychochirurgie." *Wiener Zeitschrift für Nervenheilkunde und deren Grenzgebiete* 3: 425–39.

———. 1953. "Begutachtung von Neurosen, vegetativer Dystonie und Psychopathien." *Mitteilungen der österreichischen Sanitätsverwaltung* 54: 143–45.

———. 1971. "Die Klinik psychischer Verfolgungsschäden." In *Spätschäden nach Extrembelastungen, II. Internationale Medizinisch-Juristische Konferenz in Düsseldorf, 1969*, edited by H.-J. Herberg, 285–89. Herford: Nicolaische Verlagsbuchhandlung.

Hoff, Hans, with the cooperation of G. Benedetti, R. Brun, M. Gschwind, H. Krayenbühl, H. Meng, and W. A. Stoll (eds.). 1956. *Lehrbuch der Psychiatrie: Verhütung, Prognostik und Behandlung der geistigen und seelischen Erkrankungen. 2 Bände*. Basel: Benno Schwabe & Co.

Holzer, W. 1948. "Gegenwartsfragen der physikalischen Therapie." *Wiener klinische Wochenschrift* 60: 122.

Hubenstorf, Michael. 1987. "Österreichische Ärzteemigration." In *Vertriebene Vernunft I. Emigration und Exil österreichischer Wissenschaft 1930/1940*, edited by Friedrich Stadler, 359–415. Wien.

Huk, Benedikt. 1955. "Reihenuntersuchung ehemaliger KZ-ler." In *Gesundheitsschäden durch Verfolgung und Gefangenschaft und ihre Spätfolgen*, edited by Max Michel, 82–83. Frankfurt am Main: Röderberg-Verlag.

Jütte, Robert, Wolfgang U. Eckart, Hans-Walter Schmuhl, and Winfried Süß. 2011. *Medizin und Nationalsozialismus. Bilanz und Perspektiven der Forschung*. Göttingen: Wallstein Verlag.

Kauders, Otto. 1945. "Zur Psychologie der Terrorwirkung." *Der Turm* 1: 51–53.

———. 1946a. "Der psychiatrische Unterricht innerhalb des medizinischen Bildungsganges: Antrittsvorlesung an der Psychiatrisch-neurologischen Universitätsklinik in Wien am 29. Oktober 1946." *Wiener klinische Wochenschrift* 58(44): 709–14.

———. 1946b. *Vegetatives Nervensystem und Seele*. Wien: Urban und Schwarzenberg.

Kloocke, Ruth, Heinz-Peter Schmiedebach, and Stefan Priebe. 2005. "Psychisches Trauma in deutschsprachigen Lehrbüchern der Nachkriegszeit—die psychiatrische 'Lehrmeinung' zwischen 1945 und 2002." *Psychiatrische Praxis* 32(7): e1–e15.

Kranebitter, Andreas. 2018. "Jenseits des Zählbaren: Quantitative Auswertungen zur jüdischen Bevölkerung Österreichs zwischen 1938 und 1945." *Jahrbuch des Dokumentationsarchivs des österreichischen Widerstandes*: 31–52.

Moser, Jonny. 1999. *Demographie der jüdischen Bevölkerung Österreichs 1938–1945*. Wien.

Nagy, K. 1959. "Neue biochemische Aspekte in der Pathogenese psychiatrischer Erkrankungen." *Wiener klinische Wochenschrift* 71(37): 702–5.

Neugebauer, Wolfgang. 1989. "Das Opferfürsorgegesetz und die Sterilisationsopfer in Österreich." *Jahrbuch des Dokumentationsarchivs des österreichischen Widerstandes*: 144–50.

———. 2002. "Juden als Opfer der NS-Euthanasie in Wien 1940–1945." In *Von der Zwangssterilisierung zur Ermordung: Zur Geschichte der NS-Euthanasie in Wien Teil II*, edited by Eberhard Gabriel and Wolfgang Neugebauer, 99–111. Wien/Köln/Weimar: Böhlau.

Neugebauer, Wolfgang, and Peter Schwarz. 2005. *Der Wille zum aufrechten Gang: Offenlegung der Rolle des BSA bei der gesellschaftlichen Reintegration ehemaliger Nationalsozialisten; Herausgegeben vom Bund sozialdemokratischer AkademikerInnen, Intellektueller und KünstlerInnen (BSA)*. Wien: Czernin Verlag.

Patka, Marcus G. 2001. "Das Rothschild-Spital in Wien." In *"Displaced": Paul Celan in Wien 1947–1948 (Katalog zur gleichnamigen Ausstellung im Jüdischen Museum Wien)*, edited by Peter Goßens and Marcus G. Patka, 46–50. Frankfurt am Main: Suhrkamp.

Präsidium der Israelitischen Kultusgemeinde Wien. 1948. *Bericht des Präsidiums der Israelitischen Kultusgemeinde Wien über die Tätigkeit in den Jahren 1945 bis 1948*. Wien: Verlag der Israelitischen Kultusgemeinde Wien.

Priebe, Stefan, Marion Nowak, Heinz-Peter Schmiedebach. 2002. "Trauma und Psyche in der deutschen Psychiatrie seit 1889." *Psychiatrische Praxis* 29(1): 3–9.

Pytell, Timothy. 2000. "The Missing Pieces of the Puzzle: A Reflection on the Odd Career of Viktor Frankl." *Journal of Contemporary History* 35(2): 281–306.

———. 2005. *Frankl: Ende eines Mythos?* Innsbruck/Wien/Bozen.

———. 2015. *Viktor Frankl's Search for Meaning: An Emblematic 20th-Century Life*. New York: Berghahn Books.

Ringel, Erwin. 1953. *Der Selbstmord: Abschluß einer krankhaften psychischen Entwicklung; Eine Untersuchung an 745 geretteten Selbstmördern*. Düsseldorf: Maudrich.

Schaller, Anton. 2000. "Das medizinische Ischl. Solebad, kaiserliche Sommerresidenz, Lazarettstadt." *Mitteilungen des Ischler Heimatvereines*: 10–16.

Schwarz, Peter. 2002. "Mord durch Hunger: 'Wilde Euthanasie' und 'Aktion Brandt' in Steinhof in der NS-Zeit." In *Von der Zwangssterilisierung zur Ermordung: Zur Geschichte der NS-Euthanasie in Wien Teil II*, edited by Eberhard Gabriel and Wolfgang Neugebauer, 113–41. Wien/Köln/Weimar: Böhlau.

Sheffer, Edith. 2018. *Asperger's Children: The Origins of Autism in Nazi Vienna*. New York: W. W. Norton & Company.

Söhner, Felicitas, and Gerhard Baader. 2018. "The Impact of Dealing with the Late Effects of National Socialist Terror on West German Psychiatric Care." *Psychiatric Quarterly* 89: 475–87.

Spring, Claudia. 2002. "Schickt mir Gift, das kostet nicht viel: Gesundheitspolitische Verfolgung während des NS-Regimes und die legistische, medizinische und gesellschaftliche Ausgrenzung von zwangssterilisierten Frauen und Männern in der Zweiten Republik." In *Medizin im Nationalsozialismus: Wege der Aufarbeitung*, edited by Sonia Horn and Peter Malina, 185–210. Wien: Verlag der Österreichischen Ärztekammer.

Watzka, Carlos. 2016. "Die 'Fälle' Wolfgang Holzer und Hans Bertha sowie andere 'Personalia': Kontinuitäten und Diskontinuitäten in der Grazer Psychiatrie 1945–1970." *Virus—Beiträge zur Sozialgeschichte der Medizin* 14: 103–38.

CHAPTER 16

"TO PREVENT FURTHER UNFOUNDED ALY CONSTRUCTIONS"

Götz Aly
Translated by Jefferson Chase

In his day, Julius Hallervorden (1882–1965) was one of world's leading brain researchers. On 16 July 1941, he wrote to his former boss, the psychiatrist Hans Heinze, "Enclosed I'm sending a report and the images of Ursula Kriesch, which have just been finished. Give my regards to Miss Pusch, who is particularly interested in this case. I'm very curious about how far we can realize our plans. In the short terms, it seems uncertain whether Miss Pusch can be part of them."[1]

Heinze was the director of the Brandenburg-Görden Sanatorium and Nursing Home and is considered one of the founders of the discipline of child and youth psychiatry. Back then, he worked as an evaluator for *Aktion T4*, rendering thousands of death sentences on the basis of short questionnaires over usually adult, long-term patients in German mental asylums. He also ran a so-called child specialty department at his clinic. As was also the case at some thirty similar institutions throughout the Third Reich, it carried out what were known as "interruptions of life" of children with moderately serious to serious handicaps. Moreover, Heinze had a leading position in conjunction with child euthanasia, in which he was one of the three evaluators responsible for the entire Reich. Together the evaluators sent at least five thousand children and young people to their deaths between 1939 and 1945.

The Miss Pusch to whom Hallervorden sent his special regards was Dr. Friederike Pusch. Under Heinze, she was responsible for the hospital ward in Brandenburg-Görden at which handicapped children were murdered. Ursula Kriesch was one of her patients, and Pusch received sixteen photographs of her brain. Kriesch was one of the many victims of Hans Heinze und Julius Hallervorden. On 28 October 1940, she was taken together with thirty-four other children and young people to a nearby gas chamber and killed in the interests of scientific research. Hallervorden came to Brandenburg-Görden specially from Berlin-Buch to remove the victims' brains immediately after they were murdered.

Details about the plans Hallervorden had with Heinze are contained in an application for financial support Hallervorden sent to the German Research Society on 8 December 1942: "The material is constantly being made more complete by the autopsy division of the Brandenburg State Welfare Institute at Görden bei Brandenburg.... Additionally, I was able over the course of the summer to autopsy 500 brains of imbeciles and prepare them for analysis."[2] Hallervorden was researching the causes of congenital imbecility and the difference between traumatic and so-called genuine epilepsy, which was at the time considered hereditary. Heinze added his own special area of interest: the "abnormal character."

In order to compare the insights derived from autopsying brains with the clinically determined level of imbecility of a child before he or she was murdered, Dr. Pusch and her team at the death ward drew up lists of findings. They contain statements that give us an idea of what sort of a child Ursula Kriesch was:

> Ursula was transferred here from the Buch Mental Hospital. During the admissions process, she made a reserved impression. She opened up when she discovered a young female friend of hers in the ward, whom she greeted with tight embraces. Ursula continued to maintain her affection for the other little patient. She was more helpless than Ursula, which is why the latter took care of her. Ursula was always there when the young girl lacked something. She helped her with her daily needs. Ursula enjoyed talking about her relatives and was very grateful every time she received a package. She liked looking at the enclosed postcard and showed it to everyone with great joy.... She quickly found her bearings in the ward and soon understood its daily routines. She knew the rules of the board game Parcheesi and was capable of explaining them to others. She played with respect for others and an overview of the greater situation. She added the sums of the rolls of the dice for everyone and recognized the advantages and disadvantages of her playing partners. When she talked for longer intervals, her unclear speech became noticeable . . .

After Ursula Kriesch was murdered in the name of science, Hallervorden himself removed her brain, had it cut into razor-thin slices, and had sixteen extremely sharp photographs made. He subsequently determined that they contained small "marrow-bearing scars" that probably resulted from a trauma at birth as well as a few other irregularities.

Hallervorden added the results of his investigation and the brain sample to his collection. It represented the empirical foundation of the Kaiser Wilhelm Institute for Brain Research in Berlin-Buch. From 1938 to 1956, Julius Hallervorden served as the director of its Histopathologic Department and specialized in collecting the brains of victims of Nazi crimes up until 1945. (This was well known in specialist circles.) In 1944, amid the bombardment of Berlin, the institute was relocated to Dillenburg in the state of Hessen. It later became the Max Planck Institute in Gießen before moving to Frankfurt am Main in 1961. It still exists there today as part of the city university's neuropathological Edinger Institute.

In June 1945, Julius Hallervorden admitted to Major Leo Alexander of the US military that he had prepared numerous brains of victims of the Nazi euthanasia program for scientific experimentation. In early 1946, he confirmed to the president of the International Criminal Court at Nuremberg that among the "brains of deceased mentally ill people and idiots were those who had been victims of the euthanasia program."[3] Before that, on 9 March 1944, he remarked to Paul Nitsche, the medical director of the organization responsible for the euthanasia murders, "In total I have received 697 brains including those I removed myself in Brandenburg. That also includes those from Dösen. A significant number of them have already been examined. It's unclear whether I will subject them all to histologic examination."[4]

This document too has been part of the public record since the Nuremberg Doctors Trial. But amid the enthusiasm of the German Economic Miracle of the 1950s, the public conveniently forgot facts that had often been established directly after World War II. The presidents, general secretaries, and institute directors of the Max Planck Society, founded in 1949, behaved much the same. They forgot whatever they wanted to forget and denied whatever could be denied. At the same time, almost without exception, they took over the institutes and personnel from the Kaiser Wilhelm Society unchanged. Working from this foundation, which was morally rotten from its very inception, neuro-anatomists continued for four decades to use the huge collection of brain cross-sections that Julius Hallervorden systematically brought together between 1939 and 1945.

Nonetheless, in 1962, the institute declined to publish, as was customary, a special journal in honor of Hallervorden's eightieth birthday. His long-time colleague and successor Wilhelm Krücke advised against it because the Nuremberg Doctors Trial had determined that his former boss had "taken possession of 600 brains from euthanasia facilities," and Krücke considered it "likely that this information was true." The document in question had been part of the famous compilation of source materials *Diktat der Menschenverachtung* (Dictate of contempt for human beings), published and commentated by Alexander Mitscherlich and Fred Mielke in 1947. Both the compilation and the quoted document have been studiously ignored but had been reissued by the Fischer publishing house in 1960 under the title *Medizin ohne Menschlichkeit* (Medicine without humanity). Only then had this historic work found a broad echo in the media, attracting broad attention to the doctors who had been complicit in medical crimes, including Julius Hallervorden. For that reason, and because the general prosecutor's office in Frankfurt had begun investigating the euthanasia murders, Krücke advised against honoring Hallervorden's name.

A third reason not to celebrate Hallervorden's career related directly to Mitscherlich himself, who had made himself into a persona non grata of the medical guild as a young man in 1946, when he had published the report about the Doctors Trial at Nuremberg. In 1960, Krücke had spoken out against Mitscherlich, as is detailed in a confidential note made by the then-president of the Max Planck Society:

> The author of the book that has just appeared in the Fischer publishing house, Professor Mitscherlich, is at present the director of the State Institute for Psychotherapy and Psychoanalysis in Frankfurt a.M. He received this position, Mr. Krücke says, over the objections of the School of Medicine. According to his information, efforts are being made within the state government and ministry of culture of Hessen to incorporate Mr. Mitscherlich into the University of Frankfurt. The school of medicine will resist this under Mr. Krücke, who will become the dean at the start of next semester. Since Mr. Krücke is of the opinion that Mitscherlich will pursue this battle with every means at his disposal, Mr. Krücke thinks that it would be counterproductive to go out on a limb in the Hallervorden affair.[5]

Krücke's maneuvering proved successful. The institute Mitscherlich had founded in 1960, which since 1964 had born the name of Sigmund Freud, was not made part of the university. Instead, it existed in the unusual form of an independent state institution. In 1973, when Alexander Mitscherlich, who had published his postdoctoral thesis all the way back in 1946, finally received a full professorship at the age of fifty-nine, it was not from the University of Frankfurt School of Medicine but rather from the philosophy department.

"Arbitrary and Illegal" Obstruction by the Max Planck Society

In 1984, after overcoming persistent resistance, I became the first historian to view the Hallervorden Collection. Almost thirty years later, I was revisited by this chapter from my past. In May 2013, Gerhard Kalb, the former director of the legal division of the Max Planck Society, tried to get a legal injunction against a passage in my book *Die Belasteten: Die "Euthanasie"-Morde 1939–1945* (Morally compromised: The "euthanasia" murders 1939–1945). In 1983, Kalb had brusquely rejected my application to look at the documents in the Hallervorden Collection, citing physicians' general responsibility for patient confidentiality. Thirty years later, he didn't want to admit that this had been the case. In response to Kalb's ultimately unsuccessful legal threats, I turned to the Max Planck Society's historical archive. It contains more than two thousand pages of documents that were generated from 1983 to 1990 as a result of my applications. The following text, in which the lines blur between biography and scientific and social history, deals with this mountain of paperwork.

In late 1982, having learned of the documents cited above, I asked the director of the German Federal Archive to have the brain cross-sections from the Hallervorden Collection, insofar as they came from victims of National Socialism, transferred to the archive in Koblenz together with all the accompanying written documentation. That request followed the procedure established with the academic estate of the Tübingen anthropologist and "gypsy researcher" Sophie Ehrhardt. One year earlier, after a public scandal, her collection was transferred to the Federal Archive.

I justified my suggestion by invoking "political, moral and also legal perspectives." My goal was to remove the many thousands of samples from Hallervorden's neuro-anatomical estate from further research while investigating, in the interests of the history of science, what interests had led the respected brain researcher to attach himself to the euthanasia murders and how their cooperation had functioned on a practical level.[6]

Six weeks later, the president of the Federal Archive, Hans Booms, forwarded my suggestion to the president of the Max Planck Society with a note: "Naturally I cannot judge whether all aspects of Mr. Aly's account are correct, but I believe that you should definitely follow up on the matter." Edmund Marsch, general secretary of the Max Planck Society, immediately charged the deputy director of the society's historical archive in Berlin-Dahlem, Marion Kazemi, "with discretely dealing with this matter." In a priority letter Kazemi alerted the director of the Frankfurt Institute, Wolf Singer, who immediately reacted with one purpose in mind: to get rid of this morally contaminated burden from the past.

He recommended that "the files and all the paperwork" be transferred to the historical archive and the "samples and cross sections from the collections be destroyed" to prevent any further experimentation with them. Singer wrote me, however, claiming that he had spoken with Professor Wilhelm Krücke (a student of Hallervorden), who had assured him that the collection didn't contain "brains, samples or documents connected with the 'euthanasia' action against physically and mentally handicapped children from 1939 to 1945." Singer definitively stated, "There is no material at out institute connected with this 'children's action.'"[7]

In contrast to Singer, I recommended that the samples be "temporarily preserved" until a neuro-pathologist could determine the methods Hallervorden had used. Equally caught up in the prevailing values of the times, I too wanted to see the samples "destroyed" and not laid to rest. It was only several months later that my friend from Hamburg Martin Schmidt, a scholar of Ancient Greece and a Green Party politician, asked me during a conversation, "What is to be done with things like this?" He answered himself: "'Destruction' is out of the question. They must be buried."[8] That was what happened, although not until May 1990.

Following General Secretary Marsch's wishes, Marion Kazemi traveled to Frankfurt in late March 1983, inspected parts of the collection, and reported that samples "were still being used, if not often." She added that she had not found "indications of killings in the 'cases' being ordered."[9] Following her hasty and mistaken judgment, the Max Planck Society's legal division reviewed two case histories and the photographs of brain cross-sections to determine whether "viewing them was permissible." Gerhard Kalb subsequently rejected my request, citing Paragraph 203 of the German Criminal Code, according to which physicians become liable to prosecution if they pass along patients' personal data and thus violate their duty to maintain confidentiality. Kalb even contended that the permission "of the specific deceased person could not be presumed."[10] To spread responsibility, General Secretary Marsch asked the person within the society responsible for data privacy to review my application while explicitly ordering that the Hessen commissioner for data protection, who was responsible for the Frankfurt Institute and was considered quite liberal, "should not be involved," as I had suggested. A handwritten remark by Marsch read, "In my opinion, these are not questions of data protection but patient confidentiality etc."[11]

When I learned that my application had been rejected, I once again approached the president of the Federal Archive, who inquired of the Max Planck society "under what circumstances" those responsible "would consider inspection permissible."[12] The addressees insisted that "as a matter of principle photographs of brain cross sections and patient files cannot be viewed for purposes other than medical research." In the meantime, Wolf Singer had asked two Frankfurt professors of medicine to evaluate the collection. Only one of them fulfilled that request, concluding that the collections had nothing to do with the euthanasia murders.[13]

I was given crucial help by Spiros Simitis, the commissioner of the Hessen data protection authority. Without knowing that Marsch had intentionally bypassed him, I informed Simitis in early 1984 about the Max Planck Society's position. Simitis began to pursue the matter immediately and energetically.[14] The result was an official statement, written by Simitis's expert on legal principles, Eckard Hohmann, who doubted whether "physicians' duty to maintain patient confidentiality includes such cases in which from the very start it is not intended to treat patients, but rather physically destroy tissue." From this perspective, the Max Planck Society was misusing paragraph 203 of the Criminal Code.

Hohmann employed an argument that was particularly unpleasant to the society. Because the brain samples had been used for decades for medical research, he proposed, the society was obliged to permit their use by other equally valid academic disciplines. Consequently a refusal to let me as a political scientist inspect this material was "arbitrary and illegal." The evaluation continued: "Because of the historical circumstances, there is an objective interest of the humanities to inspect material possibly connected with the euthanasia program. Given the nature of the case, it can only be determined after inspection how relevant the material in fact is." Summarizing the case, the data protection commission instructed the Max Planck Institute: "Establishing the historical facts surrounding the euthanasia program cannot impinge upon the human dignity of its victims; on the contrary, it prevents collective forgetting and establishes respect for mentally ill people by investigating the National Socialist past."[15]

First Impressions of the Hallervorden Collection

The Max Planck Society was unable to reject the force of this argument, even if Kalb noted on the first page of Hohmann's letter, "Almost nothing in this is correct!" (Someone else added a question mark after this marginal note.) Whatever the precise circumstances, on 21 May 1984, a year and a half after I filed my application, I was finally allowed to view the Hallervorden Collection in Frankfurt am Main. The decision had been made by Kalb and Günter Preiss, the person in the general administration responsible for the Frankfurt Institute for Brain Research. Director Singer didn't insist upon being present and allowed me to make unlimited copies. He would later have to justify this decision, declaring that he had "by no means expected" me to make and take home hundreds of photocopies.[16] Several weeks later, I dictated a report to Heinz A. Staab, then president of the Max Planck Society, which I will quote at length here:

> From 23 to 24 May 1984 I inspected and copied parts of the Hallervorden Collection. The files are stored at the Neurological Institute of the University of Frankfurt a.M. (Edinger Instituté) in the hallway behind some wooden paneling. The way the collection is stored doesn't reflect its historical and perhaps neuro-anatomical value.
> My work was supported in very welcoming fashion by Professor Wolf Singer, the director of the Max Planck Institute for Brain Research, Neurophysiological Division, Professor Ekkehard Thomas, the managing director of the Neurological Institute, and Helge Gräfin Vitzthum, who gave me a very vivid account of the history of the institute.
> I inspected the following files:
>
> Sektionen (autopsies) 1936; 1937, 1–90; 1939, 1–70, 71–111; 1940, 1–60, 61–110, 111–170; 1941, 1–60, 61–119, 120–185, 186–282; 1942, 1–60, 61–102; 1943, 76–130; 1944, 1–83.
>
> The reports and the accompanying correspondence are kept in upright ringed binders and are occasionally missing. In the short time I had I didn't note which particular files are missing. In light of the historical, medical and ethical value of this collection, albeit in a negative sense, it seems appropriate to me to look for the missing files in order to recomplete the collection.
> I evaluated a Leitz binder labeled "Neural Muscular Atrophy, Cracow E. and Cracow W." and several suspension files which were stored in a separate room un-

der the rubric "Hallervorden Collection": They seem to have been removed from the upright binders because they're of particular interest and seem to display signs of current usage. The suspension files in question are as follows (the names refer to the people from whom the brains were removed):

Vierhub, Fischer, Horcher, Porcher, Giesel, Woitha, Kutschke Alfred, Kutschke Günter, Kutschke Herbert Henning, Behrendt, Maue, Brauns, Fischer, Lehmann, Schulze, Kiewert, Bartel, Milbredt, Witschel, Geissler, Beyer, Seburg, Bernau, Fröde, Hiller, Gaus, Hoffmann, Schulze, Rothkegel.

The brains of all these people were removed in the period between 1940 and 1945. The written documents were without doubt originally filed in the upright binders.

In total I made some 700 copies. I would like to specifically express my gratitude for being allowed to do so since the copies have greatly assisted and accelerate my historical evaluation. They form a representative sample, although I paid special attention to personal names and places that seemed important in light of my working hypothesis.

My working hypothesis is that the Kaiser Wilhelm Institute (KWI) for Brain Research in Berlin-Buch knowingly procured brains and the accompanying clinical findings in conjunction with the "euthanasia project" of the Third Reich, scientifically examined these brains, and later published the results. This hypothesis has been confirmed by my evaluation of the Hallervorden Collection in Frankfurt. It has in the past been repeatedly and even legally disputed by the legal successor of the Kaiser Wilhelm Society, the Max Planck Society.

The Hallervorden Collection, which bears noticeable traces of later cleaning, yields three important indications of collusive knowledge and—where brain research is concerned—organizational participation by the Brain Research Institute of the Kaiser Wilhelm Society in Berlin-Buch in the institutional killing of the Third Reich:

1. The file "Selektionen (Autopsies) 1941, 1–60" contains reports on a large number of murdered children from the Brandenburg-Görden Mental Hospital, all of whom died on 28 October 1940. The age of the children is given in parentheses: Annelise Rotzoll (14), Werner Zimmermann (17), Günther Dietrich (11), Heinz Böhm (11), Heinz Pietack (10), Heinz Piescher (8), Hubert Falkenberg (9), Irmgard Dörr (16), Willy Venz (13), Günther Schiemann (12), Ursula Krabbe (16), Wolfgang Fengler (10), Dora Zech (16), Elisabeth Jarosch (15), Marie Kretschmer (?), Werner Przadka (13), Willy Schemel (16), Margarete Korioth (13), Henry Herzog (17), Erika Höhne (10), Berta Handrich (10), Herbert Schade (18), Willy Bading (16), Horst Friedrich (9), Renate Wringe (17), Hellmuth Lesniewske (11), Vera Böhlke (14), Werner Böttger (15), Günther Nitschke (7), Siegfried Gaida (9), Rolf Pfunfke (12), Hildegard Eckert (17), Emmy Kunz (17).[17]

As the reports indicate, these 33 children and adolescents were not "empty husks" or "mentally dead"—terms later employed in court by their murderers. They were children who, in some cases, attended the special school in Brandenburg-Görden, and were often from difficult social backgrounds. They were obviously killed for scientific reasons. At the time, Hallervorden was researching the causes of "congenital imbecility" and the difference between "traumatic" and "genuine hereditary epilepsy," to use the terminology of the period. Added to this was the main focus of research by the director of the Brandenburg-Görden mental hospital, Prof. Hans Heinke—"the abnormal character." In all three studies, anatomical examinations of brains were used to determine and describe any regular scientifically verifiable changes in the brain that would correspond to these deviations from the norm.

A statement by one of the examination doctors, Heinrich Bunke, before an interrogating judge in Frankfurt am Main on 16 April 1962 supplies the background of the scientific massacre of children on 28 October 1940. Beginning in August 1940, Bunke worked in the Brandenburg extermination center, housed in a prison, and was transferred to its successor institution at Bernburg at the end of October 1940. The statement reads:

> Children between the ages of approximately 8 and 12, perhaps 14, were also gassed in Brandenburg. The children were transferred to us from Görden by Professor Heinze—either directly or through an intermediate institution—for the express purpose of killing them. During the period that I worked at Brandenburg, this involved about 100 children, Medical histories and documents with the consultants' decisions were sent along with the patients. You could tell what intermediary institution the children came from by the advisory opinions in the files. They were the only cases that can be said to have been examined as we would have expected in all cases, I mean that in those cases, a non-psychiatrist could also have understood the reasons for the consultants' decisions. In all other cases, the decision was clear, but not the reasoning, aside from a general psychiatric diagnosis. Some of the bodies were autopsied by Prof. Hallervorden of Berlin (histologist at the Kaiser Wilhelm Institute) and taken along for scientific evaluation. I assume this was based on an agreement with Professor Heinze, I do not know if Prof. Heinze himself also took part in the killings at Görden. In any case, the abovementioned children came from the mental hospital. I believe there was a total of two transports. Prof. Heinze himself was at Brandenburg at the time.

According to his testimony, Bunke had gotten to know Hallervorden better on this occasion. In mid-May 1941, he spent four to six weeks in training at Berlin-Buch, after which he removed brains from patients gassed at Bernburg that he assumed "would be of interest in Buch." During this short training period he lived in the home of the director of brain research for the Kaiser Wilhelm Institute, Hugo Spatz.

There is no doubt that the abovementioned files from the Hallervorden Collection about the above-named children and young people were based on these murders and that Hallervorden was himself present when their brains were removed.

2. The files on autopsies carried out in 1940 and 1941 contain many similar descriptions of brain removals that point to the extermination centers at Brandenburg and Bernburg. The very short report forms were almost all typed on the same typewriter, with a "Be Nr." on the upper left-hand corner and a "Z Nr." on the up-

per right-hand corner. The Be and Z numbers are definite evidence that the killings took place in the context of the euthanasia operation. The Z number was the central number in the Berlin index; it designated the patient questionnaires that the asylums sent to the Reich Association of Mental Hospitals. The Be number designated the current number of murders. The date of death is generally unspecified. Autopsy followed very shortly after death, within one to four hours. These short descriptions were dictated by Bunke at the extermination center and transported to Berlin-Buch along with the brains and pertinent medical records.

The first of these reports is reprinted here as an example:

> Be Nr. 23 828; Z Nr. 55 150; Name: Kothe, Arthur, Born: 11 June 1912 in Berlin. Dissection after 2 hours. Diagnosis: imbecility, Height: 1.52 meters, Body Type: Thin, Bone Type: Fine; Circumference of Head: 55 cm.; Lengthwise Diameter: 17.5 cm.; Widthwise Diameter: 14 cm. Brain Weight ..., Autopsy: Brain; Macroscopic Findings: Strikingly small, soft brain. Soft tissues normal. The left hemisphere is better developed than the right. In the area of the right parietal brain, there are changes in convolutions reminiscent of microgyria. Nothing remarkable at the base of the cerebellum. During removal, the right pedunculus tore off, and the left was torn. Brief patient report: A family report could not be obtained. The patient was placed in institutional care in 1929. Is described as a completely impassive idiot who reacted to neither threats nor loud noises. No verbal expression was heard from him; he only uttered animal noises from time to time. Spastic paralysis on the left side. Strong rigor in the musculature of the left arm. Slight rigor of the left leg. Tendon reflexes are pronounced on both sides. The patient apparently survived polio, after which the left-side paralysis appeared.

These brief reports were apparently written by Bunke in the summer of 1941 after his training at the Kaiser Wilhelm Institute. During this period, Bunke resided at the house of the director Hugo Spatz.

As a result of my research I will reconstruct exemplary life stories of the above-named patients. This is possible since the autopsy documents allow conclusions to be drawn about the institutions from which they were transferred, and because deportation lists and patient files there have in part been made available for historical research. But on the basis of external indicators, it can already be said with near certainty that the above-named people were victims of the Brandenburg and Bernburg extermination centers and that the cooperation between these centers and the Brain Research Institute in Berlin-Buch was not secret, but rather took place by mutual agreements. (The protocols of the autopsy were apparently not filed by the victims' dates of death but rather by the dates on which their brains were processed in the institute.)

3. . . . . In addition to the Görden files, I also evaluated files from the Sanatorium and Nursing Home Berlin-Buch and the Ludwig Hoffmann Hospital, a part of the Kaiser Wilhelm Institute in Berlin-Buch, as well as the Children's Clinic in Berlin-Frohnau, which was run by the second evaluator in the "Reich Committee," Ernst

Wentzler, whose research focus was "Little's Disease." Conspicuous are the relatively frequent deliveries of brains from the Sanatorium and Nursing Home Lörchingen in occupied Lorraine by Dr. Rudolf Leppien. I have not evaluated deliveries to Berlin from various autopsies in the field of an obviously military nature.[18]

That was what I knew in May 1984. Unlike back then, the files concerning the children murdered in Görden are now available at the Brandenburg State Archive, and since the 1990s, almost half of the files concerning people who died in the gas chambers of the Action T4 until the summer of 1941 are kept at the Federal Archive. I was able to locate the files of more than 60 percent of the people I identified in 1984 and prove definitively that they were murdered. By extension we can assume that nearly all of the samples in the collection came from people murdered as unworthy of life in the euthanasia program. In 2013, I used the files to write short biographies of several of the children and young people autopsied by Hallervorden himself in the immediate proximity of the gas chambers.[19]

Archive Director Henning and the Max Planck Society's "Good Name"

Back in 1984, my report attracted the disapproval of Eckart Henning, the recently appointed director of the historic archive of the Max Planck Society in Berlin. "I regret the decision" of the general administration of the Max Planck Society to grant usage, he wrote, especially as it "only resulted from a kind of 'own goal' by internal lawyers." He then turned personal, adding that, "when the whole affair began," he himself was not in his post, but that the president of the Federal Archive at the time, Hans Boom, had spoken "negatively about academics who tried to find source evidence to prove their pre-existing conclusions." Boom had included me in this category, "which from the current perspective doesn't seem to be entirely mistaken."[20] Subsequently, Henning formulated a "response to the report by Götz Aly of 16 September 1984 and his letter to the president of the Max Planck Society of 17 September 1984." It read:

> When reading the report, I got the impression that author's main purpose was to promote his preformed opinion ("working hypothesis") as proven after a brief look at the Hallervorden Collection. The fact that this opinion was preconceived can be gleaned from a letter by Aly of 15 December 1982 to Archive Director Dr. Oldenhage (Federal Archive), in which he already contended that Prof. Hallervorden "was, according to the results of my research thus far, involved of his own initiative in the euthanasia action." The moral zeal of the author of this letter, further encouraged by the fact that he is the father of a handicapped child, seems to get in the way of his academic honesty.

In 2013, when I discovered this document in the Max Planck Society archive, I ran across Henning, who had by then retired but still served the society in a reduced capacity, in the hallway. I confronted him with his response and asked, "Do you have anything to say about this?" "Yes," he answered, "I had no choice but to assume you were biased." I said, "My discoveries back then all proved correct." He replied, "I had no way of knowing that." I said, "Would you like to apologize for doubting my academic honesty because I have a handicapped daughter?" He said, "No!"

Henning behaved with the same self-confidence thirty years before in 1984. Without any knowledge of his own, he asserted that it was hardly possible to prove from a Frankfurt collection of patient histories and autopsy protocols that "the Kaiser Wilhelm Society had 'knowingly procured brains' for research within the context of the Third Reich's euthanasia program." Quite rightly, he noted that my thesis pointed in the direction of "the accusation of killing on demand and the assertion that the institute had been actively involved in these actions." Such an accusation, he wrote, was to be "rejected until it can be proven beyond a shadow of a doubt—the suggestion so-and-so 'apparently killed in the interests of science' is by no means enough."[21]

In late 1985, my report appeared in slightly revised form in the second volume of essays concerning research into National Socialist health and social policies. The title of the volume was *Reform und Gewissen* (Reform and conscience), and my seventy-page contribution on the various health-based political utopias and research projects of the euthanasia murderers was called "Der saubere und der schmutzige Fortschritt" (Clean and dirty progress). Subsequently, General Secretary Marsch contacted Professor Heinz Wässle, the managing director of the Frankfurt Institute for Brain Research, requesting a response. "Although this article contains shattering assertions for our institute and the Max Planck Society as a whole," Wässle answered, "and although Aly writes at best half-truths on many points, we would advise against a legal confrontation." Legal proceedings, he added, "would only cause a public discussion about the activities of the Kaiser Wilhelm Institutes for Brain Research and Psychiatry during the euthanasia program," which would be "exploited to the fullest by certain organs of the press." That danger seemed all the greater to Wässle because the Max Planck Institute for Brain Research in Frankfurt had "already received a lot of negative publicity because of the euthanasia program, the psycho-surgery of our predecessors and experiments on animals."[22]

In the response Henning sent to the general secretary of the Max Planck Society on 6 January 1986, he complained, "Just like last year, this all starts with Götz Aly. From one of his collaborators, I got a copy of the collection of essays 'Reform und Gewissen,' in which I have been reading the past few days." The agitated Henning listed the passages in which I—"expressis verbis"—asserted unambiguous connections between research and murder. "Monstrosities," he called them.

Henning continued: "Apparently G. Aly is trying to provoke the Max Planck Society and cast aspersions on it with the following sentence, which I would like to cite: 'In 1974, the Max Plack Society, represented by Professor Adolf Butenandt, forbade a Munich journalist from saying that the Institutes of the Kaiser Wilhelm Society had carried out brain research in the context of the euthanasia program.'" Henning asked, "How did he come to see the court files?" continuing, "He dares to presume that the Max Planck Institute would shy away from the publicity of a court case against him to the extent that he publishes his suspicions, without any evidence, as facts." Henning concluded with the sentence: "I cannot judge to what extent an appeal by the Max Planck Society's legal department or its subsidiary institutes would ward off further damage or at least prevent further unfounded Aly constructions that hurt our good name."[23]

For Archive Director Henning, things went from bad to worse. Acting on an initiative by Anna Bergmann, on 15 September 1987, Gabriele Czarnowski, Annegret Ehmann, Susanne Heim, and I affixed a memorial plaque to the building at the free University of Berlin, which had originally been used for the discipline of "racial studies" and which since the 1970s had been part of the Otto Suhr Institute (OSI). The plaque's inscription read:

> From 1927 to 1945 this building housed the Kaiser Wilhelm Institute for Anthropology, Human Heredity and Eugenics of the Kaiser Wilhelm Society (today Max Planck society). Its directors, Prof. Eugen Fischer (1927–1942) and Prof. Otmar v. Verschuer (1942–1945), and their research assistants provided the foundation for the racial and birth policies of the Nazi state. By training SS doctors and lawyers, by providing legal evaluations and using their expertise for compulsory sterilizations, they actively contributed to persecution and murder of minorities.
>
> In 1943, as an SS doctor in the Auschwitz concentration camp, Dr. Josef Mengele, an assistant to Verschuer, continued the research on twins supported by the German Research Society with horrific experiments upon prisoners and provided the institute with the blood and bodily organs of the murdered subjects of these experiments as research samples.
>
> After 1945, with few exceptions, the perpetrators of these crimes continued their scientific careers. Those crimes were never punished. The medical sciences continue to use the results of their research to this day.

In the middle of the day after the plaque had been affixed, only around three hundred meters from the archive of the Max Planck Institute, Archive Director Henning appeared and reported to the society's general directorship in Munich: "Today at around 1:30 PM as I was about to copy the 'inscription,' which is located to the right of the front door of the former Kaiser Wilhelm Institute for Anthropology etc. . . . and consists of black letters on white painted metal plaque in roughly DIN-A3 format, Mrs. Wickert (Otto Suhr Institute) happened to address me." Christl Wickert, who taught in the university's political science department, told Henning that the faculty council had distanced itself from the plaque "because of factual inaccuracies" and that in her opinion "the whole second paragraph would have to go." Subsequently, the two of them spoke with the dean, Professor Ulrich Albrecht. Henning summarized: "He and Mrs. Wickert opined that the OSI was now under pressure to install an official plaque. They didn't want to take down the 'foreign' plaque for fear they would be accused of trying to lessen that pressure."[24]

In 1988, the "official" plaque was put up. Cast in bronze, it was difficult to read and contained a partly identical, partly watered-down, and partly morally inflated inscription.

In response to a request by General Secretary Marsch, the Max Planck Society's legal division, in the person of the department director Michael Weidmann, responded to my article. After discarding all other legal options against me, he suggested the following course of action, which, too, would prove to be unsuccessful: "We might consider, in this one specific case, to put Mr. Aly under pressure to defend himself with a likewise drastic criticism of his scholarship (along the lines of 'worthless work, incompetent research, unproven assertions'—I'm sure more would occur to me) in order to provoke him into seeking a cease-and-desist and recantation order. But in the interests of the Max Planck Institute, I wouldn't advise anyone to cause such a spectacle."[25] In any case, the society's leadership had already decided not to take "any contrary measures at the moment so as to avoid blowing up the matter into something even more serious."[26]

Hallervorden's student and successor, Professor Krücke, railed against the "disgusting pamphlet by Aly Götz," while his own successor, Professor Wässle, opined that (1) "with Prof. Krücke a certain 'phenomenon of repression' had to be reckoned with"; (2) there was "at least a suspicion that brains from euthanasia victims" might also be found at the institute; and (3) that he regretted "not having any better news."[27]

"Destruction versus Dignified Burial"

It wasn't until four years later, in January 1989, seven years after my original letter to the Max Planck Society, that Henning thought it necessary to write about "material" in the Hallervorden Collection that should not be used in any form—at least not as long as "suspicions have not been cleared up that it might have originated in the euthanasia action of the Nazi period."[28] Nonetheless, he reacted with great irritation when the Hessen Ministry of Science suggested "burying in dignified form such morally compromised material." He noted, "Worrying suggestion. No Kaiser Wilhelm Society plaque if you please. Warned the president verbally on 24 January 1989." The mention of the plaque was typical of Henning's strict rejection of the idea that the Max Planck Society had any historical responsibility as the successor of the Kaiser Wilhelm Society. Since 1984, the society's president had been the chemist Heinz A. Staab. Unlike Henning, after repeatedly consulting my report, he came to the conclusion: "The conclusions Mr. Aly has reached after looking through the Hallervorden files give reason to believe that brain cross sections from euthanasia victims are part of the collection."[29]

There was no way Benno Müller-Hill and I could have changed attitudes at the head of the Max Planck Institute by ourselves. Ultimately, that change was down to the fact that colleagues, doctors, and journalists in the United States, Israel, Canada, and England publicized the results of our research and began to ask questions. Professors William E. Seidelman and Arthur Caplan put the society under particular pressure. English-language articles, like the one by Steven Dickman in *Nature* magazine, caused a domestic political stir in Germany.[30] In the end, the US TV station ABC even requested an interview with the Max Planck Society.

In January 1989, after international attention had reached a critical mass, the Israeli minister of religion Zevulun Hammer wrote to German chancellor Helmut Kohl demanding that the bodily remains of Nazi victims in the anatomic collections be given a dignified burial. Kohl reacted immediately, saying he was horrified that this hadn't happened forty years ago. On 11 January 1989, he called the use of samples from the Nazi era "completely unbearable and intolerable." At the same time, the chairman of the Central Committee of Jews in Germany, Heinz Galinski, spoke of a "monstrous incident" that was shaking the ethical foundations of the Federal Republic of Germany. Former chancellor Helmut Schmidt also had a word with Munich.[31] Within fourteen days, on 25 January 1989, the Conference of Culture Ministers (KMK) ordered those in possession of all anatomic collections throughout Germany to "immediately remove all samples taken from Nazi victims and of uncertain origins, to deal with them in dignified fashion and to report back without delay to the secretary of the KMK."

Around this time, the weekly newspaper *Die Zeit* asked me to report about my research. The article appeared on 3 February 1989. The headline was essentially based on two quotes from Hallervorden and read, "'It wasn't my business where the brains came from' / 'The more the better' / On the treatment of samples taken from Nazi victims before and after 1945." I told the story of my research between 1982 and 1984, naming the Max Planck Society six times, as Henning noted on his copy of the article. On 8 February 1989, the Bavarian State Ministry for Science and Art, which was responsible for the general directorship of the Max Planck Society, demanded that "any remaining samples from the bodies of Nazi victims and samples of indeterminate origin be immediately removed from the collections."[32]

International pressure and the reaction it elicited from German politicians made those who had previously refused responsibility take swift action. Henning still wasn't willing to store the written documents about the murdered victims in his archive (he referred to them as "not genuine archive material" or "material foreign to the archive"), but he did advise that the questionable collections be "kept separately" so as at least to "protect them from use as long as suspicions cannot be dismissed" that the samples "partly came from the euthanasia actions of the Nazi era." As if in defiance, Henning wrote atop the copy of this letter for his files, "This is uncertain."[33]

Among those who pressed for a worthy burial of "materials obtained under criminal conditions (murder)" was the entire Max Planck Society employees' committee. The resolution it passed was quickly followed by censure from the society's administrative board. Even in the spring of 1989, the society's leaders found it "incomprehensible" that "the committee would start a public discussion of this topic without taking account of the interests and good name of the Max Planck Society."[34]

And the administrative board wasn't the only part of the society that long had trouble acknowledging the truth. For example, the director of the Max Planck Institute for Psychiatry (formerly the German Research Institute for Psychiatry), Professor Georg W. Kreutzberg, vehemently denied that a single brain from euthanasia victims was "incorporated" into the institute's collection "from the incriminated years." The institute may have run a morgue at the München-Eglfing-Haar Sanatorium and Nursing Home, Kreutzberg said, but nothing specific was known about it, and the director of this facility, a Professor Schleussing, seemed not to have been a member of the institute's academic personnel. If this relatively unknown figure "could not definitively rule out victims of the euthanasia program having been autopsied in Eglfing-Haar," that was part of the "entanglements of the Nazi era."[35]

In fact, the later professor for pathological anatomy Hans Schleussing had been an academic member of the German Research Institution for Psychiatry, and thus the Kaiser Wilhelm Society, since 1936. His letterhead read, "Autopsy facility / German Research Institution for Psychiatry / (Kaiser Wilhelm Institute) / Chairman: Prof. Dr. med. Schleussing / Eglfing b. München." His assistant Barbara Schmidt often signed his correspondence. In 1945, Schleussing was fired "upon the demands of the American military government because of his membership in the NSDAP," although he continued to practice and regularly wrote evaluations using institute stationery. In 1948, he was officially rehired as a coroner, and the Max Planck Society paid monthly contributions toward his pension. In 1961, Schleussing was still listed in Kürschner's Register of German Men of Learning as "Chairman of Autopsies at the German Research Institution for Psychiatry of the Max Planck Institute, Munich." He also identified himself as a member of that organization in his scientific publications.[36]

In order to avoid having to admit any wrongdoing while still getting rid of the annoying, increasingly frequent questions, Kreutzberg now only wanted to "bury all the brains from the years in question that are present in the collection" as quickly as possible. By the end of 1989, Kreutzberg had "removed six macro- and 2.4 meters of micro-tissue samples from the years 1933–45 (no individual list)."[37] According to the protocol, President Staab reported somewhat pompously to the Max Planck Society senate, "Should closer examination turn up samples from the period from 1939 to 1945, whose origins cannot be determined beyond the shadow of a doubt, they will be removed from the collections and buried in an appropriate manner."[38]

Slowly, Archive Director Henning was coming around to the idea that the Hallervorden Collection contained a large number of samples that could be assigned to hundreds of victims of euthanasia murders. Nonetheless, not for that reason but because the samples were considered "scientifically worthless" by the head of the Frankfurt institute at the time, Henning wrote that "destroying all of them or burying them in dignified form could be considered."[39]

Under pressure, he decided to remove "all medical samples from the Nazi era" from the institutes, "regardless of what the evidence said." This was the most radical solution, an attempt to banish the repeatedly appearing ghost of "history of science research projects." He justified his decision as follows: "The sort of quick cleansing of the collection that people abroad demand cannot be expected from such a (lengthy) process."[40]

In a draft press statement, the Max Planck Society continued to dispute the basic facts. "More recent investigations," wrote the society, had concluded that "samples which could be from euthanasia victims were contained within at least one of the collections." Because their provenance could not be proven "beyond the shadow of a doubt," they were to be "removed and—in line with the federal culture ministers' conference's suggestion—buried in dignified form."[41]

Following that lead, the society under President Staab's leadership agreed upon a "removal action" of all anatomic samples from the Nazi era whose provenance was obviously homicidal or deemed to be unclear.[42] A summary by General Secretary Marsch about the Frankfurt Max Planck Institute for Brain Research read, by the fall of 1989 "84,300 samples from 1,540 cases were removed from the Hallervorden Collection, and 30,650 samples from 1,400 cases were removed from the Spatz Collection. That's a total of 114,950 samples from 2,940 cases."[43] Henning was caught up in the spirit and began to search for samples from the Nazi era in an institution that "Götz Aly has thus far never mentioned." Obsequiously, he reported to General Secretary Marsch, "I mention this solely for your information. I wanted to communicate this, in case you were asked about it."[44]

Under the new atmosphere, discovering samples from the Nazi years was no longer a source of shame but a sign of success. Nonetheless, in light of the numbers, Hessen's minister of science, Wolfgang Gerhardt (FDP), was still shocked that the head of the Max Planck Society had done nothing for so long. "I find it telling that those responsible in Frankfurt knew about these samples for years and thought it proper to keep them under lock and key," Gerhardt wrote. "That's not at all acceptable."[45]

Slowly but surely, the heads of the society gave in to the inevitable, but the president, who had read my report, still asserted that "the 33 cases that are known could be identified to a high degree of probability by an external historian as Nazi victims because of their identical dates of death."[46] He meant me. But I had listed a far greater number of suspicious cases in my report.

Buried at Munich's Waldfriedhof Cemetery

On 7 November 1989, the vice president of the Max Planck Society addressed, as he called it, the burial question. A short time before, he had received two calls from "Mr. Boutsenin the chancellor's office," who had asked to be called back as soon as possible. Under discussion was whether the human remains should be buried de-centrally or centrally, and whether intact brains should be cremated. It was decided to carry out the burials centrally and not to cremate the many tissue samples of glass microscope slides, but to "leave them in their present condition."[47]

After the samples were packed in "24 metal and wooden containers," the heads of the society were faced with the task of how to make body parts used by science disappear in halfway dignified fashion. That was done without fanfare and away from the public eye on 21 February 1990 at 7:45 AM. There are no photos or descriptions of the event. No one was intended to see the "containers." The Max Planck Society didn't arrange for a ceremonial interment. They were simply buried at dawn at Munich's Waldfriedhof Cemetery.

An official ceremony was scheduled for 25 May. By then, the "unfortunately somewhat bleak location" was to be "cleaned up as much as possible." For that reason, it "was recommended," as Marsch noted on the day the containers were buried, that the gravesite "be enclosed in a box hedge."[48] In the interval, stonecutters had made a headstone with an inscription, which had been thought up in January 1990: "In memory of the victims of National Socialism and their abuse by medicine. Let this be a warning to all researchers to limit themselves responsibly. Erected by the Max Planck Society in 1990."

The inscription didn't mention the individual victims or how they were abused "by medicine." The abusers were people—researchers, doctors, and professors who were highly respected before and after 1945—exploiting the chances Hitler's government gave them to arrive more quickly at scientific discoveries by using illegal means. They participated in murder because of their desire for knowledge and professional ambition, developing carefully considered methods of a fatal science. Those who were murdered and the scientists involved all had names. But the Max Planck Society chose to draw an obscuring veil of anonymity over everything. They developed a new, respectable seeming form of silence.

According to their plan, the heads of the society celebrated their memorial ceremony at 2:00 PM on 25 May 1990 in the cemetery chapel to the strains of a largo for string quartet by Dmitri Shostakovich. The service concluded with Jewish, Protestant, and Catholic prayers after which a wreath was laid at the memorial site. The phrase "mass grave" was studiously avoided. The main speaker was Professor Kreutzberg, who read out a statement that did more to conceal than it did to reveal: "You all know that some time ago microscopic brain tissue samples that we had to assume came from victims of the National socialist dictatorship were found at the Max Planck Institute." Nothing about that statement was true. "Some time ago" was actually six years earlier. "That we had to assume" should have read, "that we denied for years could have anything to do with the murders." And the supposed "microscopic samples" were not tiny objects that could only be seen under a microscope but rather full-sized cross-sections of human brains. Kreutzberg acted as if all of this had only happened recently, as if the Max Planck Society had immediately and voluntarily reviewed "their scientific collections from the time before 1945" and as if the samples hadn't been repeatedly loaned out for examination by scientists.

The *Frankfurter Allgemeine Zeitung* newspaper reported much the same in October 1989. The samples, the paper wrote, had been "discovered last year in the Max Planck Institute for Brain Research." The *FAZ* even dug out the information that the samples came from thirty-three children and young people, adding, "The archivist [presumably Henning] noticed that all the children died on the same day. He interpreted this to mean that they had died violent deaths. But there is no definitive proof even to this day."[49] Of course, in the minds of the *FAZ* and the "archivist" it could have been just accidental that thirty-three children died on the same day in one mental home for young people.

The Murders of Three Relatives for Science

In 2013, after reading up on everything again, I decided to investigate the fate of the three Kutschke boys. The Kutschkes also suffered from the same, apparently genetic, degenerative illness and were also murdered in Brandenburg-Görden between 1942 and 1944. I had noticed their files all the way back in 1984 and had described them extensively in my report to the president of the Max Planck Society:[50]

> Among the "interesting cases" collected in Görden, I would like to highlight what happened to the three Kutschke boys. Alfred Kutschke died at the age of seven on 6 April 1942 from a "feverish bacterial infection"; six weeks previously his brother Günter, who had just turned three, died of "bronchial pneumonia"; at that point the cousin Herbert was not yet born, He died aged fifteen months on 25 April 1944

of "pneumonia localized in the lower right lung." All three boys suffered from the same apparently hereditary illness, which involves the decay of the medulla fiber in nerve cells and, over a period of years, leads to a child's death. It's possible that the oldest Kutschke boy died of natural causes. His autopsy showed that his illness was quite advanced in any case. The report on the examination of his younger brother stated that "the loss of medulla is not yet very far advanced."

Because this finding was somewhat similar to the one concerning the older brother, it didn't provide any important indications of the course of the illness. The case was different concerning the 1944 autopsy of the younger cousin Herbert, who had died at the age of one year, three months. "Much more informative are the samples from the younger cousin, Herbert K.," the autopsy report read.[51] "A Spielmayer incision through the stem ganglia clearly reveals the medulla, though diminished." The files on these three boys show signs of recent scientific use.

Back then, in 1984, I was only acquainted with the results of the neuro-anatomical examinations, not the history of the three boys' illnesses. Documents from the clinic that have become available in the meantime allow us to rule out the possibility that Alfred Kutschke died a natural death. Back in 1984, I also didn't know that Franz Seitelberger had earned his academic degree with a study of the brains of the Kutschke boys. This essay, which was published in 1954 in the Viennese *Zeitschrift für Nervenheilkunde*,[52] begins with the sentence "From the Max Planck Institute for Brain Resrach in Gießen, Neuropathological Department (Prof. J. Hallervorden)." The essay's title is "Pelizaeus-Merzbacher Disease: Clinical-Anatomical Investigations about Its Status among the Various Scleroses." On the second page, the author thanks "Hr. Prof. Heinze" for being nice enough to provide the patient files and examination material from the three cases from the holdings of the state institution in Potsdam—meaning Brandenburg-Görden. In 1938, Seitelberger had joined the SS in Vienna and had written his postdoctoral thesis in 1954 under Hallervorden. Later, between 1976 and 1978, he was president of the University of Vienna.

In his 1954 essay, he compared the three brains. He was particularly interested in the brain of the youngest boy because it allowed him to "encounter the very slowly progressing degeneration at an early stage." The opportunity to observe visible neuroanatomical stages of one disease at three different stages was what made Seitelberger's study special. He put it this way: "The youngest case [i.e. the boy who was murdered at the age of fifteen months] allows us to gain insight into an early stage of medulla loss that makes it easier for us to reconstruct and evaluate the entire process." In his summary, he wrote, "We have discussed the case histories of and anatomical findings on three brothers aged seven, three, and one year, who suffered since their earliest childhoods of an identical sort of illness and came to their deaths because of intercurrent afflictions."

Günter Kutschke was admitted to Brandenburg-Görden on 17 January 1942. This was one of the most important observation, research, and homicide centers of the euthanasia program. The director was Professor Hans Heinze. Hallervorden maintained a separate autopsy facility there for his own institute, and conversely Heinze sat on the board of the Kaiser Wilhelm Institute for Brain Research. Heinze signed Günter Kutschke's death sentence nine days after his admission to the hospital. Heinze wrote, "In terms of intellect, physical coordination and language not even at the level of a two-year-old child." The following week Günter allegedly contracted the flu and died on 18 February 1942 of a lung infection at the age of two years, nine months. Because of the "suspicion of an ailment contracted to the brain tissue," his body was autopsied by the senior physician Karl Brockhausen. At this point, the doctors thought that a hereditary illness was unlikely and assumed that Günter K. had contracted a brain defect.

One month after Günter's death, on 21 March 1942, seven-year-old Alfred Kutschke was admitted to the institution. Like his brother, he was hospitalized on the basis of the decree of 18 August 1939 from the official physician of the Ost-Sternberg district in Zielenzig (Neumark). The decree was designed specially to allow the murder of permanently handicapped children. The official physician was named Dr. Kober. In his admission diagnosis, Heinze's senior physician Ernst Illing, who would soon direct a hospital ward of his own in Vienna for murdering children, described the new patient as entirely fit physically. But some two weeks later, on 6 April 1942, Alfred Kutschke, too, was dead, allegedly of heart or circulatory collapse or, as was also imaginatively put forward in another section of his lengthy file, of "bronchopneumonia" or "chronic catarrh-like bronchitis" with "extended, overlapped pneumonias localized to the upper and lower lobes of both lungs."

The morning of Alfred K.'s death, Brockhausen autopsied the body on account of "suspicion of a contracted organic brain ailment with idiocy, marasmus, and hyptertonic tetraplegia." Brockhausen also recorded exact information about the state of Alfred K.'s inner organs. Apparently Heinze also summoned his colleague Julius Hallervorden to look at the body. In any case, the autopsy contains handwritten corrections he made. Hallervorden made the first correct diagnosis of Pelizaeus-Merzbacher disease. He wrote a question mark behind these words and noted, "Extreme loss of medulla. Unclear picture." But more precise histological examinations would soon confirm his hypothesis.

Two years after the violent deaths of Günter and Alfred Kutschke, their cousin Herbert, who had only been born on 22 January 1943, was admitted to the institution on his first birthday. He, too, was physically healthy, but unlike his cousins he was diagnosed correctly: "Familial diffuse scleroses, Pelizaeus-Merzbacher disease." Hallervorden had confirmed his hypothesis in the interval. Herbert K. would also die after a short time of a lung infection. But ten weeks passed until his death on 25 April 1944 because, unlike his cousins, he had to endure extensive, and very painful, diagnostic operations.

Heinze himself made the detailed neurological diagnosis in this case. Spinal fluid was drawn, stool and urine were examined, a second spinal tap was made, cholesterol levels in the blood were determined, and Herbert K.'s eyes were checked by an ophthalmologist. On 2 February, the research doctors had Herbert's hands and lower arms X-rayed and determined, "Bone development is that of a five to six-month old boy." The same day, X-rays were also made of Herbert's chest and skull. The following morning, the doctors injected a contrast medium into the carotid artery of a one-year-old child, who was destined to be murdered in the name of science, in order to be able to make an encephalogram. The doctors had gone without such a procedure with Herbert's cousins because his parents refused, but this time they didn't bother to ask for permission. On 14 and 18 April, ward doctor Friederike Pusch subjected Herbert Kutschke to "blood and sugar stress tests." Within five hours, she carried out nine spinal taps on the child, who weighed eight kilograms. To her regret, the examination had to be broken off because of "suspension of the flow of spinal fluid." The final three spinal taps were mixed with blood and thus unusable. Until her retirement in 1972, Pusch worked as a senior physician in psychiatry in Communist East Germany. Although the responsible authorities knew about her past, she was never punished for what she had done.

After the fall of the Berlin Wall, the case files on the three Kutschke boys, which had been kept in Brandenburg-Görden, were transferred to the Main Brandenburg State Archive. Alfred Kutschke's file contains a complete copy of the neuropathological investigation results. In 1954, as a gesture of cordiality, Hallervorden had sent them to his former colleagues in Görden so that they could share in the scientific results of the murders they had jointly carried out. The date stems from a handwritten reference to Seitelberger's work. There is one difference between the copy and the original in Frankfurt. In the copy, the last paragraph is concealed, which in the original contained Hallervorden's handwritten corrections and initials.[53]

Jürgen Peiffer's Faulty Memory

After the anatomical samples from the Hallervorden Collection had been laid to rest in the Munich Cemetery, the Max Planck Society made initial plans for an "academic investigation" of this chapter of the Nazi past, which kept cropping up. Society president Staab had increasingly warmed to the idea of a research project into the behavior of members of the Kaiser Wilhelm Society in the Nazi era. But Henning resisted, arguing that no one could take an interest "à la Aly in such a project."[54]

Nonetheless in 1990 Jürgen Peiffer (1922–2006), a professor emeritus of neuropathology and a senator of the Max Planck Society, was semi-publically tasked with investigating the practices of Hallervorden during the Third Reich. Peiffer visited me, we corresponded on numerous occasions, and I provided him with whatever he wanted from my collection of documents. In the end, he published two impressive supplementary studies and an edited edition of modern correspondence in his discipline, which focused in part on the Nazi years.[55] When I mentioned the murder of the three boys and Seitelberger's monograph, he waved me off: "Yes, yes, colleague Seitelberger, he too. I know." But Peiffer never mentioned this so obvious criminal case in his published work. Why not?

In the meantime, since 2014, I think I know the reason why. I found it by accident, as I was looking up the correct German spelling for Pelizaeus-Merzbacher disease on the internet. I happened to discover an essay from 1963 by Peiffer titled "On the Spectrum of Variations of Pelizaeus-Merzbacher Disease: A Contribution to Familial Multiple Sclerosis."[56] At the time, the author had worked at the Max Planck Institute in Munich. The coauthor of the essay was Edith Zerbin-Rüdin, the daughter and true heir of Ernst Rüdin, who had been the director of the institute from 1931 to 1945 and a Nazi who was highly active in the areas of genetic and racial health. In 1942 Rüdin had written to the Reich Research Council, arguing that children classified as "undoubtedly of lesser worth" were "worthy of elimination."

In his essay, Peiffer directly referenced the study by Seitelberger and the obviously murdered Kutschke boys and cited two additional cases: Luise Adl., who had died in 1954 at the age of fifty-six "apparently of a 'concussion'" in the Klingenmünster Clinic in Western Germany and Brigitte Ment., who had died in 1955 at Munich's Haar Clinic in a state of serious malnutrition.[57]

In the tradition of Rüdin, Peiffer addressed his study primarily to questions of heredity ("Half-sister born out of wedlock who still wets the bed at age 14," "paternal grandfather very 'nervous,'" uncle with "multiple sclerosis," younger brother "is careless and incurs debts"). The study was dedicated to "Professor J. Hallervorden on his 80th birthday." In his autobiography, Peiffer mentions neither Seitelberger nor Zerbin-Rüdin nor their mutual work. Memory is always selective. Peiffer wrote honestly of his past as being a "broken mirror."

Professor Peters's Theft

In early 2014, while investigating Peiffer's earlier research at the Munich Max Planck Institute for Psychiatry, I ordered the index of files kept at the Max Planck Archive at this institution. The holdings are scant and consist mainly of "results of examinations of brain samples that were buried on 25 May 1990 at the Waldfriedhof Cemetery in Munich" (numbers 1–19). That description isn't quite accurate. As we've seen, the "containers" with the samples were buried on 21 February 1990. The files contained nothing about Peiffer's essay.

But I did take notice of the title of the final file, number 23: "Sanatorium and Nursing Home Bruckberg b. Ansbach: Autopsy results from children, 1942–1944." That made me remember a story from my past. On 1 April 1985 I went to the Max Planck Institute for Psychiatry to track down brain samples from victims of the euthanasia murders. In advance, the general administration of the Max Planck Society had repeatedly prepared the directors of the institute for my visit.[58] The director at the time, Professor Gerd Peters (1906–87), a member of what he called "the generation that had experienced everything," gave me quite a friendly reception. It turned out that he had worked at the Institute for Aviation Medical Pathology of the Aviation Ministry at the beginning of World War II and had been transferred to its External Department for Brain Research in Berlin-Buch in 1941. There he researched, among other things, the effects of hypothermia on the human brain. On 26 and 27 October 1942, he took part in the conference "Medical Questions of Emergencies at Sea and Deadly Exposure to Cold in Winter," where participants had reported on experiments carried out upon concentration camp inmates. The doctors Sigmund Rascher and Ernst Holzlöhner, for example, had described fatal experiments with ice-cold water: "Rigor ceases immediately, when death arrives." According to information given to me by the archivist of the Max Planck Institute for Psychiatry in 2014, Peters had done everything in his power during his time as director there (1961–74) to erase any written traces that could lead back to medical crimes committed in the Nazi period.

On 1 April 1985, this very Professor Peters led me into the institute's archival space and tied his tongue in knots assuring me that nothing illegal or immoral had taken place in the institution he had directed for so many years. This demonstratively cordial old Nazi was telling me a pack of lies, as soon became apparent. For my part, I had brought along two thick ring binders full of photocopied case reports of children who had been murdered in a sanatorium and nursing home near Ansbach and whose brains had often been sent to the following address: "German Research Institution for Psychiatry (Kaiser Wilhelm Institute) for personal delivery to Dr. Schleussing." I tried to convince Peters that the documents were authentic and asked to see the corresponding proof of receipt from his institute. In vain.

After we had taken leave of one another, I noticed in the street that my bag was much lighter. One of the ring binders was missing. I ran back; the secretary informed Peters and apologized ten minutes later, saying, "Professor Peters looked everywhere, but couldn't find anything." When I was back in Berlin, I sent Peters a few documents he had asked for and concluded my letter with the sentences: "On 1 April I forgot a ringed binder labeled 'Ansbach II' at your institution. I would ask you to return this binder by this summer."[59] Peters never got back to me.

In 2014, I took a closer look at what Peters had written about my visit at the time and immediately discovered something interesting. In February 1986, he had prepared a commentary about my essay "Clean and Dirty Progress," published late the previous year, and worked himself into a state of agitation. In that commentary, he wrote about the "files Aly had put at my disposal during his visit" concerning case histories from Ansbach.[60] Two years later, Professor Detlev Ploog dealt with the estate of his by then deceased colleague Peters. He wrote to his institutional director, Kreutzberg: "I found an important ring binder that contains among other things autopsy results from children at the Sanatorium and Nursing Home Bruckberg bei Ansbach. I don't think that this binder can be destroyed so I am transferring it to your hands."[61]

Kreutzberg immediately forwarded the binder to the Max Planck Society Archive in Berlin, where I ordered it on 3 February 2014.[62] It still contained the Post-it Notes I had put there in 1984. Four days later, the society restored the property that one of their institute directors had stolen from me twenty-nine years earlier.

Götz Aly, PhD, studied journalism, political science, and history. He has worked for the German dailies *tageszeitung* and *Berliner Zeitung*, as a visiting lecturer, and as a freelance historian. His books have been translated into various languages. His latest publications include *Into the Tunnel: The Brief Life of Marion Samuel, 1931–1943*; *Hitler's Beneficiaries: Plunder, Racial War, and the Nazi Welfare State*; *Why the Germans? Why the Jews? Envy, Race Hatred, and the Prehistory of the Holocaust*; *Die Belasteten: "Euthanasie" 1939–1945; Eine Gesellschaftsgeschichte*; and *Europa gegen die Juden, 1880–1945*. Götz Aly was also one of the founders and was from 2004 to 2010 an editor of the ongoing sixteen-volume source edition *Die Verfolgung und Ermordung der europäischen Juden durch das nationalsozialistische Deutschland 1933–1945*. For his work he has received the following prizes: Heinrich-Mann-Preis, Marion-Samuel-Preis, Order of Merit of the Federal Republic of Germany, National Jewish Book Award, Ludwig-Börne-Preis, Estrongo-Nachama-Preis.

Notes

First published in Aly 2015, 201–39, 255–59, under the German title "Weitere Elaborate Alys verhindern." Parts of my 1984 report have previously been published in English in Aly 1994, 156–237.

1. Archive of the Max Planck Society (Max-Planck-Gesellschaft, MPG), Abt. III, Rep. 55, 21-2, Bl. 274–76.

2. Quoted in Pfeiffer 1997, 38.

3. Hallervorden to the International Military Tribunal in Nuremberg, 11 February 1946; "Die Geschichte der Kaiser-Wilhelm-Gesellschaft/Max-Planck-Gesellschaft 1945–1949" [The history of the Kaiser Wilhelm Society/Max Planck Society 1945-1949] (manuscript, MPG archive), contains: J. Hallervorden, "Die Pathologische Abteilung des Max-Planck-Instituts für Hirnforschung" [The pathological department of the Max Planck Institute for Brain Research], 130–41, see p. 134.

4. German Federal Archives (Bundesarchiv, BArch), R96I/2/127898.
5. Note to the president (Butenandt), signed Seelinger, 27 August 1962.
6. Aly to BArch (Oldenhage), 15 December 1982; BArch (Trumpp) to Aly, 11 January 1983.
7. Aly to Singer, 29 January 1983; Singer to Aly, 3 February 1983.
8. On my initiative, Martin Schmidt (1933–2011) then wrote the article "Hephaistos lebt—Untersuchungen zur Frage der Behandlung behinderter Kinder in der Antike" (Schmidt 1983/84, 133–61).
9. Note (Kazemi), 24 March 1983, and Kazemi to Marsch, 29 March 1983.
10. Statement by Kalb, 15 May 1983, his letter to Aly, 24 May 1983, and his notes to Aly's request, 15 April 1983 and 4 July 1983.
11. Aly to Singer, 21 March 1983; telephone call, Marsch with Kazemi, 25 March 1983; Kazemi to Singer, 29 March 1983.
12. BArch (Boberach) to MPG (Kalb), 23 June 1983; BArch (Oldenhage) to Aly, 5 August 1983 ("Der Vorstoß des Bundesarchivs bei der Max-Planck-Gesellschaft ist leider erfolglos geblieben.") [The request by the Bundesarchiv at the Max Planck Society has unfortunately been unsuccessful].
13. Note (Kalb), 4 July 1984.
14. Aly to Simitis, 9 June 1983; Simitis to Aly, 16 June 1983; Simitis to Singer, 4 August 1984.
15. Data protection officer of the federal state of Hesse (Hohmann) to MPG (Kalb), 9 April 1984.
16. Note (Preiß) on a conversation with Singer, 3 October 1984.
17. Individual names and dates corrected and extended: Aly 2013, 120–38, 163–69. According to my new count, not thirty-three but thirty-five children and adolescents were murdered in the gas chamber for scientific reasons.
18. Götz Aly, report, "Zeitgeschichtliche Erforschung der 'Sammlung Hallervorden' im Max-Planck-Institut für Hirnforschung in Frankfurt" [Contemporary historiographic research on the Hallervorden Collection at the Max Planck Institute for Brain Research], 16 September 1984 and cover letter, 17 September 1984.
19. Aly 2013, 163–69. Previously, I had published details about the Hallervorden Collection and its connection to euthansia in the following texts: Aly 1985; Aly 1989b; Aly and Pross 1989; Aly 1989a; Aly 1997, 73–93.
20. BArch (Booms) to MPG archive (Henning), 19 November 1984; MPG archive (Henning) to MPG-GenV (Marsch), 12 December 1984. Henning was referring to the advisory committee meeting on 16 March 1983.
21. Note (Henning), 26 September 1984.
22. Wässle to Marsch, 5 February 1986.
23. Henning to Marsch, 6 January 1986.
24. Henning to Gutjahr-Loeser (Administrative Headquarters), 16 September 1987.
25. Marsch to Peters (Max Planck Institute for Psychiatry), 27 January 1986, with Weidmann's handwritten note, 9 May 1986.
26. Marsch to Peters, 25 March 1986.
27. Krücke to Marsch, 1 April 1986; Wässle to Marsch, 12 March 1986; Wässle to Marsch (note of a telephone call, signed O. Schulz), 17 March 1986.
28. Henning to Wässle, 19 January 1989.
29. Staab to Singer, 28 February 1989.
30. Dickman 1989; Walsh 1989; Seidelman, 21 September 1989; Seidelman 1989; "Call for Commemoration and Burial of Nazi Victims" 1990.
31. Report by the German news agency *ddp*, printed for instance in the *Stuttgarter Zeitung*, 12 January 1989.
32. Office of the Standing Conference of the Ministers of Education and Cultural Affairs of the States in the Federal Republic of Germany, final report "Präparate von Opfern des Nationalsozialis-

mus in anatomischen und pathologischen Sammlungen deutscher Ausbildungs- und Forschungseinrichtungen" [Tissue samples of victims of National Socialism in anatomical and pathological collections of German educational and research institutions], 25 January 1994; Bavarian State Ministry for Sciences, Research and the Arts (Weininger) to MPG (Administrative Headquarters), 8 February 1989.

33. Henning to Wässle, 19 January 1989.

34. "Resolution des Gesamtbetriebsrats der MPG zur Problematik noch vorhandener Euthanasie-Präparate im MPI für Hirnforschung" [Resolution of the joint works council concerning the problem of still existing euthanasia samples at the Max Planck Institute for Brain Research], 9 March 1989; works council (Kleinschmidt) to Marsch, 13 March 1989; Protokoll der 146. Sitzung des Verwaltungsrates der MPG [Protocol of the 146th meeting of the board of administration of the MPG] 16 March 1989. In the discussion that was carried out "in agreement," Wolfgang Hasenclever (former general secretary of the MPG), Benno Hess (vice president of the MPG), Alfred Herrhausen (spokesman of the Deutsche Bank board, treasurer and senator of the MPG), Eberhard von Kuenheim (chairman of BMW), general secretary Marsch, and president Staab participated.

35. Kreutzberg to Staab, 24 February 1989.

36. Archive of the MPG, Berlin, personal file Schleußing.

37. Kreutzberg to Staab, 24 February 1989; report Henning ("Abschlussbericht") [final report], 3 November 1989.

38. Report given by the president (Staab) at the 121st meeting of the MPG senate, 17 March 1989, p. 9 (statements concerning "an article written by Götz Aly in *Zeit*").

39. Research at the Max Planck Institute for Brain Research, "Bericht Henning 4" [Report Henning 4], 9 March 1989.

40. Henning to Staab, 23 March 1989, and "Bericht Henning 1" [Report Henning 1].

41. Draft of a press release by the MPG, 2 May 1989, is much clearer than the press release from 13 October 1989.

42. Staab to Singer, 31 May 1989.

43. Note by Marsch, 6 October 1989.

44. Henning to Marsch on the Max Planck Institute for Neurological Research in Cologne, 16 May 1989.

45. MPG archive to MPG Administrative Headquarters, 17 October 1989.

46. MPG (Staab) to the State Minister for Sciences, Research and the Arts of Hesse (Gerhardt), 17 October 1989.

47. Note (for Marsch), 16 October 1989; Note "Umgang mit NS-Präparaten" [Handling of NS preparations] (H.-G. Husung), 7 November 1989.

48. Note "Hirnpräparate" [brain specimens] by Marsch, 21 February 1990.

49. *Frankfurter Allgemeine Zeitung*, 18 October 1989.

50. Today, the files can be found in the MPG archive, Abt. III, Rep 55, 26-24, 26-25, 29-41 (1942/101, 1942/102, 1944/79).

51. In fact, only Arthur and Günther were brothers—Herbert was their cousin. Of this I was unaware during my 1984 research.

52. The article can be found in vol. 9, pp. 228–89.

53. The autopsy files of the Kutschkes can be found in the MPG archive, Abt. III, Rep. 55, 26-44, 26-25, 29-43, the patients' records in the Brandenburgian State Main Archive in Potsdam, Rep. 55C, Brandenburg-Görden, 2475, 3180, 9772.

54. Henning to Marsch, 5 March 1990.

55. Peiffer 2004; Peiffer 2005.

56. Peiffer 1963, 87–107.

57. In the book of arrivals (1949–55) of the former histopathological department of the MPI of Psychiatry in Munich, there are brief notes on the deceased patients whose brains Peiffer had exam-

ined at the time. He had recorded the arrival of the brain of Brigitte Ment on 9 August 1955 himself. The medical records, epicrises, and specimens could not be found in 2014.
  58. Marsch to Ploog, 8 February 1985; Marsch to Peters, 5 March 1985.
  59. Aly to Peters, 23 April 1985.
  60. Peters to Henning (February 1986) "Stellungnahme zu den Ausführungen von Herrn Dr. Götz Aly in 'Reform und Gewissen' und im Bericht (an den Präsidenten der MPG) vom September 1984" [Statement concerning the remarks by Dr. Götz Aly in 'Reform und Gewissen' and in his report (to the president of the MPG), September 1984]; already in the beginning of 1985, Peters had given Henning, the director of the archive, a table of the "Brain material send from Ansbach, 1936–1945," with regard "to Mr. Aly's research project." Peters must have evaluated the stolen file quickly. Note by Hennings on his visist to the MPI for Psychiatry on 18 January 1985.
  61. Ploog to Kreutzberg, 29 December 1988.
  62. Archive of the history of the MPG, I Abt., Rep. 0038, formerly Bd. 23. The previous users, noted on the file's cover, were Jürgen Peiffer, Thomas Beddies, and Volker Roelcke.

References

Archival Sources

Archiv der Max-Planck-Gesellschaft, Berlin.
Archiv des Max-Planck-Instituts für Hirnforschung, Frankfurt am Main.
Bundesarchiv, Berlin.

Books and Articles

Aly, Götz. 1985. "Der saubere und der schmutzige Fortschritt." In *Reform und Gewissen: "Euthanasie" im Dienst des Fortschritts*, edited by G. Aly, K. F. Masuhr, M. Lehmann, K. H. Roth, and Ulrich Schultz, 9–78. Berlin: Rotbuch Verlag.
———. 1989a. "Hirnforschung im Dritten Reich: Bericht an die Max-Planck-Gesellschaft zur Förderung der Wissenschaften vom 16. September 1984." *die tageszeitung*, 21 October.
——— (ed.). 1989b. *Aktion T4, 1939–1945: Die "Euthanasie"-Zentrale in der Tiergartenstraße 4*. Berlin: Edition Hentrich.
———. 1994. "Pure and Tainted Progress." In *Cleansing the Fatherland: Nazi Medicine and Racial Hygiene*, edited by G. Aly, P. Chroust, and Christian Pross, 156–237. Baltimore: John Hopkins University Press.
———. 1997. "Im Gehirn liegt die Führung." In *Macht, Geist, Wahn: Kontinuitäten deutschen Denkens*, edited by G. Aly, 73–93. Berlin: S. Fischer.
———. 2013. *Die Belasteten: "Euthanasie" 1939–1945; Eine Gesellschaftsgeschichte*. Frankfurt am Main: S.Fischer.
———. 2015. *Volk ohne Mitte: Die Deutschen zwischen Freiheitsangst und Kollektivismus*. Frankfurt am Main: S. Fischer.
Aly, Götz, and Ch. Pross (eds.). 1989. *Der Wert des Menschen: Medizin in Deutschland 1918–1945*. Berlin: Edition Hentrich.
"Call for Commemoration and Burial of Nazi Victims." 1990. Jewish News, Cleveland, Ohio, 30 March.
Dickman, S. 1989. "Scandal over Nazi Victims' Corpses Rocks Universities." *Nature*, 19 January.
Pfeiffer, Jürgen. 1963. "Zur Variationsbreite der Pelizaeus-Merzbacherschen Krankheit: Zugleich ein Beitrag zur familiären Multiplen Sklerose." *Acta Neuropathologica* 3(2): 87–107.
———. 1997. *Hirnforschung im Zwielicht: Beispiele verführbarer Wissenschaft aus der Zeit des Nationalsozialismus; Julius Hallervorden, H.-J. Scheerer, Berthold Ostertag*. Husum: Matthiesen Verlag.

———. 2004. *Hirnforschung in Deutschland 1849 bis 1974: Briefe zur Entwicklung von Psychiatrie und Neurowissenschaften sowie zum Einfluss des politischen Umfeldes auf Wissenschaftler.* Berlin: Springer.

———. 2005. *Wissenschaftliches Erkenntnisstreben als Tötungsmotiv? Zur Kennzeichnung von Opfern auf deren Krankenakten und zur Organisation und Unterscheidung von Kinder-'Euthanasie' und T4-Aktion: Ergebnisse des Forschungsprogramms 'Geschichte der Kaiser-Wilhelm-Gesellschaft im Nationalsozialismus'* 24. Berlin: Max-Planck-Institut für Wissenschaftsgeschichte.

Schmidt, M. 1983/84. "Hephaistos lebt—Untersuchungen zur Frage der Behandlung behinderter Kinder in der Antike." *Hephaistos* 5–6: 133–61.

Seidelman, W. E. 1989. "Legacy of the Nazis." *Nature*, 21 September.

———. 1989. "In Memoriam Medicine's Confrontation with Evil." *Hastings Center Report*, November/December.

Walsh, M. 1989. "Nazi Research under the Microscope." *Time*, 27 January.

CHAPTER 17

BANEFUL MEDICINE AND A RADICAL BIOETHICS IN CONTEMPORARY ART

Andrew Weinstein

That many Nazi medical researchers were both notorious criminals *and* excellent scientists raises an urgent question.[1] If ethical responsibility happens to be irrelevant to the systematic methods of research, then what, if anything, can we do to anchor it more securely to medical science? After the Nuremberg Doctors Trial in 1947–48, American jurists addressed this question with the Nuremberg Code, which emphasized informed consent for human research subjects and laid the foundations of what would later become the field of bioethics.[2] Since that time, bioethicists have expanded and modified the ethical principles.[3] All will surely agree that these are indispensable achievements. Still, regarding the unprecedented challenges posed today by genomics and bioengineering, fields that could radically transform humanity and civilization, I believe that contemporary artists can make a unique contribution. The startling artworks they create have the potential to turn public attention to bioethical issues in a way that written arguments seldom do. Beyond publicity, some promote ethical frameworks defined by an expanded notion of responsibility that might serve as models for medical professionals to follow. What's more, some artists even go so far as to question the very methods and assumptions of science. They reject the conviction that rational, systematic thinking and testing can exhaust the mystery of an object of study; in other words, they reject the notion that any such object can ever be totally defined or understood.

Philosophical Articulations against Positivism

I imagine that some scientists, and anyone committed to instrumental rationalist and positivist thought, will have a hard time taking seriously this last, most radical position among artists engaged with medical ethics. What has guided my own appreciation of that position are studies of Holocaust representation, which have led me to recognize an affinity between the antipositivist perspective of such artists and of many scholars and artists focused on Holocaust history and memory. In Holocaust studies, this perspective appears in the way that scholars and artists generally reject the prospect of making sense of the Holocaust, which they see as intrinsically senseless. For example, Holocaust historian Saul Friedländer rejects the genre of conventional history writing, typically characterized by interpretive arguments that drive toward neat conclusions. In contrast, he champions a humbler mode of historical writing that accepts "two contradictory moves: the search for ever-closer historical linkages and the avoidance of a naive historical positivism leading to . . . closures."[4] Particularity without comprehension is the strategy, and it likewise describes the approach of Claude Lanzmann, director of the riveting nine-and-a-half-hour filmic oral history *Shoah* from 1985. Convinced of "the obscenity of the very project of understanding," Lanzmann instead emphasizes minutiae ("Did the driver sit in the cab of the van?" "Did he race the motor?" "Was it a loud noise?").[5]

In the philosophy of the thinker most often associated with Holocaust representation, Theodor W. Adorno, positivism similarly comes under fire. Adorno's famous quote of 1949, "To write poetry after Auschwitz is barbaric," offers a good point of entry to his challenging thought.[6] As I understand it, writing poetry in the wake of the Holocaust is barbaric because doing so demands that the poet regard the Holocaust as something that can be characterized by a few defining words, which is to say made sense of, and consequently subject to closure. In the act of writing, therefore, the poet overcomes the debilitating legacy of the incomprehensible inhumanity of the Holocaust. This attitude, writes Adorno, expresses "the coldness, the basic principle of bourgeois subjectivity, without which there could have been no Auschwitz."[7] Adorno suggests that this coldness became preeminent with the rise of the bourgeoisie during and since the Enlightenment (though he also explains it began long before that time). In particular, he explains that it appeared in the calculating desire "to dispel myth, to overthrow fantasy with knowledge" as a means of "liberating human beings from fear." Central to this "disenchantment of the world," Adorno contends, was the development of a manner of thinking that defined things in terms of equivalences.[8] Whether in business, science, or other domains, this way of thinking "makes dissimilar things comparable by reducing them to abstract quantities."[9] For example, the manufacturer, marketer, and consumer appraise the value of objects no longer by their use value or other means but by their monetary exchange value. The worth of dissimilar objects is reduced to the same terms.

In this way, "exchange society" fosters what Adorno calls "identitarian thinking" or simply identity thinking.[10] This kind of thinking misleads a person, a subject, to believe that a defining concept in mind entirely describes an object of consideration. The result: "identity of the mind and its correlative," which is one form of assumed equivalence.[11] Here is another: with an assumption of total understanding, the thinker, exemplified by the scientist, presumes for example that one atom or one laboratory rabbit is the same as, and interchangeable with, another. "Representation gives way to fungibility. An atom is smashed not as a representative but as a specimen of matter, and the rabbit suffering the torment of the laboratory is seen not as a representative but, mistakenly, as a mere exemplar."[12] Inferring interchangeability of what are in fact only similar objects, each with a particular and mysterious being, the thinking subject assumes a magisterial position to evaluate any particular specimen or exemplar. Appraisal may include whether that specimen or exemplar is valuable or valueless, and, at its extreme, worthy or unworthy to exist at all. To Adorno, "Auschwitz confirmed the philosopheme of pure identity as death."[13] One need only consider Dr. Josef Mengele, the so-called "Angel of Death," momentarily assessing each arrival at Auschwitz with a word and a gesture of the hand, right or left, life for another day or immediate annihilation.

Adorno's antidote for positivism is the substance of his "negative dialectics," which "says no more . . . than that objects do not go into their concepts without leaving a remainder. [This] contradiction . . . indicates the untruth of identity, the fact that the concept does not exhaust the thing conceived."[14] Meanwhile, a desire to find the true name for a thing propels the philosopher forward. In response to specific evidence, the thinker rigorously poses questions in a process that requires the thinker's "self-relinquishment" of preconceived ideas in acquiescence to the particulars. In other words, the subject seeks to learn from the object of study, not to impose a concept on it.[15]

Adorno's method for the discovery of truth is almost mystical. The thinking subject strives to unriddle the riddle of an object of study in its historical particularity. "The function of riddle-solving is to light up the riddle-*Gestalt* like lightning. . . . Authentic philosophical interpretation does not meet up with a fixed meaning which already lies behind the question, but lights it up suddenly and momentarily, and consumes it at the same time."[16] The goal: unlocking the "unintentional truth" of an object, which, coming from the object itself, is distinct from a concept originating in the thinker's mind.[17] The method: "exact fantasy," in which the thinker examines a range of particularities in conjunction with the right "key" to unlock meaning from the riddle (one supposes that Marxism, Freudian psychoanalysis, and an infinity of other methodologies might provide a basic shape for crafting a particular key).[18] Riddles present all the clues for their own solution, but to figure them out, the clues must be recombined. Adorno imagines a "combination of numbers" or "changing constellations" like a formation of stars that congeal through imagination into an image of the object and reveal, in an epiphanic and utopian flash, the unintentional truth, which is also its true name.[19] Then, instantly, the name of the object transforms into a concept, an example of identity thinking, leaving the conscientious nonidentity thinker no choice but to reject that name and start the quest for another. "This is the font," writes Adorno, "the determinable flaw in every concept makes it necessary to cite others."[20]

Adorno contends that after the fall of the Nazi regime, the fundamentals of society did not change, largely because identity thinking has remained the prevalent mode of cognition. A present-day example: the reductive public discourse about what has been called "the quintessential bioethics topic," abortion.[21] An internet meme equating abortion with the Holocaust, shorthand for the most egregious evil, inflames partisan emotions while obfuscating the particulars that differentiate abortion and the Holocaust (figure 17.1).

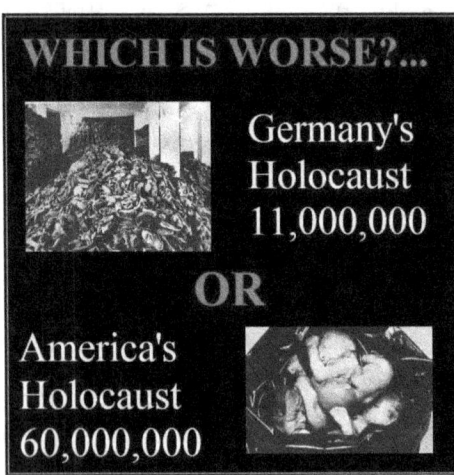

Figure 17.1. Internet meme, ca. 2019.

In contrast to such reductive images, many contemporary artworks that are engaged with medical ethics present imagery that is shaped by intellectual frameworks like the ones we have considered from the field of Holocaust studies. And far from abortion, they address bioethical challenges that scarcely enter the arena of public debate. Genomics and bioengineering have opened a proverbial Pandora's box, beginning in the 1980s with corporate property claims to naturally occurring genes and continuing now with the disturbing reality of modification to the human genome with CRISPR-Cas9 technology.[22] There is a lot to worry about, something that BioArt pioneers Oron Catts and Ionat Zurr, known as the Tissue Culture & Art Project, understood acutely in 2000 when they created their Guatemalan-influenced *Semi Living Worry Dolls*, in which living tissue from the commercially available human-derived McCoy cell line grew over biodegradable/bioabsorbable polymer frames (figure 17.2). In Guatemalan Indian tradition, children whisper troubling concerns to worry dolls, which are supposed to resolve the worries overnight. With their own adult-sized worries in mind, TC&A created seven dolls instead of the traditional six and associated them with alphabetized letters for specific concerns: A "for the worry from Absolute truths, and of the people who think they hold them"—absolute truths being the product of identity thinking; B for "the worry of Biotechnology, and the forces that drive it"; C for those forces, "Capitalism, Corporations"; D for "Demagogy, and possible Destruction"; E for "Eugenics and the people who think they are superior enough to practice it"; F for the "fear of Fear"; and H for the "fear of Hope"

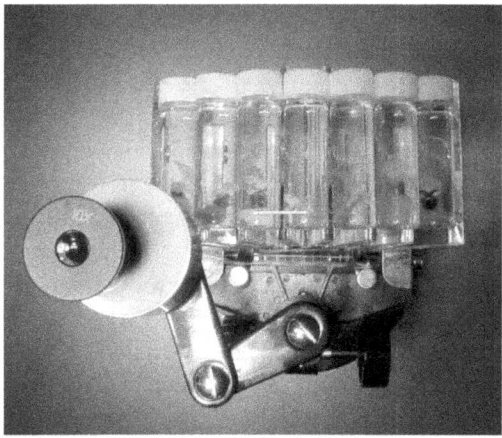 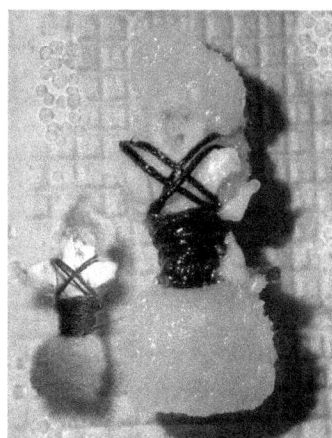

Figure 17.2. The Tissue Culture & Art Project (Oron Catts and Ionat Zurr), *Semi Living Worry Dolls*, 2000. From *The Tissue Culture & Art(ificial) Wombs Installation*, Ars Electronica, 2000. Living cells, biodegradable/bioabsorbable polymers, and surgical sutures, dimensions variable. *Left:* Seven dolls, shown here in microscope display. *Right:* Detail of doll before and after cell growth. Courtesy the artists.

(they passed over G, which in referencing "genes" was general to all the dolls). In the spirit of nonidentity, they also invite the viewer to "find new worries and new names" for each of the letters. Most importantly, by engaging with a premodern, non-Western tradition, they invoke a realm of mystery and enchantment in their lab-created worry dolls. TC&A asks, "Will they take our worries away?"[23]

There are reasons for hope. Personally I am comforted and moved by the small, dedicated community of high-minded medical professionals who, through personal conviction and often in their spare time, organize and attend bioethics conferences and contribute to the creation of books like this one. Moreover, some medical schools have enriched their curriculum with humanistic learning to foster sensitivities in their students so that they may go forth in their careers and self-regulate. Still, to make sure that they do self-regulate, an informed and engaged public will have to keep watch and demand more stringent legal regulation of medical research. How to nurture the development of such a public? One answer: through artworks as potent as the abortion poster but that are wary of the intellectual risks of identity thinking.

Bioethicists on Board

Beginning around 2005, bioethicists took note of the power of art to communicate concerns about developments in genomics and biotech. Tod Chambers writes, "How can people visualize a future at risk? The dangers ... have not deeply aroused the American public, and one reason has been a lack of images appropriate to the problem." Chambers contends that art can achieve what bioethical arguments cannot. First, because artists deal by definition with frameworks of representation, they are well equipped to recognize, explore, and critique the cultural means with which science gains its rhetorical authority (these, I suggest, might include medical jargon, white lab coats, high-tech equipment, etc.). Secondly, by presenting a personal and often autobiographical perspective on the issues of science, artists can offer a vividly human dimension. Finally, by creating arresting images, artists can seize public attention.[24]

Writing at the same time, the bioethicist Paul Lauritzen asks the larger question of whether bioethics itself possesses the conceptual tools to grapple with new challenges, which include addressing such fundamental questions as what it means to be human. Medical technologies may well realize the dream of transhumanism, that is, of genetically enhancing the human being. What consequences may there be for society? The prospect that science would deliver transhumanist technology only to the financially and culturally privileged "does not bode well" for cultivating compassion across societal dividing lines.[25] What's more, if assumptions of a universal and eternal "species-typical" human nature are the foundation of societal principles of human rights, then biotechnology may threaten "the very basis of human morality as we know it."[26] To stimulate broad public dialog about matters of biotechnology, Lauritzen, like Chambers, believes that art can accomplish more than bioethics. For an example of an artwork that has done just that, Lauritzen cites the well-known *GFP Bunny*, made in 2000 by artist Eduardo Kac (figure 17.3).[27]

To create *GFP Bunny*, Kac explains that at his direction, two scientists in a French laboratory engineered a being that possessed the DNA of two species, in this case a rabbit and the *Aequorea victoria* jellyfish.[28] (The green fluorescent

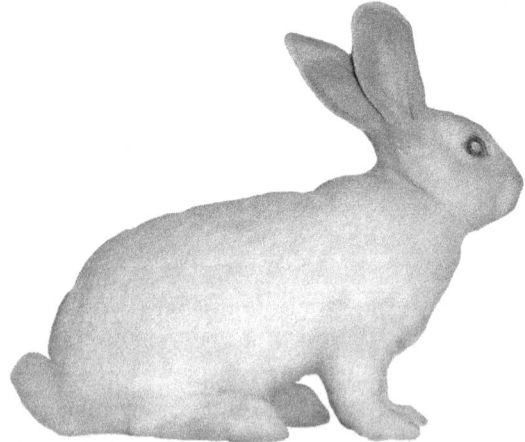

Figure 17.3. Eduardo Kac, *GFP Bunny*, 2000. Transgenic rabbit. Courtesy the artist.

protein or GFP gene introduced into the rabbit's DNA is a synthetic mutation of a naturally occurring jellyfish gene and is commonly used in research to monitor gene expression.) Kac and his family chose the name Alba for the transgenic rabbit to call attention to her albino characteristics, the result of a long history of breeding, precursor of transgenic manipulation.[29] The artist planned to bring Alba home as a family pet, but the lab director, learning of the project, refused to release her. In response, Kac launched a worldwide media campaign on Alba's behalf, which he promoted with a series of art actions and artworks (including those in figures 17.4, 17.5, and 17.6) to publicize the story of her creation and captivity and to foster what he calls an "ongoing debate" about transgenic life.[30]

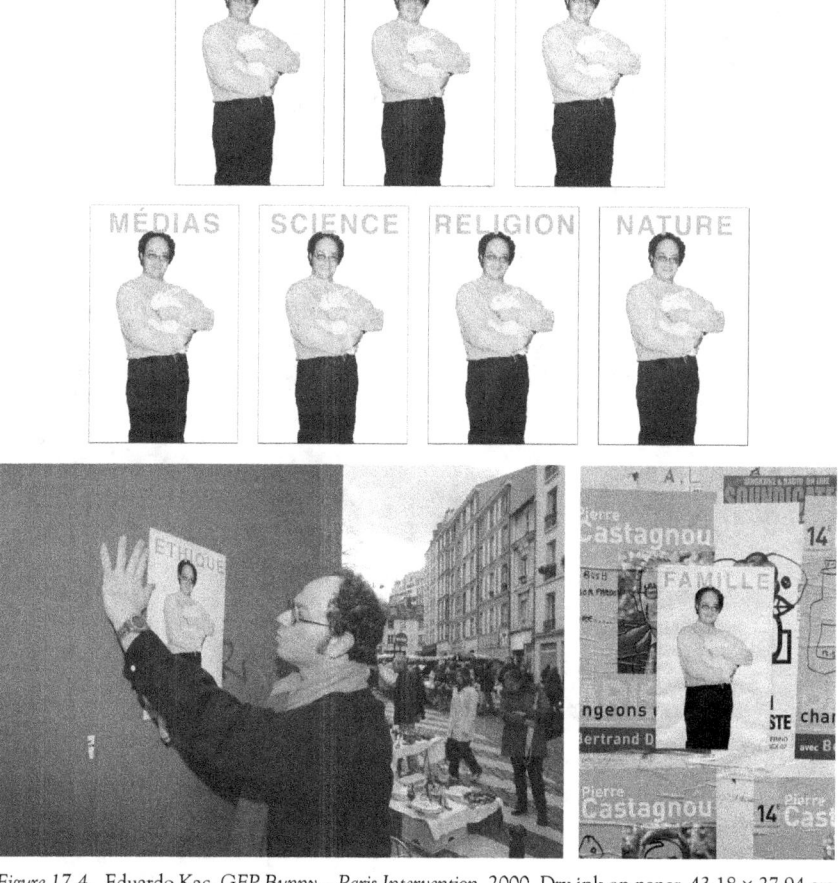

Figure 17.4. Eduardo Kac, *GFP Bunny—Paris Intervention*, 2000. Dry ink on paper, 43.18 × 27.94 cm (17 × 11 in.) each. *Bottom left:* Eduardo Kac in Montparnasse. *Bottom right:* Poster in Montparnasse. Courtesy the artist.

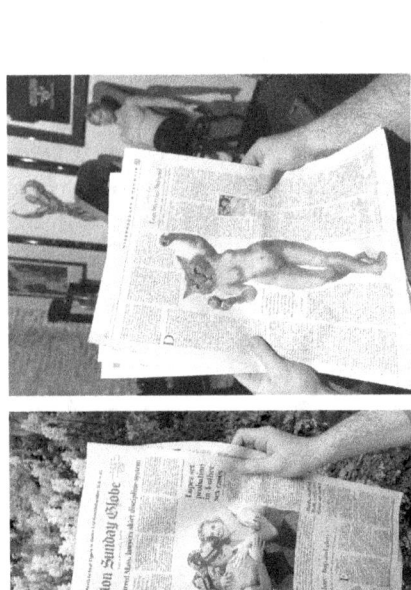
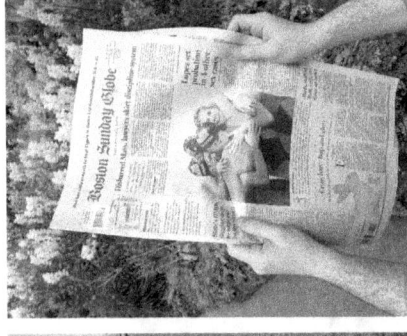
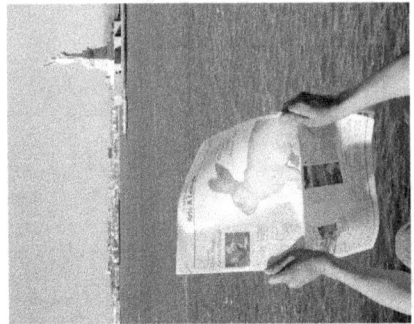
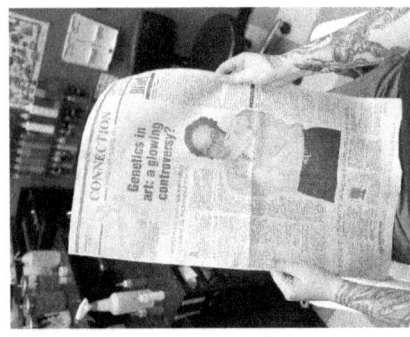
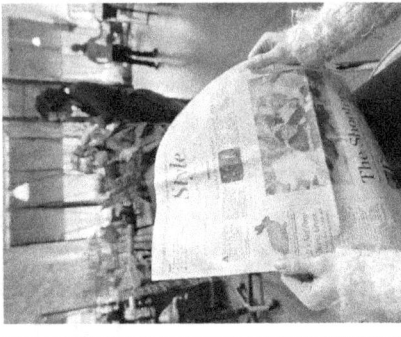
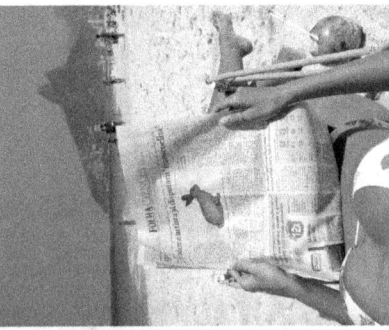
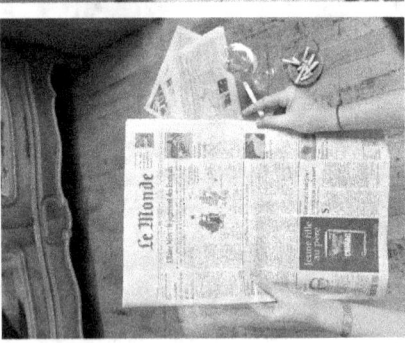

Figure 17.5. Eduardo Kac, *Free Alba!*, 2001–02. Color photographs mounted on aluminum with plexiglas, 91.4 × 118 cm (36 × 46.5 in.) each. Courtesy the artist.

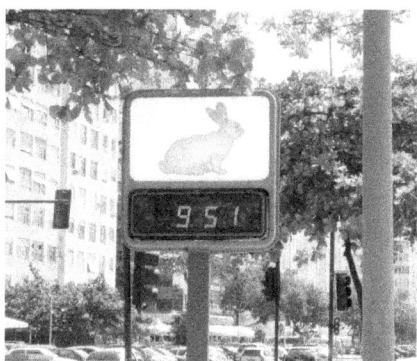
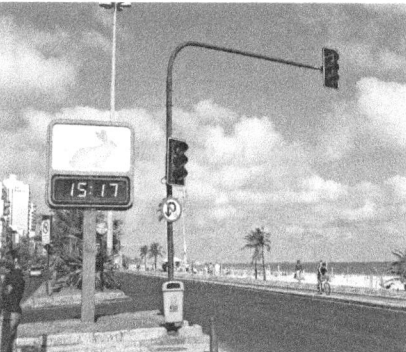

Figure 17.6. Eduardo Kac, *Rabbit in Rio*, 2004. Rio de Janeiro, Brazil. Photos by Nelson Pataro. Courtesy the artist.

Narrative, Love, and Responsibility

Kac draws a larger lesson from GFP Bunny and her story: art that manipulates or creates life must be pursued "above all, with a commitment to respect, nurture, and love the life created."[31] This commitment suggests the possibility of fostering responsibility and even love within the bioengineer as one means of preventing ethical transgressions. Through his activist work, Kac implies that art can serve as a means of demonstrating moral action and even inspiring it in others, and in this position he is not alone. The philosopher Martha Nussbaum (following Henry James) celebrates certain novels as works of moral philosophy for their wise, subtle, and evocative renditions of real-life moral conduct, which offer readers "training in a tender and loving objectivity that we can also cultivate in life."[32] Such artworks are, according to Nussbaum, not only "representations of moral achievement, they are moral achievements."[33] Remarking more broadly about the power of narrative, Nussbaum suggests that the meaning of love, and ethical understanding in general, is learned not by "sitting in an ethics class" but by hearing and contemplating stories from earliest childhood on. "Stories first construct and then evoke (and strengthen) the experience of feeling."[34]

What a seemingly wonderful basis for nurturing ethics in medical science: love learned through stories, including Kac's narrative about Alba and his devotion to taking responsibility for her. This idea of narrative as a source of moral instruction has influenced medical school curriculum to adopt studies of literature. It has also inspired what physician and literary scholar Rita Charon calls "narrative medicine," where practicing physicians may cultivate an empathic connection to their patients by listening to the stories they tell of their lives and plights; doctors, she contends, like literary critics, should employ "close reading" and other narrative skills in response to those stories for an understanding of the state of their patients' holistic well-being.[35]

Stories give resonance to Verena Kaminiarz's art, which calls attention to the service of laboratory animals, and also calls longstanding scientific and bioethical protocols into question. Documented through photographs, her 2008 *may the mice bite me if it is not true*, was an installation artwork in a laboratory at the University of Western Australia that she created for her master's degree in biological arts (figures 17.7, 17.8, and 17.9). It focused on four mice that had been bred to serve as human disease models but, as excess, had been slated for euthanasia. Kaminiarz conceived not simply of rescuing these mice but of honoring them for their availability to serve. She provided them with enhanced living conditions for the rest of their natural lives, which she arranged would be lived in the lab, where their difference from other mice would call attention to their story. Also, she replaced their identification numbers with proper names taken from famous human beings who had died of the diseases the mice would have modeled: Joseph Beuys for natural causes (Beuys died of congestive heart failure), Gilles Deleuze and Franz Kafka for lung cancer, and Felix Gonzalez-Torres for compromised immune system (Gonzalez-Torres died of AIDS). Human names for the mice, and photos of the mice paired with their human namesakes in similar poses and situations (both Gilleses alongside

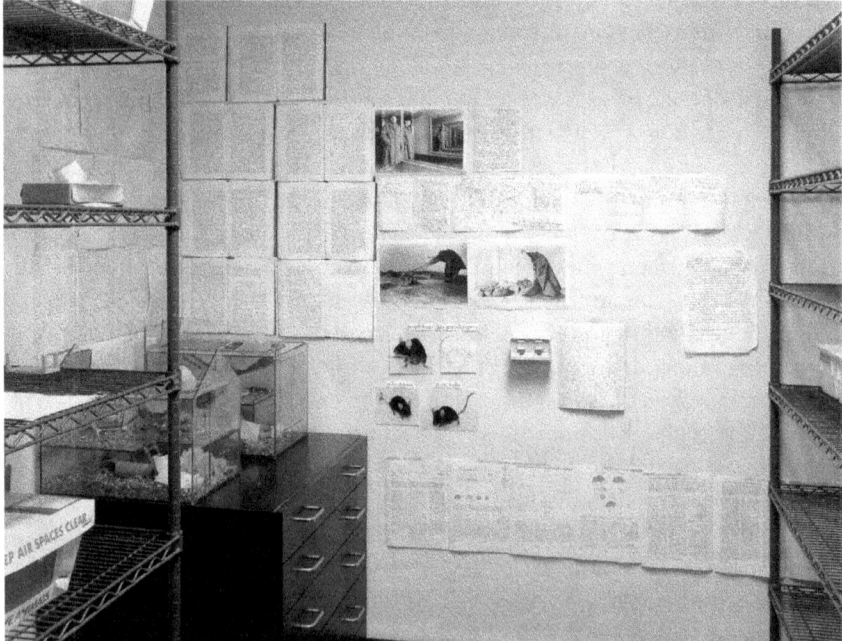

Figure 17.7. Verena Kaminiarz, *may the mice bite me if it is not true*, installation detail: *Habitat*, 2008. Inkjet print, dimensions variable. Courtesy the artist.

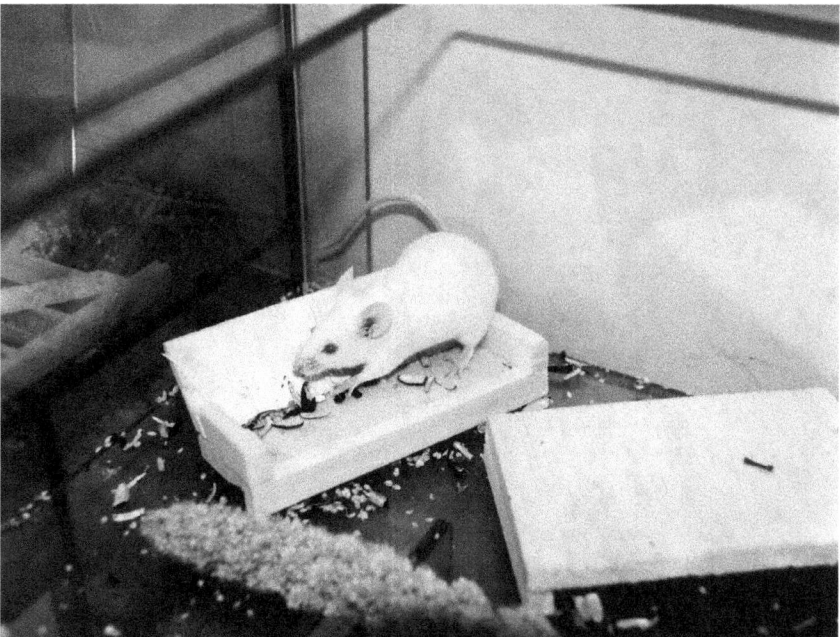

Figure 17.8. Verena Kaminiarz, *may the mice bite me if it is not true*, installation detail: *Felix*, 2008. Inkjet print, dimensions variable. Courtesy the artist.

mirroring surfaces, for example) hint at an equivalent value of life, whether human or murine, and clarify the artist's determination to expand moral concerns that have been traditionally reserved only for human beings, a posthumanist perspective.[36]

Reviewing Kaminiarz's proposal for her artwork, the university Animal Ethics Committee became, in the artist's words, "very concerned" about how the naming would affect the objectivity and morale of scientific researchers working in the same facility. The committee also initially insisted that the artwork conclude by euthanizing the mice, for two reasons: (1) ongoing artworks and experiments were not permitted past a student's graduation; (2) Kaminiarz's plan to let the mice grow old violated a bioethical guideline in subjecting the mice to "potentially suffer some 'old age malady,'" as the artist puts it.[37] Kaminiarz eventually prevailed in convincing the committee to allow the project to continue past her graduation, provided that the laboratory animal care staff periodically check the four mice for health problems. (In old age, when health problems did in fact develop, the mice were euthanized.) By featuring Kaminiarz's rescue of these mice and respectful care for them in implicit contrast to the treatment of other mice in the same laboratory facility, the artwork starkly spotlights what Adorno

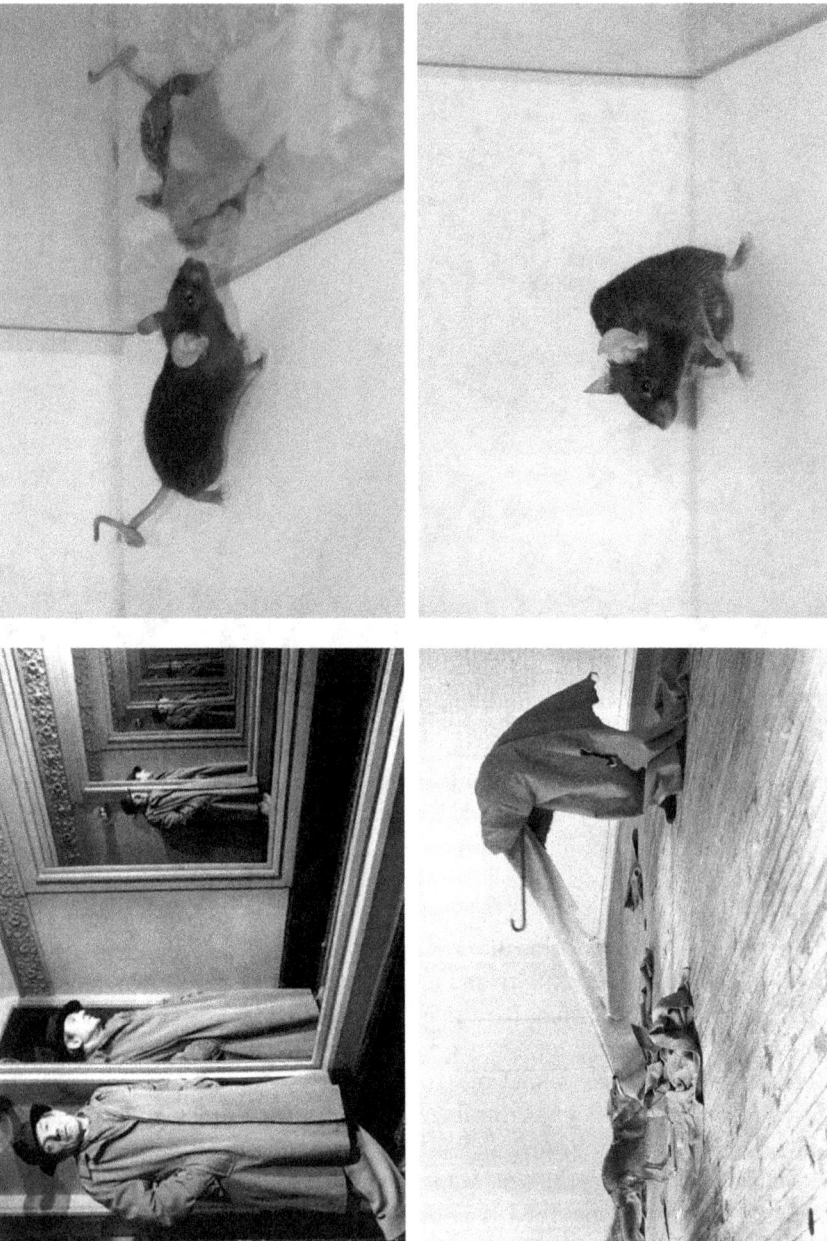

Figure 17.9. Verena Kaminiarz, *may the mice bite me if it is not true*, installation detail: *Gilles and Joseph*, 2008. Courtesy the artist.

might call the coldness of scientific protocols, even when modified by bioethical considerations.

In a companion piece, *death masks (mus musculus)*, Kaminiarz collected the remains of seventy-eight mice that research scientists at UWA had euthanized after a muscular dystrophy study, then made plaster casts of their anterior bodies to record their faces in keeping with a long tradition of remembering and honoring eminent people (figure 17.10). Kaminiarz suggests her own humility in light of the service and sacrifice of the lab mice with her lowercase titles, the longer of which, *may the mice bite me if it is not true*, sounds like a personal pledge or promise to promote a non-human-centered ethic of responsibility and something of a narrative in itself.[38]

As inspiring as it is, however, narrative has a problem, at least in light of identity thinking. Whether documentary or invented, all stories are representations, constructions of the storyteller's mind. So are all images; selected from an infinity of possible images, every image encodes and reveals its maker's point of view. Therefore, notions of love and responsibility that are promoted in Western literature and art may traffic in culturally determined concepts and universalizing assumptions about emotion, illness, personhood, etc. For a medical professional who draws moral instruction from studies of such literature and art, these concepts may have little or nothing to do with the experience of the patients or research subjects in that doctor's charge. This general problem with literature and art relates to Adorno's objection to poetry after Auschwitz for its "bourgeois subjectivity." Distinct from advancing narrative with its problematic promotion of feeling, some artworks present models of *thinking* that focus self-critically on avoiding the conceptual pitfalls of thinking itself.[39]

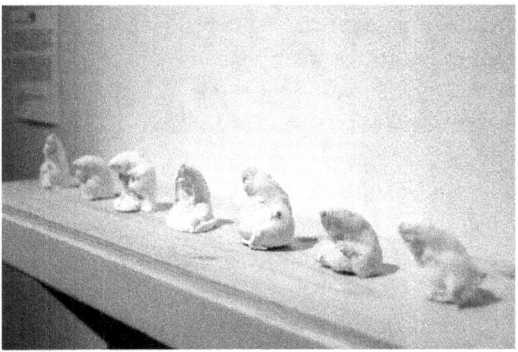 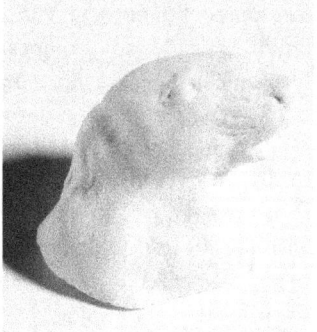

Figure 17.10. Verena Kaminiarz, *death masks (mus musculus)* (details), 2008. Seventy-eight plaster casts, dimensions variable. Courtesy the artist.

Uniqueness

When Kaminiarz gave proper names to four mice that previously had been identified only with numbers, she sought to demonstrate how "individualization breaks a conventional understanding of these animals" as multiples of "an endless 'set of tools'"—Adorno's "interchangeable exemplars."[40] A type of linguistic sign, a proper name possesses the quality of uniqueness: "not transferable and not reusable, ... the proper name completes, exhausts itself, in the act of reference. Aside from labelling the object that is its bearer, it has no further meaning," writes art theorist Rosalind E. Krauss.[41] Through proper naming, Kaminiarz gives a mouse identity without identity thinking. Similarly, each plaster cast that Kaminiarz made represents only the one particular body whose form it indexically preserves. In both of these ways, Kaminiarz presents the viewer with the irreducible uniqueness of every mouse. By leaving each undefined except in terms of its uniqueness, Kaminiarz encourages the viewer to appreciate the ultimate mystery of its being. This radical particularity resembles Friedlander's emphasis on "ever-closer historical linkages," Lanzmann's focus on minutiae, and Adorno's advocacy of exactitude in "exact fantasy."

In their own distinct way, Jake and Dinos Chapman also champion uniqueness. The brothers have become world famous for transgressive depictions of the human body, including sexually provocative representations of what appear to be bioengineered or mutant children. Generating controversy, media attention, and large crowds in London, Berlin, and New York, the 1997–2000 *Sensation* exhibition of the YBAs (Young British Artists) included the Chapman brothers' 1995 *Zygotic Acceleration, Biogenetic Desublimated Libidinal Model (Enlarged × 1000)* (figure 17.11). It depicts a humanoid creature (or rather, as the title specifies, a model of one) with innumerable legs and heads, independently expressive childlike faces, and a composite torso. Except for wearing many pairs of identical black sneakers, it is naked, exposing crotches with no genitals. Where noses and mouths should be, some of the heads display erect penises and anus-like orifices. Vaginas appear between several of the fused faces.

To critics of the piece who accused the Chapman brothers of celebrating or at least making light of the sexual abuse of children, Jake Chapman counters with an interesting defense: "I've never seen a child look like one of our mannequins—abused or not."[42] He sounds cheeky, but he makes an important point: the piece depicts a unique being. Even though its appearance may suggest certain meanings to a viewer, its uniqueness ultimately means that it stands only for itself. There is, for example, no reason for a viewer to assume that this creature is a juvenile; in fact, the brothers describe it as "mature."[43] Anyone who identifies sexualized children in its non-normative body, they suggest, approaches it with a preconceived idea of sexualized children already in mind, one that is piqued by the sculpture's unspecific prompts (for example, the word "libidinal" in the title,

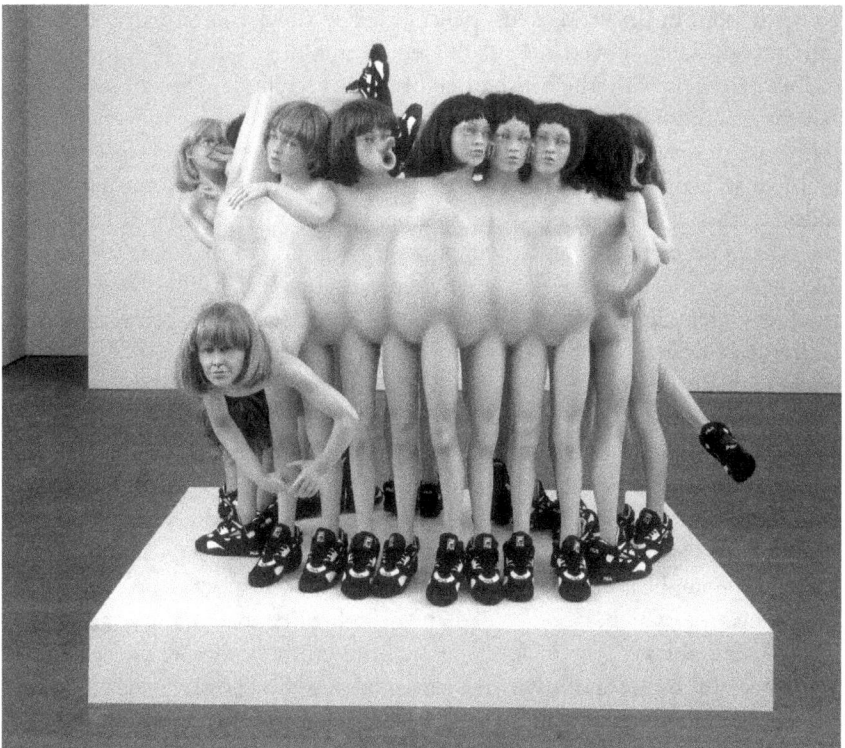

Figure 17.11. Jake and Dinos Chapman, *Zygotic Acceleration, Biogenetic Desublimated Libidinal Model (Enlarged × 1000)*, 1995. Mannequin, mixed media, wigs, and trainers, 150 × 180 × 140 cm (59.06 × 70.87 × 55.12 in.). Courtesy the artists.

the childlike faces and the sexual organs on display). As such, the provocative piece functions as a sort of snare for identity thinkers. Directing a suspicion of pedophilia back against critics of the sculpture, Jake Chapman remarks that "moral outbursts are as effective in discharging libidinal energy as any other corporeal eruption."[44]

Excess

Most dramatically, the art of Jake and Dinos Chapman exhibits excess. Some people regard their subject matter as excessive in transgressing standards of decorum, but by excess I mean something else. These artists infuse their works with an excess of meanings. They employ text in conjunction with image to generate an overload of signification to the extent that their art appears to refuse fixed or consistent definition in the manner of postmodernist complexity and contradiction. In this way, excess typically serves them as a formal strategy and intellectual tool to subvert the risk of identity thinking.

Take, to begin with, the title of their disturbing sculpture. *Zygotic Acceleration, Biogenetic Desublimated Libidinal Model (Enlarged × 1000)* offers an overwhelming mishmash of scientific-sounding jargon. In its excess—a string of terms invoking multiple and contradictory associations, including a reference to the discredited scientific theory of biogenesis—the title becomes uninterpretable. It caricatures the culture of science and tacitly impugns it for failing to articulate its methods and objectives in language that the public can understand. In other words, the title does what Chambers expects art to do—to critique the often intimidating authority of science.

Individually considered, some words in the title also suggest troubling associations. "Enlarged × 1000" indicates that the actual creature this model represents would have a height just shy of one and a half millimeters (about a sixteenth of an inch). Its offensive details would be too tiny to detect with the naked eye. The general public, uninformed about scientific developments, would invariably overlook the very details that offend were they to encounter such an organism in person. The implication: the public fails to recognize the microscopic offenses of bioengineering, which, if confronted, might well strike that public as perverse.

With the phrase "zygotic acceleration," the brothers conjure generative developments in biotechnology with increasing speed and possibly out of society's control. Yet in a self-parodic twist, Jake Chapman introduces an entirely different interpretation based on the sound of the same two words: "psychotic acceleration."[45] From this perspective, the work becomes evidence of the artists' delusional and racing imaginations—a depiction of their own misguided concept of bioengineering and failure to reveal truth.

Nor do the brothers stop at that self-subversion. As a scientific term, "desublimation" seems irrelevant, referring to a material phase change from gas to solid without the intermediary phase as a liquid; however, its appearance in the Chapman brothers' title as "desublimated libidinal model" resonates within the context of culture critique. In *One-Dimensional Man*, Herbert Marcuse, once a colleague of Adorno's at the Frankfurt Institute, discusses what he calls "repressive desublimation." This involves the undoing of what Freud called "sublimation," by which he meant the redirection of instinctual sexual impulses into socially acceptable activities like art making. Marcuse explains that our technologically oriented culture, which demystifies, rationalizes, and circumscribes sexual experience, fosters repressive desublimation: "Compare love-making in a meadow and in an automobile. . . . In the former . . . , the environment partakes of and invites libidinal cathexis and tends to be eroticized." In the latter, however, instinctual sexual impulses are discharged only as themselves in one-dimensional terms, simultaneously "diminishing erotic and intensifying sexual energy."[46] The Chapman brothers' sculpture exaggerates these tendencies. To listen to the brothers talk about the work, it would seem to illustrate still another of Marcuse's ideas of one-dimensionality. No longer sublimating sexual impulses as in earlier, sexually repressed times, art in contemporary commodity culture, argues Marcuse, becomes simple entertainment, "its commercial release for business and fun . . . replacing mediated by immediate gratification."[47] Slyly echoing Marcuse to undermine any presumption that they are qualified to speak as authoritative critics of medical technology, the Chapman brothers say that they themselves "fantasize about producing things with zero cultural value . . . art to be consumed and then forgotten."[48]

Through carefully chosen titular words, the Chapmans prompt a viewer's uneasy response to contemporary science in ways that bear on ethical questions, yet they simultaneously undermine their own critique. Put another way, the sculpture as a whole teases a viewer to leap to conclusions based on preconceptions, something that the brothers themselves will not do. Ultimately all they will vouch for is the uniqueness of the being that the sculpture represents. In this way, the sculpture presents what can be called a productive tension between excess and uniqueness, one that engages a viewer to probe the dangers and ethical limits of identity.

Much the same can be said of the Chapman brothers' *Ubermensch*, a sculpture from 1995 (figure 17.12). *Ubermensch* features a re-created craggy mountain peak of a sort that the Nazi filmmaker Leni Riefenstahl might have been proud to climb to prove her Aryan mettle. On its summit sits a life-size representation of the eminent British scientist Stephen Hawking, lodged and seemingly stranded precariously in his wheelchair. An *Übermensch* (superman)? The title conjures Nazi eugenics in a viewer's mind. As the Nazis defined the so-called master race through idealized physical characteristics, the representation of Hawking's "imperfect," non-normative body poses a contradiction. Yet who can question what the Chapman brothers themselves call Hawking's "perfect mind?"[49] For his superior intellect, Hawking might legitimately be described as a superman. The term originates with Friedrich Nietzsche, who meant something rather different from what the Nazis did: a person who could bring the empowering illusion of meaning to the meaninglessness of existence through promoting big lies, science among them. By this definition, Hawking might again be an *Übermensch*. The Chapmans' sculpture calls up these many concepts in a viewer's mind; however, at some point, the viewer notices that the title lacks the requisite umlaut over the u. As written, *Ubermensch* is not a word. In the end, the title seems to mean nothing. All that the sculpture presents for sure is a portrait of Stephen Hawking. Again, excess and uniqueness jostle together in a productive tension, freeing the work from identity thinking even as it grounds it in identity.

In 2000 the Chapman brothers completed an expansive installation incorporating some sixty thousand customized toy figures in a work unironically called *Hell*, critically celebrated as a masterpiece and accidentally destroyed in

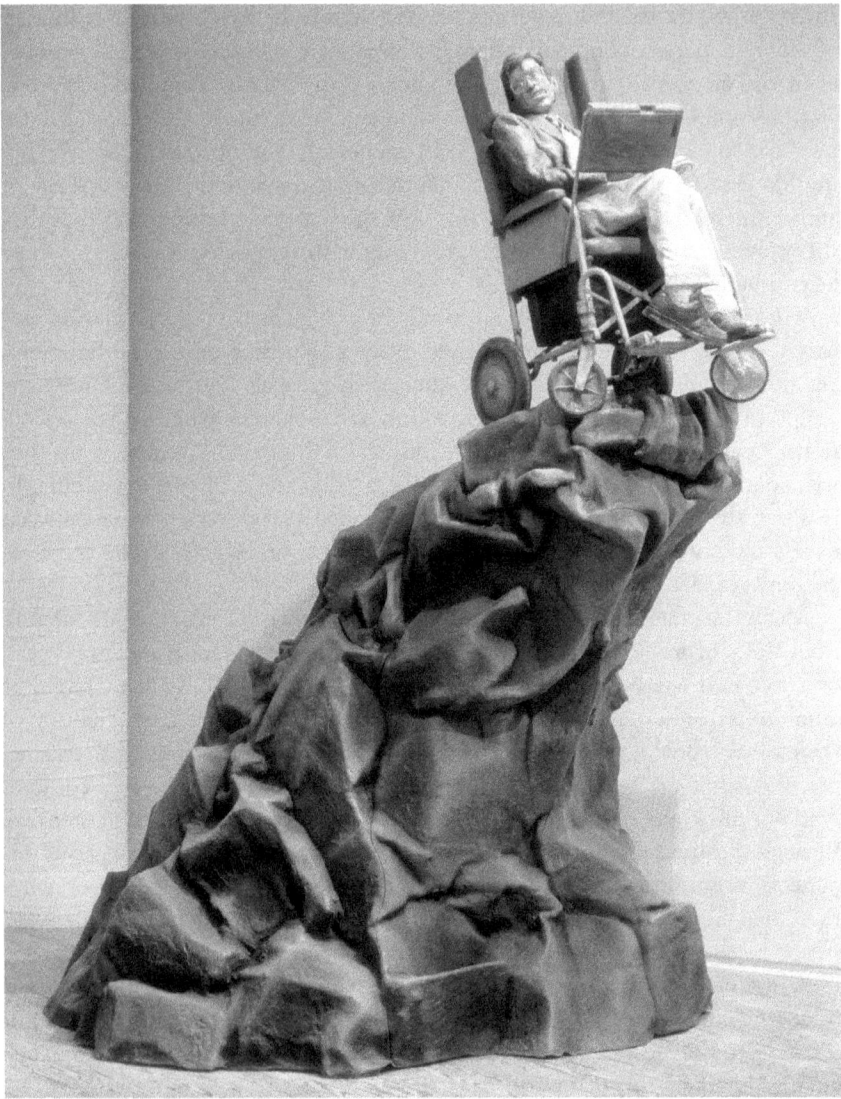

Figure 17.12. Jake and Dinos Chapman, *Ubermensch*, 1995. Fiberglass and mixed media, 366 × 183 × 183 cm (144.09 × 72.05 × 72.05 in.). Courtesy the artists.

a warehouse fire in 2004.[50] Four years later, in 2008, the brothers recreated the piece as *Fucking Hell*. They displayed it like the original in nine vitrines arranged in the configuration of a backward Nazi swastika (figure 17.13). These works, along with smaller related pieces, present swastika flags and armbands along with a panoply of deathly horrors, including a mass grave in *Hell*, and a pile

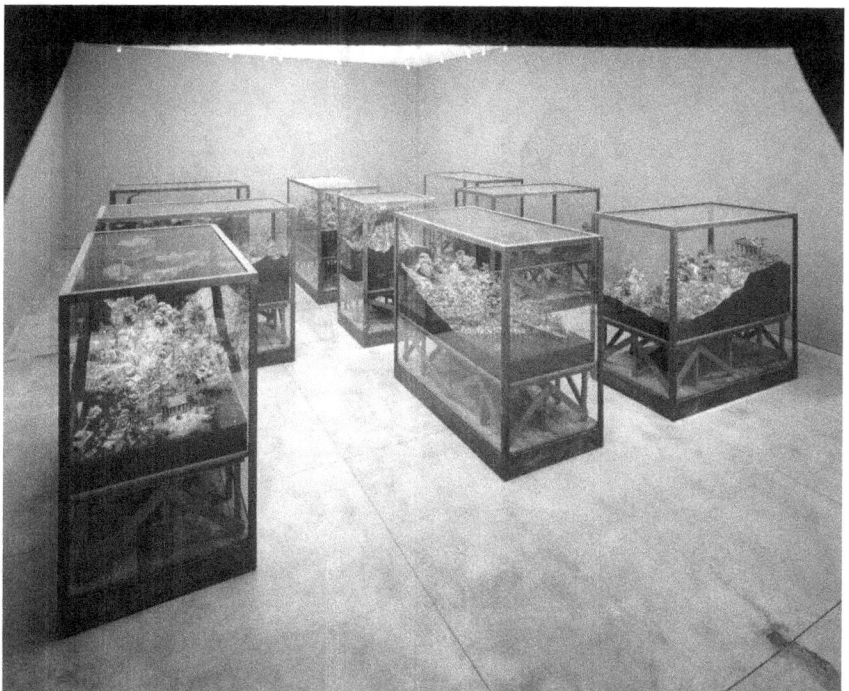

Figure 17.13. Jake and Dinos Chapman, *Fucking Hell*, 2008. Mixed media, eight parts, each 215 × 128.7 × 249.8 cm (84.65 × 50.67 × 98.35 in.); one part, 215.4 × 128 × 128 cm (84.80 × 50.39 × 50.39). Courtesy the artists.

of teddy bears that suggests the industrial-scale murder of their absent owners (figure 17.14). These direct the viewer to thoughts of the Holocaust, notwithstanding the inclusion of a mushroom cloud, Ronald McDonald, heads on stakes, etc. There are clones of Adolf Hitler, and mutants that are multiheaded or have multiple arms that are sometimes twisted in the shape of a swastika. By suggesting bioengineering, such images lead a viewer to think of Nazi eugenics (figure 17.15). But because the figures are grotesque, "really small and really pathetic," they are anything but exemplars of an imagined master race.[51] "Less historical than . . . hysterical," the works depict what the Chapman brothers describe, in fact, as genocide targeted against the Nazis themselves by skeletons, aliens, and mutants.[52] The brothers explain: "Nazis killing Jews is the historical truth. Nazis getting the shit kicked out of them is so science-fictionally wrong that there might as well be Martians in there."[53] Nazis fill the mass grave. Teddy bears seem to lunge at Nazis and bite them.

One realizes that these sculptures, like previous works, present a test of a viewer's tendency to label based on preconceived ideas—i.e., that they dare the viewer to identify their depictions as representations of the Holocaust. But there

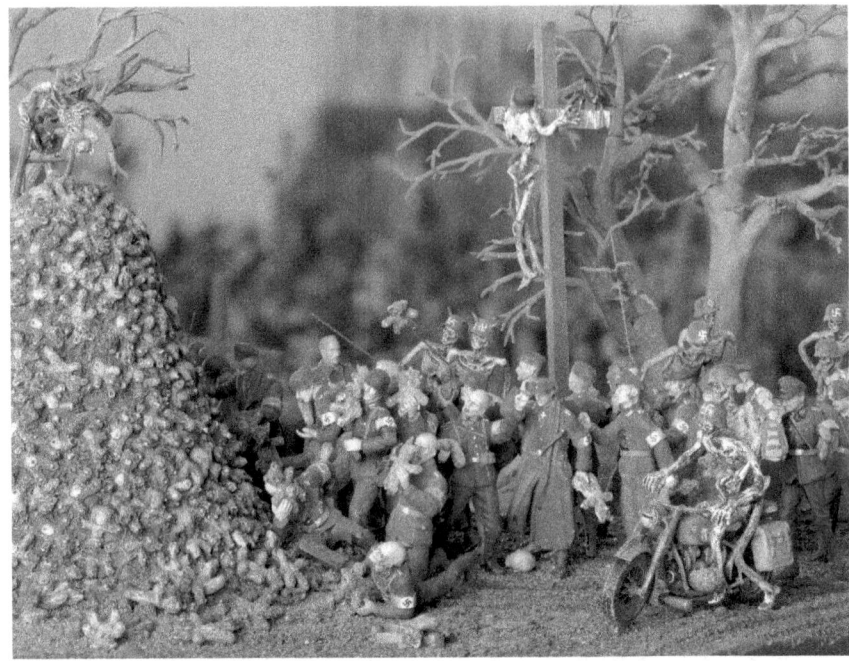

Figure 17.14. Jake and Dinos Chapman, *The Sum of All Evil* (detail), 2012–13. Mixed media, four parts, each 215 × 128.7 × 249.9 cm (84.65 × 50.67 × 98.39 in.). Courtesy the artists.

is more to this case of the Chapman brothers' excess. They *do* in fact represent something of the Holocaust, I believe, because, in short, the Holocaust itself is a topic that also "carries an excess," as Friedlander puts it. In that excess, Friedlander recognizes "something which is not determined," not subject to definition or closure.[54] Following Friedlander, Dinos Chapman asks, "How can you possibly approach such a subject and expect to be able to do it any justice?" Apparently with the indeterminacy of the Holocaust in mind, the Chapman brothers chose to "do exactly the opposite" of attempting to represent it. Through an ongoing series of smaller sculptures that explore the seemingly infinite possibilities for inflicting harm on their plastic soldiers, they determined to "never finish" the work, to never bring closure to its topic.[55] In short, they aimed to "make the grand narrative into a grand failure." Further describing their efforts, Jake Chapman remarks, "We missed it miserably, and that's the point. Proximity not mimicry. The idea of verging upon something obliquely, to achieve proximity to this 'thing' that betrays representation . . ."[56] And elsewhere: "It has everything to do with nothing."[57]

This negativism is *nonidentity* thinking, but of a special sort. Unlike Friedlander, Lanzmann, and Adorno, the Chapman brothers don't "verge upon" the Holocaust through mimicry by marshaling documentary facts. Instead, "obliquely,"

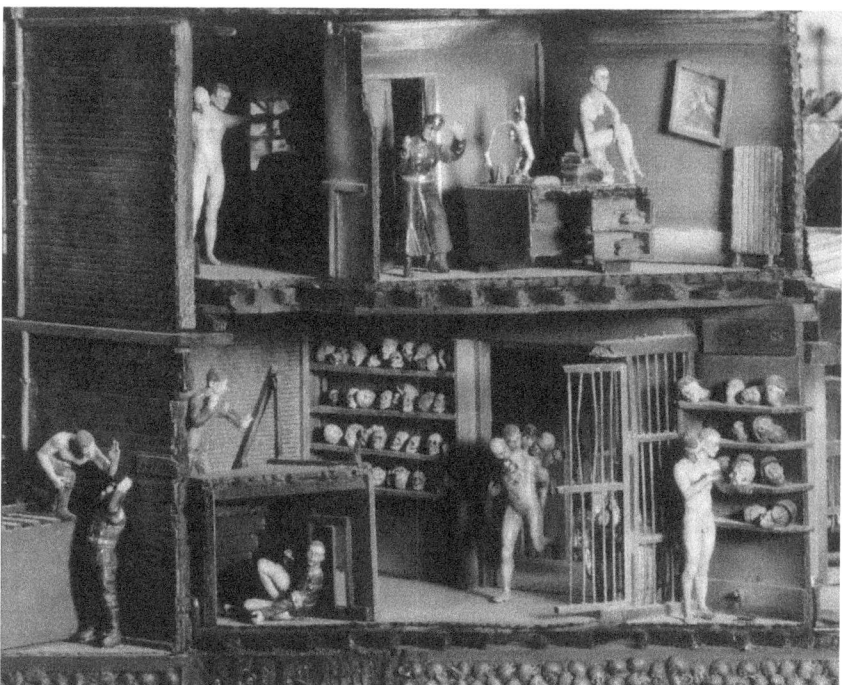

Figure 17.15. Jake and Dinos Chapman, Hell (detail), 1999–2000. Mixed media, eight parts: 215 × 128.7 × 249.8 cm (84.65 × 50.67 × 98.35 in.); one part: 215.4 × 128 × 128 cm (84.80 × 50.39 × 50.39 in.). Courtesy the artists.

their effort at proximity offers the *spirit* of the Holocaust. A world in which skeletons kill and teddy bears bite is a world of violated understandings bearing on death. The Chapmans' Holocaust-suggestive sculptures can appropriately be called abject, but not (only) for their graphic depictions of blood and filth. Rather, it's for the way that the philosopher Julia Kristeva discusses the abject, as something first recognized by our ancient ancestors in "the threatening world of animals or animalism, . . . imagined as representatives of . . . murder"—an anarchic and violent world from which human society long ago separated itself by creating "borders, positions, rules."[58] A challenge to those rules, and consequent reversion to the abject, comes precisely from those who do not respect them: "the liar, the criminal with a good conscience, . . . the killer who claims he is a savior." Kristeva posits that the Holocaust is abject not for its filth or disease but for its demonstration of "the fragility of the law," which it violated: "The abjection of Nazi crimes reaches its apex when death . . . interferes with what . . . is supposed to save me from death: childhood, science, among other things."[59]

The Chapman brothers' *Arbeit McFries* of 2001, another related Holocaust-suggestive sculpture, provides a particularly clear example of the abject (figure 17.16). It features a structure that is part McDonald's restaurant, a place whose exterior (before being ransacked) would have offered the enticement of presumptive pleasures for those who enter, but which simultaneously presents a deathly contradiction: another part of the structure resembles a Nazi crematorium chimney and hints at horrors inside. In a viewer's mind, the title recalls the Nazi slogan *Arbeit Macht Frei* (work sets you free) displayed on the entrance gate to Auschwitz and other Nazi concentration camps, but as with other works, its parodic turn means that it falls short of identifying in an Adornian sense what a viewer may presume to see: an aspect of the Holocaust. Now, however, through the strategic second turn of the abject, the Chapmans *do* meaningfully present the deceitful spirit of the Nazi slogan's comforting reassurance to nervous new arrivals, an absurd lie that masked a sinister agenda behind the gates. In other words, proximity not mimicry. Using the abject as a "key" to unlock an "unintentional truth" of the Holocaust, these works by the Chapman brothers create a kind of Adornian "riddle-*Gestalt*" that offers an image of the Holocaust even as they simultaneously negate it through their nonidentity. By so doing, they manifest yet another sort of productive tension between excess and identity without identity thinking.

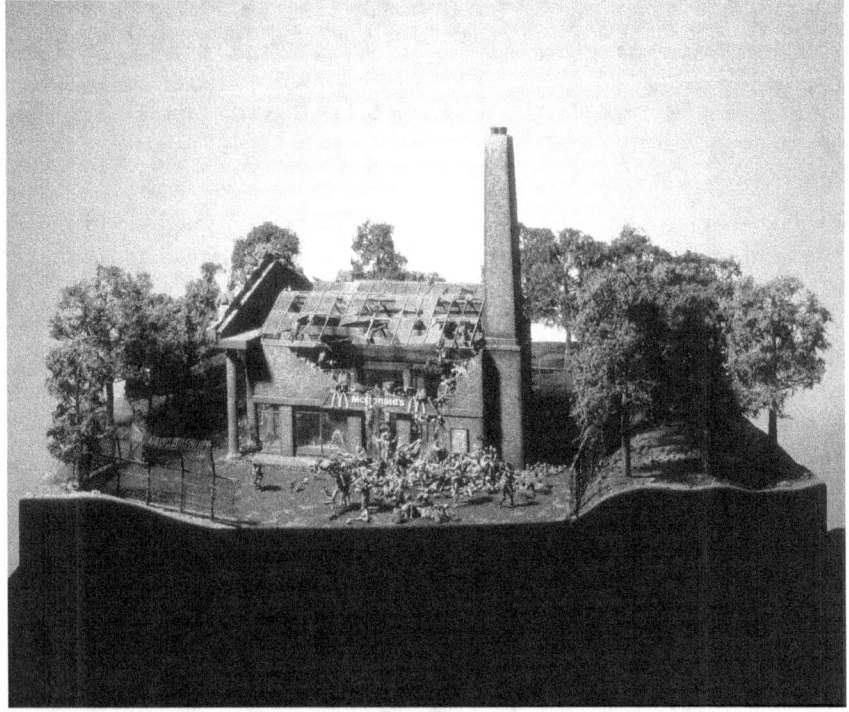

Figure 17.16. Jake and Dinos Chapman, *Arbeit McFries*, 2001. Mixed media, 195 × 121 × 121 cm (76.77 × 47.64 × 47.64 in.). Courtesy the artists.

Conclusions

To try and save ourselves from the challenges of medical science, challenges posed years ago by Nazi doctors and arguably still characteristic of scientific structures of thought and practice, we need to create a new kind of human being, one changed from within by means that have nothing to do with genomics and biotechnology. Arrayed in front of us is a set of tools with which we can do this. Philosophy teaches how to develop a keen awareness in thinking and feeling. While Friedlander for one is gloomy about the prospects, he, reminiscent of Nussbaum, holds out hope in the "growing sensitivity in literature and art."[60]

In his actions as an artist, Eduardo Kac promotes love through empathic connection, together with responsibility. Verena Kaminiarz performatively accepts responsibility for the nonhuman other and recognizes an antidote to reductive thinking in a particularity so extreme that labels become meaningless except in describing uniqueness. The Chapman brothers exploit both uniqueness and excess to confront a viewer with the ethical risks and possibilities of different manners of thought. By a variety of means, these thinking subjects remain humbly aware of the limits of understanding; consequently, the beings, objects, and circumstances in their gaze retain their mystery—a consequence that is vividly evoked by the mystical sensibility of Oron Catts and Ionat Zurr of the Tissue Culture & Art Project. In the performative content and the conceptual structures of their artworks, the most perceptive artists present models of ethical action and responsibility.

Andrew Weinstein is professor of art history at the Fashion Institute of Technology, State University of New York, and a curator of exhibitions of contemporary art, most recently *Baneful Medicine* at John Jay College of Criminal Justice, City University of New York. His academic writing focuses mostly on Holocaust representation in art.

Notes

1. Seidelman 2010, 29.

2. American jurors based much of the Nuremberg Code on regulations from the 1931 Reichsrundschreiben, which many Nazi doctors failed to follow. See Sass 1983. For a study of ethical teaching in Nazi-era German medical schools, see Bruns and Chelouche 2017.

3. Subsequent codes for human research include the Declaration of Helsinki (1964–2013); the Belmont Report (1979); the Common Rule (1991); the CIOMS/WHO Council for International Organizations of Medical Sciences: International Ethical Guidelines for Biomedical Research Involving Human Subjects International Guidelines (1993, 2002); the ICH/GCP International Conference on Harmonization—Good Clinical Practice (1996); and the Ethical for Biomedical Research in Human Subjects (ICMR) (2000). In the United States, considerations for the bioethical treatment of ani-

mals emerged in the mid-1960s with the American Association for the Accreditation of Laboratory Animal Care (AAALAC), and the Animal Welfare Act (1966), and were further codified by the US Public Health Service as the "Policy on the Humane Care and use of Laboratory Animals" (1985), based on the "US Government Principles for the Utilization and Care of Vertebrate Animals Used in Testing, Research and Teaching."

4. Friedlander 1993, 131.
5. Lanzmann 1991, 480; Lanzmann 1985, 77–78.
6. Adorno 1981, 34. Adorno later qualified his judgment: "Perennial suffering has as much right to expression as a tortured man has to scream; hence it may have been wrong to say that after Auschwitz you can no longer write poems." Adorno 1990, 362.
7. Adorno 1990, 363.
8. Adorno and Horkheimer 2002, 1. Adorno and Horkheimer borrow the phrase "disenchantment of the world" from Max Weber.
9. Adorno and Horkheimer 2002, 4.
10. Adorno and Horkheimer 2002, 9; Adorno 1990, 149.
11. Adorno and Horkheimer 2002, 8.
12. Adorno and Horkheimer 2002, 7.
13. Adorno 1990, 362.
14. Adorno 1990, 5.
15. Adorno 1990, 13.
16. Adorno 1977, 127. This 1931 essay makes explicit what Adorno keeps obscure in his 1966 *Negative Dialectics*. In the later work, Adorno makes no mention of "exact fantasy," "imminent criticism," and "unintentional truth," though he does describe how "as a constellation, theoretical thought circles the concept it would like to unseal, hoping that it may fly open like the lock of a well-guarded safe-deposit box." Adorno 1990, 163. The opaque and complicated form of the 1966 text repels all but the most dedicated thinkers who can, through praxis, make Adorno's system their own, even as it resists cooptation by casual readers.
17. Adorno 1977, 128.
18. Adorno 1977, 131, 128.
19. Adorno 1990, 163; Adorno 1977, 127.
20. Adorno 1990, 53.
21. Adelaide Centre for Bioethics and Culture 2018.
22. Patenting of naturally occurring genes was legal until the unanimous decision of the US Supreme Court on 13 June 2013 in the case of *Association for Molecular Pathology, et al. v. Myriad Genetics, Inc., et al.* (Kolata, Lee-Wee, and Belluck 2018).
23. "Semi Living Worry Dolls," The Tissue Culture and Art Project 2018.
24. Chambers 2005, 3.
25. Lauritzen 2005, 30.
26. Lauritzen 2005, 28.
27. Laurtizen 2005, 31.
28. Kac 2003, 18. Louis-Marie Houdebine, one of the two scientists in question at France's National Institute of Agronomic Research, claims that he merely arranged for Kac to take an already-created GFP rabbit from among several in the lab (Philipkoski 2002).
29. While Alba's "whiteness . . . is intensely visible and yet remains politically or culturally invisible to most viewers . . . as a mutation engineered by humans . . . her phosphorescence . . . is invisible to the naked eye and yet becomes hyper-visible to . . . those who . . . are scandalized" by Kac's project (Blocker 2003, 209).
30. Kac 2003, 97. Not all scholars celebrate *GFP Bunny*. Joanna Zylinska suggests that Kac may have done more to promote the authority of science and the interests of the biotech industry than to raise a healthy debate, given the public fascination with Alba as an appealing would-be pet (Zylinska

2009, 151). Suzanne Anker and Dorothy Nelkin question whether Kac should have had the freedom to orchestrate the creation of a transgenic animal without the oversight and constraints that scientists must negotiate, and they accuse Kac of circulating a doctored image of Alba colored fluorescent green; they contend she would glow under certain conditions only if her fur were shorn, Anker and Nelkin 2004, 95.

31. Kac 2003, 97.
32. Nussbaum 1985, 516 and 527.
33. Nussbaum 1985, 529.
34. Nussbaum 1988, 233–34.
35. Charon 2001, 1897, 1901.
36. See Miah 2008, 71–94.
37. Verena Kaminiarz, email message to author, 16 May 2019.
38. Kaminiarz's approach to human-animal relations recalls the philosophy of Emmanuel Levinas, who proposes relations between the self and the human Other that are not based on love and who are not imagined as equal. The self recognizes that the Other exists in the shadow of the divine and possesses unknowable infinity associated with the divine (Levinas 1991b, 194–95). In the presence of the Other, whose face is "a source from which all meaning appears," the subject takes responsibility in answer to the demands of the Other (Levinas 1991a, 299).
39. With this in mind, bioethicist Claire Hooker proposes that doctors adopt a specifically postmodernist mode of relativist thought as a corrective to narrative absolutism and that they simultaneously maintain these two approaches in a "productive, dialectical tension" (Hooker 2014, 220–21).
40. Kaminiarz 2017.
41. Krauss 1981, 8.
42. Chapman and Chapman 2011, 16.
43. Chapman and Chapman 2015.
44. Chapman and Chapman 2015.
45. Chapman and Chapman 2011, 16. Jake Chapman employs the phrase in describing the "unhygienic claim" by critics who charge that the piece either glorifies or makes light of pedophilia.
46. Marcuse 1964, 73.
47. Marcuse 1964, 72.
48. Chapman and Chapman 1997, 149.
49. Chapman and Chapman 1997, 152.
50. Chapman and Chapman 2015. The Chapman brothers' depictions of horror in miniature and with a profusion of detail has a precedent in four museum models that depict scenes at Auschwitz. Sculpted between 1947 and 1949 with almost three thousand tiny figures, a plaster model of the Auschwitz gas chambers by Mieczyslaw Stobierski has long been on display at the Memorial and Museum Auschwitz-Birkenau. The sculptor made copies for the United States Holocaust Memorial Museum, Washington, DC, which opened with its model on display in 1993, and for the German Historical Museum, Berlin, in 1994. For the Imperial War Museum London, sculptor Gerry Judah similarly incorporated some three thousand tiny figures in a rendition of the selection ramp at Auschwitz between 1998 and 2000, when it went on display.
51. Dinos Chapman in Chapman and Chapman 2013.
52. Jake Chapman in Chapman and Chapman 2011, 86. The Chapman brothers' hysteria justifies a psychoanalytic reading of their work in terms of Freudian notions of acting out and working through. Chapman and Chapman 2015.
53. Chapman and Chapman 2015.
54. Friedlander 1993, 133.
55. Dinos Chapman in Chapman and Chapman 2013, 10.
56. Jake Chapman in Chapman and Chapman 2013, 11.
57. Jake Chapman in Chapman and Chapman 2011, 86.

58. Kristeva 1982, 13 and 4.
59. Kristeva 1982, 4.
60. Friedlander 1993, 134.

References

Adelaide Centre for Bioethics and Culture. 2018. "Abortion." Retrieved 21 September 2018 from http://www.bioethics.org.au/Resources/Resource percent20Topics/Abortion.html.

Adorno, Theodor W. 1977. "The Actuality of Philosophy." *Telos* 31 (Spring 1977): 113–33.

———. 1981. "An Essay on Cultural Criticism and Society." *Prisms*. Translated by Samuel Weber and Shierry Weber, 17–34. Cambridge: MIT Press.

———. 1990. *Negative Dialectics*. Translated by E. B. Ashton. London: Routledge.

Adorno, Theodor W., and Max Horkheimer. 2002. *The Dialectic of Enlightenment: Philosophical Fragments*. Translated by Edmund Jephcott. Stanford, CA: Stanford University Press.

Anker, Suzanne, and Dorothy Nelkin. 2004. *The Molecular Gaze: Art in the Genetic Age*. Cold Spring Harbor, NY: Cold Spring Harbor Laboratory Press.

Blocker, Jane. 2003. "This Being You Must Create: Transgenic Art and Witnessing the Invisible." *Cultural Studies* 17(2): 193–210.

Bruns, Florian, and Tessa Chelouche. 2017. "Lectures on Inhumanity: Teaching Medical Ethics in German Medical Schools under Nazism." *Annals of Internal Medicine* 166(8): 591–96.

Chambers, Tod. 2005. "Another Voice: The Art of Bioethics." *Hastings Center Report* 35(2): 3.

Chapman, Jake, and Dinos Chapman. N.d. Interview by Maia Damianovic. *Journal of Contemporary Art*. Retrieved 14 January 2015 from http://www.jca-online.com/chapman.html.

———. 1997. "Revelations: A Conversation between Robert Rosenblum and Dinos & Jake Chapman." Interview by Robert Rosenblum. In *Unholy Libel: Six Feet Under*, edited by Jake Chapman and Mollie Dent-Brocklehurst, 147–53. New York: Gagosian Gallery.

———. 2011. Interview by Nick Hackworth. In *Flogging a Dead Horse: The Life and Works of Jake and Dinos Chapman*, 15–16, 128, 142, 180. New York: Rizzoli.

———. 2013. Interview by Julia Peyton-Jones, Hans Ulrich Obrist, et al. October. Retrieved 14 January 2015 from https://www.serpentinegalleries.org/sites/default/files/downloads/Chapman percent20interview percent20transcript.pdf.

———. 2015. "Jake and Dinos Chapman: How We Made Hell." Interview by Kate Abbott. *The Guardian*, 16 June 2015. https://www.theguardian.com/artanddesign/2015/jun/16/jake-and-dinos-chapman-how-we-made-hell.

Charon, Rita. 2001. "Narrative Medicine: A Model for Empathy, Reflection, Profession, and Trust." *Journal of the American Medical Association* 286(15): 1897–902.

Friedlander, Saul. 1993. *Memory, History, and the Extermination of the Jews of Europe*. Bloomington: Indiana University Press.

Hooker, Claire. 2014. "Ethics and the Arts in the Medical Humanities." In *Ethics and the Arts*, edited by Paul Macneill, 213–24. Dordrecht: Springer.

Kac, Eduardo. 2003. "GFP Bunny." *Leonardo* 36(2): 97–102.

Kaminiarz, Verena. 2017. *"death masks (mus musculus)."* Retrieved 22 December 2017 from http://www.aedc.ca/verena/may_the_mice_bite/main_deathmasks.htm.

Kolata, Gina, Sui Lee-Wee, and Pam Belluck. 2018. "Chinese Scientist Claims to Use Crispr to Make First Genetically Edited Babies." *New York Times*, 26 November 2018. https://www.nytimes.com/2018/11/26/health/gene-editing-babies-china.html.

Krauss, Rosalind E. 1981. "In the Name of Picasso." *October* 16: 5–22.

Kristeva, Julia. 1982. *Powers of Horror: An Essay on Abjection.* Translated by Leon S. Roudiez. New York: Columbia University Press.

Lanzmann, Claude. 1991. "The Obscenity of Understanding: An Evening with Claude Lanzmann." *American Imago* 48: 473–95.

———. 1985. *Shoah: An Oral History of the Holocaust; The Complete Text of the Film.* New York: Pantheon.

Lauritzen, Paul. 2005. "Stem Cells, Biotechnology, and Human Rights: Implications for a Posthuman Future." *Hastings Center Report* 35(2): 25–33.

Levinas, Emmanuel. 1991a. "Conclusions." In *Totality and Infinity*, 287–307. Translated by Alphonso Lingis. Dordrecht: Springer.

———. 1991b. "Ethics and the Face." In *Totality and Infinity*, 194–219. Translated by Alphonso Lingis. Dordrecht: Springer.

Marcuse, Herbert. 1964. *One-Dimensional Man: Studies in the Ideology in Advanced Industrial Society.* Boston: Beacon.

Miah, Andy. 2008. "A Critical History of Posthumanism." In *Medical Enhancement and Posthumanity*, edited by Bert Gordijn and Ruth Chadwick, 71–94. Dordrecht: Springer.

Nussbaum, Martha. 1985. "'Finely Aware and Richly Responsible': Moral Attention and the Moral Task of Literature." *Journal of Philosophy* 82(10): 516–29.

———. 1988. "Narrative Emotions: Beckett's Genealogy of Love." *Ethics* 98(2): 225–54.

Philipkoski, Kristen. 2012. "RIP: Alba, the Glowing Bunny." *Wired*, 12 August. Retrieved 11 November 2018 from https://www.wired.com/2002/08/rip-alba-the-glowing-bunny/.

Sass, Hans-Martin. 1983. "Reichsrundschreiben 1931: Pre-Nuremberg German Regulations Concerning New Therapy and Human Experimentation." Journal of Medicine and Philosophy: A Forum for Bioethics and Philosophy of Medicine 8(2): 99–112.

Seidelman, William. 2010. "Academic Medicine during the Nazi Period: The Implications for Creating Awareness of Professional Responsibility Today." In *Medicine after the Holocaust: From the Master Race to the Human Genome and Beyond*, edited by Sheldon Rubenfeld, 29–36. New York: Palgrave Macmillan.

Tissue Culture and Art Project. 2018. "Semi Living Worry Dolls." Retrieved 16 August 2018 from http://lab.anhb.uwa.edu.au/tca/semi-living-worry-dolls/.

Zylinska, Joanna. 2009. *Bioethics in the Age of New Media.* Cambridge, MA: MIT Press.

CHAPTER 18

THE HISTORY OF THE VIENNA PROTOCOL

Sabine Hildebrandt, Rabbi Joseph Polak,
Michael A. Grodin, and William E. Seidelman

> [He] set me in the center of a valley—
> Full of bones!
> ... Very many on the face of the valley, and here!—utterly dry.
> ... can these bones live?
> —Ezekiel 37, from translation by Rabbi Arthur Waskow

The Vienna Protocol is a 2017 guideline that prescribes steps for properly dealing with recently discovered Holocaust-era human remains and includes not only considerations of medical ethics but also a religious grounding for its advice. The guidelines are part of a more general set of recommendations for dealing with Holocaust-era human remains that were formulated at a 2017 symposium held at Yad Vashem, the World Holocaust Remembrance Center in Jerusalem.[1] At this conference, an international group of scholars came together to devise a response to the discovery on the Dahlem campus of the Free University of Berlin of human skeletal remains from possible victims of experiments carried out at the Auschwitz concentration camp by Dr. Josef Mengele.

In this chapter, the final document, named the Vienna Protocol, will be placed not only within the relevant historical context of the study of medicine after the Holocaust but also within the history of the development of other guidelines on how to deal with human remains from mass violence and genocide. The Vienna Protocol is discussed as unique among similar recommendations in its representation of the voice of those having suffered violence and being targeted as victims. It will be argued that the Vienna Protocol is formulated in such a general and practical manner that it can be adapted to other specific contexts of human rights abuses and crimes against humanity.

Berlin-Dahlem, Summer 2014

On 1 July 2014, during routine construction of a drainage ditch next to the University Library of Freie Universität Berlin (FU Berlin) in Harnackstrasse, Berlin-Dahlem, bones were discovered. This is a common enough event in a city with a history of violent death from sustained carpet bombings and killings in the general chaos of World War II. Following standard legal procedure, the excavation work was stopped and the Berlin police department notified. The police then initiated the investigation of the human bones (as well as small plastic specimen tags and glass vials found with them) by transferring them to the forensic authorities for elucidation of origin and age of these specimens. Up to this point, the various accounts of the incident concur.[2] However, the following sequence of events cannot be fully reconstructed from the differing and variously disputed reports by the parties involved. It appears that in the communications between FU Berlin, the police, the Department of Legal Medicine of the university hospital Charité, and the forensic institute of the state of Berlin, crucial information on the historic significance of this particular excavation site was lost.

This particular construction area was located in close proximity to the former Kaiser-Wilhelm-Institut für Anthropologie, Menschliche Erblehre und Eugenik (KWIA, Kaiser Wilhelm Institute for Anthropology, Human Heredity, and Eugenics). According to then-president of FU Berlin, Professor Peter-André Alt, this location was mentioned in messages by mail and phone between FU Berlin, the police, and what he calls "the Forensic Medicine department at Charité."[3] However, according to Professor Michael Tsokos, these communications never explicitly mentioned the Holocaust or the potential origin of these bones from victims of the National Socialist (NS) regime. Tsokos is the director of the Department of Legal Medicine at Charité Hospital Berlin as well as of the Landesinstitut für gerichtliche und soziale Medizin in Berlin-Moabit (Berlin State Institute for Forensic and Social Medicine),[4] and was responsible for the further handling of these human remains and plastic tags. It is also unclear whether either the police or the forensic specialists could have been immediately aware of the very specific historic significance of this particular site: the director of the KWIA from 1942 on was Professor Otmar von Verschuer, an internationally renowned twin researcher with a postwar career as chairman of genetics at the University of Münster. Often less well known to the general public is the fact that Verschuer was also the mentor of Josef Mengele, MD PhD, the infamous medical experimenter and murderer of Auschwitz. Financed through a research grant by the German Research Foundation, Mengele's work was subsidized by Verschuer as principal investigator, and Mengele sent specimens from his medical experiments on children and other NS victims from Auschwitz to the KWIA.[5] Mengele's prisoner assistant, the Hungarian forensic pathologist Dr. Miklos Nyiszli, had to perform autopsies for Mengele, remove specimens such as the eyes of twins murdered in May 1944, which he then had to send to the researcher Karin Magnussen, a member of Verschuer's group.[6] There is also evidence that Nyiszli may have sent bone specimens to the anthropologist Wolfgang Abel, who directed the Division of Ethnography at the KWIA.[7]

The crucial information: that the bone specimens unearthed in the summer of 2014 might have been those of Auschwitz victims was clearly lost somewhere in the trail of communications between FU Berlin, the police, and the Department of Legal Medicine at Charité, as otherwise the resulting series of events would be inexplicable. The bones were examined following a standard protocol, but the final forensic report described them as "in poor condition following a great deal of weathering," consisting mostly of fragments that had been in the ground for a long time and deemed to be unidentifiable.[8] The FU Berlin online magazine reported about the findings in November 2014, and announced the transfer of the bones, apparently following standard protocol, to the Berlin State Institute for Forensic and Social Medicine for a "dignified burial."[9] Nowhere in this account was the historic significance of the discovery site discussed. Two months later, the magazine described a ceremony for the German Holocaust memorial day, 27 January 2015, which took place in front of the former KWIA and included the lighting of candles at the excavation site, and only then was the possibility mentioned that the bones could have been those of NS victims.[10]

However, just a day earlier, on 26 January 2015, the Berlin newspaper *Tagesspiegel* had reported that the human remains had been sent to Ruhleben crematory, where they had been cremated and the ashes buried in the Christian cemetery Ruhleben.[11] The actions by the FU Berlin and others involved were criticized as "mindless and insensitive" by Berlin historian Götz Aly, who informed his international colleagues.[12] The general public—especially the Jewish community—was scandalized by the handling of these human remains from potential NS victims[13]: once again another set of human remains from potential victims of the Holocaust had "gone up in smoke"—just like the millions of Jews who had been murdered and incinerated in the NS extermination camps. In response to these events, the participants of a March 2015 academic conference on Medicine after the Holocaust in Houston, Texas, sent a letter to the leadership of the FU Berlin and the Max-Planck-Gesellschaft (Max Planck Society, MPG), the postwar successor of the Kaiser-Wilhelm-Gesellschaft, requesting an investigation into the events of summer 2014. They demanded "the appropriate identification of future discoveries of human remains" and suggested "that a formal protocol of standard procedure be established for the handling of human remains that might originate from unethical academic conduct such as during the periods of Imperial Germany and National Socialism."[14]

FU president Alt responded, recounting his version of the incidents, and the fact of internal discussions on proper memorialization and deliberations by a committee including experts from FU Berlin, MPG, and the Berlin State Monument Department concerning "further investigations."[15] An external evaluation of the events was not planned, and a follow-up concerning the announced "further investigations" did not occur, even though the FU did in fact start an archeological exploration at this site (see postscript below). Apart from a formal confirmation of receipt of the letter, MPG president Martin Stratmann never replied; but then, he may have been rather busy with the planning of a separate urgent investigation of another discovery of human remains from NS victims within the Max Planck Institute (MPI) system.[16] The emeritus director of the MPI for Brain Research, Professor Heinz Wässle, had come across brain sections from "euthanasia" victims in an MPG archive, within the neuroanatomical collection of specimens assembled by neuroanatomist Julius Hallervorden.[17] This came as a surprise to Wässle, the MPG leadership, and the general public, as all suspect specimens from the NS period were supposed to have been buried in 1990 following investigations by medical historian Götz Aly.[18]

At this juncture, a group of medical historians and cosigners of the letter to Professors Alt and Stratmann felt that the response to their letter was unsatisfactory. Under the leadership of Professor William Seidelman,[19] they decided that the events at the FU Berlin and MPI archives demanded a concerted effort to formulate a protocol for the handling of human remains that might originate from NS victims. It was felt that such a protocol should be created with the input of representatives from the various disciplines potentially involved in the handling of such remains, and, most importantly, it should include an authoritative "voice of victims," as such a "voice" has been missing from most similar sets of guidelines. To facilitate this process, historian Professor Dan Michman[20] and other leaders of Yad Vashem, the World Holocaust Remembrance Center, agreed to host a one-day symposium, which took place on 14 May 2017.[21]

Meanwhile in St. Louis

On Holocaust Remembrance Day, 16 April 2015, anatomist Sabine Hildebrandt gave a presentation on the history of anatomy in NS Germany at the Medical School of Washington University in St. Louis, Missouri. Following this lecture, surgeon Susan Mackinnon[22] and her associate Andrew Yee started a conversation with Hildebrandt and Seidelman on the ethicality of the use of an atlas of human anatomy that was created by a proponent of NS ideology and potentially depicted bodies of NS victims. Mackinnon had been using the so-called

Pernkopf atlas since 1981. The book had been created between 1937 and 1955 by the Austrian Eduard Pernkopf, chair of anatomy at the University of Vienna. She knew about the book's background, i.e. Pernkopf's NS convictions and his use of NS victims in his work, and included this historical example of his unethical research practices in her teaching on medical ethics.[23] In her surgical practice she had found that only this atlas gave her the detailed visual information necessary to understand certain procedures, and that specific illustrations from the Pernkopf atlas had enabled her to alleviate her patient's suffering or even save a patient's life.[24] Her team had created an online video platform for global education on rare and difficult nerve reconstruction surgery and had plans to use images from the Pernkopf atlas, including its history, in this educational venue. The conversation intensified, when in 2016 Mackinnon and Yee asked the publisher Elsevier[25] for the right to use some of the Pernkopf images for their teaching platform, and were refused. As a reason, Elsevier cited the connection of the atlas with the Holocaust, and the publisher's upholding "the highest ethical and business standards."[26]

At this point, the question arose whether Elsevier could be urged to grant the copyright for ethical reasons on grounds of saving human lives. It was strongly felt that any valid answer to this query needed to be addressed by an authority who not only had knowledge of ethics and the history of medicine during the Holocaust but also could represent the voice of the victims of NS atrocities. Thus it was decided to send a formal request to Rabbi Joseph Polak and Professor Michael Grodin of Boston, which asked for an opinion on the ethical, religious, and ritual aspects of the use of Pernkopf images from the Jewish perspective, under consideration of the concept of *pikuach nefesh*, the saving of human life.[27] Rabbi Polak, the chief justice of the Rabbinical Court of Massachusetts, is an authority on Jewish law and medical ethics and the Holocaust, and is a child survivor of the Westerbork and Bergen-Belsen concentration camps.[28] His expertise extends to questions surrounding the handling of human remains of Holocaust victims, a subject rarely systematically explored in twenty-first-century Jewish religious case rulings (responsa).[29] Professor Grodin, of the Elie Wiesel Center for Jewish Studies and director of the Project on Ethics and the Holocaust at Boston University, is an internationally noted expert on the history of medicine and the Holocaust and on health and human rights. Polak and Grodin not only agreed to take on the task of considering the dilemma of using the Pernkopf images but also, given the developments following the discovery of human remains in Berlin-Dahlem in 2014, decided to widen the scope of their deliberations and response. The resulting document was called the Vienna Protocol due to its origins in the Pernkopf inquiry, and it addresses the strict conditions under which it might be permitted to use the images (i.e. data) derived from potential NS victims' bodies, as well as formulating a set of guidelines on what to do with the physical remains of possibly Jewish persons.[30]

Why Another Set of Guidelines?

The significance of the recommendations from the Yad Vashem symposium and the Vienna Protocol can only be discussed within the context of the history of the search for and discovery of human remains from NS victims, which will be briefly outlined here. Also, a look at existing relevant recommendations and guidelines on the care of human remains is necessary. First, the term "NS victim" needs to be defined, which has differed over time, and between places and authors.[31] While Jews were the foremost targets of NS persecution, there were other groups of victims, namely Sinti and Roma, Jehovah's Witnesses, homosexuals, forced laborers, deserters, and political opponents of the NS regime of all religions, as well as persons killed in the so-called "euthanasia" program, and the many persecuted who committed suicide.[32] Furthermore, there were those executed following the extended NS legislation on capital punishment, whose bodies were delivered in great numbers to the anatomical departments for teaching and research purposes.[33] Directly after the war the search for these victims' bodies began and was led not only by their friends and families but also by the Allied Occupation Forces. They searched in the cemeteries of concentration camps, in graves near their home communities, in anatomical departments, and for many the search has still not ended to this day.[34]

In the decades following the war there were also many inadvertent discoveries reported of human remains from the NS period. These findings gained especial notoriety when they were connected to university collections, as some German and Austrian anatomical departments continued to use NS victims' bodies that were still stored in their facilities for several years after the war.[35] Anatomists had also included specimens of tissues from NS victims in their macroscopic and microscopic research collections and teaching materials. When this was revealed in 1989, Israeli minister for religion Zevulun Hammer sent a letter of inquiry to Federal Chancellor of Germany Helmut Kohl. On 11 January 1989, Kohl ordered—via the Council of Secretaries of Culture (Kultusministerkonferenz)—that all state ministries require universities to investigate the matter of retained specimens from NS victims. The universities, including their anatomical departments, followed this request with more or less extensive investigations of their collections.[36] The self-study at the University of Tübingen remains exemplary,[37] followed by the *Senatsprojekt* of the University of Vienna, which came to pass as a consequence of international pressure in 1998.[38]

While these various efforts of discovery were ongoing, it appears that, despite the horrific scale of the murder of Jews in the Holocaust, there was no systematic search for their remains through excavations of potential sites of mass murder. Archeologist Caroline Sturdy Colls identified multiple reasons for this phenomenon, which she saw rooted in the perceptions of the various stakeholders. These include local communities who might wish to either hide or at least not be implicated in crimes against humanity, the cultural and religious beliefs of the various groups of victims potentially involved, and ultimately considerations of the costs of such investigations.[39] Apart from the, as Sturdy Colls formulated, unrealized potential of locating human remains through systematic archeological investigations of Holocaust killing fields, incidental discoveries such as the one in Berlin-Dahlem and at the MPG continue to occur. Furthermore, there still exist collections that hold human tissues from a potential NS background, collections owned by universities and other institutions in Germany and the former NS-occupied territories. Some are currently under investigation, while others still need to be examined.[40] The existence of questionable specimens is often only revealed when personnel changes occur and the new persons in charge of the collections start having a closer look.[41]

Given the multitude of postwar searches and findings of human remains from NS victims, several efforts have been made to develop guidelines for the handling of such specimens. They come in the global context of an apparent evolving sensitivity surrounding the dignity of human remains in academic collections and other settings, and their potential origin from contexts of mass violence.[42] The so-called Vermillion Accord was formulated at the World Archaeological Congress in 1989 and was declared to be the first international ethical code on the care of human remains, followed in 1990 by the Native American Graves Protection and Repatriation Act (NAGPRA). Since then, various groups of archaeologists, anthropologists, museum administrators, and government organizations have created guidelines and policies for their specific context,[43] and many discussion revolve around the repatriation of human remains from colonial contexts.[44] Notable in the German context of National Socialism is that the 1989 Kultusministerkonferenz request had demanded the removal of any questionable specimens from collections and their "dignified handling," but had left it open to the interpretation of each individual institution to decide what "dignified handling meant." In some cases, the suspect specimens were simply removed without further investigation or effort at identification of potential victims.[45] It was only in 2003 that the German General Medical Council created a set of "recommendations on the treatment of human remains in collections, museums and public places," which included practical advice, such as that relating to removal of questionable specimens, transparency of origin, and commemoration. The need for relevant legislation was also identified.[46] Since then, administrators of museums in Germany and elsewhere have risen to the task of creating codes of ethics and guidelines for the care of human remains,[47] but no new legislation was introduced in Germany. Except for the Recommendations by the German General Medical Council, specimens from NS victims are rarely discussed in any of the guidelines; and while respect for local religious, ethnic, and cultural customs is mentioned, there are no indications that any of these recommendations were authorized or endorsed by representatives of the potential groups of victims involved. Furthermore, none of the various guidelines appear to be the result of an interdisciplinary discussion. And, most importantly, none of them prevented the incident at the FU Berlin in 2014. The university leadership, the police, and the forensic specialists followed their standard procedure, presumably with the best of intentions, which ended with the cremation of the unidentified human remains and the interment of their ashes in a Christian cemetery. This result was felt to be a cruel insult to the potential victims by many observers, Jews and non-Jews among them, and ignited the active discussion that ultimately led to the organization of the symposium at Yad Vashem in May 2017.

The recommendations from the symposium and the Vienna Protocol differ decisively from all previously formulated guidelines. Given the specific complexity of the repeated inadvertent discovery of human remains from NS victims, it was felt that all professional disciplines potentially involved in the handling of these tissues needed to add their expertise to any set of recommendations to be considered valid. A request for expert information was sent to the Anatomische Gesellschaft, whose leadership decided that this matter needed the expertise of anthropologists. The chairman of EVAN—the European Virtual Anthropology Network—Dr. George McGlynn was then kind enough to collate a set of recommendations for procedures in the handling of human remains from contexts of injustice, which served as a point of reference for the deliberations at the symposium.[48] Participating in the conference were scholars with expertise in the area of the NS history of anthropology, anatomy, and medicine, as well archaeologists who had practical experience in the excavation of NS sites and scholars of Jewish history and religion. The recommendations demand an interdisciplinary approach to the handling of such human remains, which includes historians, archaeologists and anthropologists who are tasked to focus on the foremost need of identification of the potential victims. The demand for a quest for identification was considered crucial, as giving identity back to these human remains will allow for an appropriate burial, e.g. of Jewish remains in a Jewish cemetery, and not a Christian one. Thus dignity may be restored to the dead, and they may in some cases even be remembered by name. The recommendations also emphasize the foremost need for documentation of the history of these victims, as well as what was done with their remains after discovery, as part of the dignified commemoration. One excellent example of such commemorative work is the website that historian Hans-Joachim Lang has created for the victims of anatomist August Hirt, victims whose names and biographies Lang has been able to restore on the basis of their camp tattoo numbers.[49]

This theme of the dignity of the dead is picked up once again in Rabbi Polak's Vienna Protocol, and he extends it from the treatment of physical human remains to the use of their images in the Pernkopf atlas. Rabbi Polak makes very clear that the use of these images from potential victims is only permissible if the dire need arises in the saving of a human life, and even then it is permitted only under the condition that the historical context of the atlas is revealed to all involved. Only then, according to Rabbi Polak, can the dead be "accorded at least some of the dignity to which they are entitled."[50] Indeed, the dignity of the dead stood at the center of all deliberations for the formulation of the recommendations and the protocol.

Conclusion: What to Do with the Vienna Protocol

As far as can be ascertained, the recommendations from the symposium at Yad Vashem present the first interdisciplinary approach to the problem of handling human remains from the Holocaust with an emphasis on identification, and it is the first that includes a strong Jewish voice. Also, the Vienna Protocol appears to be the first specific responsum on the subject, and certainly the first to comment on images from NS victims. Given that these images can also be interpreted as data, the Vienna Protocol could contribute to the longstanding discussion on whether to use or not to use data from NS medical experiments.[51] Furthermore, it is believed that the stipulations in the Vienna Protocol are so simply and practically formulated that they should be applicable beyond the Jewish context, in other situations of human rights violations and mass violence.

What remains to be done is to make the Recommendations/Vienna Protocol known to one and all. For this purpose, the next step will need to be a translation into other languages so that the text can be distributed not only to universities and other academic institutions but also to police stations and other potential "finders" of human remains.

Postscript

New and systematic archaeological excavations have taken place in the garden of the former KWIA and revealed another cache of human remains. The archaeologists involved are still deliberating whether they will use so-called invasive procedures for the further identification of the bone fragments, and detailed results have not been published yet. They are in contact with the Central Council of German Jews and the Central Council of the Sinti and Roma.[52] Meanwhile at the MPG, the investigations were extended to the MPI for Psychiatry in Munich. In early 2016, historian of science Florian Schmaltz and colleagues were allowed for the first time to visit the archives in the basement of this institute, where they discovered many more specimens and documents on "euthanasia" victims.[53] Since then, the MPG has financed another scholarly investigation into the history of these specimens.[54]

Somehow, it does not feel that this will be the last one.

Appendix: Excerpts from Recommendations for the Handling of Future Discoveries of Human Remains from Victims of Nazi Terror and Vienna Protocol[55]

Recommendations

Given the likelihood of future discoveries, it is imperative that there be clearly defined policies and guidelines regarding any possible future discoveries. The enactment and implementation of such policies and guidelines are ultimately the responsibility and jurisdiction of the state or region or institution in whose jurisdiction such discoveries occur.

The basic principles for handling of such discoveries must include:

1. Immediate securing and protection of the specimens and the surrounding site, including, where appropriate, excavation.
2. The identification and securing of any and all available archival records and materials related to the discovery, including, where possible, the provenance of the specimen and the identity of the victim. Ensuring unrestricted access to these archival records for research.
3. Notification of the legal and institutional authorities.
4. Where possible, notification of the relevant religious authorities.
5. Engagement of historians with expertise in the history of the institution, the era, and the specific program, e.g. anatomy, "euthanasia," experimentation, etc.
6. The engagement of expert archaeologists and anthropologists or other such persons with expertise in the identification of human remains.
7. Where possible, notification of family or relatives of the victim. Or, if these cannot be determined, relevant representatives of potential victim groups. Addendum: Vienna Protocol.
8. Determination of final resting place for the remains, based on any potentially known wishes of the victim, and wishes of victim's family or representative.
9. Documentation of the history and identification of the remains, including biographies of victims. Also exact documentation of the handling of the remains since their discovery.
10. Institutional commemoration of the victim(s) based on documentation of the history of events that led to the demise of the victim; including that of the institutions and organizations involved.

Vienna Protocol
Rabbi Joseph Polak and Professor Michael A. Grodin, MD

The Ensuing Preamble to the Protocol:
Whereas:
1. The classic Jewish legal tradition requires burial of its dead,
2. and requires burial without delay,
3. and maintains that such burial is of benefit to the mourners permitting them to grieve,
4. and because such burial is also of benefit to the dead:
    a. since the remains are now putrefying and ugly and should therefore not be seen by others
    b. because burial is part of the process of forgiveness for the sins of deceased,
5. and since it is prohibited to derive any BENEFIT from both corpses and objects on them or in their immediate vicinity,
6. and since all cremation is strictly prohibited,
7. and since bodies burned at the request of the deceased may not be interred in a Jewish cemetery,
8. but bodies cremated against the will of the deceased, must be buried in a Jewish cemetery,
9. and since, while body parts smaller than the size of an olive need not be buried, but are still prohibited from benefit,
10. and whereas the remains of anonymous dead discovered inadvertently assume the halakhic status of *metay mitzvah*—imposing the obligation of incumbent, immediate burial upon its finder—to the extent that the discovered anonymous Jewish deceased legally acquires deed and title to the earth upon which he is found.

The Protocol and Recommendations
1. When human remains are (inadvertently) found, local legal (forensic) civic and religious authorities need to be consulted immediately.
2. If there is even a remote chance that such remains may be of Jewish origin, the nearest Jewish rabbinic authorities need to be consulted immediately.
3. If a full cemetery or killing field is come upon, marked or unmarked, then except under the rarest circumstances, reinterment to another site is not recommended, and ignoring these remains so as to, for example, construct real estate (e.g. the shopping center in Vilnius) over them, is extraordinarily offensive to Jewish custom, life, traditions, and values and to the memories of victims, if victims they be, and should be vociferously avoided. Under no circumstances should they be either cremated, or buried in a gentile cemetery.

4. Since not all rabbis are expert in these matters, a copy of these Protocols should be forwarded to the local rabbinic administration in which the remains are discovered, and a central clearinghouse established.
5. The remains should be immediately covered and kept covered, and where humanly possible, buried the same day, in a Jewish cemetery close to where discovered, or sent for burial in Israel.
6. It is permitted to delay reinterment in order to do the forensic investigation to identify some or all of the victims or their persecutors.
7. Survivor families who would normally mourn such victims need to observe *shiva* rites on the day itself of reinterment.
8. If the discoveries are likely a mixture of gentiles and Jews, all may be buried in a demarcated area of a Jewish cemetery.
9. If the remains found are smaller than the size of an olive, the obligation for immediate burial is lifted, but the prohibition against benefit is not, and so all such discoveries should, in fact, be buried, not forgetting the Untermann Protocol discussed above.
10. There is a rich Jewish legal literature on the impermissibility of photographing the dead, for reasons already cited. Moreover, according to some authorities including Strashun and others, this might extend to histology slides and similar minute samples so as to preclude violating the prohibition of "benefit." Where no issues of *pikuach nefesh* or medical education are involved, competent local halakhic decisors should be consulted regarding their disposition.
11. All graves of reinterred remains, or of remains of this type buried for the first time, need to bear elaborate explanatory markings as to their nature ("the Untermann Protocol").
12. In a far-ranging discussion on the permissibility of human autopsy in Jewish Law, Rabbi Doctor Abraham Steinberg speaks about the permissibility of autopsy for the purposes of discovering the cause of death that could save the lives of others, as in a plague, and of its permissibility in teaching medicine, and his study is too nuanced and lengthy to summarize here. But the drawings in the Pernkopf Atlas, drawn by artists and scientists mostly with Nazi sympathies, based on corpses of prisoners executed by rogue civilian and military courts of the Third Reich, would normally fall under the prohibition of benefit from the dead. They might also likely fall under the prohibition of photographing the dead, which R. Grunwald prohibits, and of gazing at the dead, which is also prohibited. Yet the use of cadavers would certainly be permitted by most authorities to help save lives (*pikuach nefesh*), as during surgery, and, following other authorities, even for medical education. In all cases where using the Pernkopf Atlas becomes permissible, I would invoke the Untermann Protocol, which requires making it known to one and all

just exactly what these drawings are. In this way, the dead are accorded at least some of the dignity to which they are entitled.
13. If the remains found have been burned, and appear to be the result of unsought violence, then their charred or cremated remains must be buried in a Jewish cemetery.
14. If fresh remains are found, not yet buried, which were clearly the result of a murder, then there is no need for a tahara (ritual washing of the body). A killing field or large mass grave should probably not be disturbed but formally designated as a Jewish cemetery, a ritual procedure familiar to many rabbis and Jewish burial societies. This ritual would include establishing unambiguous formal perimeters for all the graves in the area (for purposes of establishing sacred space and for tziyun la Kohanim). A broad, fully descriptive plaque detailing the events that took place on this site should be erected at once, following the Untermann Protocol.

Sabine Hildebrandt, MD, is an associate professor of pediatrics at Boston Children's Hospital and an anatomy educator at Harvard Medical School. Her research interests are the history and ethics of anatomy. She also works on the restoration of biographies of victims of the Holocaust. Her book *The Anatomy of Murder: Ethical Transgressions and Anatomical Science during the Third Reich* was published in 2016, paperback in August 2017, and is the first systematic study on this topic. The biography *Käthe Beutler, 1896–1999: Eine jüdische Kinderärztin aus Berlin* was published in June 2019.

Rabbi Joseph Polak, a child survivor of two Nazi concentration camps, is the chief justice of the Rabbinical Court of Massachusetts and adjunct associate professor of health law at the Boston University School of Public Health. His memoir, *After the Holocaust the Bells Still Ring* (Urim, 2015), won the National Jewish Book Award and is scheduled to appear in a Hebrew translation being prepared by Yad Vashem. For almost half a century he was a university chaplain, mostly at Boston University.

Michael A. Grodin, MD, is professor of health law, bioethics, and human rights at the Boston University School of Public Health, and professor and director of the Project on Ethics and the Holocaust at the Elie Wiesel Center for Jewish Studies. Dr. Grodin has served on national and international commissions focusing on medical ethics, human rights, and the Holocaust. He has received a special citation from the United State Holocaust Memorial Museum for "profound contributions—through original and creative research—to the cause of Holocaust education and remembrance," and is the author of over two hundred articles and the editor or coeditor of seven books.

Dr. William E. Seidelman, an emeritus professor of family medicine at the University of Toronto, has been involved for the past four decades in researching the role of academic and scientific elite medical institutions associated with the crimes of the Third Reich. His focus has been on the exploitation of the bodies of victims of Nazi terror, some of which remained in institutional collections for decades after the war. In 1995, Professor Seidelman joined Professor Howard Israel, a specialist in oral and maxillofacial surgery in New York, who together with Yad Vashem: The World Holocaust Remembrance Center, brought pressure to bear on the University of Vienna for a full examination of their collections of human specimens after the Anschluss. Professor Seidelman chaired the 17 May 2017 Special Symposium at Yad Vashem on the subject of discovered remains of possible victims of the Holocaust.

Notes

1. Seidelman et al. 2017.
2. Position FU Berlin, 2015: Freie Universität Berlin 2015a; also: Letter Präsident FU Berlin Univ.-Prof. Peter-André Alt to Professor Dr. Paul Weindling, 2nd April 2015, personal archive S. Hildebrandt; Position Prof. Dr. Michael Tsokos, Director of the Department of Legal Medicine at Charité Hospital Berlin and of the Landesinstitut für gerichtliche und soziale Medizin in Berlin-Moabit: Aulich and Bischoff 2015; Kühne 2015a.
3. Letter Präsident FU Berlin Univ.-Prof. Peter-André Alt to Professor Dr. Paul Weindling, 2nd April 2015, p. 1.
4. Kühne 2015a.
5. On Verschuer, Mengele, and the KWIA, see Müller-Hill 1984; Müller-Hill 2001; Sachse and Massin 2000; Benzenhöfer 2012; Schmuhl 2008; Ehrenreich 2007; Kröner 1998; Weiss 2010. As an eyewitness to Mengele's activities in Auschwitz, see Nyiszli 1993.
6. Sachse and Massin, 2000: 23–24.
7. Sachse and Massin, 2000: 27
8. Letter Präsident FU Berlin Univ.-Prof. Peter-André Alt to Professor Dr. Paul Weindling, 2nd April 2015, p. 2.
9. Freie Universität Berlin 2014.
10. Freie Universität Berlin 2015b.
11. Kühne 2015b.
12. Götz Aly, personal communication via electronic mail, 2 February 2015; Berliner Zeitung 2015.
13. E.g. Kühne 2015; rbb Fernsehen 2015; Spohd 2015.
14. Statement Re: Discovery of Human remains in Berlin, letter sent on 9 March 2015 by Professor Paul Weindling for the paticipants of the First International Scholarly Workshop on Medicine, Houston, to President FU Peter-André Alt and MPG president Martin Stratmann, personal archive S. Hildebrandt.
15. Letter Präsident FU Berlin Univ.-Prof. Peter-André Alt to Professor Dr. Paul Weindling, 2 April 2015, p. 3.
16. The archives of the MPG, the umbrella organization of the network of the Max Planck Institute, have been subject of critical investigation since the first studies by historian Götz Aly in the early 1980s—see his chapter in this volume—and are currently under investigation by an external commission, including additional findings at the MPI for Psychiatry, Munich. See also Gannon 2017.

17. MPI Brain Research 2015; Wässle 2017.
18. See Götz Aly's account of this history in chapter 16 of this volume.
19. Correspondence via electronic mail between Bill Seidelman and Paul Weindling, 6 and 8 November 2015, personal archive S. Hildebrandt.
20. Professor Michman is head of the International Institute for Holocaust Research and incumbent of the John Najmann Chair in Holocaust Studies, Yad Vashem; and chair, the Arnold and Leona Finkler Institute of Holocaust Research, Bar-Ilan University.
21. Participants were: William E Seidelman, chair, Beer-Sheva, Israel; Dan Michman; historian Götz Aly, Berlin, Germany; anthropologist Margit Berner, Vienna, Austria; anatomist Sabine Hildebrandt, Boston, United States; historian Miriam Offer, Akko, Israel; archeologist Yoram Heimi, Jerusalem, Israel; Rabbi Joseph Polak, Boston, United States; neurologist Heinz Wässle, Frankfurt, Germany; historian Paul Weindling, Oxford, United Kingdom; and an archeologist cognizant of the Berlin excavations. See Seidelman et al. 2017.
22. Susan Mackinnon is the Sydney M. Jr. and Robert H. Shoenberg Professor and chief of the Division of Plastic and Reconstructive Surgery at Washington University.
23. On the Pernkopf atlas, see Williams 1988; Hildebrandt 2006.
24. For a case study of Mackinnon's work, see Yee et al. 2018.
25. The original publisher of the atlas was Urban and Schwarzenberg, and after a series of acquisitions the copyright is now in the hands of Elsevier.
26. Cathrin Korz to Susan Mackinnon, electronic mail, 14 September 2016. Personal archive S. Hildebrandt.
27. Letter Hildebrandt and Seidelman to Professor Michael Grodin MD, Rabbi Joseph Polak, 20 November 2016, Re: The Ethical Challenge of Using Paintings from *Pernkopf Anatomy* and Saving the Life of a Human Being: *Pikuach Nefesh*; personal archive S. Hildebrandt.
28. Polak 2015.
29. Polak 2001; on the history of Jewish opinions concerning the handling of human remains from the Holocaust, see Deutsch 2016; Sturdy Colls 2015; Sturdy Colls 2016; Finder 2015.
30. Polak 2018.
31. For a fuller discussion of this topic, see Hildebrandt 2016, 15–16.
32. Berenbaum 1990.
33. Hildebrandt 2013.
34. Dreyfuss 2015; Finder 2015, "Final chapter"; see Hildebrandt 2013.
35. Czech 2015; Noack 2012; Oehler-Klein et al. 2012.
36. Weindling 2012.
37. Universität Tübingen 1990.
38. Seidelman 2012.
39. Sturdy Colls 2016.
40. Example of ongoing investigation: Blechschmidt collection of embryos, University of Göttingen, retrieved 27 June 2018 from https://www.uni-goettingen.de/en/provenance+research+"blechschmidt+collection"/575416.html.
41. E.g. Redies et al. 2012.
42. Jones and Whitaker 2009.
43. Anderson and Lane 2016. This text gives a good overview of the variety of laws, recommendations, and guidelines developed over the last two decades.
44. E.g. Feikert 2009; Stoecker et al. 2013.
45. Weindling 2012.
46. Bundesärztekammer 2003.
47. E.g. Deutscher Museumsbund 2013; Department of Culture, Media and Sport UK 2005; ICOM Code of Ethics for Museums 2013.

48. Dr. McGlynn's EVAN memo is part of the Recommendations/Vienna Protocol, retrieved 28 June 2018 from http://www.bu.edu/jewishstudies/research/medicine-and-the-holocaust/project-of-the-discovery-of-jewish-remains/.
49. Lang 2007; also at https://www.die-namen-der-nummern.de/index.php/en/ (retrieved 2 July 2018).
50. See appendix in this chapter.
51. Hildebrandt and Seidelman 2018.
52. Bernbeck 2015; Kirchner 2017; Pollock and Cyrus 2018.
53. Berndt 2017.
54. Neumann 2017; and Max-Planck-Gesellschaft 2019: https://www.mpg.de/victims-research-project.
55. The full text of the Recommendations/Vienna Protocol is hosted by the Boston University Elie Wiesel Center for Jewish Studies: http://www.bu.edu/jewishstudies/research/project-on-medicine-and-the-holocaust/recommendations-for-the-discovery-of-jewish-remains-project/.

References

Personal Archive Sabine Hildebrandt

Letter Präsident FU Berlin Univ.-Prof. Peter-André Alt to Professor Dr. Paul Weindling, 2 April 2015.
Letter sent on 9 March 2015, by Professor Paul Weindling for the participants of the First International Scholarly Workshop on Medicine, Houston, to President FU Peter-André Alt and MPG president Martin Stratmann: Statement Re: Discovery of Human remains in Berlin.
Letter Hildebrandt and Seidelman to Professor Michael Grodin MD, Rabbi Joseph Polak, 20 November 2016, Re: The Ethical Challenge of Using Paintings from *Pernkopf Anatomy* and Saving the Life of a Human Being: *Pikuach Nefesh*.
Correspondence via electronic mail between Bill Seidelman and Paul Weindling, 6 and 8 November 2015.

Books and Articles

Anderson, David M., and Paul J. Lane. 2018. "The Unburied Victims of Kenya's Mau Mau Rebellion: Where and When Does Violence End?" In *Human Remains in Society: Curation and Exhibition in the Aftermath of Genocide and Mass-Violence*, edited by Jean-Marc Dreyfuss and Élisabeth Anstett, 14–37. Manchester: Manchester University Press.
Aulich, Uwe, and Katrin Bischoff. 2015. "Michael Tsokos wehrt sich: 'Wir haben rechtzeitig informiert.'" *Berliner Zeitung*, 27 February 2015.
Benzenhöfer, Udo (ed.). 2012. *Mengele, Hirt, Holfelder, Berner, von Verschuer, Kranz: Frankfurter Universitätsmediziner der NS-Zeit*. 2. Unveränderte Edition 2012. Fredersdorf: Verlag Klemm und Oelschläger.
Berenbaum, M. (ed.). 1990. *A Mosaic of Victims. Non-Jews Persecuted and Murdered by the Nazis*. New York: New York University Press.
Berliner Zeitung. 2015. "Zur Kolumne 'Geistlos und roh an der FU Berlin': Richtigstellung," 4 February. Retrieved 26 June 2018 from http://www.berliner-zeitung.de/meinung/zur-kolumne—geistlos-und-roh-an-der-fu-berlin—richtigstellung,10808020,29750314.html.
Bernbeck, Reiner. 2015. "Die Opfer nicht erneut zu Objekten machen." *Tagesspiegel* 18 February 2015. Retrieved 26 June 2018 from https://www.tagesspiegel.de/wissen/position-die-opfer-nicht-erneut-zu-objekten-machen/11385976.html.

Berndt, Christina. 2017. "Was ich gesehen habe, hat meine Befürchtungen noch übertroffen." Sueddeutsche.de 14 March 2017. Retrieved 26 June 2018 from http://www.sueddeutsche.de/muenchen/max-planck-institut-was-ich-gesehen-habe-hat-meine-befuerchtungen-noch-uebertroffen-1.3417758-2.

Bundesärztekammer. 2003. "Recommendations on the Treatment of Human Remains in Collections, Museums and Public Places." *Deutsches Ärzteblatt*, C1532–36.

Czech, Herwig. 2015. "Von der Richtstätte auf den Seziertisch: Zur anatomischen Verwertung von NS-Opfern in Wien, Innsbruck und Graz." *Jahrbuch des Dokumentationsarchiv des österreichischen Widerstandes*: 141–90.

Department of Culture, Media and Sport UK. 2005. Guidance for the Care of Human Remains in Museums. Retrieved 26 June 2018 from https://collectionstrust.org.uk/resource/guidance-for-the-care-of-human-remains-in-museums/.

Deutsch, David. 2016. "Exhumations in Post-war Rabbinical Responsas." In *Human Remains in Society: Curation and Exhibition in the Aftermath of Genocide and Mass-Violence*, edited by Jean-Marc Dreyfuss and Élisabeth Anstett, 90–111. Manchester: Manchester University Press.

Dreyfuss, Jean-Marc. 2015. "Renationalizing Bodies? The French Search Mission for the Corpses of Deportees in Germany, 1946–58." In *Mass Violence, Genocide, and the Forensic Turn*, edited by Élisabeth Anstett and Jean-Marc Dreyfuss, 129–45. Manchester: Manchester University Press.

Deutscher Museumsbund. 2013. "Recommendations for the Care of Human Remains in Museums and Collections." Retrieved 26 June 2018 from https://www.museumsbund.de/wp-content/uploads/2017/04/2013-recommendations-for-the-care-of-human-remains.pdf.

Ehrenreich, Eric. 2007. "Otmar von Verschuer and the 'Scientific' Legitimization of the Nazi Anti-Jewish Policy." *Holocaust and Genocide Studies* 21(1): 55–72.

Ezekiel 37. Translated by Rabbi Arthur Waskow. Retrieved 29 June 2018 from https://theshalomcenter.org/node/248.

Feikert, Clare. 2009. "Repatriation of Historic Human Remains: Australia." Retrieved 28 June 2018 from https://www.loc.gov/law/help/repatriation-human-remains/australia.php.

Finder, Gabriel. 2015. "Final Chapter: Portraying the Exhumation and Reburial of Polish Jewish Holocaust Victims in the Pages of Yizkor Books." In *Mass Violence, Genocide, and the Forensic Turn*, edited by Élisabeth Anstett and Jean-Marc Dreyfuss, 34–58. Manchester: Manchester University Press.

Freie Universität Berlin. 2014. "Gerichtsmedizinischer Bericht zu den Knochenfunden auf dem Campus: Knochen lagen mehrere Jahrzehnte in der Erde." Campus.leben, 19 November 2014. Retrieved 26 June 2018 from https://www.fu-berlin.de/campusleben/intern/2014/20141119_knochenfunde/index.html.

———. 2015a. "'Unhaltbare Vorwürfe': Ein Interview mit Universitätspräsident Peter-André Alt zu den Anschuldigungen im Umgang mit den Knochenfunden auf dem Campus." Campus.leben, 4 February 2015. Retrieved 30 May 2018 from http://www.fu-berlin.de/campusleben/campus/2015/150204_interview-alt-knochen/index.html.

———. 2015b. "'Ihr, die ihr gesichert lebet . . .': Freie Universität gedenkt der Befreiung des Vernichtungslagers Auschwitz mit einer Kranzniederlegung." Campus.leben, 27 February 2015. Retrieved 26 June 2018 from https://www.fu-berlin.de/campusleben/campus/2015/150127-kranzniederlegung/index.html.

Gannon, M. 2017. "Germany to Probe Nazi-Era Medical Science: Overlooked Brain Tissue Slides Prompt Another Look at 'Euthanasia' Victims." *Science* 355(6320): 13–14.

Hildebrandt, Sabine. 2006. "How the Pernkopf Controversy Facilitated a Historical and Ethical Analysis of the Anatomical Sciences in Austria and Germany: A Recommendation for the Continued Use of the Pernkopf Atlas." *Clinical Anatomy* 19: 91–100.

———. 2013. "Current Status of Identification of Victims of the National Socialist Regime Whose Bodies Were Used for Anatomical Purposes." *Clinical Anatomy* 27: 514–36.

———. 2016. *The Anatomy of Murder: Ethical Transgressions and Anatomical Science during the Third Reich.* New York: Berghahn Books.

Hildebrandt, Sabine, and W. E. Seidelman. 2018. "To Use or Not to Use: The Legitimacy of Using Unethically Obtained Scientific Human Tissue from the National Socialist Era." *Wiener Klinische Wochenschrift*, 130(3): S228–31.

ICOM Code of Ethics for Museums. 2013. Retrieved 28 June 2018 from http://icom.museum/filea dmin/user_upload/pdf/Codes/code_ethics2013_eng.pdf.

Jones, David G., and Maya I. Whitaker. 2009. *Speaking for the Dead: The Human Body in Biology and Medicine.* Farnham: Ashgate.

Kirchner, Annett. 2017. "Knochenfunde auf FU-Gelände." *Tagesspiegel*, 5 February 2017. Retrieved 28 June 2018 from https://www.tagesspiegel.de/berlin/bezirke/steglitz-zehlendorf/steglitz-zehlen dorf-knochenfunde-auf-fu-gelaende-in-dahlem/19341158.html.

Kröner, Hans-Peter.1998. *Von der Rassenhygiene zur Humangenetik.* Stuttgart: Gustav Fischer Verlag.

Kühne A. 2015a. "Neue Widersprüche bei Skelettresten auf dem FU-Campus." *Tagesspiegel.* 6 February 2015. Retrieved 26 June 2018 from http://www.tagesspiegel.de/wissen/heikler-fund-neue-widersprueche-bei-skelettresten-auf-dem-fu-campus/11333914.html.

———. 2015b. "Umgang mit den Skeletten in Dahlem: Einfach eingeäschert." *Tagesspiegel*, 26 January 2015. Retrieved 26 June 2018 from https://www.tagesspiegel.de/wissen/umgang-mit-den-skel ettfunden-in-dahlem-einfach-eingeaeschert/11278454.html.

Lang, Hans-Joachim. 2007. *Die Namen der Nummern: Wie es gelang, die 86 Opfer eines NS-Verbrechens zu identifizieren; Überarbeitete Ausgabe.* Frankfurt am Main: S. Fischer Verlag.

MPI Brain Research. 2015. "Full Transparency about Institute's History—New Traces of Third Reich Atrocities Discovered." 9 April 2015. Retrieved 26 June 2018 from http://brain.mpg.de/news-events/news/news/archive/2015/april/article/additional-traces-of-former-institute-directors-crim es-discovered.html.

Müller-Hill, Benno. 1984. *Tödliche Wissenschaft.* Reinbek bei Hamburg: Rowohlt Taschenbuch Verlag.

———. 2001. "Genetics of Susceptibility to Tuberculosis: Mengele's Experiments in Auschwitz." *Nature Reviews-Genetics* 2: 631–34.

Neumann, Conny. 2017. "Grausige Funde." *Spiegel*, 3 April 2017. Retrieved 26 June 2018 from http://www.spiegel.de/spiegel/euthanasie-im-ns-funde-im-max-planck-institut-muenchen-a-1137219 .html.

Noack, Thorsten. 2012. "Anatomical Departments in Bavaria and the Corpses of Executed Victims of National Socialism." *Annals of Anatomy* 194: 286–92.

Oehler-Klein, Sigrid, Dirk Preuss, and Volker Roelcke. 2012. "The Use of Executed Nazi Victims in Anatomy: Findings from the Institute of Anatomy at Giessen University, Pre- and Post-1945." *Annals of Anatomy* 194: 293–97.

Polak, Joseph A. 2001. "Exhuming Their Neighbors: A Halakhic Inquiry." *Tradition: A Journal of Orthodox Jewish Thought* 35(4): 23–43

———. 2015. *After the Holocaust the Bells Still Ring.* Jerusalem: Urim Publications.

———. 2018. "Vienna Protocol for When Jewish or Possibly-Jewish Human Remains Are Discovered." *Wiener Klinische Wochenschrift* 130(3): S239–43.

Pollock, Susan, and Georg Cyrus. 2018. "Skelettreste unklarer Herkunft: Untersuchungen in Berlin-Dahlem." In *Archäologie in Berlin und Brandenburg 2016*, edited by Archäologische Gesellschaft in Berlin und Brandenburg e.v., 140–42. Konrad-Theiss Verlag.

rbb Fernsehen. 2015. *Entsorgte Erinnerung- Knochenfunde in Berlin.* TV Program: Stilbruch, das Kulturmagazin 12 March 2015.

Redies, Christoph, Rosemarie Fröber, Michael Viebig, and Susanne Zimmermann. 2012. "Dead Bodies for the Anatomical Institute in the Third Reich: An Investigation at the University of Jena." *Annals of Anatomy* 194: 298–303.

Sachse, Carola, and Benoit Massin. 2000. "Biowissenschaftliche Forschungen an Kaiser-Wilhelm-Institute and die Verbrechen des NS-Regimes: Informationen über den gegenwärtigen Wissensstand." Retrieved 1 June 2018 from https://www.mpiwg-berlin.mpg.de/KWG/Ergebnisse/Ergebnisse3.pdf.

Schmuhl, Hans-Walter. 2008. *The Kaiser Wilhelm Institute for Anthropology, Human Heredity and Eugenics, 1927–1945: Crossing Boundaries*. Dordrecht: Springer Science and Business Media B.V.

Seidelman, William E. 2012. "Dissecting the History of Anatomy in the Third Reich—1989–2010: A Personal Account." *Annals of Anatomy* 194: 228–36.

Seidelman, William E., Lilka Elbaum, and Sabine Hildebrandt (eds.). 2017. "How to Deal with Holocaust Era Human Remains: Recommendations Arising from a Special Symposium. Recommendations/Guidelines for the Handling of Future Discoveries of Human Victims of Nazi Terror / 'Vienna Protocol' for When Jewish or Possibly-Jewish Human Remains are Discovered, by Rabbi Joseph A. Polak." Elie Wiesel Center for Jewish Studies. Retrieved 30 January 2020 from https://www.bu.edu/jewishstudies/research/medicine-and-the-holocaust/recommendations-for-the-discovery-of-jewish-remains-project/.

Spohd, E. 2015. "Das Rätsel von Dahlem." *Jüdische Allgemeine*, 5 March 2015. Retrieved 26 June 2018 from https://www.juedische-allgemeine.de/article/view/id/21649.

Stoecker, Holger, Thomas Schnalke, and Andreas Winkelmann (eds.). 2013. *Sammeln, erforschen, zurückgeben? Menschliche Gebeine aus der Kolonialzeit in akademischen und musealen Sammlungen*. Berlin: Ch. Links Verlag.

Sturdy Colls, Caroline. 2015. *Holocaust Archaeologies: Approaches and Future Directions*. New York: Springer.

———. 2016. "'Earth Conceal Not My Blood': Forensic and Archaeological Approaches to Locating the Remains of Holocaust Victims." In *Human Remains in Society: Curation and Exhibition in the Aftermath of Genocide and Mass-Violence*, edited by Jean-Marc Dreyfuss and Élisabeth Anstett, 163–96. Manchester: Manchester University Press.

Universität Tübingen. 1990. "Berichte der Kommission zur Überprüfung der Präparatesammlungen in den medizinischen Einrichtungen der Universität Tübingen im Hinblick auf Opfer des Nationalsozialismus." Manuscript, personal archive Sabine Hildebrandt.

Wässle H. 2017: "A Collection of Brain Section from 'Euthanasia' Victims: The series H of Julius Hallervorden." *Endeavour* 41(4): 166–75.

Weindling, Paul J. 2012. "'Cleansing' Anatomical Collections: The Politics of Removing Specimens from Anatomical Collections 1988–1992." *Annals of Anatomy* 194: 237–42.

Weiss, Sheila. 2010. "After the Fall: Political Whitewashing, Professional Posturing, and Personal Refashioning in the Postwar Career of Otmar Freiherr von Verschuer." *Isis* 101: 722–58.

Williams, David J. 1988. "The History of Eduard Pernkopf's Topographische Anatomie des Menschen." *Journal of Biocommunication* 15(2): 2–12.

Yee, Andrew, Ema Zubovic, Jennifer Yu, Shuddhadeb Ray, Sabine Hildebrandt, William E. Seidelman, Joseph A. Polak, Michael A. J. Grodin, Henk Coert, Douglas Brown, Ira J. Kodner, and Susan E. Mackinnon. 2019. "Ethical Considerations in the Use of Pernkopf's Atlas of Anatomy: A Surgical Case Study." *Surgery* 165(5): 860–67.

Conclusion
The Past in the Present and the Future

Sabine Hildebrandt, Miriam Offer, and Michael A. Grodin

The chapters collected in this volume explore a dynamic spectrum of new studies on the role and importance of medicine within the wider history of the Holocaust. They reveal new insights into fields that have seen substantial research in the past, such as racial hygiene theory and the practice of different Nazi perpetrator groups and individual biographies. However, even within these well-established areas of research, the variety and extent of alignment and nonalignment of actors with the NS regime and its ideology is surprising. On the other hand, the two articles focusing on the underresearched area of Jewish medicine in the first decades of the twentieth century give a first glimpse into the as-yet-untapped wealth of information that can be gained through a closer study of this history. Jewish medicine and ethical practice is presented here as a counterimage to Nazi medicine, wherein Jewish medicine retained the traditional medical ethics of care for the individual, whereas at the center of Nazi medical ethics stood the care for the group, the German *Volk*. Another underdeveloped field of research is the Nazis' war against women, and the two chapters contained in this volume give first insights into the extent of the gendered violence wrought by the Nazis.

While postwar legacies of medicine during the Holocaust have recently come into focus,[1] the studies in this collection look at never-before-investigated continuities of suffering in the decades after the war, not only in Germany but also in the formerly occupied territories of Poland and Austria. In these chapters the victims of NS violence are at the center of the narrative in a move away from "perpetrator history." These survivors were often re-traumatized by the many professionals, doctors among them, who continued in their positions after the war in institutions of power. The latter included the Max Planck Institutes as successors of the Kaiser Wilhelm Institutes, which—as is elaborated in one essay—were not only responsible for the decades-long silence and obstruction of research into the history of medicine during the Holocaust but also guilty of continuing to hold on to physical remains of Nazi victims. More physical remains of victims are still found inadvertently or in university collections, and the chapter on the Vienna Protocol describes how a set of guidelines on their handling was developed, integrating insights from Jewish medical ethics. How then can we deal not only with the physical remains of medicine and the Holocaust but also with its moral, aesthetical, and political aftermath? This question is addressed in examples from recent artwork that reflects the artists' engagement with bioethics and innovative medical technology.

The chapters in the second half of the volume clearly show that the past, as addressed in the studies of the first half, is very much alive in the present and needs to be studied, described, and reflected upon. As editors we believe that this set of new studies on medicine and the Holocaust is testament to the fact that not only has scholarship become more specific but also that the field of research has widened and thus needs much more attention. Many of the contributors to this volume have pointed out areas of future research.

Firstly, the continuity of "racial theory and thinking" from the past into the present needs further attention worldwide in terms of the meaning of individual choice and social justice in the field of modern genetics. Closer examination of this topic might help understand the recent reemergence of overt anti-Semitism globally, and specifically in Germany. Ideally, researchers in biology and genetics would work here together with historians, sociologists, political scientists, and philosophers on a common theory.

Secondly, Miriam Offer pointed out that despite the fact that we have much to learn from them, writings of Jewish physicians from the Holocaust period still have to be located and, once found, systematically study. Very often this will need multilingual researchers or research collaborations to cope with the different languages usually encountered in these writings.

Thirdly, the systematic investigation of gendered victimization is an important area of research also for the time frame of the Holocaust and may in the future produce even more results through the support of feminist theorists.

Fourthly, the exploration of the motivation of perpetrators, individuals, and groups may lead to a better understanding of the historical development of the Holocaust and current streams of thinking about it.

Fifthly, the effect of wartime experiences in medicine on victims, perpetrators, and the society in general is still in need of further investigation. One area that remains completely unexplored is the effect on medical students who were trained on and who trained with the bodies of victims of the Nazi regime in preclinical and clinical disciplines between 1933 and 1945, and who served the German population for decades after the war. Likewise not studied is the effect of the confrontation between postwar medical students and the academic teachers, those who had served in the same position under the Nazis, who educated them.

Sixthly, we don't know how much of the past still exists in the present. Ongoing investigations of university and institutional collections of specimens show that even physical human remains from this period are still with us. How much more then is this true for data from these specimens?

As to the latter point, efforts are underway in several areas. The Pernkopf atlas and its use—as an example of "data" from Nazi victims—is at the center of a new debate that was the topic of an interdisciplinary and international group of scholars in Toronto, Canada, in November 2019.[2] Furthermore, investigations of the history of Nazi medicine and its physical remains are ongoing at a number of institutions in Germany and the former occupied territories, foremost among them a comprehensive historical investigation of the Reichsuniversität Strassburg.[3] However, much more work is ahead of us, which has never been more important than in this current time, when we see a global resurgence of nationalism, anti-Semitism, and racism; a time of increasing "othering"[4] and dehumanization that has left many in our societies looking for safe spaces—be they spaces of thought and belief or physical spaces of refuge. And all the while we do not fully understand the experiences and events of the past, because much of the historical work and reflection has not been done. This failure is exemplified in the role of medicine in the history of Nazi Germany and the Holocaust, but it extends to such histories as slavery in the United States or genocide in the Balkans, Cambodia, Rwanda, Myanmar, the ongoing war in Syria or the persecution of certain ethnicities in China. The lasting effect of these histories and their legacies can only be understood and then remedied by research, public discussion, commemoration, and political action on a worldwide scale.

What then is needed to enable and facilitate such future research? At a minimum two prerequisites must be fulfilled: funding and researchers. The former will depend on the political will of governments and institutions. The latter rests very much on the continued interest of a new generation of researchers in history generally, and in the history of the Holocaust specifically. To engender such interest, this history must be researched, known, and taught, as widely as possible. This volume hopes to make a contribution to this effort.

Sabine Hildebrandt, MD, is an associate professor of pediatrics at Boston Children's Hospital and an anatomy educator at Harvard Medical School. Her research interests are the history and ethics of anatomy. She also works on the restoration of biographies of victims of the Holocaust. Her book *The Anatomy of Murder: Ethical Transgressions and Anatomical Science during the Third Reich* was published in 2016, paperback in August 2017, and is the first systematic study on this topic. The biography *Käthe Beutler, 1896–1999: Eine jüdische Kinderärztin aus Berlin* was published in June 2019.

Miriam Offer, PhD, is an expert on Jewish medicine in the Holocaust. Her book *White Coats inside the Ghetto: Jewish Medicine in Poland during the Holocaust* was published in Hebrew in 2015 by Yad Vashem; English edition forthcoming. Miriam has researched the history of medicine (organization, science, ethics) in ghettos in Poland and Lithuania. Her current focus is Jewish medical activity immediately before, during, and after the Holocaust, and medicine/Holocaust gender issues. Miriam is a senior lecturer in the Holocaust Studies Program, Western Galilee College, and teaches medicine and the Holocaust in the Sackler Faculty of Medicine, Tel Aviv University.

Michael A. Grodin, MD, is professor of health law, bioethics, and human rights at the Boston University School of Public Health, and professor and director of the Project on Ethics and the Holocaust at the Elie Wiesel Center for Jewish Studies. Dr. Grodin has served on national and international commissions focusing on medical ethics, human rights, and the Holocaust. He has received a special citation from the United State Holocaust Memorial Museum for "profound contributions—through original and creative research—to the cause of Holocaust education and remembrance," and is the author of over two hundred articles and the editor or coeditor of seven books.

Notes

1. E.g. Roelcke et al. 2015; Topp 2013; Weindling 2015.
2. Seidelman et al. 2019.
3. Communiqué de Presse de L'Université Strasbourg 2017.
4. Morrison 2017.

References

Communiqué de Presse de L'Université Strasbourg. 2017. "Historical Commission for the Medical Faculty of the Reichsuniversität Straßburg, 1941–1944." 6 July 2017. Retrieved 12 December 19 from https://dhvs.unistra.fr/fileadmin/uploads/websites/dhvs/Manifestations/CP-GB_Commission-historique-Reischuniversitat_20170706.pdf.
Morrison, Toni. 2017. *The Origin of Others*. The Charles Eliot Norton Lectures (Book 56). Cambridge: Harvard University Press.
Roelcke, Volker, Sascha Topp, and Etienne Lepicard (eds.). 2014. *Silence, Scapegoats, Self-Reflection: The Shadow of Nazi Medical Crimes on Medicine and Bioethics*. Göttingen: V&R unipress.
Seidelman. W. E., S. Hildebrandt, S. Mackinnon, J. A. Polak, P. Berger, A. Agur, L. Lax. "The Vienna Protocol: Medicine's Confrontation with Continuing Legacies of Its Nazi Past." Sarah and Chaim Neuberger Holocaust Education Centre's Holocaust Education Week Program, "The Holocaust Then and Now," 3–10 November 2019; symposium held at University of Toronto, Faculty of Medicine, 10 November 2019. https://www.holocaustcentre.com/hew-2019/the-vienna-protocol.
Slaughter, Karin. 2017. *The Good Daughter*. New York: HarperCollins.
Topp, Sascha. 2013. *Geschichte als Argument in der Nachkriegsmedizin: Formen der Vergangenheitsbewältigung der nationalsozialistischen Euthanasie zwischen Politisierung und Historiographie*. Göttingen: V&R unipress.
Weindling, Paul J. 2015. *Victims and Survivors of Nazi Human Experiments: Science and Suffering in the Holocaust*. London: Bloomsbury Academic.

Index

Abderhalden, Emil, 145, 147
Abel, Wolfgang, 53, 356
abortion: as criminalized, 105; ethics and, 330; as forced, 104, 106, 108, 110–11, 115–16, 119n89, 129, 133; Freilich on, 109–10, 117n49; gendered violence and, 103; Jewish law on, 107–8, 113, 117n38; Jewish medical professionals and, 110, 117n59; for mother's life, 85, 93, 106–7, 109–10, 112–14, 117n38; numbers, 109–10, 112–14, 118n78; Oshry on, 108, 117n38; survivors on, 115, 119m89; as taboo, 106–7, 116n23
Abramczyk, Rachel, 112
accessories to murders, 213
accomplices in medical atrocities, 213
Adelsberger, Lucie, 110–11
Adorno, Theodor W., 330, 337–40, 342, 346; positivism and, 328–29, 350n6, 350n8, 350n16; on stereotype identity, 11–12
Africans, 51
Aichel, Otto, 4
Aichhorn, August, 292n53
Aktion Reinhard, 141–42, 149n4
Aktion T4: Austrian patients in, 279; departments and secrecy of, 176–77; extermination camps from, 177, 276; Hitler discontinuing, 177–78; killed patients by, 176; real estate administration and, 177; Süß on mentally ill and, 174; T4 Planning Commission and, 105, 141, 172–84, 261, 270, 276, 279, 281, 298, 308
Albrecht, Hans, 128
Alt, Peter-André, 234, 355, 357
Aly, Götz: on bones, 356; Boom on, 302, 308; on child euthanasia, 223, 298–322, 323n17; on euthanasia victim remains, 11; on euthanized children, 304–8, 323n17; as German historian, xvi, 11, 173–74, 233, 356–57; on German medical professionals, xvi; on Hallervorden, 301, 304–6; Henning disapproval of, 308–14, 316, 319, 323n20, 325n60; Kalb on, 301, 303–4; on KWI, 305, 309; MPG investigation and, 11, 356–57, 367n16; 'Reform und Gewissen' from, 309, 311; Simitis helping, 303; Wässle on, 309, 311, 357, 368n21
"ambiguity of good," 140–41
Améry, Jean, 250, 254n65
anatomical dissection, 131, 143–48
anesthesia, xiii, 132, 136n39
Anker, Suzanne, 350n30
anti-Semitism, xvii; by Gerstein, 141, 148; Hitler goal of, 2–6; racial medicine as, 154; racial theory and, 374; Verschuer and, 227; Wastl and, 44
Apper (doctor), 70–71. *See also* Lensky, Mordechai
applied biology, 5
Arbeit Macht Frei (work sets you free), 348
Arbeit McFries (Chapman, J., and Chapman, D.), 347–48
Arendt, Hannah, 149, 172–73, 184, 204–5, 251
artists: animal death masks and, 339; bioethics and, 327, 331–32; Chapman, J., and Chapman, D., as, 340–49, 351n45, 351n50, 351n52; on genomics and bioengineering, 330, 350n22; on Holocaust, 328; Kaminiarz as, 336–40, 349, 351n38; Nussbaum on, 335, 349; against positivism, 328–31; trauma and, 268
Aschenauer, Rudolf, 243, 248–50, 254n68
Asperger, Hans, 288, 293n60
Auschwitz, 351n50; blood and bones from, 226, 229; eyes from, 225–28; Frankfurt Auschwitz Trial on, 11, 241; KWI and research of, 223–24; Lucas and, 247, 253n44; Mengele and, 222, 226–27, 232; research at, 225, 229; selections at, 246;

Weindling on research and, 222–34; Wirths at, 227, 242
Austria: *Aktion T4* and, 279; Holocaust and Jews of, 277–78; NS euthanasia in, 276; Pernkopf of, 51, 358; psychiatry in, 276, 278–81; racial investigations in, 46–48; Victim Welfare Law of, 288–90; Vienna and, 276–84, 286. *See also* Vienna Protocol
aviation experiments: Dachau with, 205; deliberate death in, 207, 215n24; Göring and, 207; Holzlöhner leading, 210–12, 321; as legacy, 218n69; mobile decompression chamber in, 208–9, 211; overlapping interests in, 213–14; Peters and, 321–22, 325n60; Pfannenstiel and, 211, 217n45; Rascher and, 10, 207–14, 216n28, 216nn35–38, 217n45, 217n57, 321; Rein and, 216n42; Romberg and, 208–9, 211, 213, 216nn35–37; Ruff and, 208–9, 213, 215n22; since late 1880s, 207; Strughold and, 211–12, 216n25; Weltz and, 208–10, 212–13, 216n38, 216n40, 217n62
Axmann, Artur, 164, 168n63

Baader, Otto, 53
backshadowing, 100n37
Baeyer, Walter von, 246, 250
BÄK. *See* Bundesärztekammer
"banality of evil," 173, 204–5
Bauer, Karl Heinrich, 5–6, 129, 132, 136n24
Baur-Fischer-Lenz text, 5–6
Becker, Herbert, 178, 180, 182
BEG. *See* Federal Compensation Law
Begleitarzt (personal physician), 155, 166n6
Bendorf-Sayn, 261–62
Berlin-Dahlem institute, 6, 229, 232–33, 355, 358, 360
Berner, Peter, 285
Bernhardt, Heike, 174
Bernstein, Michael Andre, 100n37
Bert, Paul, 218n69
Bertha, Hans, 281
bioengineering, 11, 330, 344–45, 350n22, 350n28, 351n52
bioethics, 12; animals and, 337, 339–40; art and, 327, 331–32; bioengineering and, 11; ethics and, 330; Kac on transgressing, 335; Kaminiarz on, 336–40, 349, 351n38; scientists for, 331; *Semi Living Worry Dolls* and, 330–31, 349; uniqueness and, 340–41
biological anthropology, 29, 36, 38n1, 54
Bláha, František, 211–12
blood: from Auschwitz, 226, 229; diagnoses from, 226; from Mengele, 231–32; Nyiszli on, 229; tests and transfusions of, xiii; Verschuer receiving, 223, 231–32
body parts, xiii; burial of, 144, 315, 364–65; plaster casts of, 45, 49; receipt of, 223, 225, 227, 230–31; Vienna Protocol on, 364
bones, 8; from Auschwitz, 226, 229; cremation of, 356; at FU Berlin, 354–56; of Holocaust victims, 1, 11–12; Jewish skeletons and, 44–45, 356; KWI and, 355–56; Nyiszli on, 229
Boom, Hans, 302, 308
Bormann, Martin, 155, 162–64, 168n63
Borst, Maximilian, 212
Bosnians, 49
brains: Brandenburg-Görden hospital and child, 223, 298–99, 305–8, 316–17, 319; Bunke on children, 306–7; burial of children, 302, 315–16; of children, 1, 223, 227, 279, 298–300, 302–21, 357; of decompression experiments, 211; destruction versus burial of, 311–15; Hallervorden and child, 298–300, 357; Hallervorden and mentally ill, 223, 227; Henning on burials and, 311–12, 314; Kohl and Hammer on burial and, 312, 359; KWI and hypothermia, 211; MPG finding, 357; numbers of, 314–15
Brandenburg centers, 261
Brandenburg-Görden psychiatric hospital: child brains and, 223, 298–99, 305–8; Kutschke boys death at, 316–17, 319
Brandt, Karl, 155, 162–63
Brandt, Rudolf, 216n40
British Mandate policy, 63, 76n24
British soldiers, 47, 49
Browning, Christopher, 204, 251
Bruns, Florian, 165
Büchner, Franz, 207, 212, 217n57, 217n60, 217n62
Bundesärztekammer (BÄK), xv–xvi
Bundesentschädigungsgesetz (Federal Compensation Law, BEG), 241, 244–45
Bunke, Heinrich, 306–7
burial: of body parts, 144, 315, 364–65; brains and, 311–15; of children brains, 302, 315–16; concentration camps and, 359; Gerstein on, 142–43, 145, 148, 150n9, 150n19; Jewish people on, 364–65; Kohl and Hammer on, 312, 359
Burkhardt, Anika, 174, 177

Caplan, Arthur, 12
Carnegie Foundation, xiii–xiv
Catts, Oron, 330–31, 349
Chalmers, Beverly, 104, 116n4
Chamberlain, Houston Stewart, 27, 39n20

Chapman, Dinos and Jake (aka. Chapman brothers, 340–49
Charon, Rita, 335
Chełm, 261, 271n20
children: brains of, 1, 223, 227, 279, 298–300, 302–21; Brandenburg-Görden and, 223, 298–99, 305–8, 316–17, 319; Bunke on brains and, 306–7; congenital imbecility and, 299; euthanasia of, 223, 278, 298–322, 323n17; of Goebbels, 155, 163, 168n61; Grosskind, Friedmann, and Oesterreichischer as, 287; Heinze and psychiatry for, 298; Kriesch as, 298–99; KWI and euthanasia of, 223; KWI with brains of, 299; Mikulicz-Radecki for sterilization and, 130; psychiatry or curative pedagogy for, 287; Pusch and euthanasia of, 298–99, 319; scandal on Jewish, 278–79; Spiegelgrund institution for, 279; worth proven by, 288, 293n60
Chirurgensondergruppe beim Kommandostab des RfSS (special surgeons' unit), 159
Ciechocinek, 68
circumcisers (*Mohalim*), 67–68
Clauberg, Carl, 105, 129, 225
Clauß, Ludwig Ferdinand, 8, 22–40
cleft palates and lips, 193, 196–97
collusion, 244–46
color perception, 51
compensation: BEG for, 244–45; as cigarettes, 49; information sources for, 251; for invisible ravages, 250; for de la Penha, 225, 248; struggle for, 246, 282, 284, 289, 293n68; twin experiments and, 225
concentration camps: *Arbeit Macht Frei* on, 348; body parts from, 227; criminals in, 207, 216n32; dental surgeons in, 193, 199; experiments in, 48, 53, 213; fates and, xvi–xvii; former prisoners from, 282–83; graves of, 359; Kantorowicz in, 194–95; "Kapo" in, 209, 216n32; killing fields and, 9, 104, 360, 364, 366; Lenz on, 226; medical experiments in, 54, 213; Mengele suitability for, 232; de la Penha in, 247; prisoner doctors in, 249, 253n61; racial studies in, 44–45; survivors of, 267, 277, 283, 285–86. *See also* Auschwitz; Dachau research; Ravensbrück concentration camp; selections
congenital debility, 132, 229, 235n46, 299, 305–6
constitutional defects, 282, 285, 288, 292n48
Craemer, Hans-Dietrich, 211
crimes: abortion and, 105; accessories to murders and, 213; concentration camps and, 156, 159–62, 207, 216n32; of German medical profession, 242; Gerstein on convicts and, 147; of Mengele, 9; Nuremberg Doctors Trial on, 1; of Stumpfegger, 156, 159–62
curative pedagogy (*Heilpädagogik*), 287–88, 293n60
Czerniaków, Adam, 263–64

Dachau research: aviation medicine and, 205; Diringshofen and, 211; Neff as Kapo and, 209, 216n32; Nuremberg Doctors Trial and, 205; overlapping interests in, 213–14; Pfannenstiel and, 211, 217n45; Rascher in, 10, 207–14, 216n28, 216nn35–38, 217n45, 217n57, 321; Romberg and, 208–9, 211, 213, 216nn35–37; Ruff and, 208–9, 213, 215n22; Sievers and, 216n26, 216nn36–37, 217n57; SS-Ahnenerbe and, 53, 207, 210, 213–14, 216n26, 227–28; Weltz and, 208–10, 212–13, 216n38, 216n40, 217n62
Darwinism, 5, 22, 44, 104, 131, 149
Davidson, Noach, 63–64
"death asylums for expired cases," 182
death to protect others, 92–94, 108
defendants, 208, 243–45, 247
Demjanjuk, John, 204
dental profession: concentration camps and, 193, 199; emigration and, 194; eugenics and, 191; gold taken by, 193, 196; Jewish people and, 191, 193–94, 197; mass murder and, 196; Nazism and, 10, 199; NS cooperation by, 190–91, 196, 199; skilled dentists in, 192, 197–99; as surgeons, 191–99; wages in, 191–92
Department of Anthropology of the Natural History Museum Vienna, 44–46
Deutsche Dienststelle (WASt), 156, 166n8
Deutsche Forschungsgemeinschaft (German Research Fund, DFG), 223, 226
Dictate of contempt for human beings (*Diktat der Menschenverachtung*), 300
Diehl, Karoline "Nini," 207–8, 216n28, 217n57
Diktat der Menschenverachtung (Dictate of contempt for human beings), 300
Diringshofen, Heinz von, 211
displaced persons (DPs): Friedmann as, 287; as Jewish, 277–79, 291nn11–13; Rothschild DP hospital with, 277–78, 281; social adjustment lack by, 286
dissection, 307; Mengele and, 146–47, 229; of mentally ill people, 131, 143–44; Nyiszli on numbers and, 229–30
Der Doktor (Lensky), 68–71

380 • INDEX

doubling, 145–48
DPs. *See* displaced persons
Düx, Heinz, 247
dwarves, 224, 227, 230

Efrati, Shimon (rabbi), 92–95, 100n49, 108
Ehrhardt, Sophie, 302
Eichmann, Adolf, 100, 104, 172, 174, 204–5, 247
Eicken, Carl Otto von, 163
Einhorn, Moses, 67, 263
Elias, Ruth, 110
Elkes, Elchanan, 98n14
Elsevier, 358, 368n25
"e-measure" (euthanasia), 181, 186n85
"engaged followership," 205–7, 213–14
The Epidemic of Influenza (Lensky), 65
Eretz, Israel, 62, 64, 76n24
ethics, 54, 150n8; Abderhalden and, 145, 147; abortion and bioethics in, 330; artists for bioethical, 327; of bioengineering, 11; Chapman brothers and, 343; for German citizens, 142; for German medical profession, 327; Gerstein on anatomy and, 9–10, 142–44, 149, 150n9; lack of, 182; Lerner and Caplan on, 12; Lifton on German doctors and, 105, 145–46, 148, 22; NS and, 8, 141, 143, 147–48; Nussbaum on, 335, 349. *See also* bioethics
eugenics: British Mandate on, 76n24; Darwinism to, 5; dental surgeons and, 191; Fischer, E., and, 4–5; Fraenkel on, 135n16; German medical profession on, 131, 136n39; Law for the Prevention of Hereditarily Diseased Offspring and, 125, 164, 196, 242; Lensky on, 63; racial hygiene for, 154; sterilization and, 127; study of Nazi, 222
Euler, Hermann, 193
euthanasia, 1; administration visits for, 180; Austria and NS, 276; Brandenburg centers for, 261; Brandenburg-Görden and, 223, 298–99, 305–8, 316–17, 319; Büchner against, 212; bureaucracy and administration in, 172; Chełm and, 261, 271n20; children and, 223, 278, 298–322, 323n17; cleft palates for, 197; "e-measure" as, 181, 186n85; Frankl on, 292n52; genocide and, 174; of Jewish mental patients, 261–62, 271n19; Klee on, 173–74; KWI and child, 223; mass murder within, xv, 6, 105; medicalized killing and, 3; of mentally ill people, 10, 175, 183–84; of mice, 337, 339–40; Müller on, 182; NS and, 183–84, 257, 276; NSDAP and, 177;

NS victims from, 359; numbers in, 261, 271n21, 271n23, 272n35; planned law for, 182; racial medicine as, 154; Rüdin on, 5–6, 180, 320; Schmuhl on, 38n1, 53, 174, 224; T4 Headquarters employees and, 172, 176, 183; T4 program numbers of, 261, 271n21, 271n23, 272n35; Trieb and, 10, 182; victim remains and, 11; Yad Vashem on victims and, 269; at Zofiówka, 264–65
excess, 336, 341–42, 348–49
Exner, Robert, 51–54
Exner, Willi, 178
experimental medical studies, 53–54
extermination medicine, 154, 207, 215n24
eyes: from Auschwitz, 225–28; color perception of, 51; death for, 228–29, 231; genetics of, 225; Helmerstedt and, 225; Liebau and, 225–26, 228, 231; Magnussen on, 225, 228, 231–32, 356; Mengele and gypsy, 224, 226, 229–30, 302; Nachtsheim and, 223, 225, 233–34; Nyiszli on tumors and, 224, 226–31; Verschuer receiving, 223, 231–32

fatigue, 282–84
Faulstich, Heinz, 174
Federal Compensation Law (*Bundesentschädigungsgesetz*, BEG), 244–45
Fiderkiewicz, Alfred, 111
Final Solution, 103–4, 115–16, 119n92
Finke, Erich, 210
Fischer, Eugen, 4–6, 52–53
Fischer, Fritz, 160–62
Fischer, Martin, 283
Flexner, Abraham, xiv
"following orders": Eichmann pleading, 100, 104, 172, 174, 204–5, 247; German defense lawyers using, 208, 215n3, 244; Gröning pleading, 204; by special interest groups, 209
Forman, Paul, 38n11
Foucault, Michel, 217n66
Fraenkel, Ludwig, 135n16
Frank, Willy, 196
Frankfurt Auschwitz Trial, 11, 241
Frankl, Viktor, 277, 285–86, 292n52
Freie Universität Berlin (Free University, FU Berlin), 134, 233–34, 310, 354–57
Freilich, Bernard, 109–10, 117n49
French soldiers, 47, 50, 53
Freud, Sigmund, 285–86, 301, 329, 342, 351n52
Friedlander, Henry, 174, 260, 340, 346, 349
Friedländer, Saul, 140, 142, 328
Friedmann, Moische, 287
Fröwis, Babette, xv–xvi

FU Berlin. *See* Freie Universität Berlin
Fucking Hell (Chapman, J., and Chapman, D.), 344–45, 351n52

Galilee Declaration, xvii
gangrene, 160, 226
Gaum, Max, 178
Gebhardt, Karl, 155–62, 164–65, 166n13
Gedda, Luigi, 6
gendered violence: abortions and, 103; avoidance on, 105–6; German medical profession with, 9, 131–34; in Holocaust, 7–9, 103; in Kovno Ghetto, 108–10. *See also* women
General SS, 156–57, 166n10
genetics: artists on, 330, 350n22; of dwarfism, 230; of eyes, 225; Günther rejecting, 29; Müller-Hill on, xvi, 223, 226; Nazi emphasis on, 8, 22; Nordic vision of, 39n19; science of, 23–24, 32, 37, 374; of twins, 222; Verschuer and, 233, 355
genocide, 375; Chapman brothers and, 345; euthanasia and, 174; extermination medicine as, 154; foreknowledge of, 91, 100n37; Frankfurt Auschwitz Trial and, 241; as gynecological, 103–4, 106, 113–16, 119n92; Jewish doctors on, 74–75; Kahane Shapiro on, 90–91; Lucas and trial for, 253n46; Mengele and, 223, 226; pesticide for, 141, 226–27, 229, 235n40, 242–43; rabbinical responsa on, 90; Vienna Protocol and, 354. *See also* mass murder
German academia, 213–14, 218n69
German Association for Psychiatry and Psychotherapy, xvi
German citizens: Aly as historian and, xvi, 11, 173–74, 233, 356–57; ethics for, 142; "following orders" and, 208, 215n3, 244; Günther on physiognomics and, 23, 28; investigations by, 7; race of, 32; resistance by, 198–99, 217n68, 231, 289–90; resistance hindered by, 181, 213, 301; *Volk* as healthy, 4, 6, 38n1, 134, 373; *Volksdeutsche* as, 46, 68; *Volkskörper* as, 104, 131, 154
German medical profession: administration and, 172–73, 175, 177, 180, 182–84; Albrecht as, 128; Aly on, xvi; anatomical dissection and, 131, 143–48; BÄK acknowledging, xv–xvi; biological anthropology and, 29, 36, 54; Bruns on, 165; careers preserved for, xv, 10, 213, 224, 246, 276, 279, 310, 319, 321, 355; collective forgetting and, 304; crimes of, 242; death exploitation by, 315; as defendants, 208; dentists in, 10; doubling for, 145–48; emigration and, 194; ethics for, 327; on eugenics, 131, 136n39; forced sterilization with narcotics, 132–33; gendered violence of, 9, 131–34; on hereditary health policies, 131; on Hippocratic Oath, xiii–xiv, xviii; Holocaust and, 1–3; investigations opposed by, 7; Jewish persecution by, 191, 193–94; Jewry destruction by, 2–3, 144–49, 257, 260; Lifton on, 105, 145–46, 148, 222; for medical certainty, 132–34; medicalized killing by, 3; Mikulicz-Radecki as gynecologist and, 125–38; Mitscherlich on human material and, 242, 252n7; moral downfall of, 154–55; Müller-Hill on geneticists and, xvi, 223, 226; NSDAP, SS membership by, 154, 192–93, 218n69; NSDAP and, 154; NS medicine in, 2–6, 368nn20–21; Nuremberg Doctors Trial on, 231, 243, 278, 327; past and slowness by, 241; pathology of power and, xviii; perpetrators in, 3; Poland atrocities by, 257; as prisoner doctors, 249, 253n61; profiting by, 6; psychiatrists in, 176; Reich leader of, 192; responsibility and, 131, 136n36, 136n39; SA membership for, 154, 192–93, 218n69; silence by, xv; social hygiene and, 5; statute of limitations for, 242; sterilization by, 1, 125–26, 128, 136n39; Stoeckel and, 126; on victim bodies, 359; on violence, 125–26, 130, 134; on war losses, 131. *See also* Dachau research
German physiognomic tradition, 28
German Research Fund (Deutsche Forschungsgemeinschaft, DFG), 223, 226
German soldiers, 292n45
Germany: aviation medicine in Nazi, 10; Bendorf-Sayn in, 261–62; Berlin-Dahlem institute in, 6, 229, 232–33, 355, 358, 360; "following orders" in, 208, 215n3, 244; Günther renovating, 29; Hitler and anti-Semitism in, 2–6; human remains laws and, 360–61; medical certainty for, 132–34; Nordification of, 27, 29–32, 39n20, 40n38, 40n40, 40n43; NS medicine and, 2–6, 368nn20–21; Nuremberg Medical Trial on, xv; science and politics in, 21–22, 38n2; sterilization and, 128; Weimar despair in, 25, 38nn10–11
Gerstein, Kurt, 9–10, 140–50
Gesetz zur Verhütung erbkranken Nachwuchses (Law for the Prevention of Hereditarily Diseased Offspring), 125, 164, 196, 242
GFP Bunny, 332–35, 350nn28–30

Goebbels, Joseph, 155, 163, 168n61
Goebbels, Magda, 155, 163, 168n61
gold, 193, 196
Goltermann, Svenja, 245
Göring, Hermann, 145, 170n19, 207
Götter, Helden und Günther: Eine Abwehr der Güntherschen Rassenkunde (Merkenschlager), 32
Grodin, Michael, 12, 358, 364–66
Gröning, Oskar, 204
Groscurth, Georg, 197–98
Gross, Heinrich, 279–81
Groß, Walter, 32–33, 36
Grosskind, Toba, 287
Grünsteinova, Katarina, 114
A Guide for Circumcisers (Lensky), 67–68
Günther, Hans F. K., 8, 22–40
Günzburg mental hospital, 10, 173–74, 178
Guttmann, Tibor, 283
gynecological fertility research, 125–38
gypsy. *See* Roma; Sinti

Halakhah (Jewish law), 83
Hallervorden, Julius: Aly on, 301, 304–6; child brains and, 298–300, 357; Heinze and, 180, 298–99, 306, 317–19; Krücke on, 223, 300–302, 311; Kutschke boys and, 317–19; mentally ill brains and, 223, 227
Hammer, Zevulun, 312, 359
handicapped people, xv, 172, 184, 298, 302, 318
Harrington, Anne, 25–26, 38n11
Havemann, Robert, 197–98, 231–32
Hawking, Stephen, 343
health dictatorship, 154
"Health of the People" (*Volksgesundheit*), xiv, 192
Heilpädagogik (curative pedagogy), 287–88, 293n60
Heinze, Hans, 180, 298–99, 306, 317–19
Hell (Chapman, J., and Chapman, D.), 343–44, 347, 351n50
Helmersen, Erwin von, 226
Helmerstedt, Ernst, 225
Henning, Eckart, 308–14, 316, 319, 323n20, 325n60
hereditary health policies, 10, 131, 154
heredity, 5–6, 8, 39n20, 76n24; as mental, 22–25, 28, 33, 45; Peiffer on, 320; phenotypic characteristics versus, 24
Herzog, Dagmar, 245
heterotopia (other), 213, 217n66
Heydrich, Reinhard, 141–42, 149n4, 160, 244
Himmler, Heinrich, 154, 161, 163, 166, 228, 244; Diehl and, 207–8, 216n28, 217n57; Gebhardt and physician for, 157, 166n13; on gold and dead people, 193; intention of, 162, 216n26; on mass sterilization, 105; as Nazi SS leader, 6, 155; Peiper and, 158, 167n22; Stumpfegger and, 155–56, 158–59, 166n17
Hippke, Erich, 207, 217n60
Hippocratic Oath, xiii–xiv, xviii
Hirt, August, 211, 214, 361
Hitler, Adolf, xiv–xvi, xviii, 2–6; on *Aktion T4*, 177–78; dental surgeons and, 192–93; Eicken and, 163; *Leibstandarte SS Adolf Hitler* for, 159, 167n31; Morell and, 162–63, 167n49; Stumpfegger and, 10, 155, 162–64, 167n49
Hoff, Hans, 277, 283–87, 292n48, 292n53, 293n54
Hohenlychen Sanatorium, 155–61
Hohmann, Eckard, 303–4
Holocaust, 2–4; abortion and, 330; artists on, 328; bureaucracy and, 172, 180, 184; Chapman brothers on, 345–48; FU Berlin and, 354–56; gendered violence in, 7–9, 103; Jewish Holocaust and, xiv–xv, xvii–xviii, 91, 100n37; on Jewish medical professionals, 73–75; on Jewish pregnant women, 103–4, 106, 108–10, 114–15, 117n49, 117n54; Lensky and, 71–73; life-for-life choices during, 9; Müller-Hill and, xvi, 223, 226; Oshry on, 86, 99nn18–19; rabbinical responsa and, 84, 96, 98n9; Rosenhügel and, 281; Tsokos and, 355; victim bones of, 1, 11–12, 354–56; Vienna and, 277–78
Holzlöhner, Ernst, 210–12, 321
Honigstein, Ingelore, 111–12
Hooker, Claire, 351n39
Horkheimer, Max, 350n8
hospitals: Günzburg as mental, 10, 173–74, 178; Königsberg Women's Hospital as, 125–31, 135n1; for mentally ill, 173–74, 177–78, 180–81, 183, 260–61, 276–300, 306–7; T4 and, 181; Zofiówka as psychiatric, 11, 257–59, 261–69, 271n7
Houdebine, Louis-Marie, 350n28
human remains: archive of, 11, 233, 302, 312–13, 357, 362–63, 374; burial of, 144, 315, 364–65; euthanasia and, 11; at FU Berlin, 354; German law and, 360–61; guidelines on, 54, 360, 368n43; KWI cache of, 362; in medical collections, 359–60, 368n40; from NS period, 359; search for, 7, 359; Untermann Protocol and, 365–66; Vienna Protocol on, 2, 12, 354–64; Yad Vashem and guidelines on, 354, 360. *See also* blood; body parts; bones; brains; eyes

Husserl, Edmund, 26, 32, 34
Hygiene Institute, 225
hypothermia experiments, 207–8, 210–12, 217n57, 217n60, 217n62, 321

identity thinking, 328–31, 339–43, 348–49, 351n45
immunization, xiii, 230
Israeli Medical Association journal, 61–62
Itzkowitz, David (rabbi), 88–89

Jacoby, Meier, 261, 271n15
Jewish Councils, 82–83, 86, 89–91, 96, 100n31, 108–10
Jewish Holocaust (Shoah), xiv–xv, xvii–xviii, 91, 100n37
Jewish law (Halakhah), 83, 107–8, 113, 117n38. See also rabbinical responsa
Jewish medical professionals, 75n2, 194, 373–74; abortion and, 110, 117n59; circumcisers and, 67–68; Fiderkiewicz as, 111; on genocide, 74–75; Holocaust ending, 73–75; Lensky as, 9, 59–60; Pik as, 113; rabbinical responsa like, 84–85; writings of, 59–60
Jewish medicine, 2–3, 7–9
Jewish mental patients, 271n15; at Bendorf-Sayn, 261–62; death investigations on, 267–68; double stigma for, 269–70; euthanasia numbers of, 261, 271n21, 271n23, 272n35; Kobierzyn commemorating, 268–69; Nazis on, 257–58, 260–61; Śrem facility deaths for, 269, 273n62; T4 euthanasia program on, 261–62, 271n19; Zofiówka sanatorium for, 257–59, 271n7; Zofiówka suicides of, 258, 264–65, 272n41. See also mentally ill people
Jewish people, 141; baby deaths and, 110–12, 114, 118n65; on bone handling, 44–45, 356; on burials, 364–65; circumcisers and, 67–68; conduct standard for, 96; death examinations of, 230; dental profession on, 191, 193–94; Der Doktor for, 68–71; DPs as, 277, 291nn11–13; Euler persecuting, 193; genocide foreknowledge of, 91, 100n37; A Guide for Circumcisers for, 67–68; on infant deaths and bunkers, 92–94, 108; interdisciplinary approach and, 361–62; Kantorowicz as, 194–95; life-for-life problems for, 85–86, 98n14; life preservation and, 86, 99n17; in Lithuania, 82; mass executions, 244–45; The Modern Family Doctor for, 59, 65–66; NS on European, 2–3, 144–49, 257, 260; NS victim as, 359; Nyiszli on, 230–31; obligations and, 74, 86–88, 91, 95, 364–65; in Poland, 11, 61–75; rabbinical responsa as resistance and, 84, 98n9; rabbinical responses for, 2, 9, 82–83; racial investigations on Polish, 46–48; ransom life for another and, 94–95; resistance as birth and, 114, 118n81; resistance by, 84, 96, 98n9, 101n54; as risking one's own life, 86–89, 99n20; "sanctification of the Divine name" and, 99n27; skeletons of, 44–45; as skilled dentists, 197; Spier as, 196–97; Stransky as, 281; Victim Welfare Law on, 289; in Vienna, 277–78, 281–82; Vienna Protocol on human remains and, 2, 12, 354–64; Vienna scandal and children of, 278–79; Wagner, R., on, 73; Yiddish press for, 64–68; Zofiówka sanatorium for, 257–59, 271n7
Jewish women: abortion and, 85, 93, 106–7, 109–10, 112–14, 117n38; Adelsberger on, 110–11; baby deaths and, 110–12, 114, 118n65; Chalmers on pregnant, 104, 116n4; Final Solution on, 103–4, 106, 113–16, 119n92; forced abortion and, 104, 106, 108, 110–11, 115–16, 119n89, 129, 133; Freilich on, 109–10, 117n49; Holocaust and pregnant, 103–4, 106, 108–10, 114–15, 117n49, 117n54; infant deaths and bunkers on, 92–94, 108; Nomberg-Przytyk and, 111; Oshry on rape and, 119n93; Perl on pregnant, 110; resistance and, 103, 114–15, 118n81, 133; resistance as birth and, 114, 118n81; sterilization of, 103–4, 110, 130; Sussmann on, 114; testimonies by, 115, 119m89

Kac, Eduardo, 332–35, 349, 350nn28–30
Kahane Shapiro, Avraham (rabbi), 90–91
Kaiser Wilhelm Institute (KWI), 373; Aly on, 305, 309; Auschwitz research and, 223–24; bones near, 355–56; brain procurement by, 305; child brains for, 299; child euthanasia and, 223; continuation of, 233–34; Fischer, E., directing, 6, 52–53; human remains cache at, 362; hypothermia brains to, 211; MPG predecessor as, xvi, 11, 300, 305, 356; plaques on, 233–34, 310–12; Rockefeller Foundation supporting, 6; Third Reich and, 305, 309; Verschuer of, 355; Weindling and, 233–34
Kalb, Gerhard, 301, 303–4
Kaminiarz, Verena, 336–40, 349, 351n38
Kantorowicz, Alfred, 194–95
"Kapo," 209, 216n32

Kauders, Otto, 276, 282–84
Kazemi, Marion, 302–3
Kellner, Bernhard, 283
Kiddush Hashem (sanctification of the Divine name), 99n27
killing fields, 9, 104, 360, 364, 366
Klapper, Sabine, 287
Klee, Ernst, 173–74
Kobierzyn, 268–69
Kohl, Helmut, 312, 359
Königsberg, 125–31, 134, 135n1, 137n52
Kottenhoff, Heinrich, 210
Kovno Ghetto: Kahane Shapiro and, 90–91; labor cards and, 82–83, 86, 89–91, 100n31; pregnant women of, 108–10
Kramer, Josef, 243, 251
Kreutzberg, Georg W., 313–14, 316, 322
Kriesch, Ursula, 298–99
Krücke, Wilhelm, 223, 300–302, 311
Kutschke, Alfred and Günter (aka. Kutschke boys), 298–99, 305, 316–20, 324n51, 324n53
KWI. *See* Kaiser Wilhelm Institute
KWIA. *See* Kaiser Wilhelm Institute for Anthropology, Human Heredity and Eugenics

labor cards: Kovno Jewish Council and, 82–83, 86, 89–91, 100n31; Oshry on Nazi, 82, 89–91, 98n3; remaining versus deportation in, 89–91; Tory on Nazi, 82, 98n1
Lang, Hans-Joachim, 361
Lanzmann, Claude, 328, 340, 346
Lauritzen, Paul, 332
Law for the Prevention of Hereditarily Diseased Offspring (*Gesetz zur Verhütung erbkranken Nachwuchses*), 125, 164, 196, 242
legal hurdles, 244–45. *See also* "following orders"
Leibstandarte SS Adolf Hitler, 159, 167n31
Lensky, Mordechai, 9, 51–74
Lenz, Fritz, 24, 36, 226; Baur-Fischer-Lenz text and, 5–6; science with politics, 28–29, 32, 39n29, 40n43
Lerner, Barron, 12
leucotomy (lobotomy), 283, 287, 293n54
Lexer, Erich, 157
Liebau, Siegfried, 225–26, 228, 231
life-for-life problems, 9, 85–86, 98n14, 99n17
Lifton, Robert Jay, 105, 145–46, 148, 222
Linden, Herbert, 178
Lithuania, 82, 86–88, 106, 108–9, 113
lobotomy (leucotomy), 283, 287, 293n54
Łódź, 72
Lozowick, Yaacov, 174

Lucas, Franz, 11, 241, 243, 248–50, 253n44, 253n46, 254n68
lumbar punctures, 51–54

Mackinnon, Susan, 357–58, 368n22
Magnussen, Karin, 225, 228, 231–32, 356
Maimonides, 89–90, 92–93, 107
Mapu, Abraham, 61
Mapu, Ida, 61, 68
Marcuse, Herbert, 342–43
Markl, Hubert, 223–24
Marsch, Edmund, 302–3, 309, 311, 314–15, 324n34
masks, 49, 56n38, 339
Massin, Benoit, 44, 53, 224–25
mass murder, 90; as administrative, 172, 180, 184; Aktion Reinhard for, 141–42, 149n4; Aktion T4 and, 176; Austrian psychiatry and, 276, 278–81; dental surgeons and, 196; within euthanasia, xv, 6, 105; Gerstein on, 141–42, 149n5; gold and, 193; of handicapped, xv, 172, 184, 298, 302, 318; human remains after, 359; of Jews, 141; of mentally ill people, xv, 172, 176, 269–70, 298–99, 305, 316; mobile killing units in, 243–44; of psychiatric patients, 281; sterilization forerunning, 105; trials on, 252n14; Ulm trial and Jews in, 244–45; Zyklon-B pesticide and, 141, 226–27, 229, 235n40, 242–43
Max Planck Institute (MPI), 312, 357, 362, 367n16, 373
Max Planck Society (Max-Planck-Gesellschaft, MPG): Aly and, 11, 356–57, 367n16; anonymity veil by, 315; Boom of, 302, 308; brains found by, 357; child brains burial by, 302, 315–16; collective forgetting and, 304; denial by, 316; forgetfulness by, 300; good name of, 308–11; Henning of, 308–14, 316, 319, 323n20, 325n60; investigation of, 356–57, 367n16; Kreutzberg of, 313–14, 316, 322; KWI replaced by, xvi, 11, 300, 305, 356; Marsch of, 302–3, 309, 311, 314–15, 324n34; obstruction by, 301–4; Peiffer of, 319–20, 324n57, 325n62; Peters of, 321–22, 325n60; plaques on, 233–34, 310–12; pressure on, 312–13; Schleussing and, 313, 321; Singer, W., of, 302–4; Staab of, 304, 312, 314, 319, 324n34; twins research apology from, 223–24; Wässle of, 309, 311, 357, 368n21
McGlynn, George, 361, 369n48
mechanistic thinking, 37
medical collections, 8, 359–60, 368n40
Mein Kampf (Hitler), 5–6

Meisels, Tzvi Hirsch (rabbi), 82–83, 94–95, 100nn48–49
Mendelian laws, 22–24
Mengele, Josef: Auschwitz and, 222, 226–27, 232; blood from, 231–32; boys deaths by, 100n49; concentration camp and, 232; DFG project and, 226; on dissection, 146–47, 229; on dwarves, 224, 227, 230; exhumation of, 222; family protection of, 224, 233; as fugitive, 224; genocide and, 223, 226; gypsy camp and, 224, 226, 229–30, 302; Liebau and, 225–26, 228, 231; as medical criminal, 9; on pregnant women, 111; Puzyna on, 227, 231; racial killing by, 224; research lack on, 2; selections by, 222, 226–28, 232; on Sinti, 225–26, 228, 230; tracking of, 233; twins research by, 224, 226–29, 231; Verschuer and student as, 6, 10, 232, 310, 355–56; Weindling on, 2, 10, 222–34; Wirths rewarding, 227, 242; Yad Vashem on, 228–29, 233
Ment, Brigitte, 320, 324n57
mental heredity, 22–25, 27–28, 30–31, 33–36, 40n49, 45, 76n24. *See also* Law for the Prevention of Hereditarily Diseased Offspring
mentally ill people: "administrative mass murder" of, 172–73, 184; *Aktion T4* on, 279; brains of, 223, 227; dissection of, 131, 143–44; euthanasia of, 10, 175, 183–84; German soldiers as, 292n45; gold and, 193; Goltermann on, 245; hospitals of, 173–74, 177–78, 180–81, 183, 260–61, 276–300, 306–7; Kobierzyn commemorating, 268–69; mass murder of, xv, 172, 176, 269–70, 281, 298–99, 305, 316; persecution and, 245–46; sterilization of, 104–5, 132; Süß on, 174; T4 Planning on, 183; trauma and, 283; Trieb on, 180; Venzlaff on, 245–46; victims as, 285–87, 290. *See also* Jewish mental patients
Merkenschlager, Friedrich, 32
Michman, Dan, 2–3, 368nn20–21
microhistory, 60, 76n11
Mielke, Fred, 252n7
Mikulicz-Radecki, Felix von, 9, 125–38
Milgram, Stanley, 10, 204–6, 208, 214, 215nn11–12
Milgram experiments, 10
Miller, Stefan, 263, 272n37
Mitscherlich, Alexander, 217n62, 242, 245, 252n7, 300–301
mobile killing units, 243–44
The Modern Family Doctor (Lensky), 59, 65–66
Mohalim (circumcisers), 67–68

Mollison, Theodor, 24–26
Morell, Theodor, 162–63, 167n49
Moscow, 61
MPG. *See* Max Planck Society
MPI. *See* Max Planck Institute
Müller, Robert, 182
Müller-Hill, Benno, xvi, 223, 226

Nachtsheim, Hans, 223, 225, 233–34
NAGPRA. *See* Native American Graves Protection and Repatriation Act
National Socialists (NS), 7, 176; anatomists and, 147–48; dental professionals with, 190–91, 196, 199; ethics and, 8, 141, 143, 147–48; for eugenic state, 4–5; euthanasia campaigns of, 183–84, 257, 276; Günther prestige in, 26–27, 39n19; human remains from, 359; on Jewish people, 2–3, 144–49, 257, 260; Mikulicz-Radecki on, 127; race defilement panic by, 260; Stransky for, 281. *See also* Nazi Party
Native American Graves Protection and Repatriation Act (NAGPRA), 360
natural sciences, 5, 26–27, 29, 33–34, 39n21
Nazi Party (NSDAP): anatomical dissection and, 131, 143–48; *Arbeit Macht Frei* of, 348; Aschenauer in, 243, 248–50, 254n68; aviation medicine and, 10; biologism and, 38n1; Claußian theory and, 36; dental profession and, 10, 199; on differences, 28, 45; eugenics study by, 222; euthanasia officials in, 177; Final Solution of, 103–4, 115–16, 119n92; forced sterilization by, 5, 76n24, 104–5, 125–35, 135n7, 136nn16–17, 154, 281, 289; General SS and, 156–57, 166n10; genetics emphasis by, 8, 22; German academia in, 218n69; German medical professionals in, 154, 192–93, 218n69; Gerstein membership in, 140–41; Günther prestige in, 26–27, 39n19; as gynecologists, 9; for health dictatorship, 154; Himmler in, 6, 155; for human experiments, 208; intention of, 90–91; Jewish mentally ill killed by, 257–58, 260–61; on Jewish standard of conduct, 96; labor card of, 82, 98n1; Law for the Prevention of Hereditarily Diseased Offspring of, 125, 164, 196, 242; Magnussen in, 225; Merkenschlager in, 32; Mikulicz-Radecki and, 129, 132–33, 136n22; Peters and, 321–22, 325n60; Poland atrocities by, 257; psychiatry influenced by, 276; psychic damages from, 245–46; rabbinical responsa and genocide of, 90; racial hygiene from, 44; Schleussing

in, 313; sterilization by, 1, 6, 9, 105, 225; Stumpfegger in, 156–57; Verschuer in, 231; Wastl in, 54n5. *See also* National Socialists
Neff, Walter, 209, 216n32
Nelkin, Dorothy, 350n30
Niederland, William, 246
Nietzsche, Friedrich, 31, 40n38, 343
Nomberg-Przytyk, Sara, 111
Nordification of German people: Clauß on, 34, 36–37; genetics and, 39n19; Günther and, 27, 29–32, 37, 39n20, 40n38, 40n40, 40n43; racial medicine as, 154. *See also* Volk
Der nordische Gedanke unter den Deutschen (Günther), 30
NS. *See* National Socialists; NS medicine; NS victims
NSDAP. *See* Nazi Party
NS medicine, 2–6, 368nn20–21
NS victims, 359
Nuremberg Code, 327, 349nn2–3
Nuremberg Doctors Trial, xv, 1, 231, 243, 278; accessories and accomplices in, 213; Brandt, R., and, 216n40; culpability and, 208–10, 215n3; Dachau research in, 205; decompression and hypothermia experiments at, 208–9, 211; Hallervorden and child brains in, 298–300, 357; Mitscherlich on, 217n62, 242, 245, 252n7, 300–301; Nuremberg Code from, 327, 349nn2–3; research guidelines from, 54; testimony during, 161–62, 212–13; twins testifying at, 228–29
Nuremberg Laws, 105
Nussbaum, Martha, 335, 349
Nyiszli, Miklós, 224, 226–31, 235n40

obedience, 10, 204–6, 208, 214, 215nn11–12
Obedience to Authority (OTA) experiments, 204–7, 215nn11–12
Oesterreichischer, Martha, 287
Ohlendorf, Otto, 243–44
Olympic Games (Winter 1936), 157–58, 164–65
The Origins of Nazi Genocide (Friedlander, H.), 174
Oshry, Ephraim (rabbi): on abortion, 108, 117n38; *Babylonian Talmud* and *Jerusalem Talmud* with, 99n23; on Holocaust, 86, 99nn18–19; on labor cards, 82, 89–91, 98n3; on resistance, 96; responsa and, 82, 86–91, 95–96, 98n3, 98n7, 98n9, 99n14; on risking one's own life, 86–89; on wives after rape, 119n93
OTA. *See* Obedience to Authority experiments

"others," 4, 12, 213, 217n66, 349
Otwock Jewish district, 11, 257–59, 262–66, 270
Overy, Richard, 204–5

pathology of power, xviii
Peiffer, Jürgen, 319–20, 324n57, 325n62
Peiper, Joachim, 158, 167n22
Penha, Abraham de la, 11, 225–54
pension neurosis, 286–87, 292n45, 292n53, 293n54
performance medicine, 154
Perl, Gisella, 110
Pernkopf, Eduard, 51, 358
Pernkopf atlas of human anatomy, xvi, 14n8; Elsevier and, 358, 368n25; Mackinnon on, 357–58, 368n22; Untermann Protocol on, 365–66; use of, xvii, 357–58, 361–62, 365–66, 375; Yee on, 357–58
perpetrators, 3, 374; careers for, xv, 10, 52, 213, 224, 246, 276, 279, 310, 319, 321, 355; continuation by, 281, 359; death exploitation by, 315; exposure of, 320–22; individual culpability by, 208–10, 215n3; investigation lack on, 10; legal hurdles loosened for, 244; moral downfall of, 154–55; obstruction by, 373; public notion of, 204; responsibility and, 131, 136n36, 136n39; statute of limitations on, 242; Sturdy Colls on, 359–60
Perry, Gina, 206–7
persecution: Frankl on, 277, 285–86, 292n52; Hoff on, 277, 283–87, 292n48; hopeless from, 285, 292n48; Kauders on victims and, 276, 282–84; mental health and, 282; of mentally ill people, 245–46; victim hierarchy and, 289–90; victims and, 245–46, 276, 282–84
personal physician (*Begleitarzt*), 155, 166n6
Peters, Gerd, 321–22, 325n60
Pfannenstiel, Wilhelm, 211, 217n45
photography, 35–36, 49
A Physician inside the Warsaw Ghetto (Lensky), 73–74
Pik, Aaron, 113
pikuach nefesh (preservation of life), 86, 99n17
Polak, Joseph (rabbi), 12, 82, 354, 358, 361–62, 364–66, 368n21
Poland: *Aktion T4* and, 177, 276; German atrocities in, 257; Jewish people in, 11, 61–75; prisoner of war studies and, 46–47; racial investigations and, 46–48; Warsaw in, 9, 11, 60–68, 72–74, 98n8, 108, 258, 263, 265; Zofiówka Jewish psychiatric hospital in, 11, 257–59, 262–66, 270

positivism, 23, 25, 28–29, 37, 327; Adorno and, 328–29, 350n6, 350n8, 350n16; artists against scientific, 328–31; identity thinking and, 328–31, 339–43, 348; interchangeability and, 329, 350n16; negativism versus, 346
post-traumatic stress disorder (PTSD), 103, 106, 246, 282, 292n45
Die Praxis der Sterilisierungsoperationen (The practice of sterilization surgery) (Bauer and Mikulicz-Radecki), 129, 132
preservation of life (*pikuach nefesh*), 86, 99n17
Prevention of Hereditarily Diseased Offspring, 5–6, 180, 320
prisoners of war: Abel researching, 53; Baader researching, 53; Bosnians as, 49; as British, 47, 49; concentration camps and, 282–83; Exner, R., researching, 51–52; experiments on, 44–45, 48, 53–54; eyes and killing of, 228–29, 231; Fischer, E., on studies and, 52–53; as French, 47, 50; hierarchy and, 46; masks of, 49, 56n38; Pernkopf on, 51, 358; Polish studies in, 46–47; punishment of, 49–50; refusals by, 47, 49–50; from Soviet Union, 46–55; Stigler researching, 50; at Vienna psychiatric clinic, 282–83; in World War I, 48
Proctor, Robert, 223
psychiatry, xvi; *Aktion T4* and Austrian, 279; in Austria, 276, 278–81; Brandenburg-Görden psychiatric hospital, 223, 298–99, 305–8, 316–17, 319; for children, 287, 298; as discredited, 278–81; as German and Austrian, 276, 278–81; German medical profession and, 176; at Günzburg mental hospital, 173; Heinze and, 298; Jewish and Polish patients in, 11; mass murder and Austrian, 276, 278–81; Nazi regime influencing, 276; NSDAP influencing, 276; racial psychology in, 33, 36, 40n49; sterilization and Austrian, 276, 278–81; T4 Planning Commission and, 105, 141, 172–84, 261, 270, 276, 279, 281, 298, 308; Third Viennese School of Psychotherapy as, 285–86; Vienna clinic on, 282–83, 286; Wehrmacht willpower and, 40n49; Zofiówka Jewish for, 11, 257–59, 261–69, 271n7
PTSD. *See* post-traumatic stress disorder
Pusch, Friederike, 298–99, 319
Puzyna, Martina, 227, 231

rabbinical responsa, 2, 9; Efrati on, 92–95, 100n49, 108; on genocide, 90; Holocaust and, 84, 96, 98n9; on infant deaths and bunkers, 92–94, 108; Itzkowitz in, 88–89; Jewish law for, 83; Jewish medical professionals like, 84–85; as Jewish resistance, 84, 98n9; of Kahane Shapiro, 90–91; Maimonides and, 89–90, 92–93, 107; Meisels with, 82–83, 94–95, 100nn48–49; obligations and, 74, 86–88, 91, 95, 364–65; Oshry with, 82, 86–91, 95–96, 98n3, 98n7, 98n9, 99n14; Palestinian Talmud and, 89–90; Polak on, 82; preservation of life in, 86, 99n17; questions and answers in, 83; on ransom life for another, 94–95; records of, 84, 98n7; risking one's own life in, 86–89, 99n20; sermons and diaries in, 84, 98n8; Zvi in, 92
race defilement panic, 260
racial anthropology, 4, 8, 44, 47
racial hygiene, 3–5, 44, 104–5, 154, 222–23
racial medicine, 154
racial psychology (*Rassenseelenkunde*), 33, 36, 40n49
racial-scholarly gaze, 27, 39n21
racial science, 8, 22–23, 44, 46–48
racial studies, 44–45, 49, 51–54
racial theory (*Rassenkunde*): Clauß on, 22–23, 35, 37, 40n55; continuity of, 374; Günther on, 8, 22–23, 26–32, 37; heredity and, 8; in interwar years, 22–23; Mengele and killing in, 224; on phenotypic characteristics, 24; Polish Jews and, 46–48; science and politics in, 21–22, 38n2; Wastl and, 8, 44–45, 54n5
ransom life for another, 94–95
Rascher, Sigmund: as academic outsider, 213–14; aviation medicine and, 10, 207–14, 216n28, 216nn35–38, 217n45, 217n57, 321; Bláha on, 211–12; Diehl married to, 207–8, 216n28, 217n57; execution of, 208, 216n28; fatal experiments by, 210–11, 321; Pfannenstiel and, 211, 217n45; in science research, 209, 216nn35–36
Rassenkunde (racial theory), 21–22, 38n2
Rassenkunde des deutschen Volkes (Günther), 26–27
Rassenseelenkunde (racial psychology), 33, 36, 40n49
Ravensbrück concentration camp, 105, 154–65, 243–44
'Reform und Gewissen' (Aly), 309, 311
Reich Association of German Dentists (Reichsverband Deutscher Dentisten, RDD), 197
Reich leader of dental surgeons (*Reichszahnärzteführer*), 192–93

Reich leader of physicians (*Reichsärzteführer*), 192
Reichsarbeitsgemeinschaft Heil- und Pflegeanstalten (T4 Planning Commission of the Reich Working Group for Psychiatric Institutions), 105, 172–73, 175, 179, 183, 270, 279, 281
Reichsärzteführer (Reich leader of physicians), 192
Reichsrundschreiben (1931), 349n2
Reichsverband Deutscher Dentisten (Reich Association of German Dentists, RDD), 197
Reichszahnärzteführer (Reich leader of dental surgeons), 192–93
Reich Working Group, 173, 176–77, 181–82
Rein, Hermann, 216n42
Reis, Shmuel, xvii
Reis/Wald/Weindling proposal, xvii
Rentsch, Paul, 197–98
resistance, 101n54, 197; Germans helping, 198–99, 217n68, 231, 289–90; Germans hindering, 181, 213, 301; by Jewish people, 84, 96, 98n9, 101n54; by Jewish women, 103, 114–15, 118n81, 133
restitution, 244, 251
re-traumatization, 11, 251, 290, 293n69, 373
Ricoeur, Paul, 270
Riefenstahl, Leni, 343
Righteous Among the Nations, 199
risking one's own life, 86–89, 99n20
Rockefeller Foundation, xiii–xiv, 6
rodef principle, 93–94
Roelcke, Volker, xvi
Roma, 224, 226, 229–30, 289, 302, 359
Romberg, Hans-Wolfgang, 208–9, 211, 213, 216nn35–37
Rose, Gerhard, 210
Rosenau, Wilhelm, 262, 271n15
Rosenhügel hospital, 281
Rothschild DP hospital, 277–78, 281
Routil, Robert, 44, 51–54
Rudaitis, Ona, 245
Rüdin, Ernst, 5–6, 180, 320
Ruff, Siegfried, 208–9, 213, 215n22

SA. *See* Sturmabteilung
Saller, Karl, 32
"sanctification of the Divine name" (*Kiddush Hashem*), 99n27
Sauerbruch, Ferdinand, 157
Schaeffer, Karl, 197–98
Schatz, Willi, 196
Scheidt, Walter, 28–29, 39n29
Schleussing, Hans, 313, 321

Schmiedek, Raoul, 286–87, 292n53, 293n54
Schmuhl, Hans-Walter, 38n1, 53, 174, 224
Scholz, Viktor, 193
Schopenhauer's postulate, 28
Schüle, Erwin, 244, 247
Schumann, Horst, 105, 225
Schutzstaffel (SS), 6, 154–57, 192–93, 218n69, 226–27
science research, 1; accessories to murders and, 213; accomplices in, 213; animals and objectivity in, 337, 339–40; Auschwitz with, 225, 229; aviation experiments and, 213; for bioethics, 331; concentration camps and, 213; "end justifies the means" defense and, 214; "engaged followership" for, 205–7; ethics of, 54; human beings and, 349; hypothermia experiments in, 207–8, 210–12, 217n57, 217n60, 217n62, 321; interchangeability and, 329, 350n16; NS politics and biology as, 5; Nuremberg Trials on, 54; overlapping interests in, 213–14; on ovulation and pregnancy, 127–29; politics and, 28–29, 32, 39n29, 40n43; on pregnant women, 128–29; on prisoners of war, 44–45, 48, 53–54; Rascher in, 209–11, 216nn35–36, 217n45; Ravensbrück and, 105, 243–44; Romberg in, 208–9, 211, 213, 216nn35–37; Sievers and, 216n26, 216n36–37, 217n57; Weindling on Auschwitz and, 222–34; on women, 127–29, 159–61
scientific positivism. *See* positivism
scientific racism, 29, 36, 73
Von Seele und Antlitz der Rassen und Völker (Clauß), 35
Seidelman, William E., xiii, xix, 312; on Vienna Protocol, 12, 354, 357, 367, 368n21
Seitelberger, Franz, 317, 319–20
selections: accuser on, 247–49; Aschenauer on, 254n68; at Auschwitz, 246; defendants over, 243–44; hiding from, 92; Lucas admitting, 247; Mengele and, 222, 226–28, 232; de la Penha on, 248; refusal fear over, 251; trauma from, 242, 246, 250; Winkelmann on, 244
Semi Living Worry Dolls, 330, 331, 349
Sewering, Hans, xv–xvi
Shapira, Kalonymus Kalman (rabbi), 84, 98n8
Shoah (Jewish Holocaust), xiv–xv, xvii–xviii, 91, 100n37
Sievers, Wolfram, 216n26, 216nn36–37, 217n57
Simitis, Spiros, 303
Singer, Ludwig, 212, 217n57
Singer, Wolf, 302–4

Sinti, xiv, 105, 242, 289, 359; Mengele on, 225–26, 228, 230
Slobodka Yeshiva, 86–89, 99n20
social obligations, 264; of Jewish religion, 74, 86–88, 91, 95, 364–65; of medical profession, 132–34; Nazi party membership and, 281
Soviet soldiers, 46–55, 356
special surgeons' unit (*Chirurgensondergruppe beim Kommandostab des RfSS*), 159
Spiegelgrund institution, 278–81
Spier, Waldemar, 196–97
sports medicine, 155–61, 164–65
Srbik, Heinrich, 51
rem facility, 269, 273n62
SS. *See* Schutzstaffel
SS-Ahnenerbe, 53, 207, 210, 213–14, 216n26, 227–28
Staab, Heinz A., 304, 312, 314, 319, 324n34
Stauffenberg group, 217n68
Steinhof institution, 276, 278–81, 283
sterilization: Austrian psychiatry and, 276, 278–81; Clauberg and, 105, 225; cleft palates for, 193, 196–97; as eugenic, 127; as forced, 5, 76n24, 104–5, 125–35, 135n7, 136nn16–17, 154, 281, 289; Fraenkel on, 135n16; German medicine and, 1, 125–26, 128, 136n39; of Jewish women, 103–4, 110, 130; Law for the Prevention of Hereditarily Diseased Offspring from, 125, 164, 196, 242; mass murder forerun by, 105; of mentally ill people, 104–5, 132; Mikulicz-Radecki and forced, 129, 132–33; Mikulicz-Radecki for child, 130; Mikulicz-Radecki lecture on, 126, 135n2, 136n17; Mikulicz-Radecki on signs and, 9, 133, 136n45; narcotics for forced, 132–33; Nazi gynecologists perfecting, 1, 6, 9, 105, 225; numbers of, 136n17; racial medicine as, 154; Ravensbrück and, 105, 243–44; Schumann for, 105, 225; victims of, 11, 242–43, 310; Victim Welfare Law on, 289; women and issues of, 9, 125–34, 136n45
Stigler, Robert, 50
Stobierski, Mieczyslaw, 351n50
Stoeckel, Walter, 126
Stransky, Erwin, 281
Strughold, Hubertus, 211–12, 216n25
Stuck, Ernst, 192–93
Stumpfegger, Ludwig, 10, 154–68
Sturdy Colls, Caroline, 359–60
Sturmabteilung (SA), 154–57, 167n31, 192–93, 218n69; Merkenschlager in, 32; Mikulicz-Radecki in, 136n22; Schaeffer in, 197–98

subhuman (*Untermenschen*), xiv
The Sum of All Evil (Chapman, J., and Chapman, D.), 346
survivors: of concentration camps, 267, 277, 283, 285–86; as Jewish witnesses, 115, 119m89; Vienna with Jewish and Holocaust, 277–78; as witnesses, 241, 245
Süß, Winfried, 174
Sussmann, Anna, 114

T4 euthanasia program: Jews in, 261–62, 271n19; numbers in, 261, 271n21, 271n23, 272n35
T4 Headquarters, 172–74, 176–77, 182–83
T4 Planning Commission of the Reich Working Group for Psychiatric Institutions (*Reichsarbeitsgemeinschaft Heil- und Pflegeanstalten*): Aktion T4 in, 105, 141, 172–84, 261, 270, 276, 279, 281, 298, 308; hospital cooperation lack and, 181; for psychiatric care reorganization, 183
Tarbut schools, 64
TC&A. *See* Tissue Culture & Art Project
Third Viennese School of Psychotherapy, 285–86
Tissue Culture & Art Project (TC&A), 330–31, 349
Tory, Avraham, 82, 98n1
trauma: artists and, 268; collusion over, 244–46; without constitutional defects, 282, 285, 288, 292n48; depression from, 285; of DPs, 286; early 20th Century and, 245, 284; fatigue and, 282; of Guttmann, 283; as ignored, 278; from politics, 292n45; PTSD and, 103, 106, 246, 282; re-experiencing of, 11, 251, 290, 293n69, 373; from selections, 242, 246, 250; victims with, 1–3, 112, 115, 214, 246, 250–51, 276
trial numbers, 252n14. *See also* Nuremberg Doctors Trial
Trieb, Ludwig, 10, 172–86
Tsokos, Michael, 355
twins research: compensation and, 225; genetics in, 222; Mengele and, 224, 226–29, 231; MPS and Markl apology on, 223–24; Verschuer and, 223–27, 229, 231–34

Übermensch (Chapman, J., and Chapman, D.), 343–44
Ulm Einsatzkommando Trial (1958), 244–45, 247
uniqueness, 340–41
United States (US), 5–6, 205
Untermann Protocol, 365–66

Untermenschen (subhuman), xiv
US. *See* United States

Venzlaff, Ulrich, 245–46
Vermillion Accord, 360
Verschuer, Otmar von: for anti-Semitism, 227; blood and eyes receipt by, 223, 231–32; genetics and, 233, 355; Helmerstedt and, 225; KWI director as, 355; Liebau and, 225–26, 228, 231; Magnussen and, 225, 228, 231–32, 356; Mengele as student and, 6, 10, 231–32, 310, 355–56; as Nazi fanatic, 231; twins and, 223–27, 229, 231–34
victims: Aichhorn and, 292n53; Aly on euthanasia and, 11; Baeyer on witnesses and, 246, 250; BEG for, 244–45; on conditions, 290, 293n66, 293n68; congenital debility and, 132, 229, 235n46, 299, 305–6; constitutional defects and, 282, 285, 288, 292n48; dignity of dead, 304, 360–62, 365–66; as forgotten, 269–70; German medical profession on, 125–26, 130, 134; Goltermann on mental, 245; hierarchy of, 289; law versus justice on, 251; lawyers accusing, 247–48; mental health of, 285–87, 290; Mikulicz-Radecki and, 130, 132, 134; Niederland on, 246; NS victim and, 359; persecution and, 245–46, 276, 282–84; PTSD for, 103, 106, 246, 282; restitution and, 244, 251; as re-traumatized, 11, 251, 290, 293n69, 373; Rosenhügel hospital on Holocaust, 281; Schüle for, 244, 247; of sterilization, 11, 242–43, 310; on torture, 250; trauma and, 1–3, 112, 115, 214, 246, 250–51, 276; trauma and fatigue for, 282; Venzlaff on, 245–46; Vienna University and, 276; women and passive, 289–90; Yad Vashem on euthanasia, 269. *See also* compensation
Victim Welfare Law, 288–90, 293n66, 293nn68–69
Vienna: former prisoners to psychiatric clinic, 282–83; on Jewish academics, 281–82; Jewish and Holocaust survivors in, 277–78; Jewish children scandal in, 278–79; psychiatric clinic of, 282–83, 286; Rosenhügel hospital of, 281; Spiegelgrund institution in, 278–79; Steinhof institution in, 276, 278–81, 283
Vienna Protocol, 2, 9, 12, 104, 354–68
Vienna University, 276, 282–84
Vieweg, August, 209
Volk: as healthy German citizens, 4, 6, 38n1, 134, 373; as *Volksdeutsche*, 46, 68;

Volkskörper as group and, 104, 131, 154; women fertility research for, 125–38
Volksgemeinschaft, 141, 147–49
Volksgerichtshof, 198
Volksgesundheit (Health of the People), xiv, 192

Waffen-SS, 141, 156, 158–59, 166n8, 166n13, 225
Wagner, Franz, 178
Wagner, Gerhard, 32, 197–98
Wagner, Richard, 73
Wald, Hedy, xvii
Warsaw: *Haynt* and *Der Moment* as Yiddish press and, 64–66; Lensky in, 61; in Poland, 9, 11, 60–68, 72–74, 98n8, 108, 258, 263, 265
Wässle, Heinz, 309, 311, 357, 368n21
WASt. *See* Deutsche Dienststelle
Wastl, Josef, 8, 44–45, 49, 51–52, 54n5
Weber, Max, 28–29
Wehrmacht, 40n49
Weimar Republic, 5, 25, 38nn10–11, 131, 164
Weindling, Paul, 368n21; on Auschwitz and research, 222–34; on chapters, 229–30, 236n53; on experimentation, 10–11; on historical analyses, 38n2; KWIA pursuit by, 233–34; on Mengele, 2, 10, 222–34; Reis/Wald/Weindling proposal with, xvii
Weltz, Georg, 208–10, 212–13, 216n38, 216n40, 217n62
Wetzel, Robert, 150n22
Who Brought Hitler to Power? (Lensky), 73
Wickert, Christl, 310–11
Wilczkowski, Eugeniusz, 269, 273n62
Winkelmann, Adolf, 244
Wirths, Eduard, 227, 242
Włocławek, 60, 68, 72
women, 374; electroshock treatments on, 283; fertility research and, 125–38; FU Berlin and hospital for, 134; gendered violence on, 7–9, 103, 105–6, 108–10, 131–34; interchangeable bodies of, 129–31; Mengele on pregnant, 111; Mikulicz-Radecki and choice by, 133–34; obstetrical genocide and, 103–4, 106, 113–16, 119n92; as passive victims, 289–90; research on ovulating, 127–28; research on pregnant, 128–29; with sterility issues, 9, 125–34, 136n45; wound research on, 159–61
work sets you free (*Arbeit Macht Frei*), 348
World Holocaust Remembrance Center (Yad Vashem), 354
Wunder, Michael, 8

Yad Vashem (World Holocaust Remembrance
    Center): on euthanasia victims, 269;
    human remains guidelines at, 354, 360;
    human remains search and, 7, 359;
    Mengele research and, 228–29, 233;
    Righteous Among the Nations by, 199;
    symposium at, 354, 357, 359, 361–62
Yee, Andrew, 357–58
Yiddish press, 64–68

Zerbin-Rüdin, Edith, 320
Zionism, 62–64, 67, 74
Zofiówka Jewish psychiatric hospital, 11,
    257–72
Zurr, Ionat, 330–31, 349
Zvi, Yitchak (rabbi), 92
*Zygotic Acceleration, Biogenetic Desublimated
    Libidinal Model* (Chapman, J., and
    Chapman, D.), 340–42, 351n45

www.ingramcontent.com/pod-product-compliance
Lightning Source LLC
Chambersburg PA
CBHW071329080526
44587CB00017B/2777